Sports and Exercise Medicine: Health and Performance

Sports and Exercise Medicine: Health and Performance

Edited by Pablo De Souza

SYRAWOOD
PUBLISHING HOUSE
New York

Published by Syrawood Publishing House,
750 Third Avenue, 9th Floor,
New York, NY 10017, USA
www.syrawoodpublishinghouse.com

Sports and Exercise Medicine: Health and Performance
Edited by Pablo De Souza

International Standard Book Number: 978-1-68286-435-7 (Hardback)

Cataloging-in-publication Data

Sports and exercise medicine : health and performance / edited by Pablo De Souza.
p. cm.
Includes bibliographical references and index.
ISBN 978-1-68286-435-7
1. Sports medicine. 2. Exercise--Physiological aspects. 3. Sports. 4. Physical education and training. 5. Physical fitness.
I. De Souza, Pablo.
RC1210 .S66 2017
617.102 7--dc23

Printed in the United States of America.

TABLE OF CONTENTS

PREFACE

Sports and exercise medicine is a branch of medicine that deals with sports injuries and its prevention through medication and exercise. This book on sports medicine deals with the overall fitness levels, performance based analysis and recurring injury prevention. This book provides comprehensive insights into the field of sports and exercise medicine. It unfolds the innovative aspects of this area of study which will be crucial for the progress of this field in the future. The text presents researches and studies performed by experts across the globe. It will serve as a valuable reference broad spectrum of readers. This book will prove to be immensely beneficial to students and researchers in this field of sports and exercise medicine.

In my initial years as a student, I used to run to the library at every possible instance to grab a book and learn something new. Books were my primary source of knowledge and I would not have come such a long way without all that I learnt from them. Thus, when I was approached to edit this book; I became understandably nostalgic. It was an absolute honor to be considered worthy of guiding the current generation as well as those to come. I put all my knowledge and hard work into making this book most beneficial for its readers.

I wish to thank my publisher for supporting me at every step. I would also like to thank all the authors who have contributed their researches in this book. I hope this book will be a valuable contribution to the progress of the field.

Editor

PREFACE

1

Carnitine Palmitoyltransferase 1B 531K Allele Carriers Sustain a Higher Respiratory Quotient after Aerobic Exercise, but β3-Adrenoceptor 64R Allele Does Not Affect Lipolysis: A Human Model

Eduardo Gómez-Gómez[1], Martín Efrén Ríos-Martínez[1], Elena Margarita Castro-Rodríguez[1], Mario Del-Toro-Equíhua[2], Mario Ramírez-Flores[1], Ivan Delgado-Enciso[2], Ana Lilia Pérez-Huitimea[3], Luz Margarita Baltazar-Rodríguez[2], Gilberto Velasco-Pineda[2], Jesús Muñiz-Murguía[1]*

1 Centro Universitario de Investigaciones Biomédicas, Universidad de Colima, Colima, Colima, México, **2** Facultad de Medicina, Universidad de Colima, Colima, Colima, México, **3** Educación Física y Deporte. Facultad de Ciencias de la Educación, Universidad de Colima, Colima, Colima, México

Abstract

Carnitine palmitoyltransferase IB (CPT1B) and adrenoceptor beta-3 (ADRB3) are critical regulators of fat metabolism. CPT1B transports free acyl groups into mitochondria for oxidation, and ADRB3 triggers lipolysis in adipocytes, and their respective polymorphisms *E531K* and *W64R* have been identified as indicators of obesity in population studies. It is therefore important to understand the effects of these mutations on ADRB3 and CPT1B function in adipose and skeletal muscle tissue, respectively. This study aimed to analyze the rate of lipolysis of plasma indicators (glycerol, free fatty acids, and beta hydroxybutyrate) and fat oxidation (through the non-protein respiratory quotient). These parameters were measured in 37 participants during 30 min of aerobic exercise at approximately 62% of maximal oxygen uptake, followed by 30 min of recovery. During recovery, mean respiratory quotient values were higher in K allele carriers than in non-carriers, indicating low post-exercise fatty acid oxidation rates. No significant differences in lipolysis or lipid oxidation were observed between R and W allele carriers of *ADRB3* at any time during the aerobic load. The substitution of glutamic acid at position 531 by lysine in the CPT1B protein decreases the mitochondrial beta-oxidation pathway, which increases the non-protein respiratory quotient value during recovery from exercise. This may contribute to weight gain or reduced weight-loss following exercise.

Editor: Giuseppe D. Norata, University of Milan, Italy

Funding: This project was funded by the Mexican government through National Council of Science and Technology (CONACYT), www.conacyt.gob.mx: project 81471 to JM. The funders had no role in study design, data collection and analysis, decision to publish, or preparation of the manuscript.

Competing Interests: The authors have declared that no competing interests exist.

* E-mail: mmurguia@ucol.mx

Introduction

A sedentary lifestyle has contributed to a substantial increase in the prevalence of overweight and obesity [1,2,3]. Although aerobic exercise can reduce excess body fat [4,5], genetic factors may determine the susceptibility of an individual to gain weight [6,7] and alter the beneficial effects of physical activity [8]. Aerobic exercise increases adipose tissue lipolysis, which releases free fatty acids (FFA) into the bloodstream, FFA uptake by active skeletal muscle, and FFA oxidation in the mitochondrial matrix [9].

Fatty acid oxidation during physical activity is strongly dependent on both the rate of lipolysis in the adipocytes [9,10] and membrane translocation of long chain fatty acids (LCFA) into the mitochondrial matrix of the muscle cell [9,11]. Corpeleijn et al. demonstrated that intramyocellular lipid oxidation depends on extracellular FFA availability as well as mitochondrial function [12]. It has been documented, that FFA concentrations increase during the recovery period after exercise at 65% of maximal oxygen uptake (VO_2max), which releases more FFA for oxidation in skeletal muscle. This is supported by the decline in non-protein respiratory quotient (RQnp) value during recovery [13].

The beta-3 adrenoceptor (*ADRB3*) gene is expressed in visceral and subcutaneous adipose tissue and encodes the catecholamine receptor that activates lipolysis [14]. A polymorphic variant of *ADRB3* is located on chromosome 8p12 [15] with the substitution of tryptophan (W) by arginine (R) at position 64 (*W64R*). The R allele has been associated with excessive abdominal fat accumulation, higher body mass index (BMI), lower high density lipoprotein (HDL) levels, and insulin resistance [14,16,17]. However, in two population studies conducted on the effect of physical activity, the results were not different between W and R allele carriers [18,19].

Carnitine palmitoyltransferase 1 (*CPT1*; chromosome 22q13.33), expressed in skeletal muscle, heart, and the testis [20], regulates long-chain acyl group entry into the mitochondria for incorporation into the beta-oxidation pathway [9,20]. Robitaille et al. found a significant association between the heterozygous *E531K* allelic variant genotype, which replaces glutamic acid (E) for lysine (K) at position 531 of muscle-type CPT1 (*CPT1B*), and indicators of obesity when the proportion of dietary fat was ≥34.4%, indicating a gene–diet interaction [11]. Another study conducted with people of African descent in Trinidad and Tobago found that K allele homozygote carriers had a lower percentage of intermuscular fat, but a higher percentage of subcutaneous fat when compared with heterozygous and homozygous E allele carriers [21]. Moreover, an association between the K allele and metabolic syndrome traits was found in an adult German population [22].

We hypothesized that under aerobic effort, R allele carriers of *ADRB3* would present lower plasma concentrations of glycerol (Gly) and FFA, whereas K allele carriers of *CPT1B* would present higher values of RQnp. Indices of lipolysis and fat oxidation can also help determine whether the R and K alleles interact to reduce the fat oxidative capacity. This study aimed to determine the influence of these genetic variations R allele on lipolysis and that of the K allele on fatty acid oxidation by comparing carriers and non-carriers during and after aerobic load. Results indicate that the *E531K* affect fatty acid oxidation regardless of *W64R*.

Methods

The Ethics and Biosafety Committee of Colima University reviewed and approved the study protocol in accordance with the Declaration of Helsinki. All participants provided written informed consent.

Participants

In total, 45 participants were included from a group of 285 individuals who had recently participated in a study of the association between markers of obesity and genetic polymorphisms. Participants had normal hemoglobin, blood glucose, blood lipid, and lipoprotein levels, and fulfilled the additional inclusion criteria of BMI values and proportions of dietary macronutrients (carbohydrates, fats, and proteins) within the average range [mean±1 standard deviation (SD)] established in the association study (unpublished data). The proportions of dietary macronutrients were obtained by 24 h recall. Data were analyzed using Diet Analyst software (Parsons Technology Inc NUTRIDATA Software Corporation). We also calculated the quantities of saturated, monounsaturated, and polyunsaturated fatty acids (SFA, MUFA, and PUFA, respectively) in the diet adjusted to the body weight.

Subcutaneous whole body fat was determined from sum of 9 skin folds (∑9P); this included triceps, subscapular, biceps, iliac crest, supraspinal, abdominal, front thigh, and medial calf in accordance with the guidelines and equipment of the International Society for the Advancement of Kinanthropometry (ISAK), [23] as well as forearm skinfold measured on the distal lateral line at maximum forearm girth [24]. Subcutaneous trunk fat was determined from the sum of 4 trunk skinfolds (Σ4S); this included subscapular, iliac crest, supraspinal, and abdominal [23], and abdominal adiposity was determined by waist circumference (WC) measured in accordance with ISAK guidelines and equipment [23]. None of the participants had undertaken an exercise program during the past year, and none had received drug or hormonal treatments during the past 6 months.

Evaluation of Cardiovascular Function

Evaluation was performed by a cardiologist. All participants were apparently healthy; however, clinical examination revealed respiratory or cardiovascular anomalies in some participants, and these underwent further review with echocardiography and electrocardiography resulting in the exclusion of 3 participants who required treatment.

Cardiopulmonary Fitness

The Tecumseh step test was used to assess fitness on a 20.3-cm high step. According to its guidelines, participants performed 24 steps/min for 3 min and maintained a constant stepping rate with the aid of a metronome and assistant. Heart rate (HR) monitors (Polar-mod A-5 902805, Kempele, Finland) [25] recorded participant HRs prior to exercise, and in the recovery phase at 1 and 3 min post-exercise. The HR value at 1 min was classified in accordance with established categories [26].

Genomic DNA

The sodium dodecyl sulfate (SDS)–proteinase K method was used to extract genomic DNA from white blood cells, using a total of 7 mL of venous blood collected in two 5 mL tubes with EDTA (Ethylenediaminetetraacetic acid, 0.25 M). Briefly, cells were washed thrice in ammonium chloride (131 mM) plus ammonium bicarbonate (0.9 mM) with intervening centrifugation (15 min, 5000 revolutions per minute (rpm), 4°C), digested in proteinase buffer (50 mM Tris, pH 7.5; 100 mM EDTA, pH 8.0; 400 mM sodium chloride (NaCl); 0.5% SDS; and 50 μL of 20 mg/mL proteinase K), and agitated for 12 h at 37°C. To separate the DNA from protein, 6 M NaCl was added under centrifugation (15 min, 10000 rpm, 4°C). The supernatant (3−4 mL) was mixed with 15 mL absolute ethanol to condense the DNA. The DNA was transferred to 1.5-mL Eppendorf tubes containing 1 mL of 70% ethanol and then centrifuged for 10 min at 7500 rpm. Ethanol was removed by evaporation using a vacuum system, and the DNA pellet was resuspended in TE solution (10 mM Tris, pH 7.5; 1 mM EDTA) at 4°C for 12 h. DNA level was quantified by absorbance spectrophotometry at 260 nm. Aliquots (100 μL) at 100 ng/μL DNA were stored at 4°C until used for genotyping.

Genotyping of Polymorphisms

The *W64R* and *E531K* were genotyped by polymerase chain reaction–restriction fragment length polymorphism (PCR–RFLP) analysis. The reference single nucleotide polymorphisms (refSNPs) for *W64R* and *E531K* are rs4994 and rs470117, respectively [27,28]. Primers were designed using Primer 4.0 (http://frodo.wi.mit.edu) as follows: F-AGCCAGGTGATTTGGGAGAC and R-GTCACACACAGCACGTCCAC for amplification of a 429-base pair (bp) fragment including *W64R* and F-GCACTTCCCTCT-TACCCACA, and R-CTTCTTGATGAGGCCTTTGC for amplification of a 311-bp fragment including *E531K*, which were synthesized by Invitrogen Custom DNA Oligos (Life Technologies).

The hybridization temperature was 60°C for *W64R* and 63°C for *E531K*. Amplification was performed in 35 cycles, each comprising 30 s denaturation at 94°C, 30 s annealing at 60°C or 63°C, and 30 s elongation at 72°C. The PCR product for *W64R* was digested for 16 h in 5 U PflMI enzyme (New England Bio Labs. R0509S. Lot: 0280905), which recognizes the tryptophan base of the W allele and cuts the product into two fragments of 252 and 177 bp. After digestion, the full 429-bp fragment is therefore from the R allele. The PCR product for *E531K* was digested for 16 h in 5 U *Taq*I (New England Bio Labs R0149S. Lot: 0540804), which recognizes the glutamic acid base of the E allele and cuts the product into two fragments of 217 and 94 bp. Thus, the full 311-bp fragment is from the K allele. Digestion products were separated by 6% polyacrylamide gel electrophoresis and stained with 0.2% silver nitrate.

Blood Chemistry Analyses

Venous blood samples were taken from the antecubital vein 12 h after fasting [29], approximately 5–6 weeks before the aerobic load. The parameters measured were (mg/dL): total cholesterol (T-Chol), triacylglycerol (TAG), high density lipoprotein cholesterol (HDL-C), and low density lipoproteins cholesterol (LDL-C) using standardized colorimetric methods (Spinreact SAU Ctra Santa Coloma, 7E-17176 Sant Esteve de Bas. GI Spain, spectrophotometer: Jenway model 6405 UV/Vis). In addition, hemoglobin (Hb) level was measured in 0.04 mL of whole blood diluted in Drabkin reagent (Hycel de México SA de CV), the hematocrit (Ht) percentage was determined by capillary tube centrifugation (10000 rpm for 5 min), and the glucose (Glc) concentration was measured from a 0.6 μL capillary blood sample using a portable glucometer (Bayer, CONTOUR TS, No Coding, Ascensia MICROLET, Japan).

Maximal Oxygen Uptake Value

VO_2max was determined using a standardized maximum exercise effort protocol on a treadmill, according to the recommendations of the American College of Sport Medicine [30]. A Quark b2. 8.0 bV oximeter (Cosmed, Rome, Italy) was used to measure oxygen (O_2) consumption and carbon dioxide (CO_2) exhalation during testing. Each participant performed a simulation of the test for 4–7 days prior to the stress test, so that they were aware of the effort required. Participants were advised to avoid consuming alcohol and caffeine as well as avoid smoking and vigorous physical activity for at least 48 h prior to testing. The stress test was performed 3–4 h after food intake.

The Aerobic Load

This consisted of a 30-min exercise on a treadmill, followed by recovery in the supine position for 30 min. To achieve greater precision in load development, the test was structured with five periods as follows: (a) Rest, 6–10 min sitting at rest; (b) Warm-up, 5-min running on the treadmill to gradually reach 40% of VO_2max; (c) Aerobic exercise, 30 min at 60% of VO_2max; (d) Cool-down, 2 min of gradually reducing the running speed to zero; and (e) Post-exercise recovery, 30 min at rest in the supine position. (Figure 1).

The CO_2 production (VCO_2) and O_2 uptake (VO_2) were measured throughout the stress test. RQnp, absolute oxygen consumption (VO_2 in mL/min), relative oxygen consumption (VO_2 in mL/kg/min), and relative CO_2 production (VCO_2 in mL/Kg/min) were calculated during all 5 aerobic load periods.

Venous blood samples were collected from the cubital vein at 4 times: sample 1, at 3−4 min before the warm-up; sample 2, at 2 min post-exercise recovery; sample 3, at 15 min post-exercise recovery; and sample 4: at 30 min post-exercise recovery (Figure 1). Blood samples were used to determine levels of the following: epinephrine (Epn), norepinephrine (Nep), insulin, glucagon, cortisol (Cor), growth hormone (GH), Gly, FFAs, beta-hydroxybutyrate (beta-HB), Glc, lactate (Lac), albumin (ALB), and Ht. Plasma hormone level measurements were performed by the UNIDAD DE PATOLOGIA CLINICA (México Av. 2341. Guadalajara, México), a laboratory certified by The College of American Pathologist (AV-ID: 1200227. LAP: 5832901). Glc and Ht (%) levels were measured as described in the blood chemistry section. Lac levels were measured using a portable lactometer (Accutrend Plus System, Roche Diagnostics, San Cugat del Vallès, Barcelona Spain). Standard colorimetric methods were used to determine beta-HB, Gly, and FFA levels (Randox Laboratories Ltd, Ardmore, Diamond Road, Crumlin, Co. Antrim, UK, BT29 4QY) and ALB levels (SAU Spinreact Ctra Santa Coloma, 7E-17176 Sant Esteve de Bas, GI Spain).

The aerobic challenge was performed 10−20 days after maximum exercise testing to determine VO_2max. Women participants performed the aerobic load test within the first 10 days of their menstrual cycle.

Blood Hormone Levels

Samples were taken once before the aerobic load challenge and thrice during recovery (2, 15, and 30 min in post-exercise recovery period) (Figure 1). At each sampling point, 16 mL of venous blood was obtained and used as follows: (a) 8 mL in 2 tubes (4 mL each) with sodium heparin to determine Epn and Nep by chemiluminescence assay, (b) 4 mL in cold EDTA for determining plasma glucagon levels by radioimmunoassay, (c) 4 mL in a dry tube for determining serum insulin and Cor levels by electrochemiluminescence immunoassay and GH by chemiluminescence assay.

Statistical Analyses

We used SPSS version 15 (IBM SPSS Software, USA) for all analyses. The effects of *E531K* and *W64R* on the oximetry values at the end of each of the 16-measurement stages and blood hormone levels were tested both separately and together (interaction). The normality and variance homogeneity of each distribution were determined by the Kolmogorov–Smirnov and Levene tests, respectively. The values are presented in tables as mean ± SD. The mean values at each stage and time point were compared between K allele carriers vs. K allele non-carriers (K+ and K−, respectively), R allele carriers vs. R allele non-carriers (R+ and R−, respectively), and, carriers of both (K+/R+), vs. carriers of K only (K+/R−) or R only (R+/K−). For normal and homogeneous distributions, one-way analysis of variance and post-hoc Tanhame tests for pairwise comparisons were used. Otherwise, the Kruskal–Wallis test was used to compare 3 distributions, and the Mann–Whitney U-test for pairwise comparisons. The statistical significance level was set at $p<0.05$.

Results

Participant Characteristics

Of the 45 individuals selected, only 37 (18 men, 19 women) successfully completed the experiment; 3 were excluded because of heart problems and 5 were lost to follow up (they relocated before the study was completed). All parents and grandparents were born in Mexico, with 35 originating from Western Mexico and two from South–Central Mexico. (Table S1 in File S1). The clinical characteristics were as follows: age range, 22.9±3.1 years; height, 162.7±7.8 cm; weight, 63.2±10.4 kg; BMI, 23.8±3.1 kg/m^2; systolic blood pressure, 115.49±13.4 mmHg; and diastolic blood pressure, 71.6±6.9 mmHg.

Data Sorting

All functional measurements were grouped and compared according to the genetic variant studied, as follows: (a) R+ (20; 10 males, 10 females) versus (vs.) R− (17; 8 males, 9 females) to assess the effect of *W64R*; (b) K+ (27; 13 males, 14 females) vs. K− (10; 5 males, 5 females) to assess the effect of *E531K*; and (c) K+/R+ (12; 6 males, 6 females) vs. K+/R− (15; 7 males, 8 females) vs. K−/R+ (8; 4 males, 4 females) to test for an interaction between alleles. Only two participants (1 male and 1 female) were K−/R−; therefore, this genotype was not included in the statistical comparison (Table S2 in File S1).

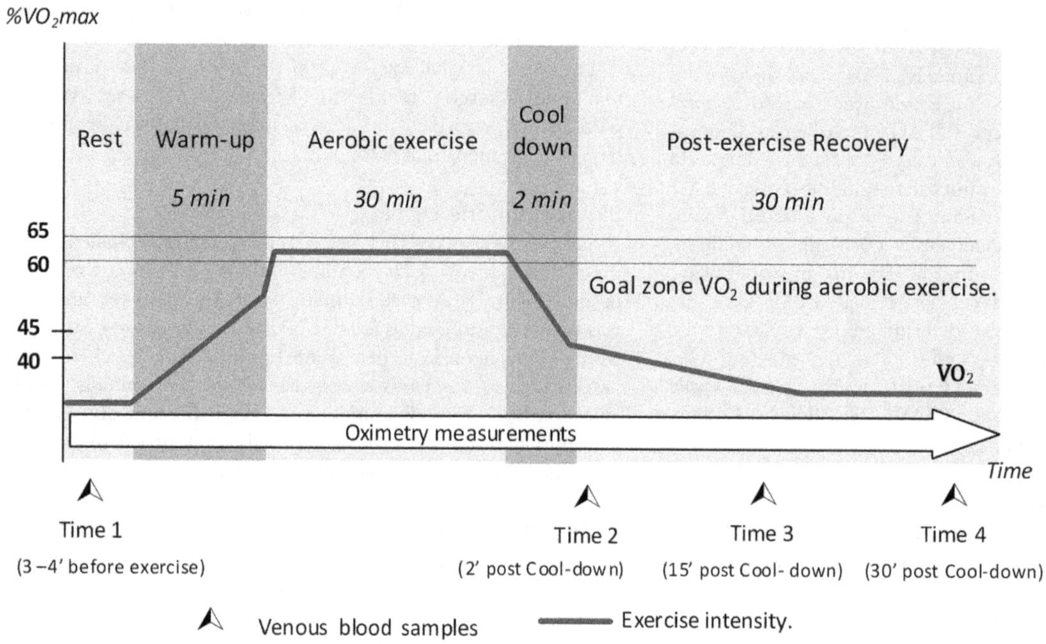

Figure 1. Aerobic load structure (5 exercise periods and 4 blood sample Times) and exercise intensity programme.

Anthropometric, Dietary, and Blood Characteristics

There were no significant differences in age or adiposity indices (BMI, WC, Σ9S, Σ4S, and WHR) between genotypes within the 3 comparison groups (R+ vs. R−; K+ vs. K−; K+/R+ vs. K+/R− vs. K−/R+; $p>0.05$) (Table 1). Furthermore, the mean dietary protein, fat, carbohydrate, dietary SFA/kg, and MUFA/kg intakes did not significantly differ between groups. The amount of PUFA/kg was marginally higher for K− than for K+ ($p<0.070$) (Table 2). Measured levels of Glc, Ht, Hb, TAG, T-Chol, HDL-C, and LDL-C were not significantly different between genotypes within the comparison groups ($p>0.05$), indicating that basal metabolic status was similar (Table 3). The mean HR values at 1 min after exercise in the Tecumseh step test did not significantly differ between any groups (Table S3 in File S1), establishing similar levels of cardiopulmonary fitness between the groups.

Oximetry Indicators

The VO_2max percentage ($\%VO_2max$) was taken as the main indicator of exercise intensity. Participants performed the warm-up phase to 35.5%±5.3% of VO_2max for 5 min, the aerobic exercise phase at 62.3%±1.1% of VO_2max for 30 min, and the cool-down phase at 42.2%±4.6% VO_2max for 2 min. A significant difference was detected between R+ and R− groups (63.1% vs. 61.3%; $p=0.027$) at 10 min into the aerobic exercise phase (Table 4). Despite similarities in baseline metabolic values, fitness levels, exercise intensity, and post-exercise hormone levels (below), there were significant differences in RQnp values between genotypes,

Table 1. Mean (SD) values of age, BMI and indicators of subcutaneous fat in each of the genetic classifications.

Genetic Classification	Groups	Age (years)	BMI (kg/m^2)	WC (cm)	∑9S (mm)	∑4S (mm)
CPT1B alleles	K+	23.1 (3.4)	24.2 (3.2)	77.3 (8.1)	150.7 (50.5)	60.2 (22.0)
	K−	22.5 (2.1)	22.7 (2.7)	75.7 (8.3)	143.9 (50.5)	55.5 (21.1)
		$^{A}p=0.663$	$^{A}p=0.182$	$^{A}p=0.618$	$^{A}p=0.720$	$^{A}p=0.562$
ADRB3 alleles	R+	22.4 (1.9)	23.6 (3.7)	76.8 (8.5)	148.2 (53.1)	57.5 (22.7)
	R−	23.5 (4.1)	24.0 (2.4)	76.8 (7.8)	149.6 (47.4)	60.6 (20.7)
		$^{A}p=0.266$	$^{A}p=0.659$	$^{A}p=0.996$	$^{A}p=0.935$	$^{A}p=0.668$
Interaction ADRB3–CPT1B	K+/R+	22.3 (1.9)	24.8 (4.1)	79.0 (8.5)	159.6 (55.8)	61.1 (23.5)
	K+/R−	23.6 (4.3)	23.7 (2.2)	75.8 (7.8)	143.5 (46.4)	59.5 (21.5)
	R+/K−	22.5 (2.1)	21.7 (1.8)	73.6 (7.8)	131.1 (46.9)	52.2 (21.9)
		$^{K\text{-}W}p=0.973$	$^{K\text{-}W}p=0.051$	$^{K\text{-}W}p=0.192$	$^{K\text{-}W}p=0.402$	$^{K\text{-}W}p=0.669$

SD: Standard deviation. *A*: One-way analysis of variance (ANOVA), significance $p<0.05$. *K-W*: Kruskal-Wallis test, significance $p<0.05$.
BMI: Body mass index. **WC**: Waist circumference. **∑9S**: Sum of triceps, subscapular, biceps, iliac crest, supraspinal, abdominal, anterior thigh, medial calf, and forearm skin folds. **∑4S**: Sum of subscapular, iliac crest, supraspinal, and abdominal skin folds. (Skinfold of trunk). **K+**: K allele carriers. **K−**: K allele non-carriers. **R+**: R allele carriers. **R−**: R allele non-carriers. **K+/R+**: K and R allele carriers. **K+/R−**: K allele only carriers. **R+/K−**: R allele only carriers.

Table 2. Mean macronutrient proportions and dietary fatty acid amounts adjusted to body weight in each of the genetic classifications.

Genetic Classification	Groups	Protein (%)	C–H (%)	Fat (%)	SFA/kg	MUFA/kg	PUFA/kg
CPT1B alleles	K+	17.3 (3.2)	53.1 (7.8)	30.7 (5.5)	0.39 (.14)	0.36 (.12)	0.17 (.06)
	K−	15.8 (3.1)	56.7 (3.6)	29.1 (2.6)	0.40 (.11)	0.40 (.14)	0.21 (.08)
		$^{A}p=0.212$	$^{U}p=0.203$	$^{U}p=0.353$	$^{A}p=0.801$	$^{A}p=0.411$	$^{A}p=0.070$
ADRB3 alleles	R+	16.6 (2.6)	54.5 (4.9)	30.2 (3.3)	0.39 (.13)	0.37 (.13)	0.18 (.08)
	R−	17.2 (3.8)	53.7 (9.2)	30.4 (6.4)	0.39 (.14)	0.37 (.12)	0.18 (.05)
		$^{A}p=0.555$	$^{U}p=0.964$	$^{U}p=0.940$	$^{A}p=0.956$	$^{A}p=0.882$	$^{U}p=0.879$
Interaction ADRB3–CPT1B	K+/R+	17.0 (2.3)	53.6 (5.7)	30.4 (3.8)	0.37 (.14)	0.33 (.12)	0.15 (.07)
	K+/R−	17.5 (3.8)	52.7 (9.4)	30.9 (6.6)	0.40 (.14)	0.38 (.12)	0.18 (.05)
	R+/K−	16.0 (3.1)	55.8 (3.3)	29.8 (2.4)	0.42 (.11)	0.43 (.13)	0.22 (.09)
		$^{K\text{-}W}p=0.719$	$^{K\text{-}W}p=0.421$	$^{K\text{-}S}p=0.567$	$^{K\text{-}S}p=0.789$	$^{K\text{-}S}p=0.178$	$^{K\text{-}S}p=0.284$

SD: Standard deviation. *A*: One-way analysis of variance (ANOVA): significance, $p<0.05$. *U*: Mann–Whitney test: significance, $p<0.05$. *K–W*: Kruskal–Wallis H test: significance, $p<0.05$.
C–H: Carbohydrates. **SFA/kg**: Saturated fatty acids per kg of body weight. **MUFA/kg**: Mono unsaturated fatty acids per kg of body weight. **PUFA/kg**: Poly unsaturated fatty acids per kg of body weight. **K+**: K allele carriers. **K−**: K allele non-carriers. **R+**: R allele carriers. **R−**: R allele non-carriers. **K+/R+**: K and R allele carriers. **K+/R−**: K allele only carriers. **R+/K−**: R allele only carriers.

Table 3. Mean fasting blood glucose, hematocrit, hemoglobin, and lipid levels in each of the genetic classifications.

Genetic Classification	Groups	Glc (mg/dL)	Ht (%)	Hb (mg/dL)	TAG (mg/dL)	T-Chol (mg/dL)	HDL-C (mg/dL)	LDL-C (mg/dL)
CPT1B alleles	K+	87.3 (9.6)	42.5 (3.8)	13.1 (1.6)	99.9 (25.5)	150.7 (24.6)	39.6 (10.8)	131.4 (49.7)
	K−	82.2 (7.2)	42.9 (4.6)	14.1 (2.1)	94.5 (45.8)	141.5 (23.9)	39.3 (7.4)	132.9 (49.6)
		$^{A}p=0.136$	$^{A}p=0.797$	$^{A}p=0.171$	$^{A}p=0.648$	$^{A}p=0.316$	$^{A}p=0.940$	$^{A}p=0.932$
ADRB3 alleles	R+	83.4 (7.9)	43.4 (3.1)	13.1 (1.5)	92.7 (33.0)	147.0 (21.8)	38.3 (9.2)	130.3 (48.5)
	R−	88.9 (10.0)	41.7 (4.7)	13.7 (2.0)	105.3 (29.5)	149.7 (27.9)	41.0 (10.7)	133.5 (51.0)
		$^{A}p=0.074$	$^{A}p=0.214$	$^{A}p=0.308$	$^{A}p=0.235$	$^{A}p=0.743$	$^{A}p=0.408$	$^{A}p=0.849$
Interaction ADRB3–CPT1B	K+/R+	83.6 (9.3)	43.6 (3.0)	12.8 (1.6)	94.8 (23.1)	151.5 (22.2)	38.7 (10.6)	134.8 (49.0)
	K+/R−	90.3 (9.1)	41.6 (4.1)	13.4 (1.6)	104.1 (27.4)	150.1 (27.2)	40.4 (11.2)	128.6 (51.8)
	R+/K−	83.3 (6.1)	43 (3.3)	13.5 (1.4)	89.6 (45.8)	140.2 (20.6)	37.7 (7.3)	123.7 (50.4)
		$^{A}p=0.091$	$^{K\text{-}W}p=0.722$	$^{A}p=0.119$	$^{A}p=0.645$	$^{A}p=0.777$	$^{A}p=0.736$	$^{A}p=0.693$

SD: Standard deviation. *A*: One-way analysis of variance (ANOVA), significance $p<0.05$. *K–W*: Kruskal–Wallis test, significance $p<0.05$.
Glc: Glucose. **Ht**: Hematocrit. **Hb**: Hemoglobin. **T-Chol**: Total cholesterol. **HDL-C**: High density lipoprotein-cholesterol. **LDL-C**: Low density lipoprotein-cholesterol. **K+**: K allele carriers. **K−**: K allele non-carriers. **R+**: R allele carriers. **R−**: R allele non-carriers. **K+/R+**: K and R allele carriers. **K+/R−**: K allele only carriers. **R+/K−**: R allele only carriers.

specifically between K+ and K− groups (Figure 2A) with either R+ or R− (Figure 2C). The RQnp values were not significantly different between genotypes within the comparison groups for the rest, warm-up, aerobic exercise, and cool-down periods, but the RQnp value in the K+ group remained significantly higher at 10 ($p = 0.003$), 20 ($p = 0.003$), and 25 min ($p = 0.048$) after exercise when compared with the K− group. Moreover, the RQnp value was significantly higher in the R− than in the R+ participants at 30 min after exercise ($p = 0.027$) (Figure 2B). The R+/K− group had an RQnp value that was significantly lower than that of the K+/R+ and K+/R− groups at 10 min after exercise ($p = 0.022$), and significantly lower than that of the K+/R− group at 20 min after exercise ($p = 0.028$) (Figure 2C) (Table 5). Mean HR were no significantly different between genotypes throughout the exercise and recovery periods ($p > 0.05$) (data not shown).

Blood Indicators of Aerobic Load

Lac levels were not significantly different between genotypes within the 3 comparison groups prior to testing and at 2, 15, and 30 min after exercise ($p > 0.05$). Lac levels exceeded 2 mM only at 2 min after exercise, and lower values were measured at 15 and 30 min. Glc levels decreased slightly during the post-exercise recovery phase, but not significant differences were observed between the genotypes. Similarly, ALB levels and Ht were not significantly different between genotypes at any stage (Table S4 in File S1). The K− group had significantly higher FFA levels than those in the K+ group at 2 min after exercise ($p = 0.044$) (Figure 3B; Table 6), whereas there were no significant differences in Gly levels between genotypes at any of the 4 measurement points. Beta-HB levels tended to increase during the post-exercise recovery phase (Table 6); however, no significant differences were found between the R+ and R− participants (Figure 4A), and levels were significantly higher at 15 min ($p = 0.022$) and 30 min ($p = 0.008$) after exercise in the K− than in the K+ participants (Figure 4B). Furthermore, a significantly higher beta-HB level was detected at 30 min after exercise in the K−/R+ group compared with either the K+/R+ or K+/R− groups ($p = 0.029$) (Figure 4C).

Plasma Hormone Levels during Aerobic Load

Insulin, Cor, and GH levels did not differ significantly between genotypes within the comparison groups at any time. Glucagon levels remained below 50 pg/mL at all 4 measurement times. Epn and Nep levels reached peak levels at 2 min after exercise (84.81 and 676.14 pg/mL, respectively) and declined thereafter. The only significant difference in Nep level was detected at 30 min after exercise between R+ and R− participants (230.6 pg/mL vs. 301.7 pg/mL; $p = 0.028$) (Table S5 in File S1). In general, the hormonal responses were as expected and were generally similar among the genotypes.

Discussion

The increasing rate of fatty acid oxidation induced by aerobic exercise is modulated by multiple factors. In this study, we therefore sought to reduce the influence of other polymorphic genes involved in the lipolysis and fatty acid oxidation pathway by including only Mexicans from only 2 generations, and primarily from the same region of Western Mexico.

Carriers of the K allele exhibited a higher mean RQnp during the post-exercise recovery phase, indicating reduced lipid beta-oxidation compared with non-carriers. In light of previous studies demonstrating an association between the K allele and obesity indices [11], this study suggests that the K allele may predispose to decreased FFA oxidation when the energy demand from lipids is increased during the recovery from effort. This can be a factor contributing to the accumulation of fat in adipose tissue given similar dietary and activity conditions to non-carriers.

The difference in RQnp between K allele carriers and non-carriers cannot be explained by differences in diet, general physical condition, or demographic valuables (sex ratio or age). Expression of the human *CPT1B* gene in transgenic mice increased 2-3-fold during both fasting and high-fat diets [31], whereas PUFA modulate the expression of genes involved in lipid metabolism, such as the peroxisome proliferator activated receptor [32]. Thus, dietary factors can influence the expression of *CPT1B* and other genes involved in fat mobilization. However, the comparison groups reported similar dietary macronutrient compositions (including SFA, MUFA, and PUFA). In addition, the level of cardiopulmonary fitness did not differ between genotypes (Table S3 in File S1); thus, obviating the differential effects of adaptation to physical activity [33,34]. Moreover, subcutaneous fat, Glc, Hb, lipid, lipoprotein, and Ht levels did not differ between the comparison groups, indicating that metabolic conditions were similar at baseline. During the development of aerobic load, there were no differences in $\%VO_2max$ among the genotypes. Moreover, blood Lac levels did not reach 4 mM at any point after exercise, which is indicative of aerobic metabolism (Table S4 in File S1). These results confirmed that exercise load was predominantly aerobic and of similar intensity among all participants.

Hormone levels involved in the modulation of lipolysis and fat oxidation did not differ significantly among the genotypes after exercise. Furthermore, ALB, Hb, and Ht levels were not significantly different. The apparent differences in lipid metabolism between K allele carriers and non-carriers was therefore unlikely to be due to differences in hormonal patterns, basal FFA, or oxygen transport and FFA transport capacity to active muscle tissue.

No significant differences were observed in plasma FFA and Gly levels between R allele carriers and non-carriers. Moreover, the similarity in catecholamine and other hormone levels before and after exercise indicates that the R allele does not affect the activation of lipolysis; these genotypes probably had similar FFA metabolism rates. There was a trend toward high values among R+ in RQnp, but only reached significant difference at 30 minute post-exercise recovery period compared to non-carriers (possibly related to the 12 K allele carriers) and a downward trend among non-carriers (possibly related to the 15 E allele carriers). In addition, it has been observed that LCFA oxidation in the mitochondria increases with FFA availability [9,35], which was similar in both groups. In addition, beta-HB levels did not differ between R allele carriers and non-carriers during recovery. These results indicate that the availability of FFA, mobilized from visceral adipose tissue was similar to its consumption by skeletal muscle tissue.

Most participants in this study were heterozygous for the R allele, which already been reported in other studies [10,14,16,18]. Thus, the gene dose may have contributed to the similarity in lipolysis indicators between R allele carriers and non-carriers. In addition, these indices were measured for only 30 min after exercise; delayed responses may therefore exist with measureable differences. Another possibility is that the effect of the *W64R* variant of *ADRB3* could be masked by the effect of other lipolysis agents, including cytokines that are activated during muscle contraction [36]. Nonetheless, several studies and meta-analyses have shown that although the R allele is associated with increased BMI and insulin resistance, its contribution to the phenotype is weak [14,17,38]. Our results indicate that the *W64R* allelic variant of *ADRB3* does not affect the activation of lipolysis.

Table 4. Mean percentage of maximal oxygen uptake during and after the aerobic load for each of the genetic classifications.

Classification		Stages of the aerobic load															
		Rest	Warm-up	5′ exercise	10′ exercise	15′ exercise	20′ exercise	25′ exercise	30′ exercise	Cool down	2′ post exercise	5′ post exercise	10′ post exercise	15′ post exercise	20′ post exercise	25′ post exercise	30′ post exercise
%VO$_2$max	**K+**	11.9	35.2	59.8	62.1	62.8	62.5	62.8	62.2	41.9	25.7	12.9	11.0	10.5	10.4	10.4	10.2
		(3.5)	(4.8)	(4.1)	(2.2)	(2.1)	(2.8)	(2.5)	(2.1)	(3.4)	(2.8)	(1.9)	(1.4)	(1.4)	(1.7)	(1.6)	(1.7)
	K-	13.3	36.1	60.8	63.9	62.4	63.1	64.0	63.8	43.2	26.1	11.9	11.9	11.6	11.4	11.2	11.2
		(2.6)	(6.6)	(8.7)	(5.5)	(7.1)	(8.2)	(7.5)	(6.7)	(7.1)	(5.4)	(4.9)	(2.9)	(2.8)	(3.2)	(3.1)	(2.7)
	p	*0.274*	*0.637*	*0.658*	*^{U}0.608*	*0.817*	*0.744*	*^{U}0.538*	*^{U}0.707*	*0.457*	*^{U}0.682*	*0.380*	*0.211*	*^{U}0.180*	*^{U}0.502*	*^{U}0.458*	*0.195*
	R+	12.4	36.3	60.8	**63.1***	63.1	63.0	63.9	63.0	42.5	25.8	12.9	11.7	11.3	11.3	11.0	11.0
		(2.7)	(5.7)	(6.3)	(4.0)	(5.2)	(6.2)	(5.6)	(4.9)	(5.6)	(4.1)	(3.6)	(2.1)	(2.0)	(2.4)	(2.3)	(2.3)
	R−	12.1	34.5	59.2	**61.3***	62.2	62.4	62.2	62.2	41.9	25.8	12.4	10.9	10.2	10.0	10.2	9.9
		(4.0)	(4.7)	(4.7)	(1.8)	(1.9)	(2.4)	(2.0)	(2.3)	(3.1)	(3.0)	(2.0)	(1.7)	(1.7)	(1.8)	(1.8)	(1.4)
	p	*0.750*	*0.319*	*0.399*	***0.027***	*0.509*	*0.688*	*0.254*	*0.537*	*0.673*	*0.989*	*0.675*	*0.213*	*0.090*	*0.081*	*0.246*	*0.116*
	K+/R+	12.1	36.5	61.1	63.2	63.4	62.8	63.3	62.2	42.0	25.5	13.5	11.2	10.8	11.0	10.5	10.6
		(2.6)	(4.6)	(2.5)	(2.0)	(2.2)	(3.3)	(2.9)	(1.9)	(3.7)	(2.9)	(1.9)	(1.6)	(1.2)	(1.8)	(1.7)	(2.0)
	K+/R−	11.8	34.2	58.8	61.2	62.2	62.3	62.3	62.2	41.8	25.8	12.5	10.9	10.2	9.9	10.3	9.9
		(4.1)	(4.9)	(4.8)	(1.9)	(2.0)	(2.5)	(2.1)	(2.4)	(3.2)	(2.8)	(1.9)	(1.6)	(1.5)	(1.5)	(1.6)	(1.3)
	R+/K−	13.0	35.9	60.3	64.4	62.5	63.3	64.7	64.1	43.3	26.2	11.9	12.3	12.0	11.7	11.7	11.5
		(2.9)	(7.3)	(9.8)	(6.1)	(8.0)	(9.3)	(8.3)	(7.5)	(7.9)	(5.7)	(5.3)	(2.9)	(2.6)	(3.1)	(3.0)	(2.8)
	p	*0.705*	*0.679*	*0.671*	*0.142*	*0.880*	*0.976*	*0.608*	*0.692*	*0.899*	*0.984*	*0.671*	*0.374*	*0.200*	*0.330*	*0.349*	*0.343*

SD: Standard deviation. One-way analysis of variance (ANOVA), significance $p<0.05$. *U*: Mann–Whitney test, significance $p<0.05$. Asterisk (*) indicates the values that significantly differ in the same stage.
K+: K allele carriers. **K−**: K allele non-carriers. **R+**: R allele carriers. **R−**: R allele non-carriers. **K+/R+**: K and R allele carriers. **K+/R−**: K allele only carriers. **R+/K−**: R allele only carriers.

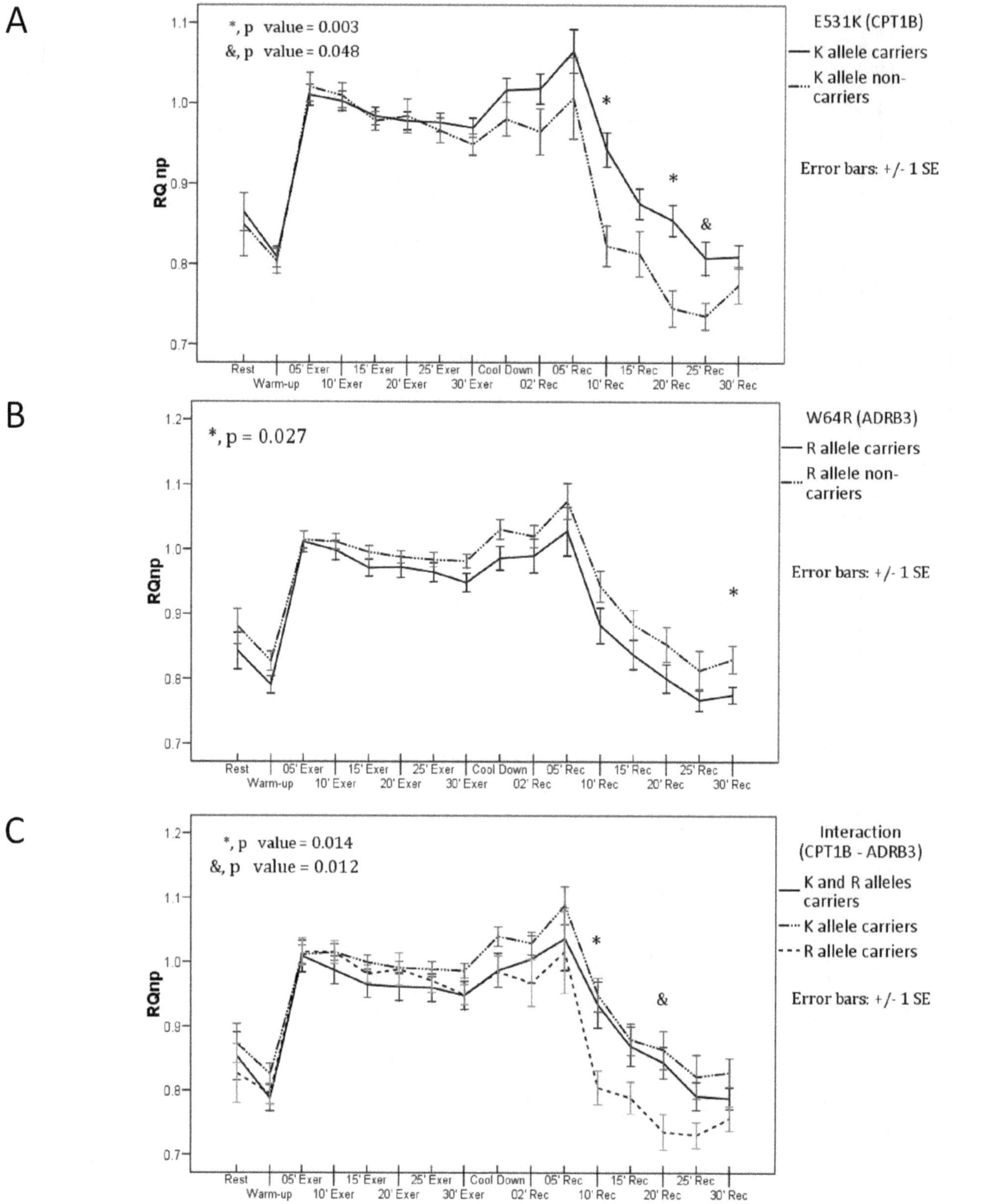

Figure 2. Non-protein respiratory quotient (RQnp) values during aerobic load. (**A**) R allele carriers (12 K and 8 E carriers) versus R allele non-carriers (15 K and 2 E carriers). (**B**) K allele carriers (12 R and 15 W allele carriers) versus K allele non-carriers (2 R and 8 W carriers) The asterisk and ampersand indicate a significant difference. (**C**) Interaction (*CPT1B–ADRB3*). The asterisk and ampersand indicate the significant difference between the R allele carrier group, with 8 carriers of the E allele, and the other groups.

Table 5. Mean non-protein respiratory quotients during and after the aerobic load for each of the genetic classifications.

Classification		Stages of the aerobic load														
		Rest	Warm-up	5′ exercise	10′ exercise	15′ exercise	20′ exercise	25′ exercise	30′ exercise	Cool down	2′ post exercise	5′ post exercise	10′ post exercise	15′ post exercise	20′ post exercise	25′ post exercise	30′ post exercise
RQnp	K+	0.864	0.809	1.010	1.002	0.984	0.978	0.976	0.969	1.016	1.018	1.065	**0.942***	0.875	**0.854***	**0.808***	0.810
		(0.12)	(0.07)	(0.07)	(0.06)	(0.06)	(0.06)	(0.06)	(0.06)	(0.08)	(0.10)	(0.14)	(0.11)	(0.10)	(0.10)	(0.11)	(0.07)
	K−	0.849	0.804	1.020	1.009	0.978	0.984	0.966	0.949	0.980	0.965	1.006	**0.823***	0.813	**0.745***	**0.735***	0.774
		(0.12)	(0.05)	(0.06)	(0.05)	(0.04)	(0.07)	(0.05)	(0.04)	(0.07)	(0.09)	(0.16)	(0.08)	(0.09)	(0.07)	(0.05)	(0.07)
	p	*0.736*	*0.818*	*0.677*	*0.758*	*0.766*	*0.790*	*0.639*	*0.335*	*0.205*	*0.143*	*0.286*	***0.003***	*0.090*	***0.003***	***0.048***	*0.210*
	R+	0.843	0.791	1.011	0.998	0.971	0.972	0.964	0.949	0.986	0.990	1.028	0.882	0.837	0.800	0.767	**0.775***
		(0.13)	(0.06)	(0.07)	(0.07)	(0.06)	(0.07)	(0.06)	(0.06)	(0.08)	(0.12)	(0.17)	(0.12)	(0.10)	(0.10)	(0.07)	(0.06)
	R−	0.881	0.827	1.015	1.011	0.995	0.988	0.984	0.982	1.030	1.020	1.074	0.943	0.883	0.853	0.813	**0.830***
		(0.11)	(0.06)	(0.06)	(0.05)	(0.04)	(0.04)	(0.05)	(0.04)	(0.06)	(0.07)	(0.11)	(0.10)	(0.09)	(0.11)	(0.12)	(0.08)
	p	*0.346*	*0.078*	*0.888*	*0.504*	*0.166*	*0.436*	*0.309*	*0.079*	*0.076*	*U0.270*	*0.343*	*0.111*	*0.160*	*0.131*	*0.173*	***0.027***
	K+/R+	0.853	0.788	1.009	0.987	0.965	0.962	0.960	0.948	0.987	1.004	1.036	0.934	0.869	0.843	0.792	0.788
		(0.13)	(0.07)	(0.08)	(0.08)	(0.07)	(0.07)	(0.07)	(0.08)	(0.09)	(0.13)	(0.17)	(0.12)	(0.11)	(0.08)	(0.08)	(0.06)
	K+/R−	0.873	0.826	1.011	1.015	0.999	0.991	0.989	0.986	1.040	1.029	1.088	0.949	0.880	**0.863***	0.822	0.828
		(0.12)	(0.06)	(0.06)	(0.05)	(0.04)	(0.04)	(0.04)	(0.04)	(0.06)	(0.07)	(0.11)	(0.10)	(0.09)	(0.11)	(0.13)	(0.08)
	R+/K−	0.827	0.795	1.016	1.015	0.981	0.989	0.971	0.949	0.985	0.968	1.015	**0.805***	0.789	**0.736***	0.731	0.757
		(0.13)	(0.05)	(0.06)	(0.05)	(0.04)	(0.07)	(0.05)	(0.04)	(0.07)	(0.10)	(0.18)	(0.07)	(0.07)	(0.08)	(0.06)	(0.05)
	p	*0.664*	*0.369*	*0.944*	*0.613*	*0.373*	*0.598*	*0.542*	*0.276*	*0.173*	*0.470*	*0.556*	***0.022***	*0.143*	***0.028***	*0.212*	*0.125*

SD: Standard deviation. One-way analysis of variance (ANOVA), significance $p<0.05$. *U*: Mann–Whitney test, significance $p<0.05$. Asterisk (*) indicates the values that significantly differ in the same stage.
K+: K allele carriers. **K−**: K allele non-carriers. **R+**: R allele carriers. **R−**: R allele non-carriers. **K+/R+**: K and R allele carriers. **K+/R−**: K allele only carriers. **R+/K−**: R allele only carriers.

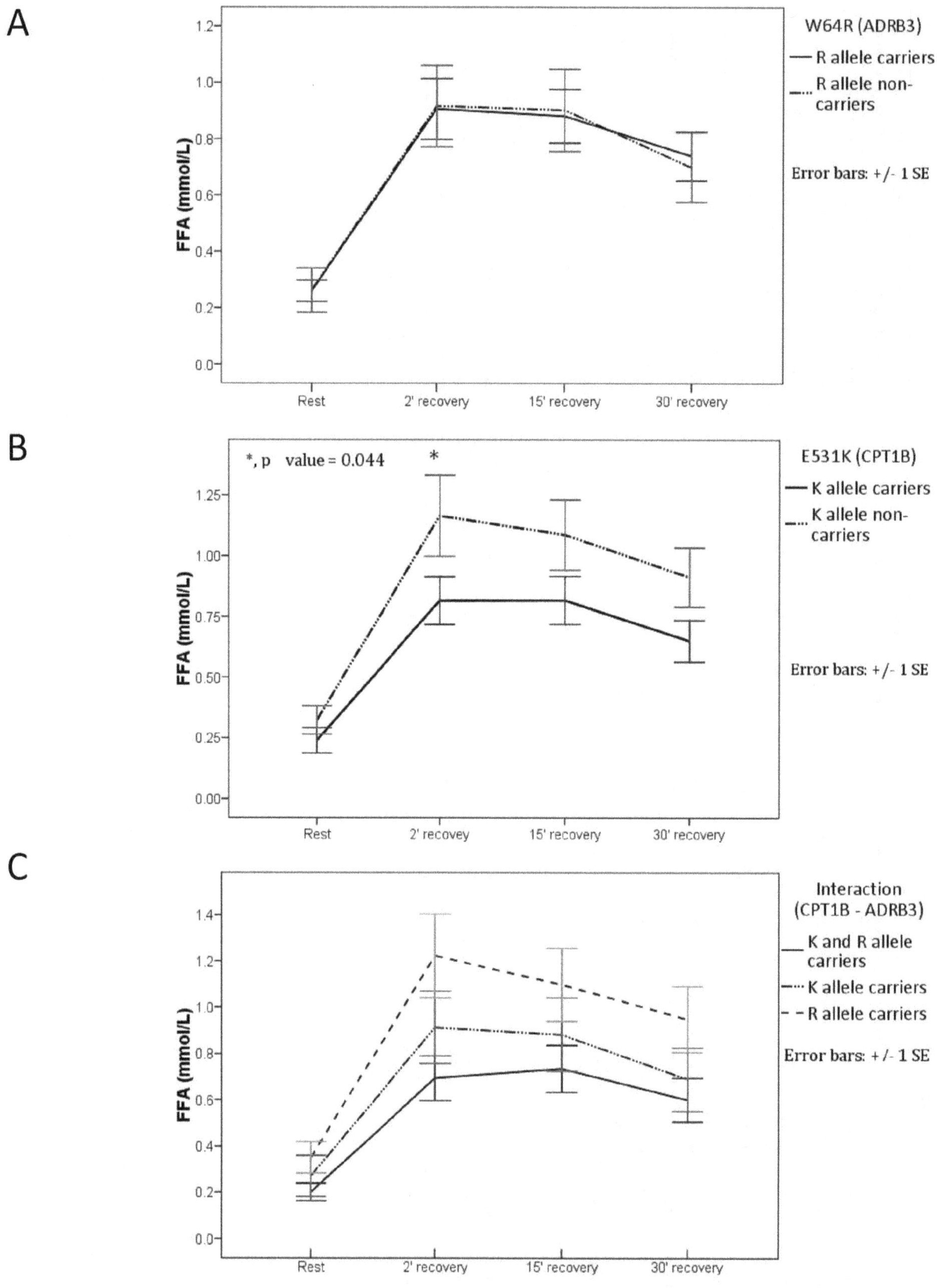

Figure 3. Free fatty acid (FFA) levels before and after the aerobic load. (**A**) R allele carriers (12 K and 8 E carriers) versus R allele non-carriers (15 K and 2 E carriers). (**B**) K allele carriers (12 R and 15 W allele carriers) versus K allele non-carriers (2 R and 8 W carriers). The asterisk indicates significant difference. (**C**) Interaction (*CPT1B–ADRB3*), carriers of both K and R alleles versus only K and only R allele carriers. Venous blood was sampled at rest and at 2, 15, and 30 min into the recovery period.

Table 6. Mean free fatty acid and beta-hydroxy butyrate at rest and at 2, 15, and 30 min post-exercise for each of the genetic classifications.

Genetic Classification		Rest	2′ post exercise	15′ post exercise	30′ post exercise
FFA (mM)	K+	0.24 (0.21)	**0.82 (0.51)***	0.82 (0.51)	0.65 (0.45)
	K−	0.32 (0.19)	**1.16 (0.53)***	1.09 (0.46)	96.2 (0.38)
		$^{U}p=0.067$	$^{U}p=\mathbf{0.044}$	$^{U}p=0.139$	$^{U}p=0.062$
	R+	0.26 (0.17)	0.91 (0.48)	0.88 (0.42)	0.74 (0.39)
	R−	0.26 (0.32)	0.92 (0.59)	0.90 (0.60)	0.70 (0.51)
		$^{A}p=0.972$	$^{A}p=0.954$	$^{A}p=0.901$	$^{A}p=0.785$
	K+/R+	0.20 (0.13)	0.69 (0.34)	0.74 (0.35)	0.60 (0.33)
	K+/R−	0.27 (0.35)	0.91 (0.61)	0.88 (0.61)	0.69 (0.53)
	R+/K−	0.35 (0.19)	1.22 (0.51)	1.10 (0.45)	0.95 (0.40)
		$^{A}p=0.627$	$^{A}p=0.189$	$^{A}p=0.464$	$^{A}p=0.414$
beta-HB (mM)	K+	0.079 (0.05)	0.089 (0.06)	**0.167 (0.09)***	**0.189 (0.11)***
	K−	0.070 (0.05)	0.090 (0.06)	**0.240 (0.08)***	**0.300 (0.09)***
		$^{U}p=0.699$	$^{U}p=0.950$	$^{U}p=\mathbf{0.022}$	$^{U}p=\mathbf{0.008}$
	R+	0.070 (0.05)	0.085 (0.06)	0.185 (0.09)	0.220 (0.12)
	R−	0.082 (0.05)	0.094 (0.06)	0.188 (0.10)	0.218 (0.11)
		$^{U}p=0.491$	$^{U}p=0.618$	$^{U}p=0.961$	$^{U}p=0.987$
	K+/R+	0.075 (0.05)	0.075 (0.06)	0.150 (0.08)	0.167 (0.11)
	K+/R−	0.080 (0.06)	0.100 (0.05)	0.180 (0.10)	0.207 (0.11)
	R+/K−	0.062 (0.05)	0.100 (0.05)	0.240 (0.09)	**0.300 (0.09)****
		$^{K}p=0.756$	$^{K}p=0.444$	$^{K}p=0.098$	$^{K}p=\mathbf{0.029}$

SD: Standard deviation. *A*: One-way analysis of variance (ANOVA). *U*: Mann–Whitney test. *K*: Kruskal–Wallis test. Significance p<0.05. Asterisk (*) indicates the values that significantly differ in the same stage. Double asterisk (**) indicates that the value differs significantly from the other values in the same stage.
FFA: Free fatty acids. **beta-HB**: Beta hydroxybutyrate. **K+**: K allele carriers. **K−**: K allele non-carriers. **R+**: R allele carriers. **R−**: R allele non-carriers.

The RQnp values during the post-exercise recovery phase were higher in K allele carriers (Figure 1-B) and independent of the R allele (Figure 1-C). This is consistent with the hypothesis that the K allele affects the translocation capacity of CPT1B, and that the effect is manifested under increased energy demands from fat that occur at the end of a prolonged workout. K allele carriers showed higher RQnp values during recovery, suggesting contributions to energy generation from fat equivalents of 19.3% at 10 min, 49.3% at 15 min, and 63.1% at 25 min compared with 59.7%, 88.0%, and 91.6% at the same post-exercise times in non-carriers [4]. Thus, K allele carriers demonstrate significantly lower fat metabolism than non-carriers. It is unlikely that the higher RQnp values among K allele carriers resulted from a reduced availability of circulating FFA because there were no differences in plasma FFA concentrations between groups after exercise, in addition the Gly values were similar, and there were no differences in hormone levels or exercise intensity. However, this is an opportunity for future research. Napal et al. [39] determined that the in vitro substitution of glutamic acid at position 590 of CPT1A increased sensitivity to malonyl coenzyme A. They concluded that the glutamic acid residue may impart structural stability to the protein, and thus affect the functional properties of the whole CPT family. In this study, we found that the substitution of glutamic acid at position 531 by lysine in the CPT1B protein had a significant effect on RQnp increase.

Notably, the sample size of this study was too small to include sufficient numbers with the rare K−/R− genotype; therefore, we could only assess the effects of allelic interaction among carriers of both alleles (K+/R+) and those carrying only one of the alleles (K+/R− and K−/R+). Consequently, the K−/R+ group also functioned as the non-carrier group for the K allele. During the recovery period, FFA levels were higher in the K−/R+ group than in the other two groups, although the difference was not statistically significant. At 10 and 20 min after exercise, this group also showed significantly lower RQnp values (Figure 2-C), and at 30 min after exercise showed significantly higher beta-HB levels (Figure 4-C). These observations indicate that the *E531K* had significant effects that were independent of *W64R*.

In this experimental design, the observation of the influence of the *E531K* SNP of *CPT1B* was facilitated because the CPT1 protein represents the only route of entry of LCFA into the beta-oxidation pathway. In contrast, ADRB3 lipolysis is modulated by the receptor as well as by several hormonal and metabolic factors. In this study, we ensured only that there were no significant differences in plasma levels of catecholamines, insulin, glucagon, Cor and growth hormone, lipids, diet (particularly PUFA content), exercise intensity, body adiposity, and cardiorespiratory fitness. Therefore, further studies are needed to strengthen and clarify the functional impact of the gene mutations involved in lipid metabolism, together with other factors such as the levels of interleukin-6 produced by muscle during contraction that can induce lipolysis within adipose tissue that peaks at the end of exercise [32,37] To this end, we have established a DNA bank with 285 participants to facilitate future cohort studies.

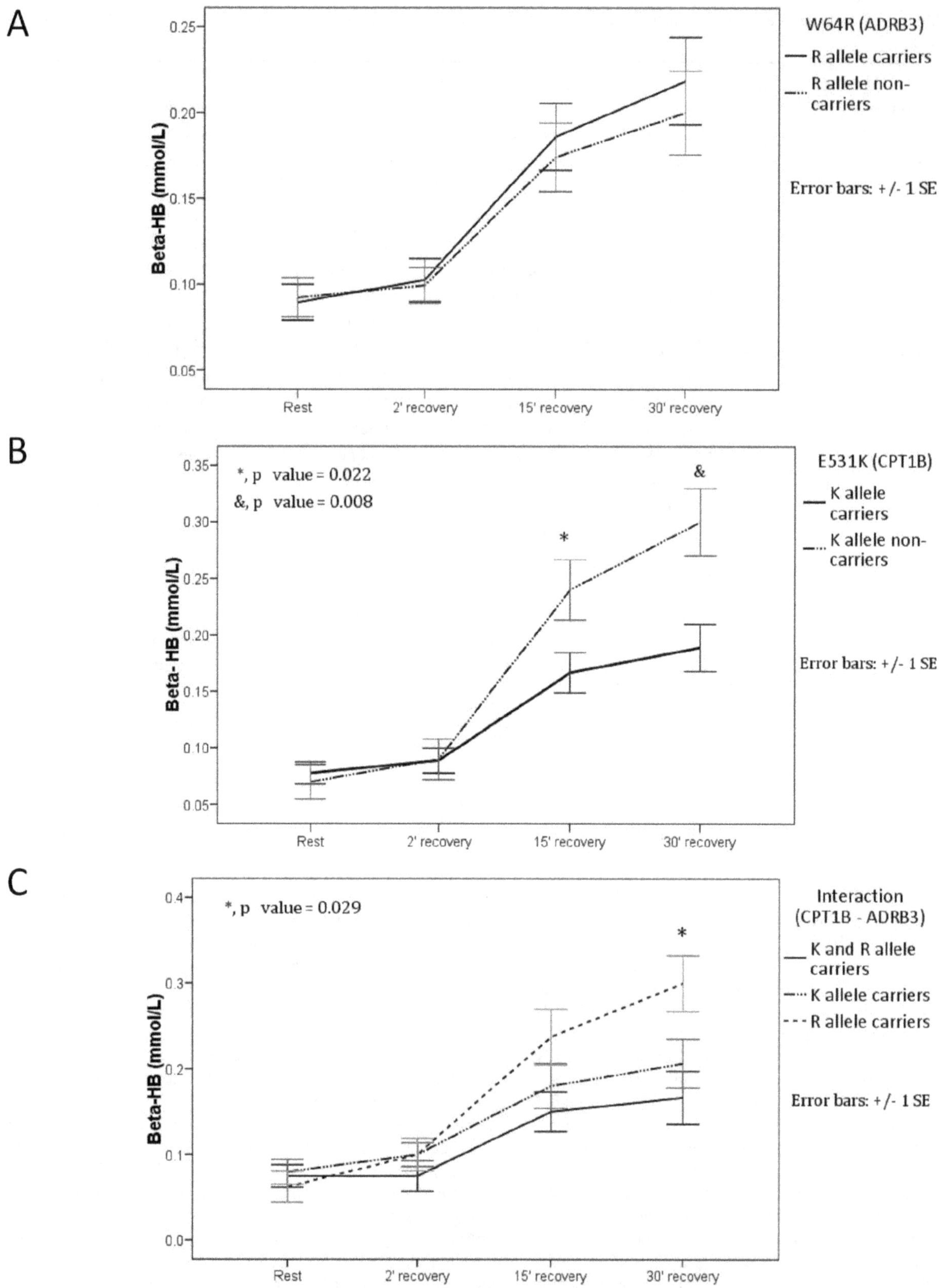

Figure 4. beta-Hydroxybutyrate (beta-HB) levels before and following the aerobic load. (**A**) R allele carriers (12 K and 8 E carriers) versus R allele non-carriers (15 K and 2 E carriers). (**B**) K allele carriers (12 R and 15 W allele carriers) versus K allele non-carriers (2 R and 8 W carriers). The asterisk indicates significant difference. (**C**) Interaction (*CPT1B–ADRB3*), carriers of both K and R alleles versus only K and only R allele carriers. The asterisk indicates a significant difference between the R allele group with 8 carriers of the E allele and the other groups. Venous blood was sampled at rest and at 2, 15, and 30 min into the recovery period.

Conclusion

The substitution of glutamic acid at position 531 by lysine in the CPT1B protein decreases the mitochondrial beta-oxidation pathway, which increases the RQnp value during recovery from exercise. This may in turn contribute to either weight gain or a reduced weight-loss following exercise.

Supporting Information

File S1 Contains Tables S1–S5. Table S1: Birthplace of the participants who completed the experimental tests. Table S2: Participants distribution in each comparison groups. Table S3: Mean (SD) values of heart rate (HR) in Tecumseh Step Test. Table S4: Means values and (SD) of blood indicators according with genetic classification. Table S5: Means and (SD) of blood hormones concentrations and hematocrit according with genetic classification.

Acknowledgments

We thank the volunteers, students and staff from the faculties of Education Sciences, Medicine and Chemical Sciences of University of Colima, for their participation.

Author Contributions

Conceived and designed the experiments: EGG JMM. Performed the experiments: EGG MRM MDTE MRF ALPH GVP JMM. Analyzed the data: EGG JMM MRM EMCR MDTE MRF IDE ALPH LMBR GVP. Contributed reagents/materials/analysis tools: JMM EMCR MDTE LMVR GVP. Wrote the paper: EGG JMM. Counseling and exposure of viewpoints to help structure discussions and conclusions: EGG JMM EMCR MDTE IDE GVP.

References

1. Nguyen DM, El-Serag HB (2010) The epidemiology of obesity. Gastroenterol Clin North Am 39: 1–7.
2. Pate RR, Mitchell JA, Byun W, Dowda M (2011) Sedentary behaviour in youth. Br J Sports Med 45: 906–913.
3. Thorp AA, Owen N, Neuhaus M, Dunstan DW (2011) Sedentary behavior and subsequent health outcomes in adults a systematic review of longitudinal studies, 1996–2011. Am J Prev Med 41: 207–215.
4. McArdle WD, Katch FI, Katch VL (2010) Exercise physiology. Nutrition, energy and human performance. Baltimore – Philadelphia: Lippincott Williams and Wilkins. 1038.
5. Shamah Levy T, Morales Ruán C, Amaya Castellanos C, Salazar Coronel A, Jiménez Aguilar A, et al. (2012) Effectiveness of a diet and physical activity promotion strategy on the prevention of obesity in Mexican school children. BMC Public Health 12: 152.
6. Bouchard C, Tremblay A, Després JP, Nadeau A, Lupien PJ, et al. (1990) The response to long-term feeding in identical twins. N Engl J Med 322: 1477–1482.
7. Ellsworth DL, Coady SA, Chen W, Srinivasan SR, Boerwinkle E, et al. (2005) Interactive effects between polymorphisms in the Beta-Adrenergic receptors and longitudinal changes in obesity. Obes Res 13: 519–526.
8. Rankinen T, Bouchard C (2012) Gene-exercise interactions. Prog Mol Biol Transl Sci 108: 447–460.
9. Hargreaves M, Spriet L (2006) Exercise Metabolism. Champaign IL: Human Kinetics. 291.
10. Zhan S, Ho SC (2005) Meta-Analysis of the association of the Trp64Arg polymorphism in the β3 adrenergic receptor with insulin resistance. Obes Res 13: 1709–1719.
11. Robitaille J, Houde A, Lemieux S, Pérusse L, Gaudet D, et al. (2007) Variants within the muscle and liver isoforms of the carnitine palmitoyltransferase I (CPT1) gene interact with fat intake to modulate indices of obesity in French-Canadians. J Mol Med 85: 129–137.
12. Corpeleijn E, Hessvik NP, Bakke SS, Levin K, Blaak EE, et al. (2010) Oxidation of intramyocellular lipids is dependent on mitochondrial function and the availability of extracellular fatty acids. Am J Physiol Endocrinol Metab 299: E14–E22.
13. Henderson GC, Fattor JA, Horning MA, Faghihnia N, Johnson ML, et al. (2007). Lipolysis and fatty acid metabolism in men and women during the postexercise period. J Physiol 584: 963–981.
14. Mirrakhimov AE, Kerimkulova AS, Lunegova OS, Moldokeeva CB, Zalesskaya YV, et al. (2011) An association between Trp64Arg polymorphism of the B3 adrenoreceptor gene and some metabolic disturbances. Cardiovasc Diabetol 10: 89.
15. Gene cards. The human gene compendium. Weizmann Institute of Science. Available: http://www.genecards.org. Accessed 2009 Nov 16.
16. Baturin AK, Pogozheva AV, Sorokina Elu, Makurina ON, Tutelian VA (2012) The Trp64Arg polymorphism of beta3-adrenoreceptor gene study in persons with overweight and obesity. Vopr Pitan 81: 23–27. [In Russian].
17. Kurokawa N, Nakai K, Kameo S, Liu ZM, Satoh H (2001) Association of BMI with the beta3-adrenergic receptor gene polymorphism in Japanese: meta-analysis. Obes Res 9: 741–745.
18. Tahara A, Osaki Y, Kishimoto T (2010) Effect of the β3-adrenergic receptor gene polymorphism Trp64Arg on BMI reduction associated with an exercise-based intervention program in Japanese middle-aged males. Environ Health Prev Med 15: 392–397.
19. Garenc C, Pérusse L, Rankinen T, Gagnon J, Leon AS, et al. (2001) The Trp64Arg polymorphism of the beta3-adrenergic receptor gene is not associated with training-induced changes in body composition: The HERITAGE Family Study. Obes Res 9: 337–341.
20. Rinaldo P, Matern D (2002) Fatty acid oxidation disorders. Annu Rev Physiol 64: 477–502.
21. Miljkovic I, Yerges LM, Li H, Gordon CL, Goodpaster BH, et al. (2009) Association of the CPT1B gene with skeletal muscle fat infiltration in Afro-Caribbean Men. Obesity 17: 1396–1401.
22. Auinger A, Rubin D, Sabandal M, Helwig U, Rüther A, et al. (2012) A common haplotype of carnitine palmitoyltransferase 1b is associated with the metabolic syndrome. Br J Nutr. 109: 810–815.
23. International Society for the Advancement of Kinanthropometry (2001) International Standards for Anthropometric Assessment. Australia: National Library of Australia. 133 p.
24. Norton K, Olds T (1996) Anthropometrica. A textbook of body measurement for sports and health courses. Australia: UNSW Press. 411 p.
25. Jekal Y, Lee MK, Park S, Lee SH, Kim JY, et al. (2010) Association between obesity and physical fitness, and hemoglobin A1c level and metabolic syndrome in Korean adults. Korean Diabetes J 43: 182–190.
26. McArdle WD, Katch FI, Katch VL (2000) Essentials of Exercise Physiology. 2nd ed. USA: Lippincott Williams and Wilkins. 365.
27. Data Base SNP, Short Genetic Variations. Pub Med NCBI. Available: http://www.ncbi.nlm.nih.gov/snp?term=rs4994 Accessed 2009 Nov 16.
28. Data Base SNP, Short Genetic Variations. Pub Med NCBI. Available: http://www.ncbi.nlm.nih.gov/snp?term=rs470117 Accessed 2009 Nov 16.
29. World Health Organization (WHO). Guidelines on drawing blood: best practices in phlebotomy. Geneva: WHO Press. 125 p.
30. American College of Sport Medicine (1991) Guidelines for exercise test administration In: Lea & Febiger. Guidelines for Exercise Testing and Prescription. 4th ed. 55–89.
31. Liu HY, Zheng G, Zhu H, Woldegiorgis G (2007) Hormonal and nutritional regulation of muscle carnitine palmitoyltransferase I gene expression in vivo. Arch Biochem Biophys 465: 437–442.
32. Sampath H, Ntambi JM (2005) Polyunsaturated fatty acid regulation of genes of lipid metabolism. Annu Rev Nutr 25: 317–340.
33. Love LK, LeBlanc PJ, Inglis JG, Bradley NS, Choptiany J, et al. (2011) The relationship between human skeletal muscle pyruvate dehydrogenase phosphatase activity and muscle aerobic capacity. J Appl Physiol 111: 427–434.
34. Egan B, Zierath JR (2013) Exercise metabolism and the molecular regulation of skeletal muscle adaptation. Cell Metab 17: 162–184.
35. Turner N, Bruce CR, Beale SM, Hoehn KL, So T, et al. (2007) Excess lipid availability increases mitochondrial fatty acid oxidative capacity in muscle: evidence against a role for reduced fatty acid oxidation in lipid-induced insulin resistance in rodents. Diabetes 56: 2085–2092.
36. Lyngso D, Simonsen L, Bülow J (2002) Metabolic effects of interleukin-6 in human splanchnic and adipose tissue. J Physiol 543: 379–386.
37. Leggate M, Nowell MA, Jones SA, Nimmo MA (2010) The response of interleukin-6 and soluble interleukin-6 receptor isoforms following intermittent high intensity and continuous moderate intensity cycling. Cell Stress Chaperones 15: 827–833.
38. Walstone J, Silver K, Bogardus C, Knowler WC, Celi FS, et al. (1995) Time of onset of non-insulin-dependent diabetes mellitus and genetic variation in the beta 3-adrenergic-receptor gene. N Engl J Med 333: 343–347.
39. Napal L, Dai J, Treber M, Haro D, Marrero PF, et al. (2003) A single amino acid change (substitution conserved Glc-590 with alanine) in the C-terminal domain of rat liver carnitine palmitoyltransferase I increases its Malonyl-CoA sensitivity close to that observed with the muscle isoform of the enzyme. J Biol Chem 278: 34084–34089.

2

Individual Responses to Completion of Short-Term and Chronic Interval Training

Todd A. Astorino[1]*, Matthew M. Schubert[2]

1 Department of Kinesiology, California State University San Marcos, San Marcos, California, United States of America, 2 School of Allied Health Sciences, Griffith University, Gold Coast, Queensland, Australia

Abstract

Alterations in maximal oxygen uptake (VO_2max), heart rate (HR), and fat oxidation occur in response to chronic endurance training. However, many studies report frequent incidence of "non-responders" who do not adapt to continuous moderate exercise. Whether this is the case in response to high intensity interval training (HIT), which elicits similar adaptations as endurance training, is unknown. The aim of this retrospective study was to examine individual responses to two paradigms of interval training. In the first study (study 1), twenty active men and women (age and baseline $VO_2max = 24.0 \pm 4.6$ yr and 42.8 ± 4.8 mL/kg/min) performed 6 d of sprint interval training (SIT) consisting of 4–6 Wingate tests per day, while in a separate study (study 2), 20 sedentary women (age and baseline $VO_2max = 23.7 \pm 6.2$ yr and 30.0 ± 4.9 mL/kg/min) performed 12 wk of high-volume HIT at workloads ranging from 60–90% maximal workload. Individual changes in VO_2max, HR, and fat oxidation were examined in each study, and multiple regression analysis was used to identify predictors of training adaptations to SIT and HIT. Data showed high frequency of increased VO_2max (95%) and attenuated exercise HR (85%) in response to HIT, and low frequency of response for VO_2max (65%) and exercise HR (55%) via SIT. Frequency of improved fat oxidation was similar (60–65%) across regimens. Only one participant across both interventions showed non-response for all variables. Baseline values of VO_2max, exercise HR, respiratory exchange ratio, and body fat were significant predictors of adaptations to interval training. Frequency of positive responses to interval training seems to be greater in response to prolonged, higher volume interval training compared to similar durations of endurance training.

Editor: Jeffrey M. Haddad, Purdue University, United States of America

Funding: The authors have no support or funding to report.

Competing Interests: The authors have declared that no competing interests exist.

* E-mail: astorino@csusm.edu

Introduction

Results from recent randomized controlled studies indicate that individual variability exists in magnitude of response to prolonged endurance training. Data from young [1] and older men and women [2] demonstrate marked variability in magnitude of change in maximal oxygen uptake (VO_2max) to endurance training. Data from the HERITAGE study [3] revealed a mean increase in VO_2max equal to 400 mL/min, yet individual responses ranged from minimal improvement to as great as 1.0 L/min. In the DREW study [4], 44.9, 23.8, and 19.3% of postmenopausal women showed no change in VO_2max in response to 6 mo of one of three aerobic exercise regimens (energy expenditure equal to 4, 8, and 12 kcal/kg/wk). More recently, Scharhag-Rosenberger et al. [5] documented similar individual variability in change in VO_2max (−0.38–0.87 L/min) and exercise HR (−22.0–2.0 b/min) in untrained individuals completing 1 yr of endurance training at 60% heart rate reserve, with 24% and 17% of participants showing no training-induced changes in these parameters. In this study, only 55% of participants (10/18) displayed meaningful increases in both parameters with training. An explanation for these results is related to genetics, as it has been reported that 47% and 34% of the change in VO_2max [3] and exercise HR [6] is heritable. In addition, baseline values of VO_2max have been shown to be associated with training-inducedchanges in some studies [4] but not others [2,7]. Clearly, there is marked heterogeneity in adaptation to chronic endurance training, which highlights the need to tailor exercise prescription to every individual to promote adaptation.

One parameter not examined in these studies is whole-body fat oxidation, which not only contributes to energy metabolism but the dysfunction of which is related to risk of obesity, insulin resistance, and diabetes [8,9]. Fat oxidation is typically increased in response to endurance training due to increased activities of carnitine acyl transferase I (CAT-1), lipase, and/or hydroxyl acyl dehydrogenase (β-HAD) [10], enhanced mitochondrial mass [11], and greater muscle fatty acid binding protein content [12]. In trained athletes, Goedecke et al. [13] demonstrated that fat oxidation during exercise, as represented by respiratory exchange ratio (RER), was determined by variables including muscle glycogen content, ratio of type I fibers, training volume, and blood lactate and free fatty acid concentration. In addition, fat oxidation is enhanced in response to low-volume sprint interval training (SIT) [14] as well as short-term [15] and more prolonged regimens [16] of high intensity interval training (HIT) characterized by completion of brief, repeated bouts of intense exercise separated by recovery.

Interval training has become a widely-employed modality of exercise training in populations including young, active men and women [17] and individuals with obesity [18], diabetes [19], and heart disease [20]. However, little is known about the magnitude of individual responses to interval training, which over the last decade has been shown to elicit similar [21,22], and in some cases, superior adaptations [20,23] versus continuous endurance training while being extremely time-efficient. Moreover, interval training has been reported [24] to be more enjoyable than continuous exercise despite exercising at higher intensities, which in the long run may promote greater adherence to training and on an individual level, superior maintenance of fitness level, health status, and quality of life. Despite over 100 studies being published in the last decade concerning effects of interval training on variables including VO_2max and body composition, no study has attempted to elucidate individual responses to interval training. Therefore, the aim of the present study was to identify individual "responders" and "non-responders" for to variables related to metabolic health (VO_2max and lipid oxidation) and cardiovascular function (exercise HR) in response to two commonly used modalities of interval training previously-employed in our lab [14,16,25]. It was hypothesized that frequency of "non-responders" would be less than that typically reported after endurance training [4,5]. Ultimately, the development of individualized exercise prescription using this novel approach may help optimize responses to training and overall health status of various individuals.

Method

Ethics Statement

Prior to providing written informed consent, all participants filled out a health-history questionnaire to ensure that they met all inclusion criteria, and all procedures were approved by the CSU–San Marcos University Institutional Review Board.

Participants

Twenty habitually-active men and women participated in study 1, which examined potential gender differences in adaptation to short-term low-volume interval training. Mean age, body fat, current physical activity, and VO_2max were equal to 24.0±4.6 yr, 20.3±4.7%, 7.9±2.0 h/wk, and 42.8±4.8 mL/kg/min, respectively. Study 2 was designed to examine the timecourse of changes in metabolic health in response to two doses of prolonged interval training in 20 non-obese sedentary women free of disease. They initially completed a validated questionnaire (Past Year Total Physical Activity Questionnaire) to confirm that they completed ≤ 1 h/wk of formal physical activity in the preceding year. Their age, body fat, and VO_2max were equal to 23.7±6.2 yr, 24.2±5.8%, and 30.0±4.9 mL/kg/min, respectively.

Design

In study 1, recreationally-active men and women underwent 2 wk of Wingate-based SIT [14,18,21]. At baseline and after completion of training, measures of VO_2max, HR, and lipid oxidation were determined on separate days at least 24 h apart. Participants were required to maintain their habitual training status which was confirmed with a training log, and time of day was standardized within subjects across all trials. In study 2, sedentary young women completed 12 wk of a more tolerable form of interval training [15,19] at intensities equal to 60–80% or 80–90%Wmax, during which these variables were assessed at baseline and every 3 wk of the study over two separate sessions. They were required to refrain from additional physical activity other than activities of daily living outside of the study. Exercise was performed at approximately the same time of day (≤60 min) within participants. In both studies, body composition was assessed pre- and post-training using waist:hip ratio and sum of three skinfolds (chest, abdomen, thigh for men and triceps, suprailiac, and thigh for women) following standardized procedures [26].

Interval Training

Following procedures described in previous studies [14,18,21], men and women in study 1 performed six sessions of low volume SIT consisting of repeated Wingate tests (4–6 per day at intensities = 200–300%Wmax) over a 2 wk period. Resistance was equal to 7.5%BW for women and 8.5%BW for men. Training was performed on the Monark peak bike (model 894e, Vansbro, Sweden) and consisted of 30 s of "all-out" cycling interspersed with 5 min of unloaded pedaling. Results [14] showed that peak power, mean power, and minimum power were increased ($p < 0.05$) with SIT, although no change in fatigue index ([peak power – minimum power/peak power] ×100) was demonstrated. In study 2, women performed 3 d/wk of interval training for 12 wk consisting of six to ten 1 min bouts of cycling at work rates equal to 60–80%Wmax or 80–90%Wmax, similar to previously performed [19]. All training was performed on an electrically-braked cycle ergometer (Velotron Dynafit Pro, RacerMate, Seattle, WA). Each week, number of bouts (+2 bouts per week) and work rate (+ 5%Wmax) were increased to promote progression [25]. By the end of training, women were training at absolute work rates 25% higher than that completed at baseline [25].

Assessment of VO_2max, HR, and Fat Oxidation

In study 1, VO_2max was assessed on a cycle ergometer (Monark 828e, Vansbro, Sweden) during which pulmonary gas exchange data were continuously obtained using a metabolic cart (Parvo-Medics True One, Sandy, UT). The system was calibrated to gases of known concentration as well as to room air, and a 3-L syringe (Hans Rudolph, Kansas City, MO) was used to calibrate volume. Work rate began at 70 W for the initial 2 min, followed by 28 W/min increases in power output until volitional exhaustion. Test duration ranged from 8–12 min [27], and attainment of a plateau in VO_2, HRmax±10 b/min of 220– age, and RERmax >1.15 were used to verify VO_2max attainment [28,29]. The coefficient of variation for VO_2max derived from controls in this study as well as other active men and women completing repeated bouts of graded exercise testing following these methods was <2.8%, comparable to other studies [29]. At least 24 h later at the same time of day and 3 h post-absorptive, participants completed 10 min of cycling at each of three intensities equal to 50, 60, and 70%Wmax, during which gas exchange data were continuously obtained. Nutritional intake was standardized for 24 h before this bout and assessed via diet records. Data were averaged every 5 min and used to calculate RER and rates of fat and carbohydrate oxidation (in kcal/min) using the Frayn equations [30]. Coefficient of variation for exercise RER at these work rates obtained from active men and women was equal to 4.3%. Intraclass correlations for RER at 50, 60, and 70%Wmax were equal to 0.63, 0.82, and 0.87, respectively, similar to a previous study in trained cyclists [13]. Heart rate was obtained continuously through telemetry (Polar Electro, Woodbury, NY) and averaged every 5 min during exercise. Coefficient of variation in exercise HR was equal to 2.1%.

In study 2, VO_2max was assessed on a cycle ergometer (Velotron DynaFit Pro, RacerMate, Seattle, WA) with simultaneous measurement of gas exchange data (ParvoMedics True One, Sandy, UT). Power output was equal to 40 W for the initial 2 min and increased in a ramp-like manner by 20 W/min until volitional exhaustion. Coefficient of variation for sedentary women completing ramp cycle ergometry in our lab is <3.0%. Similar criteria were used to confirm attainment of VO_2max [28]. Women returned at least 24 h later at the same time of day after an overnight fast and completed graded cycling (40 W for 4 min followed by 20 W/min increases in work rate every 3 min) until RER exceeded 1.0 for an entire stage. Nutritional intake was standardized for 24 h before this bout. Gas exchange data and HR were averaged from the last 2 min of each stage, with the former used to determine RER and fat and carbohydrate oxidation using the Frayn equations [30]. Coefficients of variation for these measures were equal to 4.6% for RER and 3.4% for exercise HR, respectively.

Assessing Individual Responses

In study 1, change in VO_2max (expressed as a percent as well as in L/min and mL/kg/min) was computed in response to 2 wk of Wingate-based SIT, as in some participants, body mass did change during the study. Changes in HR and lipid oxidation derived from RER were obtained from a continuous bout of cycling for 10 min at 50, 60, and 70%Wmax. Total changes in HR (b/min) and lipid oxidation (RER) were added across these three workloads and then divided by 3 to identify an average change in these variables in response to training. For example, if HR and RER were reduced by −3, −6, and −4 b/min and −0.02, −0.04, and −0.06 at 50, 60, and 70%Wmax in response to training, change in HR and RER was equal to −4.3 b/min and −0.04 (13% greater fat oxidation), respectively. In study 2, change in VO_2max was determined by comparing determinations of VO_2max before (0 wk) and after training (12 wk), and expressed as a percent change as well as in L/min and mL/kg/min, respectively. Training-induced changes in HR and lipid oxidation were obtained using similar procedures as performed in study 1. All women performed at least 4 stages of progressive cycling exercise at work rates equal to 40, 60, 80, and 100 W.

Data Analysis

Results are reported as mean ± SD and were analyzed using SPSS Version 20.0 (Chicago, IL). Confidence intervals (95%) were also computed for select variables. Multiple regression was used to determine predictors of the change in VO_2max (%), exercise HR (b/min), and fat oxidation (% change in fat oxidation according to RER) in response to SIT and HIT. Based on previous findings [4–5,7,13], variables entered in each two-predictor model included baseline values of VO_2max (mL/kg/min), exercise HR (b/min) and fat oxidation (% fat oxidation from mean RER value), age, %BF, and related parameters obtained in both studies. Responders were identified by a magnitude of adaptation greater than 1 CV for that parameter, and participants with changes from baseline less than 1 CV were labeled as "nonresponders" as previously-reported [5]. Statistical significance was established as $p<0.05$.

Results

Study 1

Individual changes in VO_2max. There was 100% compliance to training in this study. Figure 1a–c shows change in VO_2max across subjects. The mean (± SD) and 95% confidence interval for percent change, absolute, and relative increase in VO_2max was equal to 6.3±5.4% (3.7–8.8%, range = 0–20%), 0.19±0.13 L/min (0.12–0.26 L/min, range = −0.02 = 0.48 L/min), and 2.6±2.0 mL/kg/min (1.3–3.2 mL/kg/min, range = −0.65–6.25 mL/kg/min), respectively. Overall, 13 of 20 participants (65%) showed meaningful improvements (>2.8%) in VO_2max in response to 2 wk of SIT, with four individuals

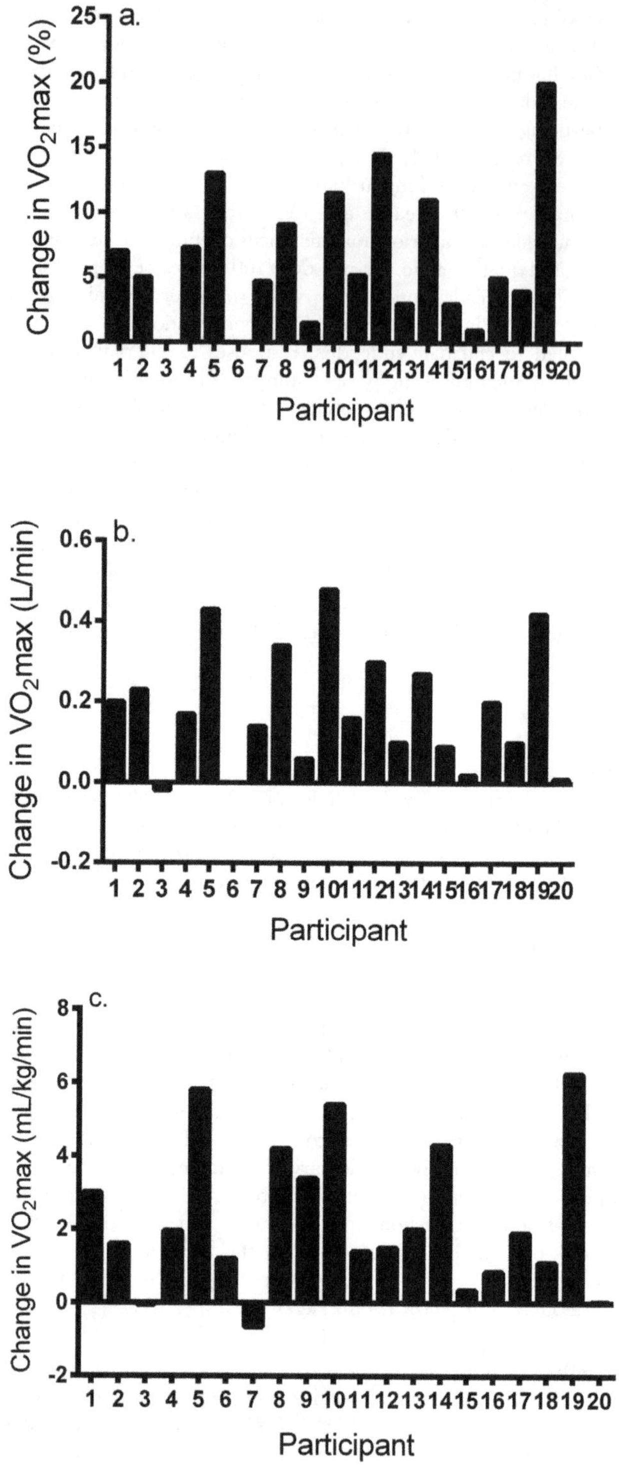

Figure 1. Individual responses for a) percent change in VO_2max; b) absolute change in VO_2max; and c) relative change in VO_2max in response to 2 wk of low-volume interval training.

(20%) showing no change and three (15%) showing insignificant increases in VO_2max.

Individual changes in exercise HR. Mean absolute and percent change in exercise HR was equal to −5±8 b/min (95%CI = −9–−1 b/min, range = −17–9 b/min) and −2.8±4.5% (−4.9 = −0.7%, range = −9.1–5.3%), respectively.

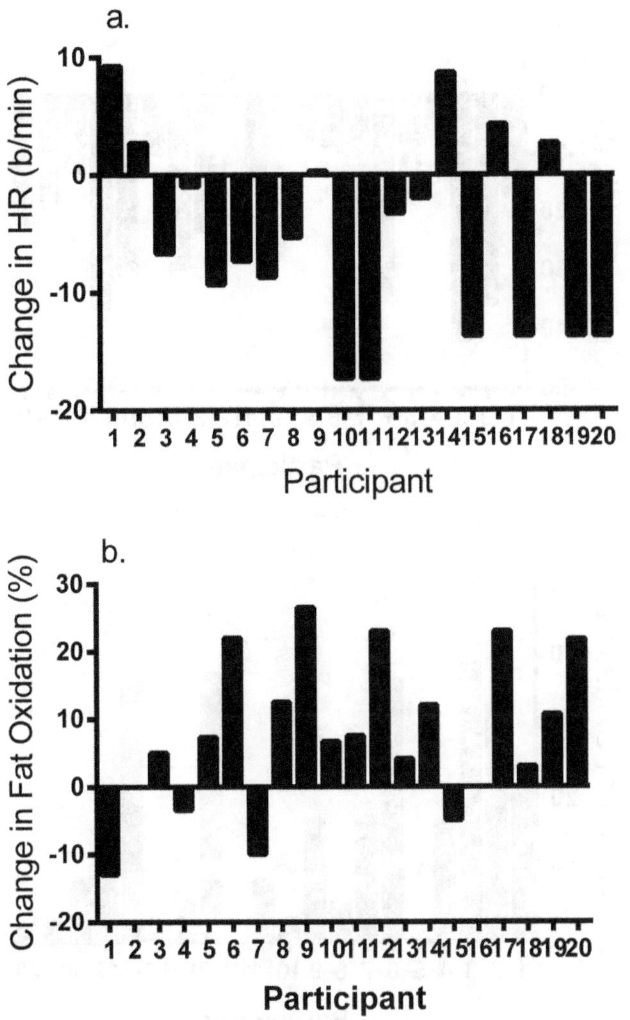

Figure 2. Individual responses for a) change in exercise HR and b) lipid oxidation in response to 2 wk of low-volume interval training.

Eleven of 20 participants (55%) showed reductions in exercise HR, with 25% showing higher HR and the remaining 20% presenting insignificant changes in HR in response to training. These data are revealed in Figure 2a.

Individual changes in fat oxidation. Mean change in fat oxidation was equal to 7.7±11.4% (2.3–13.0%, range = −13.0–26.5%). Sixty percent of men and women revealed improvements in fat oxidation; whereas, 25% showed no change and 15% demonstrated reduced fat oxidation in response to SIT (Figure 2b).

Multiple regression data. Two-predictor models were used to identify predictors of the change in each parameter in response to Wingate-based SIT. A model (R = 0.61, p = 0.03) consisting of baseline VO_2max (r = −0.44, p = 0.03) and Wingate-derived fatigue index (r = 0.50, p = 0.01) explained 36% of the percent change in VO_2max in response to training,. Age (r = 0.67, p = 0.001) and baseline HR at 30 min of cycling explained the greatest variance in change in exercise HR (R = 0.68, $R^2 = 0.46$, p<0.01), with age serving as an independent predictor of exercise HR (t = 3.84, p = 0.001). A model (R = 0.52, p = 0.03) including age (r = −0.41, p = 0.03) and current physical activity (r = −0.47, p = 0.02) explained 27% of the change (R = 0.52, p = 0.03) in fat oxidation.

Study 2

Despite somewhat different intensities of HIT performed in this study, no training-induced differences in any parameter were observed between regimens, so data were combined. Compliance to training was high (96.4% of all required sessions).

Individual changes in VO_2max. Mean change in VO_2max was equal to 25.1±9.5% (95%CI = 20.6–29.5%, range = 2.7–47.8%). Absolute and relative change in VO_2max was equal to 0.39±0.16 L/min (95%CI = 0.32–0.46 L/min, range = 0.08–0.66 L/min) and 6.4±2.3 mL/kg/min (5.3–7.4 mL/kg/min, range = 0.9−9.7 mL/kg/min), respectively. With exception of one woman, all remaining (95%) participants were classified as responders showing an increase in VO_2max via HIT. These data are revealed in Figure 3a–c.

Individual changes in exercise HR. Figure 4a demonstrates individual changes in exercise HR in response to high-volume interval training. Mean change in exercise HR was equal to −17±13 b/min (−28–−7 b/min, range = −42–3 b/min), with marked individual variability across participants. Seventeen of 20 participants (85%) showed reductions in exercise HR in response to training; whereas, 15% were classified as nonresponders.

Individual changes in fat oxidation. Individual changes in whole-body fat oxidation derived from RER are demonstrated in Figure 4b. Mean change in fat oxidation was equal to 16.8±14.4% (95%CI = 9.6–24.0%, range = 0.0–39.0%). Sixty five percent of women (13/20) revealed improved fat oxidation in response to 12 wk of HIT, and 35% showed minimal or no change in this parameter.

Multiple regression data. A model (R = 0.71, p = 0.003) consisting of baseline VO_2max (r = −0.63, p = 0.002) and body fat explained 50% of the variance in the change in VO_2max after 12 wk of training. A two-predictor model (R = 0.80, p = 0.001) consisting of baseline VO_2max and HR at 40 W significantly explained 64% of the variance in the training-induced reduction in HR. Besides VO_2max (r = 0.52, p = 0.008) and HR at 40 W (r = −0.75, p = 0.000), significant correlates of the change in exercise HR also included age (r = −0.44, p = 0.02), body fat (r = −0.44, p = 0.02) and HR at 60 (r = −0.69, p = 0.001) and 80 W (r = −0.57, p = 0.004). Many predictors were significantly related to increases in whole-body fat oxidation, including baseline VO_2max (−0.44, p = 0.03), body fat (r = 0.40, p = 0.04), age (r = 0.45, p = 0.02), waist circumference (r = 0.38, p = 0.05), waist:hip ratio (r = 0.47, p = 0.02), and RER at 40 W (r = 0.51, p = 0.01). Waist:hip ratio and RER at 60 W (R = 0.66, p = 0.008) explained the greatest variance (43%) in improvements in fat oxidation.

Overall changes in VO_2max, HR, and fat oxidation. Tables 1 and 2 show frequency of participants revealing significant changes in measured parameters in both studies. Six of 20 participants (30%) in study 1 revealed improvements in all parameters; similarly, six (30%) showed beneficial changes in two of three variables and seven (35%) revealed adaptation in only one parameter. One male participant (age = 23 yr, VO_2max = 52.3 mL/kg/min) whose VO_2max was highest in this sample was a "non-responder" for all measures. Eleven women (55%) in study 2 were classified as responders in all outcome measures; whereas, seven (35%) demonstrated adaptation in two variables and the remaining two women (10%) were classified as responders for only one measure (VO_2max).

Discussion

The primary aim of this retrospective study was to separately examine individual responses to two regimens of high-intensity

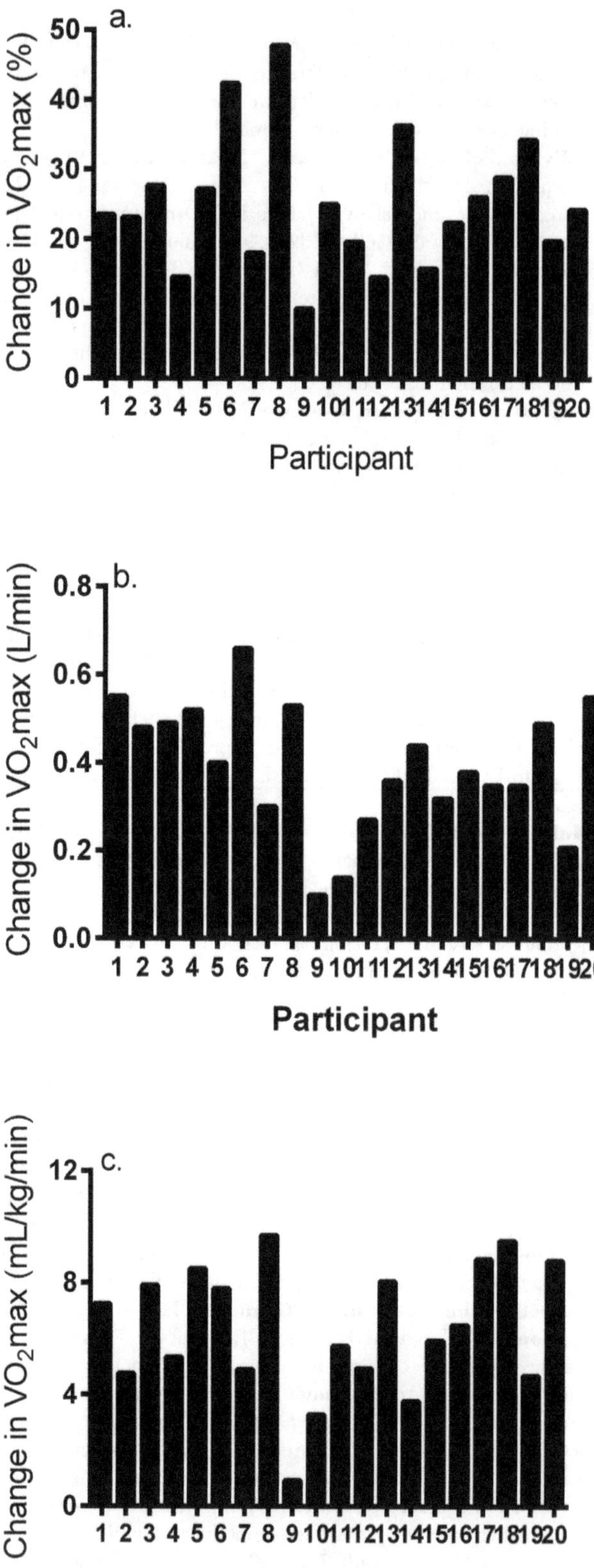

Figure 3. Individual responses for a) percent change in VO_2max; b) absolute change in VO_2max; and c) relative change in VO_2max in response to 12 wk of high-volume interval training.

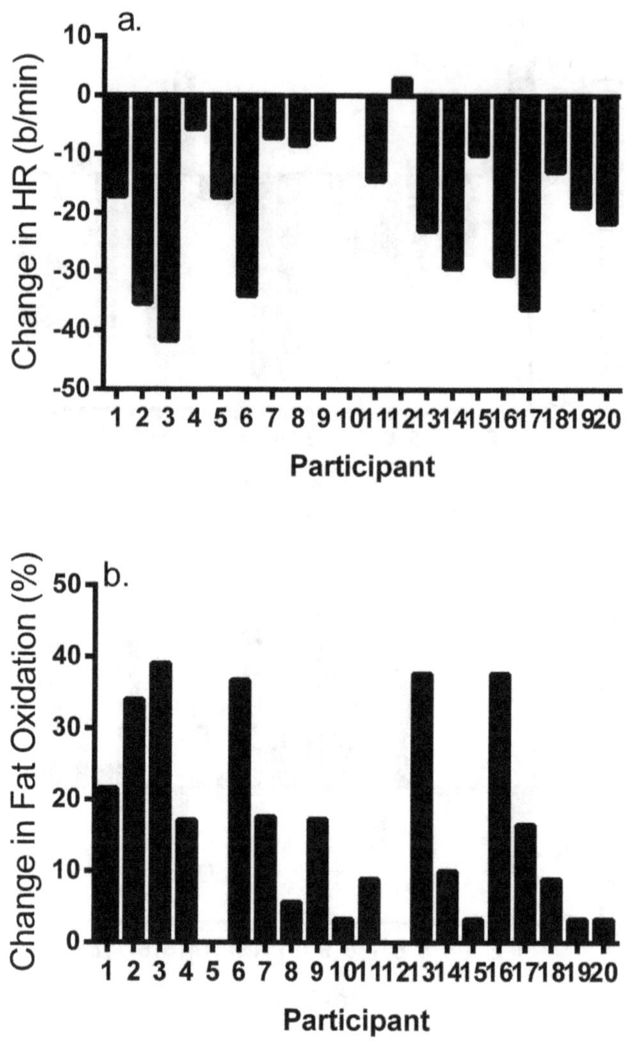

Figure 4. Individual responses for a) change in exercise HR and b) lipid oxidation in response to 12 wk of high-volume interval training.

interval training (SIT and HIT) performed by young, healthy men and women varying in fitness level. Changes in VO_2max, heart rate, and fat oxidation were identified as they are frequently assessed in response to completion of endurance [5,31]) and/or interval training interventions [14–15] and are related to cardiovascular and metabolic health. Results demonstrated that prolonged, high-volume HIT elicits greater frequency of adaptations in VO_2max and reduction in HR and lower frequency of "non-responders" compared to prolonged endurance training [4,5]. In contrast, two weeks of low-volume SIT demonstrated high frequency of non-responders (35–45%) in all variables. Predictors of change in these variables included age, baseline VO_2max and fatigue index, and current physical activity as well as waist:hip ratio and measures of HR and RER obtained during moderate exercise. Overall, participants desiring to potentially improve VO_2max through interval training may perform more prolonged, higher volume regimens of HIT as the magnitude of change in VO_2max and frequency of nonresponse are lower than those frequently reported for endurance training. Nevertheless, frequency of non-responders to all outcomes was low (1 of 40 individuals), suggesting that either HIT or SIT provides a robust

Table 1. Individual responses in VO_2max, exercise HR, and fat oxidation to low-volume HIT in active men and women.

Participant	1	2	3	4	5	6	7	8	9	10	11	12	13	14	15	16	17	18	19	20	Response Frequency
Parameter																					
VO_2max	R	R	NR	R	R	NR	R	R	NR	R	R	R	NR	R	NR	NR	R	R	R	NR	65%
eHR	NR	NR	R	NR	R	R	R	R	NR	R	R	NR	NR	NR	R	NR	R	NR	R	R	55%
Fat oxidation	NR	NR	R	NR	R	R	NR	R	R	R	R	R	R	R	NR	NR	R	NR	R	R	65%

R = responder; NR = non-responder; eHR = exercise heart rate; note that the columns refer to individual participants.
Low-volume HIT = 2 weeks (6 sessions) of Wingate-based HIT.

Table 2. Individual responses in VO_2max, exercise HR, and fat oxidation to high-volume HIT in sedentary women.

Participants	1	2	3	4	5	6	7	8	9	10	11	12	13	14	15	16	17	18	19	20	Response Frequency
Parameter																					
VO_2max	R	R	R	R	R	R	R	R	NR	R	R	R	R	R	R	R	R	R	R	R	95%
eHR	R	R	R	NR	R	R	R	R	R	NR	R	NR	R	R	R	R	R	R	R	R	85%
Fat oxidation	R	R	R	R	NR	R	R	NR	R	NR	R	NR	R	R	NR	R	R	R	NR	NR	65%

R = responder; NR = non-responder; eHR = exercise heart rate; note that the columns refer to individual participants.
High volume HIT = 12 weeks of 3 sessions/wk of 6–10 1-min bouts @ 60–90% W_{max}.

stimulus to improve cardiorespiratory fitness and metabolic health in young men and women.

Our data align with recent findings from two meta-analyses documenting effects of interval training on VO_2max in young, active adults. Gist et al. [32] demonstrated a small to moderate effect of 2–10 wk (mean duration = 4.8±2.3 wk) of Wingate-based SIT on VO_2max, as shown by 8% and 3.6 mL/kg/min improvements in VO_2max compared to controls, although the effect was similar to that of endurance training and quite heterogeneous across studies. Our lower percent change in VO_2max in response to Wingate-based SIT is likely due to its relatively brief duration, supporting data from Bailey et al. [33] revealing a 6.7% improvement in VO_2max after only 2 wk of training. Bacon et al. [34] summarized 37 studies conducted in untrained men and women (VO_2max <55 mL/kg/min) performing a minimum of 6 wk of HIT and 10 min of training per session. These authors reported larger increases in VO_2max (0.51 L/min, 95% CI = 0.43–0.60 L/min) than previously reported via interval training [15,17,21] or from the current study (0.39 L/min, see Results). In addition, they cited that studies employing longer intervals (>3 min) combined with endurance exercise producing a greater training volume typically led to greater changes in VO_2max than those characterized by shorter bouts and lower volume. This intuitively makes sense, as completion of longer duration exercise, albeit at intensities approaching or at VO_2max, is more dependent on aerobic metabolism than ≤60 s bouts more reliant on nonoxidative metabolism. Overall, these authors concluded that higher volume (>10 min of exercise) interval training increases VO_2max in most young individuals, with greater increases in VO_2max seen compared to results from large-scale training studies [3–5] revealing a high frequency of non-responders to training. Our data support this conclusion, as we show that low-volume SIT tends to elicit lower frequency of increases in VO_2max (65%) than via endurance training. The fact that low-volume SIT seems to induce mostly peripheral versus central cardiovascular adaptations [35] is a plausible explanation for this discrepancy as well as the habitually active status of the majority of individuals participating in these studies.

Results from both interval training regimens showed that baseline VO_2max was inversely related to training-induced change in VO_2max. In contrast, in the HERITAGE study [7], participants with high and low VO_2max revealed similar increases (348–419 mL/min) in this parameter. In fact, age and gender were the best predictors, with baseline VO_2max explaining only 1% of the variance in VO_2max response to training. Yet in a different subset of data from this study reported by Skinner et al. [36], a significant inverse correlation ($r = -0.38$) occurred between baseline VO_2max and percent change in this measure. Similar lack of significant associations between these baseline factors and change in VO_2max was shown in middle-aged men and women performing 1 yr of endurance training [5] and men and women aged 60–71 yr performing 9–12 mo of endurance training [2]. Differences in participants' age and baseline fitness level and mode, frequency, and duration of exercise across studies could explain these dissimilar results. For example, our participants were much younger than the individuals recruited in these aforementioned studies. In contrast, data from the DREW study [4] revealed that baseline VO_2max was a significant predictor of VO_2max response to 6 mo of continuous training in postmenopausal women. In addition to baseline VO_2max, data from the current study showed that body fat was inversely correlated to change in VO_2max in sedentary women completing 12 wk of HIT; whereas, Wingate-derived fatigue index ((peak power – minimum power)/peak power) was positively correlated with change in VO_2max in active men and women performing low volume SIT. This may suggest that body composition and fatigue resistance influences resultant changes in VO_2max to interval training, although further study is merited to confirm this assumption. Overall, it is plausible that no relationship between baseline VO_2max and resultant change in VO_2max is likely in homogeneous populations; whereas, significant relationships may be detected when participants are heterogeneous, as was the case in our studies.

Despite the robust increase in VO_2max reported by Bacon et al. [34], their results are somewhat diminished by the extensive time commitment needed to optimize VO_2max. One of the main advantages of low-volume SIT is its relative time-efficiency both in actual exercise time (~ 2–10 min/session) as well as total session time typically less than 30 min. Recent data in sedentary women [25] show that increases in VO_2max were comparable whether more (80–90%Wmax) or less intense (60–80%Wmax) regimens of HIT were performed for 12 wk, suggesting that a greater intensity of interval training following an identical regimen (mode, duration, number of bouts, frequency, etc.) may not maximize changes in VO_2max, as was revealed versus moderate exercise in athletes [37]. Moreover, HIT elicits similar adaptations as continuous exercise [21] yet has been perceived as more enjoyable [24] which in the long run may promote exercise adherence and ultimately greater gains in fitness and health outcomes. Nevertheless, does a small additional increase in VO_2max exhibited with more prolonged interval training justify the extra time allotment, based on the fact that lack of time [38] is often cited as the greatest barrier to exercise? Despite empirical data [39] showing that greater values of VO_2max reduce future risk of chronic disease, the minimal time commitment and efficacy of short-term SIT (bouts ≤1 min) described in various populations may position it as a more desirable alternative to regimens such as endurance training requiring greater than 30 min/d.

Compared to VO_2max and fat oxidation, there was lower frequency of adaptation in exercise HR in response to Wingate-based SIT. In the HERITAGE study [31], 20 wk of endurance training decreased HR during cycling at 50 W by 11 b/min, although individual responses ranged from reductions in HR as large as –42 b/min to a 12 b/min increase. Their data [7] also showed that participants with elevated pre-training HR at this workload demonstrated larger decreases in HR compared to those with a lower exercise HR (−16 b/min vs. −7 b/min, respectively). In addition, baseline HR at 50 W and gender were significant predictors of change in exercise HR, with ethnicity and age having minimal relationships. Our data support this evidence as in response to both HIT paradigms, submaximal HR obtained pre-training was a strong, significant predictor of its response to training. Recently, Rankinen et al. [6] showed that heritability of HR response to training was localized to nine single-nucleotide polymorphisms (SNPs) related to cardiomyocyte and neuronal function. Overall, practitioners should not expect marked reductions in HR in clients with an existing blunted response to exercise as typically seen in habitually active individuals.

Although predictors of change in VO_2max and exercise HR in response to endurance training have been identified, less is known regarding correlates of changes in fat oxidation. In one cross-sectional study, Stisin et al. [12] compared fat oxidation between untrained (VO_2max = 41.5 mL/kg/min) and trained women (VO_2max = 53.8 mL/kg/min) during progressive exercise. Although maximal fat oxidation (in g/min) and workload coincident with maximal fat oxidation were similar between groups, trained women showed higher fat oxidation at moderate and high intensities versus untrained women. Compared to the untrained women, trained women revealed higher ($p<0.05$) activities of citrate synthase(CS), hormone sensitive lipase, and beta-hydroxy acyl CoA dehydrogenase (B-HAD). Across all women, significant positive relationships were exhibited between CS/B-HAD and the workload coincident with maximal fat oxidation as well as fat oxidation at 150 W. In a previous study identifying determinants of RER [13], trained cyclists exercised at 25, 50, and 70%Wmax which was accompanied by measurements of blood lactate, free fatty acids, as well as substrate concentrations via muscle biopsy. Results demonstrated that training volume, muscle glycogen, percent type I fibers, and lactate and free fatty acid concentration were key determinants of exercise RER, supporting Stisin et al.'s [12] data. Our results add to the literature by showing that noninvasive, widely-obtained measures including exercise RER, waist:hip ratio, and age and volume of physical activity can also be used to predict change in fat oxidation in response to interval training. Nevertheless, VO_2max of individuals participating in our training studies was typically lower than that reported in previous studies, so generalization of our findings to more trained populations is cautioned.

One interesting finding of our study is that the frequency of improvements in whole-body fat oxidation was comparable between individuals in study 1 and 2 (see Results) despite the markedly different duration (6–9 min/wk vs. 18–30 min/wk) and intensity (200–300%Wmax vs. 60–90%Wmax) of training performed as well as discrepancies in VO_2max, gender, and body composition across participants. In addition, the protocols used to assess fat oxidation across studies slightly differed. Low-volume SIT has been reported [22,35] to induce primarily peripheral versus central cardiovascular adaptations that would increase fat oxidation, so it may be that mitochondrial signaling changes are more sensitive to the intensity of exercise rather than overall training volume. For example, mRNA content for primary regulators of mitochondrial biogenesis and lipid metabolism was similar in response to 90 min of moderate exercise compared to interval exercise at 120%VO_2max [40]. However, large variability in exercise RER has been documented in trained athletes [10,13], which suggests that training-induced changes in RER should vary across individuals. In addition, men and women in study 1 completed 30 min of cycling after a 3 h fast, yet in study 2, women underwent a 12 h fast before performing a shorter bout of progressive exercise, which may elicitt discrepancies in glycogen content and glucose/insulin levels across participants which affect substrate oxidation. All participants ingested widely divergent diets, so it is likely that circulating free fatty acid concentrations differed before exercise which may alter resultant substrate oxidation. In study 2, increases in fat oxidation peaked at 6 or 9 wk of training in many individuals and did not change or slightly declined at 12 wk, sofurther studies are needed to identify the optimal exercise regimen to sustain the improved fat oxidation observed with interval training.

There are a few implications of identifying individual responses to interval training. One, our findings corroborate data obtained from endurance-training studies [1,4] that not every individual adapts to training despite steady increases in frequency, intensity, and/or duration of training. Second, it emphasizes that assessments should be done frequently after initiation of training, and in the case of interval training, after as little as 2 wk, to ensure that anticipated adaptations are occurring. If they are not, specific training parameters should be modified to promote potential for adaptation. To our knowledge, this unique approach has yet to be instituted with interval training and may optimize adaptation, even in individuals previously identified as "non-responders." Lastly, it raises a compelling question: what can a practitioner do if, for example, VO_2max does not increase with exercise training in an individual with known risk factors for chronic disease? Potentially other factors need to be targeted such as blood pressure, waist circumference, blood lipids, or even inflammation using a more individualized approach. We encourage scientists leading large-scale training studies to attempt to "follow-up" with non-responders to examine if other modalities of exercise training are effective to improve health status.

Limitations to this study include its use of dissimilar regimes of HIT, one employing Wingate-based SIT in active men and women and the other consisting of lower intensity bouts of high-volume HIT in sedentary women, although the regimens were analyzed separately and not compared. Clearly, additional data collection is merited in untrained and active individuals completing the same interval training regimen to compare the effectiveness of each protocol. In addition, all participants were young and free of disease, so it is likely that individual responses may differ in older adults, clinical populations, as well as persons who are extremely deconditioned. Exercise was performed on a cycle ergometer which was a relatively unfamiliar mode of exercise for most participants, so adaptations to treadmill training may have varied. No mechanistic variables were obtained in either study, such as glucose tolerance (insulin sensitivity and fasting insulin), hemodynamic function (stroke volume and cardiac output), or muscle oxidative capacity (fiber type expression, citrate synthase, etc.), whose changes may parallel individual changes in VO_2max, HR, and fat oxidation. Fat oxidation is affected by habitual fat intake [13], and although dietary intake was standardized for 24 h before assessments, regular dietary practices were not considered in regards to altering the change in fat oxidation. Our use of the coefficient of variation of various measures to identify responders and non-responders has precedence [5], yet does not include random error in the measurement. Therefore, frequency of response to interval training may be slightly overestimated in the current study. However, this study is strengthened by inclusion of a large, heterogeneous sample of men and women differing in ethnicity, BMI, fitness level, and body fat as well as stringent control of workloads completed, continuous supervision of all exercise sessions, and high compliance rate.

Conclusions

Results from this retrospective analysis of 40 individuals completing different interval training regimes indicated that the frequency of non-responders was 5–45% depending upon the parameter measured and specific regimen completed. In addition, our results suggest that a 12 wk regime of HIT elicits superior individual responses in VO_2max and exercise HR compared to that reported from endurance training [5] as well as low-volume SIT [18,21]. Compared to improvements in VO_2max and exercise HR, frequency of improvement in exercise fat oxidation was typically lower, therefore further research is warranted to identify the optimal regimen of interval training to improve fat oxidation. In summary, for individuals who desire to improve their health but have low levels of cardiorespiratory fitness, beginning an exercise-based weight-maintenance or weight-loss program with HIT could increase probability of improving VO_2max before transitioning into moderate-intensity endurance exercise with the goal of improving body composition and metabolic function.

Acknowledgments

The authors thank the participants for taking part in these training studies as well as Daniel Roberson, Ryan Allen, Matthew Jurancich, Elyse Palumbo, Douglas Stirling, David W. McMillan, Rachael Gallant, Christina Cooper, and Donovan Martinez who assisted in data collection.

Author Contributions

Conceived and designed the experiments: TA MMS. Performed the experiments: TA MMS. Analyzed the data: TA. Contributed reagents/materials/analysis tools: TA. Wrote the paper: TA MMS. Designed and executed a portion of the experiments described in this manuscript: MMS.

References

1. Lortie G, Simoneau JA, Hamel P, Boulay MR, Landry F, Bouchard C (1984) Responses of maximal aerobic power and capacity to aerobic training. Int J Sports Med 5(5): 232–236.
2. Kohrt WM, Malley MT, Coggan AR, Spina RJ, Ogawa T, et al. (1991) Effects of gender, age, and fitness level on response to VO_2max to training in 60–71 yr olds. J Appl Physiol 71(5): 2004–2011.
3. Bouchard C, An P, Rice T, Skinner JS, Wilmore JH, et al. (1999) Familiar aggregation of VO_2max response to exercise training: results from the HERITAGE Family Study. J Appl Physiol 87: 1003–1008.
4. Sisson SB, Katzmarzyk PT, Earnest CP, Bouchard C, Blair SN, et al. (2009) Volume of exercise and fitness nonresponse in sedentary, postmenopausal women. Med Sci Sports Exerc 41(3): 539–545.
5. Scharhag-Rosenberger F, Walitzek S, Kindermann W, Meyer T (2012) Differences in adaptations to 1 year of aerobic endurance training: individual patterns of nonresponse. Scand J Med Sci Sports 22: 113–118.
6. Rankinen T, Sung YJ, Sarzynski MA, Rice TK, Rao DC, et al. (2012) Heritability of submaximal heart rate response to exercise training in accounted for by nine SNPs. J Appl Physiol 112: 892–897.
7. Bouchard C, Rankinen T (2001) Individual differences in response to regular physical activity. Med Sci Sports Exerc 33(6): S446–S451.
8. Blaak EE (2004) Basic disturbances in skeletal muscle fatty acid metabolism in obesity and type 2 diabetes mellitus. Proc Nutr Soc 63(2): 323–330.
9. Corpeleijn E, Saris WH, Blaak EE (2009) Metabolic flexibility in the development of insulin resistance and type 2 diabetes: effects of lifestyle. Obes Rev 10(2): 178–193.
10. Saltin B, Gollnick PD (1983) Skeletal muscle adaptability: significance for metabolism and performance. In: Peachey LD, Adrian RH, Geiger SR (Eds) The Handbook of Physiology-skeletal muscle. Baltimore, MD: Williams and Wilkins, 555–631.
11. Holloszy JO, Coyle EF (1984) Adaptations of skeletal muscle to endurance exercise and their metabolic consequences. J Appl Physiol 56(4): 831–838.
12. Stisin AB, Stougaard O, Langfort J, Helge JW, Sahlin K, et al. (2006) Maximal fat oxidation rates in endurance trained and untrained women. Eur J Appl Physiol 98: 497–506.
13. Goedecke JH, St. Clair Gibson A, Grobler L, Collins M, Noakes TD, et al. (2000) Determinants of the variability in respiratory exchange ratio at rest and during exercise in trained athletes. Am J Physiol 279(6): E1325–1334.
14. Astorino TA, Allen RP, Roberson DW, Jurancich M, Lewis R, et al. (2011) Adaptations to high-intensity training are independent of gender. Eur J Appl Physiol 111(7): 1279–1286.
15. Talanian JL, Galloway SD, Heigenhauser GJF, Bonen A, Spriet LL (2007) Two weeks of high-intensity aerobic interval training increase the capacity for fat oxidation during exercise in women. J Appl Physiol 102: 1439–1447.
16. Astorino TA, Schubert MM, Palumbo E, Stirling D, McMillan DW (2013) Effect of two doses of interval training on maximal fat oxidation in sedentary women. Med Sci Sports Exerc 45(10): 1878–1886.
17. Hazell TJ, MacPherson REK, Gravelle BMR, Lemon PW (2010) 10 or 30-s sprint interval training bouts enhance both aerobic and anaerobic performance. Eur J Appl Physiol 110: 153–160.
18. Whyte LJ, Gill JMR, Cathcart AJ (2010) Effect of two weeks of sprint interval training on health-related outcomes in sedentary overweight/obese men. Metabolism 59: 1421–1428.
19. Little JP, Gillen JB, Percival ME, Safdar A, Tarnopolsky MA, et al. (2011) Low-volume high-intensity interval training reduces hyperglycemia and increases muscle mitochondrial capacity in patients with type 2 diabetes. J Appl Physiol 111(6): 1554–1560.
20. Moholdt TT, Amundsen BH, Rustad LA, Wahba A, Lovo KT, et al. (2009) Aerobic interval training versus continuous moderate exercise after coronary artery bypass surgery: A randomized study of cardiovascular effects and quality of life. Am Heart J 158: 1031–1037.
21. Burgomaster KA, Howarth KR, Phillips SM, Rakobowchuk M, MacDonald MJ, et al. (2008) Similar metabolic adaptations during exercise after low volume sprint interval and traditional endurance training in humans. J Physiol 586(1): 151–160.
22. MacPherson REK, Hazell TJ, Olver TD, Paterson DH, Lemon PWR (2011) Run sprint interval training improves aerobic performance but not maximal cardiac output. Med Sci Sports Exerc 43(1): 115–122.
23. Nybo L, Sundstrup E, Jakobsen MD, Mohr M, Hornstrup T, et al. (2010) High-intensity training versus traditional exercise interventions for promoting health. Med Sci Sports Exerc 42(10): 1951–1958.
24. Bartlett JD, Close GL, MacLaren DP, Gregson W, Drust B, et al. (2011) High-intensity interval running is perceived to be more enjoyable than moderate-intensity continuous exercise: implications for exercise adherence. J Sports Sci 29(6): 547–553.
25. Astorino TA, Schubert MM, Palumbo E, Stirling D, McMillan DW, et al. (2013) Magnitude and timecourse of changes in maximal oxygen uptake in response to distinct regimens of chronic interval training in sedentary women. Eur J Appl Physiol 113(9): 2361–2369.
26. Heyward VH (2006) Advanced Fitness Assessment and Exercise Prescription. (5th Ed.) Champaign, IL: Human Kinetics, 202–222.
27. Astorino TA, Rietschel JR, Tam PA, Johnson SM, Sakarya CE, et al. (2004) Optimal duration of VO_2max testing. J Exerc Physiol 7: 1–8.
28. Astorino TA (2009) Alterations in VO_2max and the VO_2 plateau with manipulation of sampling interval. Clin Physiol Funct Imaging 29(1): 60–67.
29. Midgley AW, McNaughton LR, Carroll S (2006) Verification phase as a useful tool in the determination of the maximal oxygen uptake of distance runners. Appl Physiol Nutr Metab 31: 541–548.
30. Frayn KN (1983) Calculation of substrate oxidation rates in vivo from gaseous exchange. J Appl Physiol 55: 628–634.
31. Wilmore JH, Stanforth PR, Gagnon J, Rice T, Mandel S, et al. (2011) Heart rate and blood pressure changes with endurance training: the HERITAGE Family Study. Med Sci Sports Exerc 33: 107–116.
32. Gist NH, Fedewa MV, Dishman RK, Cureton KJ (2013) Sprint interval training effects on aerobic capacity: A systematic review and meta-analysis. Sports Med (in press).
33. Bailey SJ, Wilkerson DP, Dimenna FJ, Jones AM (2009) Influence of repeated sprint training on pulmonary O_2 uptake and muscle deoxygenation kinetics in humans. J Appl Physiol 106(6): 1875–1887.
34. Bacon AP, Carter RE, Ogle EA, Joyner MJ (2013) VO_2max trainability and high intensity interval training in humans: A meta-analysis. PLOS One 8(9): e73182.
35. Gibala MJ, McGee SL (2008) Metabolic adaptations to short-term high intensity interval training: A little pain for a lot of gain? Exerc Sport Sci Rev 36(2): 58–63.
36. Skinner JS, Jaskolksi A, Jaskolska A, Krasnoff J, Gagnon J, et al. (2001) Age, sex, race, initial fitness, and response to training: the HERITAGE Family Study. J Appl Physiol 90: 1770–1776.
37. Helgerud J, Hoydal K, Wang E, Karlsen T, Berg P, et al. (2007). Aerobic high-intensity intervals improve VO_2max more than moderate training. Med Sci Sports Exerc 39(4): 665–671.
38. Godin G, Desharnais R, Valois P, LePage P, Jobin J, et al. (1994) Differences in perceived barriers to exercise between high and low intenders: Observations among different populations. Am J Health Prom 8: 279–285.
39. Myers J, Prakash M, Froelicher V, Do D, Partington S, et al. (2002) Exercise capacity and mortality among men referred for exercise testing. New Engl J Med 346(11): 793–801.
40. Wang L, Psilander N, Tonkonogi M, Ding S, Sahlin K (2009) Similar expression of oxidative genes after interval and continuous exercise. Med Sci Sports Exerc 41(12): 2136–2144.

3

Effects of Exercise Training on Circulating and Skeletal Muscle Renin-Angiotensin System in Chronic Heart Failure Rats

**Igor Lucas Gomes-Santos[1], Tiago Fernandes[2], Gisele Kruger Couto[3], Julio César Ayres Ferreira-Filho[1], Vera Maria Cury Salemi[1], Fernanda Barrinha Fernandes[4], Dulce Elena Casarini[4], Patricia Chakur Brum[2], Luciana Venturini Rossoni[3], Edilamar Menezes de Oliveira[2], Carlos Eduardo Negrao[1,2]*
**

1 Heart Institute (InCor-HCFMUSP), University of São Paulo Medical School, São Paulo, Brazil, **2** School of Physical Education and Sport, University of São Paulo, São Paulo, Brazil, **3** Department of Physiology and Biophysics, Institute of Biomedical Science, University of São Paulo, São Paulo, Brazil, **4** Division of Nephrology, Kidney and Hypertension Hospital, Federal University of São Paulo, São Paulo, Brazil

Abstract

Background: Accumulated evidence shows that the ACE-AngII-AT1 axis of the renin-angiotensin system (RAS) is markedly activated in chronic heart failure (CHF). Recent studies provide information that Angiotensin (Ang)-(1–7), a metabolite of AngII, counteracts the effects of AngII. However, this balance between AngII and Ang-(1–7) is still little understood in CHF. We investigated the effects of exercise training on circulating and skeletal muscle RAS in the ischemic model of CHF.

Methods/Main Results: Male Wistar rats underwent left coronary artery ligation or a Sham operation. They were divided into four groups: 1) Sedentary Sham (Sham-S), 2) exercise-trained Sham (Sham-Ex), sedentary CHF (CHF-S), and exercise-trained CHF (CHF-Ex). Angiotensin concentrations and ACE and ACE2 activity in the circulation and skeletal muscle (soleus and plantaris) were quantified. Skeletal muscle ACE and ACE2 protein expression, and AT1, AT2, and Mas receptor gene expression were also evaluated. CHF reduced ACE2 serum activity. Exercise training restored ACE2 and reduced ACE activity in CHF. Exercise training reduced plasma AngII concentration in both Sham and CHF rats and increased the Ang-(1–7)/AngII ratio in CHF rats. CHF and exercise training did not change skeletal muscle ACE and ACE2 activity and protein expression. CHF increased AngII levels in both soleus and plantaris muscle, and exercise training normalized them. Exercise training increased Ang-(1–7) in the plantaris muscle of CHF rats. The AT1 receptor was only increased in the soleus muscle of CHF rats, and exercise training normalized it. Exercise training increased the expression of the Mas receptor in the soleus muscle of both exercise-trained groups, and normalized it in plantaris muscle.

Conclusions: Exercise training causes a shift in RAS towards the Ang-(1–7)-Mas axis in skeletal muscle, which can be influenced by skeletal muscle metabolic characteristics. The changes in RAS circulation do not necessarily reflect the changes occurring in the RAS of skeletal muscle.

Editor: Edward F. Plow, Lerner Research Institute, United States of America

Funding: This study was supported by Fundação de Amparo à Pesquisa do Estado de São Paulo (FAPESP-2010/50048-1) and, in part, by Fundação Zerbini. IL Gomes-Santos was supported by Coordenadoria de Aperfeiçoamento de Pessoal de Nível Superior (CAPES). PC Brum, DE Casarini, LV Rossoni, EM Oliveira and CE Negrao are research fellows at Conselho Nacional de Desenvolvimento Científico e Tecnológico (CNPq). The funders had no role in study design, data collection and analysis, decision to publish, or preparation of the manuscript.

* E-mail: cndnegrao@incor.usp.br

Introduction

Increased renin angiotensin system (RAS) has been consistently documented in chronic heart failure (CHF). Plasma Angiotensin (Ang) II levels are increased in CHF [1–4]. Likewise, RAS elevation in the heart, kidneys, and brain has been reported in CHF [5–8]. This scenario shows that CHF is characterized by overall RAS activation.

The classic RAS cascade depends on ACE-mediated conversion of AngI into AngII, an octapeptide binding to AT1 receptor. This ACE-AngII-AT1 axis contributes to cardiac remodeling [5,9], high sympathetic activity [7,10], and impaired vasodilation [11] in CHF. In addition, RAS exacerbation plays a role in skeletal myopathy, including reactive oxygen species generation, protein degradation, and apoptosis [12–14]. Recent studies provide evidence of an endogenous RAS axis that counterbalances the ACE-AngII-AT1 effects. ACE2, an ACE homolog enzyme [15,16], metabolizes AngII into the heptapeptide Ang-(1–7) [17], which in turn binds to the Mas receptor [18]. This ACE2-Ang-(1–7)-Mas axis causes vasodilation and improves skeletal muscle metabolism [19,20]. In addition, ACE2-Ang-(1–7)-Mas axis has antifibrotic and antiapoptotic properties, opposing the deleterious effects of ACE-AngII-AT1 overactivity [21].

Previous studies have shown that exercise training is a remarkable strategy in the treatment of CHF. This therapy reduces sympathetic nerve activity and vasoconstriction [22,23]. In addition, exercise training significantly increases exercise tolerance and quality of life in CHF patients [24]. Effects of exercise training on RAS have also been reported. Exercise training reduces plasma AngII levels [10,25]. In the cardiac muscle, exercise reduces ACE concentration, which may contribute to the reduction in hypertrophy and collagen deposition in rats with myocardial infarction [5]. More recently, we found a decrease in ACE and AngII concentrations and an increase in ACE2 and Ang-(1–7) concentration in cardiac muscle in exercise-trained rats [26]. In addition, exercise training has been shown to increase cardiac Ang-(1–7) in spontaneous hypertensive rats [27] and to normalize brain ACE and ACE2 expression in CHF rabbits [7]. However, the effects of exercise training on RAS in skeletal muscle are unknown.

To improve the understanding regarding the role of exercise training on circulating and skeletal muscle RAS, we investigated the effects of exercise training on ACE-AngII-AT1 and ACE2-Ang-(1–7)-Mas axis in rats with CHF. Our hypotheses were that: 1) Exercise training would shift the balance of RAS towards the ACE2-Ang-(1–7)-Mas axis; 2) The changes in skeletal muscle RAS would be independent of those observed in the circulation; and 3) The effects of exercise training on skeletal muscle would be influenced by muscle metabolic characteristic.

Methods

Animals

Two-month-old, male, Wistar rats from the Multidisciplinary Center for Biological Investigation on Laboratory Animal Science (CEMIB), University of Campinas, underwent surgical occlusion of the main descending branch of the left coronary artery or fictitious myocardial infarction (Sham). After a 4-week period, they were subdivided into four groups: 1) Sedentary sham-operated (Sham-S, n = 10); 2) exercise-trained sham-operated (Sham-Ex, n = 10), 3) sedentary chronic heart failure (CHF-S, n = 12); and 4) exercise-trained chronic heart failure (CHF-Ex, n = 12). Then, basal echocardiography was performed and peak oxygen consumption was measured. Finally, exercise training or follow-up began (Experimental protocol, Fig. 1). The rats were kept 3–4 per cage in a temperature-controlled room with a 12:12-hour light-dark cycle. They were fed with a standard laboratory diet and water *ad libitum*. The study was approved by the Scientific Committee of the Heart Institute (InCor-HCFMUSP) and Ethical Committee for Research Protocols of the University of São Paulo Medical School (CAPPesq 149/09). The study was carried out in accordance with the recommendations in the Guide for the Care and Use of Laboratory Animals of the National Institutes of Health, USA. The surgery and echocardiography was performed under anesthesia, and all efforts were made to minimize suffering.

Myocardial Infarction Induction

The rats were anesthetized with a single injection of ketamine (50 $mg.kg^{-1}$ body weight, Parke-Davis) and xylazine (10 $mg.kg^{-1}$ body weight, Bayer). Then, the heart was exposed through a left intercostal thoracotomy. The left coronary artery was looped by a single nylon suture (7-0) ~1 mm. The main descending branch was permanently occluded, which resulted in myocardial infarction and, subsequently, CHF. Finally, the heart was quickly repositioned into the chest [28].

Cardiac Function Assessment

The left ventricular evaluations were performed in anesthetized rats at baseline (4 weeks after surgery) and at the end of study (12 weeks after surgery). Echocardiographic studies were performed with Acuson equipment (Siemens, Mountain View, CA, EUA) with a 13 MHz transducer. Left ventricular dimensions were measured in the M-mode, and left ventricular fractional shortening (FS) was calculated by the formula $FS = [(EDD/ESD)/EDD]_x 100$, where EDD means left ventricular end-diastolic dimension and ESD left ventricular end-systolic dimension. Ejection fraction (EF) was assessed by Simpson's biplane method at 2-dimensional parasternal long-axis view. All the analyses were conducted according to the American Society of Echocardiography guidelines [29].

Exercise Capacity

Twenty-four hours after echocardiographic assessment, exercise capacity was measured, which was conducted at baseline (4 weeks after surgery) and at the end of study (12 weeks after surgery). The rats were previously adapted to treadmill exercise before testing. On a treadmill inside of a metabolic chamber coupled to a gas analyzer, rats ran progressively until exhaustion, starting at 6 $m.min^{-1}$ and 3 $m.min^{-1}$ increments every 3 minutes. Peak oxygen uptake (peak VO_2) was defined as the highest VO_2 achieved before exhaustion, calculated by the formula peak $VO_2 = [(pO_2 \text{ ambient - } pO_2 \text{ at stage})_x F]/m$, where pO_2 is the partial oxygen pressure measured in the ambient before testing and continuously through each stage inside the chamber, F is the airflow through the chamber (3500 $mL.min^{-1}$), and m is the rat's body mass in kilogram, adapted from Brooks and collaborators [30]. This procedure also provided running distance, in meters.

Exercise Training

Twenty-hour hours after exercise capacity assessment at baseline, exercise training began. Continuous moderate aerobic exercise training was conducted on a treadmill for 60 minutes at 60% of peak VO_2, 5 days a week for 8 weeks as described earlier [31]. At the end of the fourth week, training rats underwent another exercise test to adjust the intensity of exercise training. All rats kept sedentary were exposed to treadmill running for 5 minutes, once a week, to maintain their running skills.

Sacrifice and Collection of Blood and Tissues

Twenty-four hours after peak $V0_2$ assessment at the end of the experimental protocol, the rats were quickly sacrificed by decapitation with no prior anesthesia to avoid influences on RAS cascade. Trunk blood was immediately collected into dry (for serum) and cooled tubes (for plasma) with proteases inhibitor cocktail (miniComplete, Roche, USA), separated from total blood as soon as possible, and frozen for posterior analysis. The tissue samples were quickly excised, weighted, and frozen in liquid nitrogen. Thereafter, the samples were stored in a freezer $-80°$ for later analysis.

ACE and ACE2 Activity Assay

ACE activity was determined in serum, and in skeletal soleus and plantaris muscle by using fluorescent substrates [32]. Frozen skeletal muscle samples were homogenized in 0.1 M Tris-HCl buffer pH 7.0, containing 50 mM NaCl and centrifuged at 1,000×g for 10 minutes. The assays were performed at 37°C in 0.1 M Tris-HCl buffer pH 7.0, containing 50 mM NaCl and 10 µM $ZnCl_2$, and captopril 0.5 µL as inhibitor in negative samples. The hydrolysis rate of the intramolecularly quenched

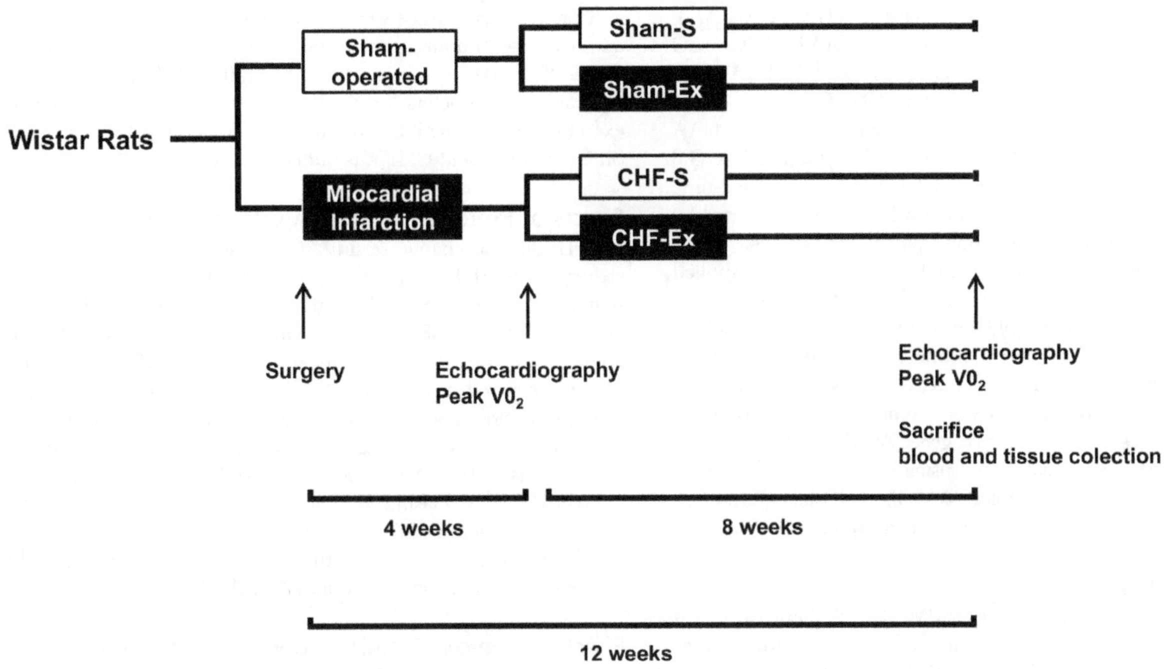

Figure 1. Experimental protocol.

fluorogenic substrate Abz-FRK-(Dnp)P-OH (10 uM) incubated with aliquots of homogenate and serum for 30 minutes at 37°C was assessed to obtain ACE enzymatic activity (420 nm λ_{em} and 320 nm λ_{ex}, read in 90 cycles). ACE2 activity was determined by the same method described above. However, Abz-APK(Dnp)-OH was used as the fluorescent peptide, in 0.2 M Tris-HCl buffer, 200 mM NaCl, pH 7.5, and DX600 1 mM as the inhibitor. ACE and ACE2 activity are expressed as uF.min^{-1}·mg^{-1} of skeletal muscle protein concentration, or uF.min^{-1}·mL^{-1} of serum.

Quantification of Angiotensins

The determination of AngI, AngII, and Ang-(1–7) was quantified by High Performance Liquid Chromatography (HPLC), as previously demonstrated by our group [26]. After centrifugation (10,000×g, 4°C, 20 min), 1 mL of plasma was filtered in Oasis C_{18} columns (Waters, USA), previously activated with methanol (5 mL), tetrahydrofuran (5 mL), hexane (5 mL), methanol (5 mL), and water (10 mL). After activation, the samples were applied into the columns, washed with water and eluted in ethanol/acetic acid/water in the proportion 90%/4%/6%. The eluted fractions were lyophilized and resuspended in 500 µL of mobile phase A (5% acetonitrile in 0.1% orthophosphoric acid) and filtered with 0.22 mm membrane for analysis (HPLC, Shimadzu System, Japan). The angiotensin of each sample was separated on a reversed phase column ODS Aquapor 300 (250×4.6 mm), 7 µ (PerkinElmer's Browlee Columns, USA) using the gradient from 5–35% of mobile phase B (95% acetonitrile in 0.1% phosphoric acid) under a flow of 1.5 mL.min^{-1} for 40 minutes. The angiotensins were identified by comparing them with the retention time of standard angiotensins. Results are expressed as pmol.mL^{-1} of plasma. Skeletal muscle soleus and plantaris samples were weighted and homogenized in 100 mM sodium phosphate buffer pH 7.2, 340 mM sucrose and 300 mM NaCl and protease inhibitor cocktail (Roche, USA). The samples were centrifuged and followed the same sequence as described for plasma angiotensins. Results are expressed as pmol.g^{-1} of tissue.

Quantification of Protein Expression

The protein expression of ACE and ACE2 in the soleus and plantaris muscles was analyzed using western blot. The frozen samples were homogenized in cell lyses buffer containing 100 mM Tris-HCl, 50 mM NaCl, 1% Triton X-100, and protease inhibitor cocktail (1:100, Sigma-Aldrich, USA). After centrifugation (10,000 × g, 4°C, 10 min), the pellet was discarded, and the samples were loaded (Laemmli 1:1, Sigma-Aldrich, USA) and underwent SDS-PAGE in 10% polyacrylamide gels. Equal loading of samples (30 µg) were applied for electrophoresis, and proteins were electro-transferred to nitrocellulose membrane (BioRad Biosciences, USA). The blot membrane was then incubated in a blocking buffer (5% BSA, 10 mM Tris-HCl, pH 7.6, 150 mM NaCl, and 0.1% Tween 20) for 2 hours at room temperature and then incubated overnight at 4°C with mouse anti-ACE (ab11734, 1:100, Abcam, USA) and rabbit anti-ACE2 (sc-20998 1:200, Santa Cruz, USA). Binding of the primary antibody was detected with the use of peroxidase-conjugated secondary antibodies, and enhanced chemiluminescence reagents (Amersham Biosciences, USA) were used to visualize the autoradiography. Quantification blot analyses were performed using Image-J software (National Institute of Health, USA), normalized to relative changes in mouse anti-GAPDH (ab9484, 1:5000, Abcam, USA).

RNA Isolation and mRNA Quantification

Frozen skeletal muscle samples were homogenized in Trizol, and RNA was isolated according to manufacturer's instructions (Invitrogen Life Technologies, USA). Following extraction, total RNA concentration was quantified using NanoDrop Spectrophotometer (Nano-Drop Technologies, USA) and checked for integrity by EtBr agarose gel electrophoresis. cDNA was synthetized using reverse transcriptase at 70°C for 10 minutes, incubation at 42°C for 60 minutes, and 95°C for 10 minutes. The mRNA expression was assessed by oligonucleotides primers (Exxtend, Brazil) for analysis of the genes AT1a (Sense: 5′-CAC AAC CCT CCC AGA AAG TG-3′; antisense:5′-AGG GCC

ATT TTG TTT TTC TG-3′), AT2 (Sense: 5′- GAA CAG AAT TAC CCG TGA CC-3′; antisense: 5′- ATG AAT GCC AAC ACA ACA GC-3′), Mas (Sense: 5′-GAC CAG CCC ACA GTT ACC AGT T-3′; antisense:5′- CCA GGG TTC CCC TTC TGA CT-3′) and reference gene Ciclophilin (Sense: 5′- TGG CAA GCA TGT TGG GTC TTT GGG AAG-3′; antisense: 5′-GGT GAT CTT CTT GCT GCT CTG CCA TTC-3′). Real-time PCRs were run separately, and amplifications were performed by ABI Prism 5700 Sequence Detection System (Applied Biosystems, USA) by using SYBR Green PCR Master Mix (Applied Biosystems, USA). Results were quantified as Ct values, where Ct is defined as the threshold cycle of the polymerase chain reaction at which the amplified product is first detected. Each sample was analyzed in duplicate. Relative quantities of target gene expressions of four groups were compared after normalization to the values of the reference gene (ΔCT). Fold changes in mRNA expression were calculated using the differences in ΔCT values between the two samples (ΔΔCT) and the equation 2-ΔΔCT. Results are expressed in percentages of control (Sham-S).

Statistical Analysis

Results are presented as mean±SEM. The Student *t* test was conducted to compare infarcted and Sham rats 4 weeks after surgery and, hence, ascertain for CHF. At the end of the protocol (12 weeks after surgery), the groups were compared by 2-way ANOVA (exercise training and CHF as the main factors), with Scheffé test for *post hoc* comparisons. *P* value ≤ 0.05 was accepted as significant.

Results

Baseline Measures

Four weeks after surgery, body weight was not significantly different between CHF and Sham rats (386±15 *vs.* 377±11.7 g). Left ventricular end-diastolic diameter (EDD), end-systolic diameter (ESD), fractional shortening (FS), and ejection fraction (EF) were significantly lower in CHF rats compared with that of Sham rats, consistent with cardiac remodeling associated with dilation and dysfunction (Table 1). Functional capacity, expressed by peak VO_2, and running distance were lower in the CHF rats, indicating exercise intolerance (Table 1). At this point, the rats were divided into sedentary and exercise-trained groups.

Effects of Exercise Training on Functional Capacity and Cardiac Function

Physiological parameters in untrained and exercised-trained Sham and CHF rats are shown in Table 2. There were no significant differences in body weight among groups. The heart and right ventricle mass were significantly increased in CHF rats, and exercise training caused no changes in these parameters (Table 2). Exercise training did not significantly change echocardiographic parameters or peak VO_2 in CHF rats. However, exercise training significantly increased running distance in both Sham-operated and CHF rats but caused no change in FS (Fig. 2).

Effects of Exercise Training on Circulating RAS

CHF did not change serum ACE activity, but caused a 25% reduction in ACE2 activity (Fig. 3, $P=0.04$). Exercise training significantly decreased ACE activity in the CHF rats ($P=0.05$), and restored the ACE2 activity towards the levels found in Sham-operated rats (Fig. 3). No significant changes in ACE and ACE2 activity occurred in the Sham-Ex. In regard to plasma angiotensins, we found no significant changes in plasma AngII levels in CHF rats. Exercise training provoked a significant reduction in AngII levels in both Sham (33%, $P=0.03$) and CHF rats (43%, $P=0.007$) (Fig. 3). Plasma AngI and Ang-(1–7) were unchanged by CHF or exercise training (Table 3 and Fig. 3). However, exercise training significantly increased the Ang-(1–7)/AngII ratio in CHF rats (Fig. 3). No changes were found in the Sham-Ex.

Effects of Exercise Training on RAS in the Soleus Muscle

CHF or exercise training did not change ACE activity and protein expression in soleus muscle (Fig. 4). CHF provoked a 2.1-fold increase in AngII concentration in the soleus muscle ($P=0.001$), and exercise training decreased it to the normal levels (Fig. 5). There were no significant differences in AngI among groups (Table 3). The AT1 receptor gene expression in the soleus muscle was significantly increased in CHF rats ($P=0.04$, Fig. 6). Exercise training normalized these levels. AT2 gene expression was not different among groups. Similarly, no changes in Ang-(1–7) concentration were found among groups (Fig. 5). Exercise training tended to increase Ang-(1–7)/AngII ratio in Sham-operated ($P=0.06$) and CHF ($P=0.08$) rats (Fig. 5). Exercise training increased Mas gene expression in both Sham and CHF rats ($P=0.02$) (Fig. 6).

Effects of Exercise Training on RAS in Plantaris Muscle

In regard to plantaris muscle, CHF and exercise training unchanged ACE activity and protein expression (Fig. 7). In contrast, AngI and AngII in the plantaris muscle were 1.5- and 2.5-fold increased of CHF rats (Table 3, Fig. 8). CHF and exercise training did not change AT1 or AT2 receptors (Fig. 9). Exercise training decreased AngI and AngII towards normal levels (Table 3, Fig. 8). Exercise training significantly increased Ang-(1–7), but caused no significant changes in Ang-(1–7)/AngII ratio (Fig. 8). There were no differences in ACE2 activity or protein expression

Table 1. Echocardiographic characteristics and functional capacity of the animals 4 weeks after surgery.

	Sham	CHF	*P*
EDD (mm)	7.36±0.16	9.92±0.22	<0.0001
ESD (mm)	4.01±0.20	9.75±0.45	<0.0001
FS (%)	46.89±1.78	11.97±1.00	<0.0001
EF (%)	80.70±2.46	28.75±2.18	<0.0001
Peak VO_2 ($mL.kg^{-1}.min^{-1}$)	68.90±2.55	59.59±1.90	0.005
Running distance (m)	390.49±23.61	276.49±15.59	<0.0001

CHF, Chronic heart failure; EDD, End-diastolic diameter; ESD, End-systolic diameter; FS, fractional shortening; EF, ejection fraction.

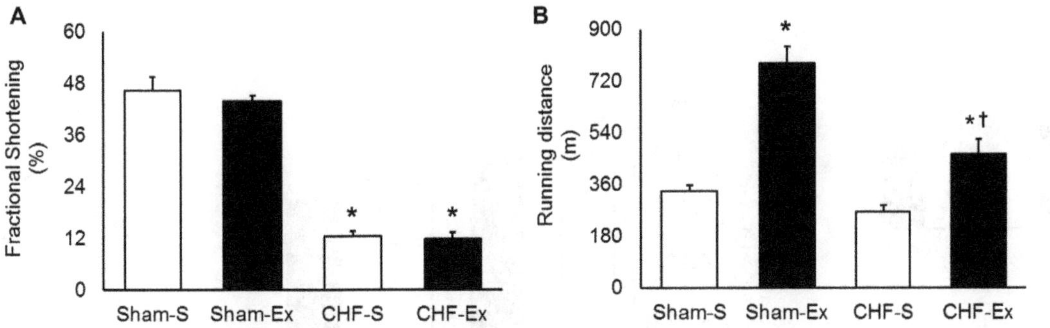

Figure 2. Ventricular function and exercise capacity in sedentary and exercise-trained Sham and CHF rats. CHF, chronic heart failure; -S, Sedentary; -Ex, Exercise-trained. A, Fractional shortening (FS); B, Running distance in Sham and CHF, sedentary and trained rats, 12 week after surgery. *$P<0.05$ *vs.* Sham-S; †$P<0.05$ *vs.* CHF-S.

among groups (Fig. 7). Exercise training significantly reduced the Mas gene expression in CHF (Fig. 9).

Discussion

The main and new findings of the present study are that exercise training in an ischemic model of CHF: 1) Normalizes AngII concentration in soleus and plantaris muscle; 2) Decreases AT1 receptors towards normal levels in soleus muscle; 3) Increases Ang-(1–7)/AngII ratio in plasma and soleus; and 4) Increases Mas receptor mRNA expression in soleus muscle.

Our study confirms previous studies [10,25] that demonstrated that exercise training causes remarkable changes in circulating RAS in CHF. The reduction in circulating ACE activity and AngII concentration in CHF rats has important implications. Firstly, the improvement in arterial baroreflex control of renal sympathetic nerve activity in CHF rats depends on the reduction in plasma AngII [31]. Mousa and collaborators [10] elegantly demonstrated that administration of AngII to maintain its levels near those found in untrained CHF restrained the amelioration in arterial baroreflex sensitivity in exercise-trained CHF rabbits. Secondly, AngII increases sympathetic nerve activity [10,33]. This knowledge may predict that exercise training decreased sympathetic outflow in our study. In fact, sympathetic deactivation has been consistently reported after exercise training in CHF [10,23,31]. Thirdly, both the improvement in baroreflex sensitivity and the reduction in sympathetic activity are associated with better prognosis in CHF [34,35].

In CHF patients, there is an association between serum ACE2 and the severity of this syndrome [36]. A possible explanation for this response is that AngII provokes ACE2 shedding mediated by TACE/ADAM-17, which increases serum ACE2 activity [37]. In conformity to a previous study on the same experimental model [38], we found that serum ACE2 activity was reduced in CHF. The contrast between serum ACE2 in humans with CHF and the experimental model of CHF is not clear. However, it could be speculated that the pharmacological inhibition of ACE usually prescribed for humans with CHF causes a compensatory increase in serum ACE2 activity. In fact, some investigators have previously observed an association between serum ACE inhibition and ACE2 increase [39]. Exercise training significantly decreased serum ACE activity and increased serum ACE2 activity. This finding reinforces the inverse association between ACE and ACE2 activity.

Despite the fact that exercise training increases serum ACE2 activity towards normal levels, no significant changes in circulating Ang-(1–7) concentration were found. Since AngII is the major substrate for the production of Ang-(1–7), it is possible to anticipate that the reduction in AngII concentration limited the formation of Ang-(1–7). All together, these findings indicate that exercise training causes a switch in circulating ACE-AngII towards an increase in ACE2-Ang-(1–7) axis in CHF rats, which may render the cardiovascular system less susceptible to the deleterious actions of AngII [40].

We hypothesized that exercise training would cause a shift in RAS in skeletal muscle towards the ACE2-Ang-(1–7)-Mas axis.

Table 2. Physiological parameters in sedentary and exercised-trained Sham-operated and CHF rats.

	Sham-S	Sham-Ex	CHF-S	CHF-Ex
Body weight (g)	452.13±11.96	424.97±7.93	451.83±17.21	423.59±13.47
Heart (g)	1.12±0.04	1.10±0.03	1.46±0.07*	1.52±0.06*
RV (g)	0.23±0.01	0.23±0.01	0.42±0.05*	0.43±0.02*
EDD (mm)	7.24±0.24	7.70±0.21	11.55±0.32*	11.30±0.32*
ESD (mm)	3.72±0.25	4.54±0.19	10.13±0.36*	9.43±0.60*
EF (%)	81.83±2.73	79.92±1.42	29.73±2.69*	28.37±3.18*
Peak VO_2 ($mL.kg^{-1}.min^{-1}$)	65.86±2.24	73.96±2.39*	55.99±2.62	62.21±2.58

CHF, chronic heart failure; -S, Sedentary; -Ex, Exercise-trained; RV, right ventricle mass; EDD, End-diastolic diameter; ESD, End-systolic diameter; EF, left ventricular ejection fraction.
*$P<0.05$ *vs.* Sham-S.

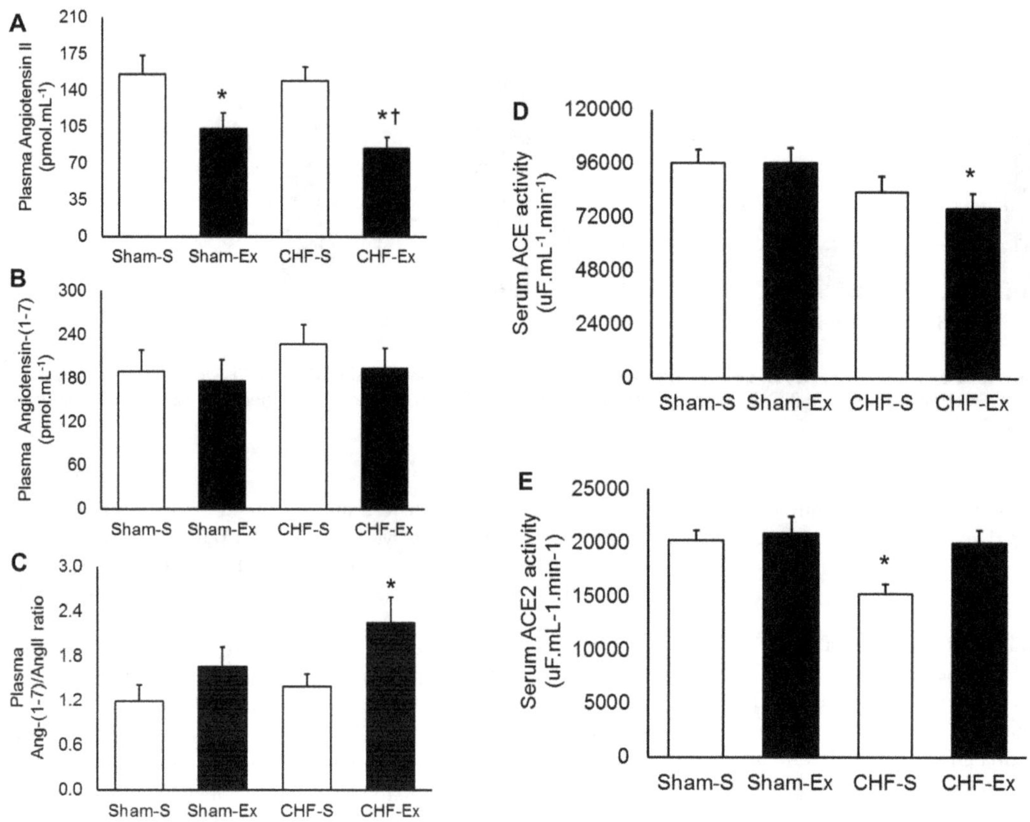

Figure 3. Circulating renin angiotensin system (RAS) in sedentary and exercise-trained Sham and CHF rats. CHF, chronic heart failure; -S, Sedentary; -Ex, Exercise-trained. A, Angiotensin II; B, Angiotensin-(1–7); C, Ang-(1–7)/AngII ratio; D, ACE activity; E, ACE2 activity. *$P<0.05$ *vs.* Sham-S; †$P<0.05$ *vs.* CHF-S.

Our findings confirm in great part this hypothesis. Exercise training decreased AngII in both soleus and plantaris muscle in the ischemic model of CHF. In addition, exercise training tended to increase the Ang-(1–7)/AngII ratio, which suggests an imbalance in the RAS towards the ACE2-Ang-(1–7)-Mas receptor axis. The reduction in the AngII concentration and AT1 receptor gene expression in skeletal muscle is an important issue. Previous studies show that AngII is involved in inflammation and oxidative stress [13,41]. These alterations contribute to muscle catabolism and apoptosis in CHF [12–14,42,43]. Our study provides no information on muscle protein synthesis and degradation. Future investigations should focus on the contribution of ACE-AngII-AT1 receptor axis in the amelioration in skeletal myopathy.

The mechanisms by which exercise training decreased AngII concentration in skeletal muscle in CHF rats is out of the scope of the present study. However, it is possible that exercise training reduced AngII uptake in the soleus muscle [44], because AT1 expression was substantially lower in the exercise-trained rats. In plantaris muscle, exercise training also reduced AngII concentration, but caused no changes in AT1 expression. These findings raise the question that the mechanisms underlying the reduction in AngII in plantaris muscle and soleus muscle are different. Someone could suggest that the reduction in AngII in the plantar muscle is due to the decrease in AngI cleavage. In fact, we found that AngI concentration in plantar muscle was significantly lower in exercise-trained CHF compared to that in untrained CHF rats.

Our data clearly demonstrate that there is a mismatch between circulating and skeletal muscle RAS. Elevation in AngII concentration was found in the skeletal muscle, but not in the circulation. These findings are consistent with those of previous studies that show that local RAS becomes activated in tissues in CHF [5–8]. The increase in the plasma AngII concentration seems to occur

Table 3. Plasma and skeletal muscle AngI in sedentary and exercise-trained Sham-operated and CHF rats.

	Sham-S	Sham-Ex	CHF-S	CHF-Ex
Plasma AngI (pmol.mL^{-1})	88.79±8.22	75.00±9.73	97.76±12.17	70.40±12.25
Soleus AngI (pmol.g^{-1})	39.18±9.68	28.50±2.96	59.79±16.98	46.46±8.44
PlantarisAngI (pmol.g^{-1})	49.19±9.01	38.88±11.76	67.70±14.90*	39.94±5.74†

CHF, chronic heart failure; -S, Sedentary; -Ex, Exercise-trained; AngI, Angiotensin I.
*$P<0.05$ *vs.* Sham-S;
†$P<0.05$ *vs.* CHF-S.

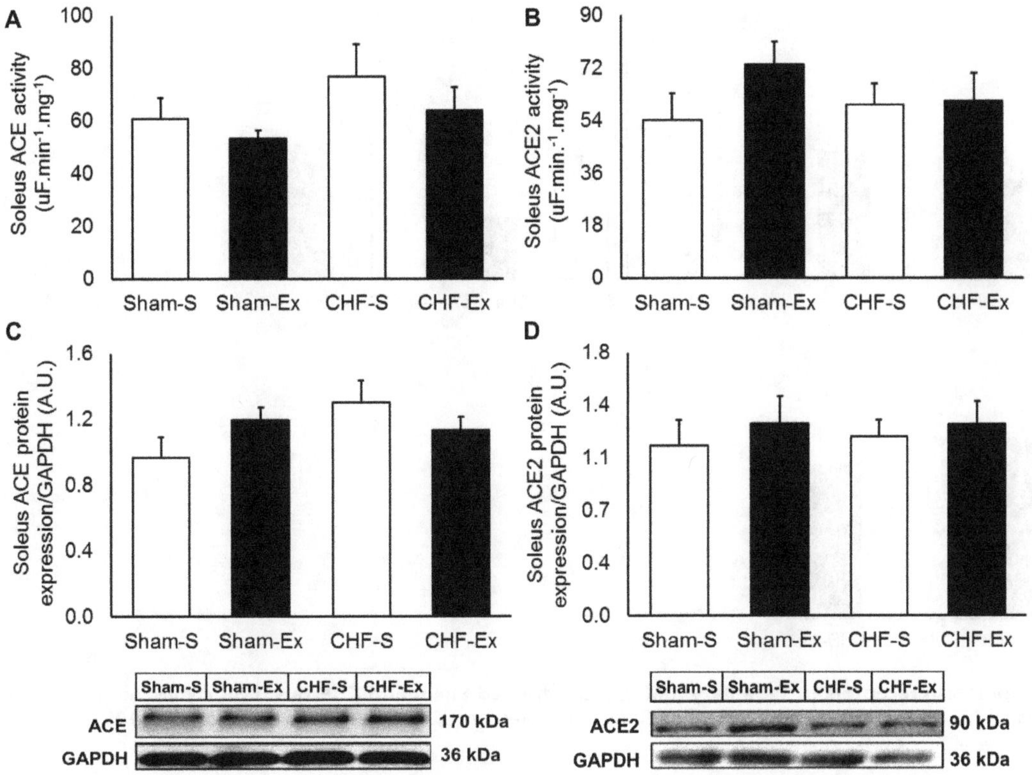

Figure 4. Soleus muscle ACE and ACE2 in sedentary and exercise-trained Sham and CHF rats. CHF, chronic heart failure; -S, Sedentary; -Ex, Exercise-trained; ACE, Angiotensin Converting Enzyme. A, ACE activity; B, ACE2 activity; C, ACE protein expression; D, ACE2 protein expression.

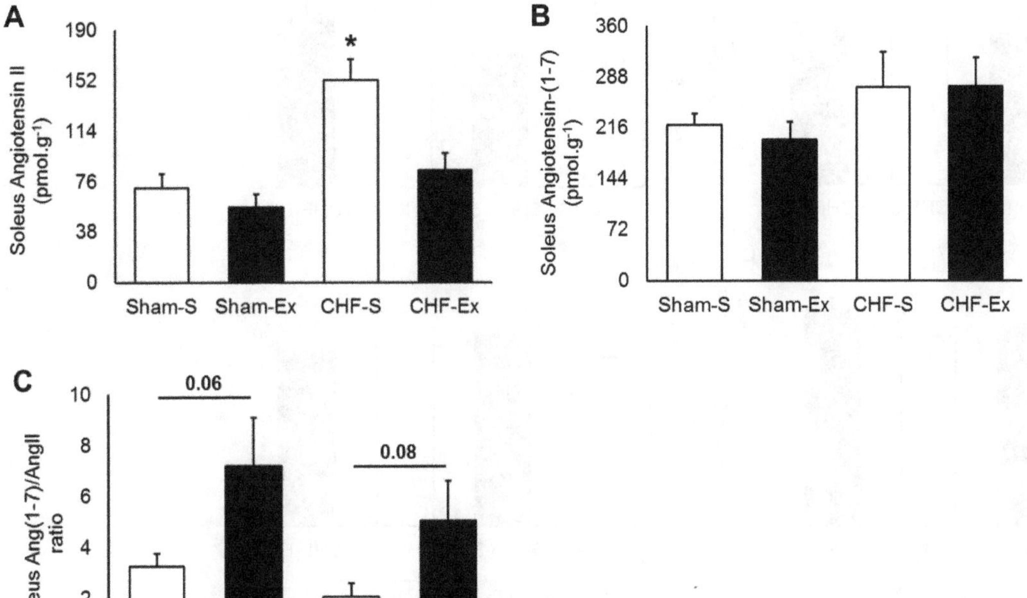

Figure 5. Soleus muscle angiotensins in sedentary and exercise-trained Sham and CHF rats. CHF, chronic heart failure; -S, Sedentary; -Ex, Exercise-trained. A, Angiotensin II; B, Angiotensin-(1–7); C, Ang-(1–7)/AngII ratio. $*P<0.05$ *vs.* Sham-S.

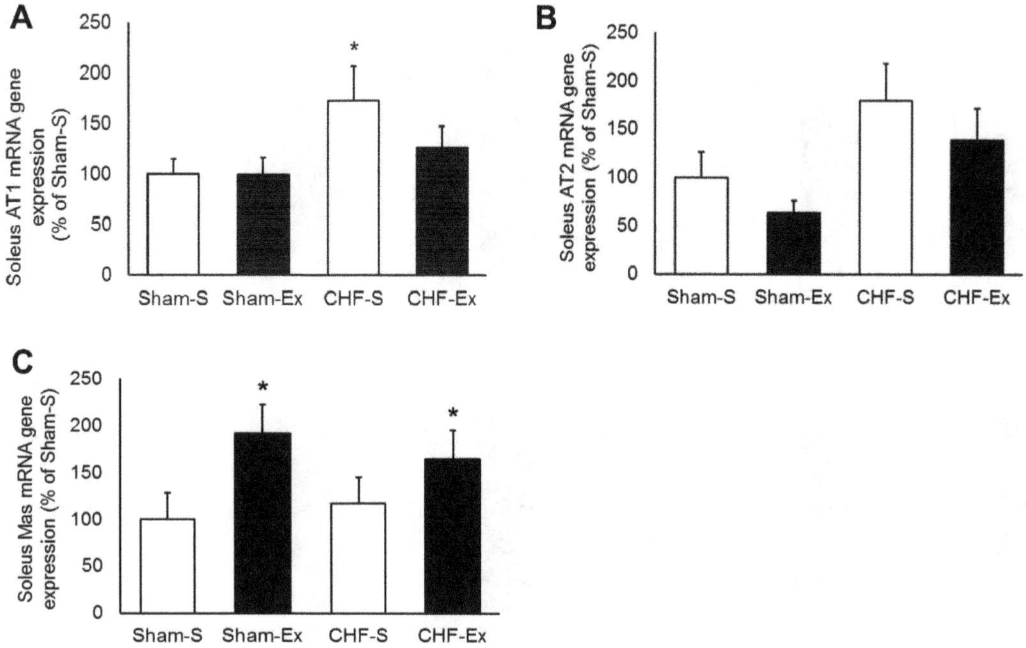

Figure 6. Soleus muscle angiotensin receptors in sedentary and exercise-trained Sham and CHF rats. CHF, chronic heart failure; -S, Sedentary; -Ex, Exercise-trained. A, AT1 mRNA gene expression; B, AT2 mRNA gene expression; C, Mas mRNA gene expression. **P*<0.05 *vs*. Sham-S.

only in the late stage of CHF [3,4]. ACE was not altered in the skeletal muscle, which suggests alternative local pathways of AngII production involving other enzymes as Prolyl-endopeptidase, Neprilysin and Chymase [45–47], especially in the plantaris muscle. Exercise training reduced AngII concentration in both plasma and skeletal muscle. Exercise training reduces ACE and

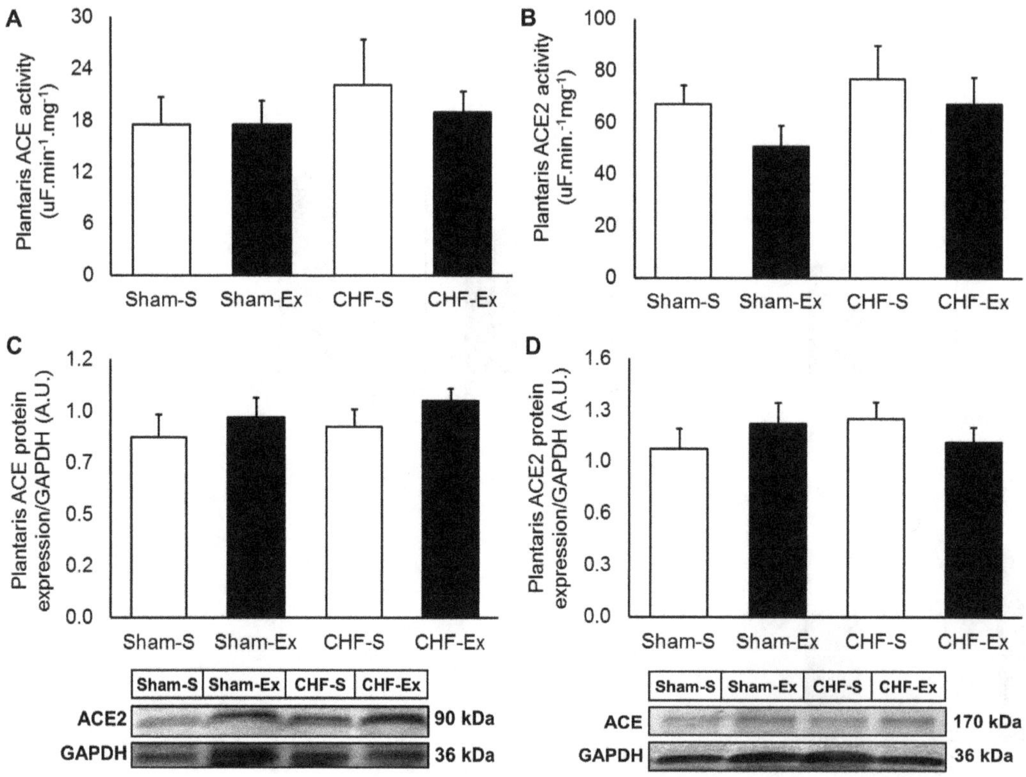

Figure 7. Plantaris muscle ACE and ACE2 in sedentary and exercise-trained Sham and CHF rats. CHF, chronic heart failure; -S, Sedentary; -Ex, Exercise-trained; ACE, Angiotensin Converting Enzyme. A, ACE activity; B, ACE2 activity; C, ACE protein expression; D, ACE2 protein expression.

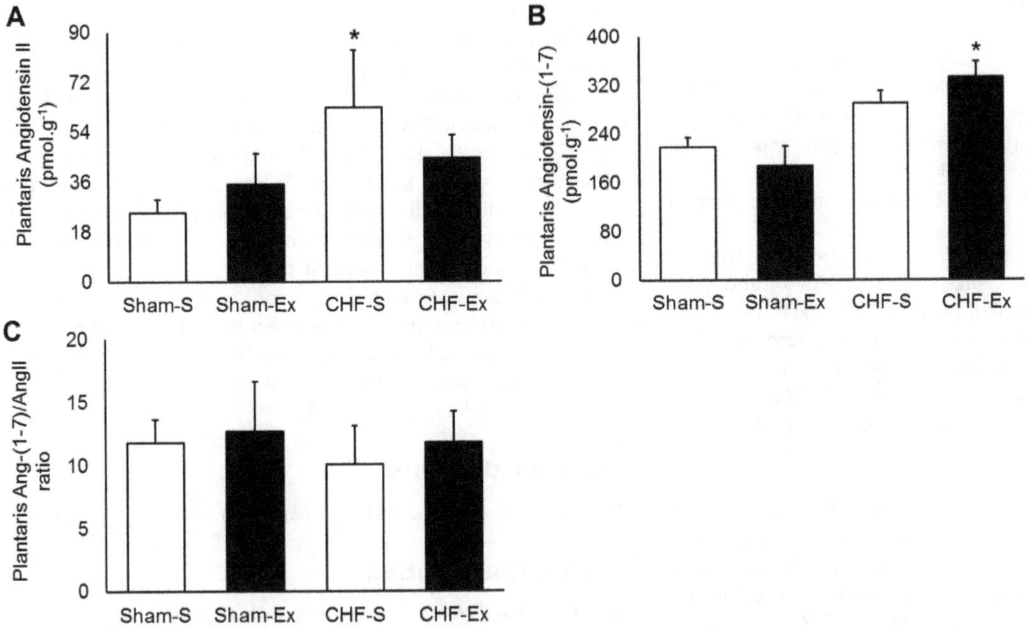

Figure 8. Plantaris muscle angiotensins in sedentary and exercise-trained Sham and CHF rats. CHF, chronic heart failure; -S, Sedentary; -Ex, Exercise-trained. A, Angiotensin II; B, Angiotensin-(1–7); C, Ang-(1–7)/AngII ratio. *$P<0.05$ *vs.* Sham-S.

restores ACE2 activity in the circulation, without changing ACE and ACE2 activity or protein expression in skeletal muscle. Other investigators reported that electric stimulated C2C12, a strategy to mimic *in vitro* exercise effects, caused no changes in skeletal muscle ACE gene expression [48].

Previous studies demonstrated that the AT1 receptor was increased in the vasculature of patients with ischemic heart disease [49], and in local tissues in experimental models of CHF [5,7,10]. In our study, we found increased AT1 receptor mRNA in soleus muscle in CHF rats. This increase in AT1 receptors may be associated with elevation in sympathetic nerve activity. In a previous study, isoproterenol administration increased AT1 receptor expression [50]. Exercise training reverted AT1 receptor gene expression towards normal levels, which may be linked to reduction in sympathetic activation. We and others have

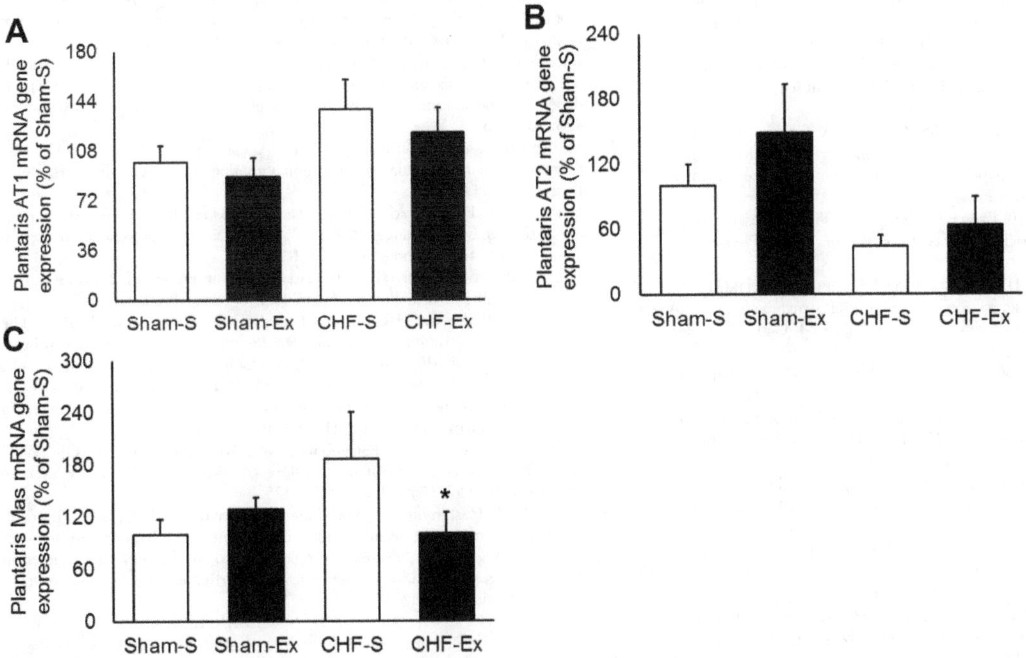

Figure 9. Plantaris muscle angiotensin receptors in sedentary and exercise-trained Sham and CHF rats. CHF, chronic heart failure; -S, Sedentary; -Ex, Exercise-trained. A, AT1 mRNA gene expression; B, AT2 mRNA gene expression; C, Mas mRNA gene expression. *$P<0.05$ *vs.* Sham-S.

consistently found a reduction in sympathetic nerve activity in heart failure [10,23,31].

We found no changes in AT2 receptors in our study. The AT2 gene expression in both soleus and plantar muscles was not altered in CHF rats. Similar findings have been reported in patients with heart failure. Some investigators found no AT2 gene expression in skeletal muscle in patients with CHF [51]. In our study, exercise training caused no changes in AT2 receptors in either normal controls or CHF rats.

Our study demonstrates for the first time that exercise training changes the Ang-(1–7) and Ang-(1–7)/AngII ratio and Mas receptor expression in skeletal muscle in CHF rats. These are remarkable effects provoked by exercise training. Ang-(1–7) is a potent vasodilator as are other interventions in the treatment of heart failure, and in the muscle level, Ang-(1–7)/Mas improves insulin sensitivity by increasing Akt phosphorilation [19].

Limitations

We recognize limitations in our study. We only studied mRNA expression of angiotensin receptors. Thus, someone could argue that there is no guarantee that the changes in gene expression have been translated into protein expression. Our study provides no direct information regarding the implications of RAS modifications in the function of skeletal muscle. The increase in running distance is suggestive of improvement in functional capacity, but not sufficient to demonstrate amelioration in skeletal muscle function.

Perspectives

The antagonism of the RAS and sympathetic outflow is the target in the treatment of heart failure. The present study shows that exercise training provokes profound changes in circulating and skeletal muscle RAS. The switch from AngII/AT1 to Ang-(1–7)/Mas axis in the skeletal muscle may have implications in the skeletal myopathy in heart failure. Growing evidence shows that AngII is involved in the skeletal muscle pathophysiology of heart failure. Finally, these findings strengthen the recommendation of exercise training in the treatment of CHF.

In conclusion, exercise training improves RAS in the Ang-(1–7)-Mas axis in skeletal muscle. This effect of exercise training seems to depend on skeletal muscle metabolic characteristics. The changes in circulating RAS do not necessarily reflect the changes occurring in skeletal muscle RAS.

Acknowledgments

We thank Katt Mattos and Marcele Coelho for technical assistance.

Author Contributions

Conceived and designed the experiments: ILGS EMdO CEN. Performed the experiments: ILGS TF GKC FBF VMCS. Analyzed the data: ILGS TF DEC FBF JCAFF. Contributed reagents/materials/analysis tools: PCB DEC LVR EMdO CEN. Wrote the paper: ILGS CEN.

References

1. Sigurdsson A, Held P, Swedberg K. (1993) Short- and long-term neurohormonal activation following acute myocardial infarction. Am Heart J 126: 1068–1076.
2. Pfeffer MA, Pfeffer JM, Steinberg C, Finn P. (1985) Survival after an experimental myocardial infarction: beneficial effects of long-term therapy with captopril. Circulation 72: 406–412.
3. Kato M, Kinugawa T, Omodani H, Osaki S, Ahmmed GU, et al. (1996) Responses of plasma norepinephrine and renin-angiotensin-aldosterone system to dynamic exercise in patients with congestive heart failure. J Card Fail 2: 103–110.
4. Roig E, Perez-Villa F, Morales M, Jiménez W, Orús J, et al. (2000) Clinical implications of increased plasma angiotensin II despite ACE inhibitor therapy in patients with congestive heart failure. Eur Heart J 21: 53–57.
5. Xu X, Wan W, Ji L, Lao S, Powers AS, et al. (2008) Exercise training combined with angiotensin II receptor blockade limits post-infarct ventricular remodelling in rats. Cardiovasc Res 78: 523–532.
6. Ferreira JCB, Bacurau A V, Evangelista FS, Coelho MA, Oliveira EM, et al. (2008) The role of local and systemic renin angiotensin system activation in a genetic model of sympathetic hyperactivity-induced heart failure in mice. Am J Physiol Regul Integr Comp Physiol 294: R26–32.
7. Kar S, Gao L, Zucker IH. (2010) Exercise training normalizes ACE and ACE2 in the brain of rabbits with pacing-induced heart failure. J Appl Physiol 108: 923–932.
8. Schunkert H, Ingelfinger JR, Hirsch a T, Tang SS, Litwin SE, et al. (1992) Evidence for tissue-specific activation of renal angiotensinogen mRNA expression in chronic stable experimental heart failure. J Clin Invest 90: 1523–1529.
9. Pfeffer JM, Pfeffer MA, Braunwald E. (1985) Influence of chronic captopril therapy on the infarcted left ventricle of the rat. Circ Res 57: 84–95.
10. Mousa TM, Liu D, Cornish KG, Zucker IH. (2008) Exercise training enhances baroreflex sensitivity by an angiotensin II-dependent mechanism in chronic heart failure. J Appl Physiol 5850: 616–624.
11. Abassi ZA, Gurbanov K, Mulroney SE, Potlog C, Opgenorth TJ, et al. (1997) Impaired nitric oxide-mediated renal vasodilation in rats with experimental heart failure: role of angiotensin II. Circulation 96: 3655–3664.
12. Dalla Libera L, Ravara B, Angelini A, Rossini K, Sandri M, et al. (2001) Beneficial effects on skeletal muscle of the angiotensin II type 1 receptor blocker irbesartan in experimental heart failure. Circulation 103: 2195–2200.
13. Russell ST, Eley H, Tisdale MJ. (2007) Role of reactive oxygen species in protein degradation in murine myotubes induced by proteolysis-inducing factor and angiotensin II. Cell Signal 19: 1797–1806.
14. Semprun-Prieto LC, Sukhanov S, Yoshida T, Rezk BM, Gonzalez-Villalobos RA, et al. (2011) Angiotensin II induced catabolic effect and muscle atrophy are redox dependent. Biochem Biophys Res Commun 409: 217–221.
15. Donoghue M, Hsieh F, Baronas E, Godbout K, Gosselin M, et al. (2000) A Novel Angiotensin-Converting Enzyme-Related Carboxypeptidase (ACE2) Converts Angiotensin I to Angiotensin 1-9. Circ Res 87: e1–e9.
16. Tipnis SR, Hooper NM, Hyde R, Karran E, Christie G, et al. (2000) A human homolog of angiotensin-converting enzyme. Cloning and functional expression as a captopril-insensitive carboxypeptidase. J Biol Chem 275: 33238–33243.
17. Vickers C, Hales P, Kaushik V, Dick L, Gavin J, et al. (2002) Hydrolysis of biological peptides by human angiotensin-converting enzyme-related carboxypeptidase. J Biol Chem 277: 14838–14843.
18. Santos RAS, Simoes e Silva AC, Maric C, Silva DMR, Machado RP, et al. (2003) Angiotensin-(1-7) is an endogenous ligand for the G protein-coupled receptor Mas. Proc Natl Acad Sci U S A 100: 8258–8263.
19. Prasannarong M, Santos FR, Henriksen EJ. (2012) Ang-(1–7) reduces Ang II-induced insulin resistance by enhancing Akt phosphorylation via a Mas receptor-dependent mechanism in rat skeletal muscle. Biochem Biophys Res Commun 426: 369–373.
20. Muñoz MC, Giani JF, Burghi V, Mayer MA, Carranza A, et al. (2012) The Mas receptor mediates modulation of insulin signaling by angiotensin-(1–7). Regul Pept 177: 1–11.
21. Santos RAS, Ferreira AJ, Verano-Braga T, Bader M. (2013) Angiotensin-converting enzyme 2, angiotensin-(1–7) and Mas: new players of the renin-angiotensin system. J Endocrinol 216: R1–R17.
22. Negrao CE, Middlekauff HR (2008) Adaptations in autonomic function during exercise training in heart failure. Heart Fail Rev 13: 51–60.
23. Roveda F, Middlekauff HR, Rondon MU, Reis SF, Souza M, et al. (2003) The effects of exercise training on sympathetic neural activation in advanced heart failure: a randomized controlled trial. J Am Coll Cardiol 42: 854–860.
24. De Mello Franco FG, Santos AC, Rondon MUP, Trombetta IC, Strunz C, et al. (2006) Effects of home-based exercise training on neurovascular control in patients with heart failure. Eur J Heart Fail 8: 851–855.
25. Braith RW, Welsch MA, Feigenbaum MS, Kluess HA, Pepine CJ. (1999) Neuroendocrine activation in heart failure is modified by endurance exercise training. J Am Coll Cardiol 34: 1170–1175.
26. Fernandes T, Hashimoto NY, Magalhães FC, Fernandes FB, Casarini DE, et al. (2011) Aerobic exercise training-induced left ventricular hypertrophy involves regulatory MicroRNAs, decreased angiotensin-converting enzyme-angiotensin ii, and synergistic regulation of angiotensin-converting enzyme 2-angiotensin (1–7). Hypertension 58: 182–189.
27. Filho AG, Ferreira AJ, Santos SHS, Neves SRS, Silva Camargos ER, et al. (2008) Selective increase of angiotensin(1–7) and its receptor in hearts of spontaneously hypertensive rats subjected to physical training. Exp Physiol 93: 589–598.
28. Gao E, Lei YH, Shang X, Huang ZM, Zuo L, et al. (2010) A novel and efficient model of coronary artery ligation and myocardial infarction in the mouse. Circ Res 107: 1445–1453.

29. Lang RM, Bierig M, Devereux RB, Flachskampf FA, Foster E, et al. (2005) Recommendations for chamber quantification: a report from the American Society of Echocardiography's Guidelines and Standards Committee and the Chamber Quantification Writing Group, developed in conjunction with the European Association of Echocardiograph. J Am Soc Echocardiogr 18: 1440–1463.
30. Brooks GA, White TP (1978) Determination of metabolic and heart rate responses of rats to treadmill exercise. J Appl Physiol 45: 1009–1015.
31. Rondon E, Brasileiro-Santos MS, Moreira ED, Rondon MUPB, Mattos KC, et al. (2006) Exercise training improves aortic depressor nerve sensitivity in rats with ischemia-induced heart failure. Am J Physiol Heart Circ Physiol 291: H2801–6.
32. Fernandes T, Hashimoto NY, Oliveira EM. (2010) Characterization of angiotensin-converting enzymes 1 and 2 in the soleus and plantaris muscles of rats. Braz J Med Biol Res 43: 837–842.
33. Liu JL, Irvine S, Reid IA, Patel KP, Zucker IH. (2000) Chronic exercise reduces sympathetic nerve activity in rabbits with pacing-induced heart failure: A role for angiotensin II. Circulation 102: 1854–1862.
34. Barretto ACP, Santos AC, Munhoz R, Rondon MU, Franco FG, et al. (2009) Increased muscle sympathetic nerve activity predicts mortality in heart failure patients. Int J Cardiol 135: 302–307.
35. Osterziel KJ, Hänlein D, Willenbrock R, Eichhorn C, Luft F, et al. (1995) Baroreflex sensitivity and cardiovascular mortality in patients with mild to moderate heart failure. Br Heart J 73: 517–522.
36. Epelman S, Tang WH, Chen SY, Van Lente F, Francis GS, et al. (2008) Detection of soluble angiotensin-converting enzyme 2 in heart failure: insights into the endogenous counter-regulatory pathway of the renin-angiotensin-aldosterone system. J Am Coll Cardiol 52: 750–754.
37. Patel VB, Clarke N, Wang Z, Fan D, Parajuli N, et al. (2014) Angiotensin II induced proteolytic cleavage of myocardial ACE2 is mediated by TACE/ADAM-17: A positive feedback mechanism in the RAS. J Mol Cell Cardiol 66: 167–176.
38. Ocaranza MP, Godoy I, Jalil JE, Varas M, Collantes P, et al. (2006) Enalapril attenuates downregulation of Angiotensin-converting enzyme 2 in the late phase of ventricular dysfunction in myocardial infarcted rat. Hypertension 48: 572–578.
39. Agata J, Ura N, Yoshida H, Shinshi Y, Sasaki H, et al. (2006) Olmesartan is an angiotensin II receptor blocker with an inhibitory effect on angiotensin-converting enzyme. Hypertens Res 29: 865–874.
40. Ferrario CM. (2011) ACE2: more of Ang-(1–7) or less Ang II? Curr Opin Nephrol Hypertens 20: 1–6.
41. Mariappan N, Elks CM, Haque M, Francis J. (2012) Interaction of TNF with angiotensin II contributes to mitochondrial oxidative stress and cardiac damage in rats. PLoS One 7: e46568.
42. Vescovo G, Volterrani M, Zennaro R, Sandri M, Ceconi C, et al. (2000) Apoptosis in the skeletal muscle of patients with heart failure: investigation of clinical and biochemical changes. Heart 84: 431–437.
43. Burniston JG, Saini A, Tan L-B, Goldspink DF (2005) Angiotensin II induces apoptosis in vivo in skeletal, as well as cardiac, muscle of the rat. Exp Physiol 90: 755–761.
44. Van Kats JP, de Lannoy LM, Jan Danser AH, van Meegen JR, Verdouw PD, et al. (1997) Angiotensin II type 1 (AT1) receptor-mediated accumulation of angiotensin II in tissues and its intracellular half-life in vivo. Hypertension 30: 42–49.
45. Uehara Y, Miura S, Yahiro E, Saku K. (2013) Non-ACE pathway-induced angiotensin II production. Curr Pharm Des 19: 3054–3059.
46. Akasu M, Urata H, Kinoshita A, Sasaguri M, Ideishi M, et al. (1998) Differences in tissue angiotensin II-forming pathways by species and organs in vitro. Hypertension 32: 514–520.
47. Ward PE, Russell JS, Vaghy PL. (1995) Angiotensin and bradykinin metabolism by peptidases identified in skeletal muscle. Peptides 16: 1073–1078.
48. Johnston APW, Baker J, De Lisio M, Parise G. (2011) Skeletal muscle myoblasts possess a stretch-responsive local angiotensin signalling system. J Renin Angiotensin Aldosterone Syst 12: 75–84.
49. Dimitrijevic I, Edvinsson M-L, Chen Q, Malmsjö M, Kimblad P-O, et al. (2009) Increased expression of vascular endothelin type B and angiotensin type 1 receptors in patients with ischemic heart disease. BMC Cardiovasc Disord 9: 40.
50. Zhang G-X, Ohmori K, Nagai Y, Fujisawa Y, Nishiyama A, et al. (2007) Role of AT1 receptor in isoproterenol-induced cardiac hypertrophy and oxidative stress in mice. J Mol Cell Cardiol 42: 804–811.
51. Malendowicz SL, Ennezat P V, Testa M, Murray L, Sonnenblick EH, et al. (2000) Angiotensin II receptor subtypes in the skeletal muscle vasculature of patients with severe congestive heart failure. Circulation 102: 2210–2213.

4

Feasibility of a Combined Aerobic and Strength Training Program and Its Effects on Cognitive and Physical Function in Institutionalized Dementia Patients

Willem J. R. Bossers[1]*, Erik J. A. Scherder[1,2], Froukje Boersma[3], Tibor Hortobágyi[1], Lucas H. V. van der Woude[1,4], Marieke J. G. van Heuvelen[1]

1 University of Groningen, University Medical Center Groningen, Center for Human Movement Sciences, Groningen, The Netherlands, **2** VU University, Department of Clinical Neuropsychology, Amsterdam, The Netherlands, **3** University of Groningen, University Medical Center Groningen, Department of General Practice, Elderly Care Medicine, Groningen, The Netherlands, **4** University of Groningen, University Medical Center Groningen, Center for Rehabilitation, Groningen, The Netherlands

Abstract

Objectives: We examined the feasibility of a combined aerobic and strength training program in institutionalized dementia patients and studied the effects on cognitive and physical function.

Methods: Thirty-three patients with dementia, recruited from one nursing home, participated in this non-randomized pilot study (25 women; age = 85.2±4.9 years; Mini Mental State Examination = 16.8±4.0). In phase 1 of the study, seventeen patients in the Exercise group (EG) received a combined aerobic and strength training program for six weeks, five times per week, 30 minutes per session, in an individually supervised format and successfully concluded the pre and posttests. In phase 2 of the study, sixteen patients in the Social group (SG) received social visits at the same frequency, duration, and format and successfully concluded the pre and posttests.

Results: Indices of feasibility showed that the recruitment and adherence rate, respectively were 46.2% and 86.3%. All EG patients completed the exercise program according to protocol without adverse events. After the six-week program, no significant differences on cognitive function tests were found between the EG and SG. There was a moderate effect size in favor for the EG for the Visual Memory Span Forward; a visual attention test. There were significant differences between groups in favor for the EG with moderate to large effects for the physical tests Walking Speed (p = .003), Six-Minute Walk Test (p = .031), and isometric quadriceps strength (p = .012).

Conclusions: The present pilot study showed that it is feasible to conduct a combined aerobic and strength training program in institutionalized patients with dementia. The selective cognitive visual attention improvements and more robust changes in motor function in favor of EG vs. SG could serve as a basis for large randomized clinical trials.

Trial Registration: trialregister.nl 1230

Editor: Terence J. Quinn, University of Glasgow, United Kingdom

Funding: These authors have no support or funding to report.

Competing Interests: The authors have declared that no competing interests exist.

* E-mail: w.j.r.bossers@umcg.nl

Introduction

Cognitive and physical function declines with dementia and the decline accelerates with disease severity. Unsurprisingly, disease severity is the most reliable predictor of institutionalization and care burden [1,2]. It is suggested that physical activity is a treatment modality which may have positive effects on dementia patients' cognitive and physical function and therefore could favorably influence the disease progression in institutionalized patients with dementia [3,4]. However, previous exercise studies with dementia patients focused mainly on aerobic-only training and the results are inconsistent and less convincing compared with studies that included healthy older subjects [5]. In those studies with healthy older subjects a combination of aerobic and strength training was most effective in improving memory and executive function (e.g. inhibition, planning, impulse control, set-shifting) [6,7]. Therefore, the emerging hypothesis is that a combined aerobic and strength exercise program for dementia patients may also be effective to improve memory and executive function.

Beneficial effects of a combined aerobic and strength training program on cognitive function may emanate from the complementariness between the neurobiological and physiological mechanisms underlying the individual exercise programs. Aerobic and strength training each can positively affect the levels of insulin like growth factor-1 and brain derived neurotrophine factors [7,8]. These proteins mediate neuronal cell growth, proliferation, survival, and differentiation. However, strength training may specifically lower the levels of the neurotoxic homocysteine, which is related to improved cognition [7,9]. Furthermore, strength training improves critical elements of physical function, such as mobility and balance [10,11]. The strength training effect could in turn allow patients to perform the aerobic exercise component at a higher intensity. Aerobic training at a moderate to high intensity level can improve cerebral blood flow [12], a factor known to mediate effects on cognitive function [13]. Altogether, there is a reasonably strong potential that a combination of aerobic and strength training could improve cognitive and physical function in patients with dementia.

A combined program of aerobic and strength activities was found feasible and effective to improve global cognitive and motor function in community dwelling patients with mild dementia [14,15]. In contrast to community dwelling patients, institutionalized patients with dementia are older and physically, cognitively, socially, and psychologically more vulnerable [2]. Therefore, an exercise program may be less feasible for this specific patient group. Although both aerobic and strength training studies with institutionalized dementia patients are available, there is no data available of how feasibility is affected by a complexity of alternating strength training with aerobic training. This complexity is important because dementia patients may perceive variation or change in activities and environment as upsetting or disruptive in daily-life routine, causing stress and leading to not attending to activities, such as exercise [16]. Last, the session-frequency in previous studies ranged between 1–7 sessions per week [5] but no extensive data on adherence rates was reported in these studies. Therefore, it remains unclear at what frequency institutionalized dementia patients are able and/or willing to exercise, which is important because the American College of Sports Medicine (ACSM) guidelines recommend 3–5 times weekly exercise at a moderate to high intensity level, with alternating aerobic and strength training, to improve physical fitness [17]. All in all, prior to investigate any potential effects of high frequency combined exercise in a frail institutionalized moderate-severe dementia population, it is required to first study the feasibility of such a training program (e.g. 5 sessions per week, alternating aerobic with strength training). Here we define an intervention feasible when adherence to the program is high (>75%), the number of drop-outs is low (<20%), there are no adverse events, and participants complete the program according to protocol.

Taken together, the purpose of the study was to determine the feasibility of a combined aerobic and strength training program and to perform an exploratory analysis concerning the effects of such an exercise program on cognitive and physical function in institutionalized patients with dementia.

Methods

Ethics statement

The Medical Ethics Committee of VU Amsterdam, The Netherlands approved the research protocol according to the principles expressed by the Declaration of Helsinki. This clinical trial is registered at the Netherlands Trial Register (trial number 1230). The protocol for this trial and supporting CONSORT checklist are available as supporting information; see Checklist S1 and Protocol S1.

Study design and procedures

This is a non-randomized, two-group, pretest-posttest, and single-blind pilot study. Between March 2010 and October 2010, a geriatrician recruited all of the participants from a psychogeriatric ward in a nursing home in Haren, the Netherlands (N = 78). The inclusion criteria were as follows: 70 years or older, a diagnosis of dementia, not wheelchair bound, and able to walk independently ten meters with or without a walking aid. All participants and their relatives were fully informed about the details of the study, including the risks, time commitment, and the possibility to be assigned to a combined aerobic and strength exercise group (EG) or a social visits group (SG). Each patient's legal representative gave written consent.

Because there are no previous studies on the feasibility of subjecting institutionalized patients with dementia residing in a psychogeriatric ward to a combined aerobic and strength training program, first we had to ascertain the feasibility that such a program can be executed at all in this specific setting with this specific population. Therefore, phase 1 of the study determined feasibility. The aim of phase 2 was to explore the effects of the program on cognitive and physical function and compare these effects to a social visits group. Figure 1 shows the flow of patient recruitment.

For phase 1 (March 2010–May, 2010), a geriatrician screened four out of eight wards in one nursing home where 35 residents with dementia were living, of whom 20 were enrolled in the study and 18 ultimately participated in the EG. Then, in phase 2 (August 2010–October, 2010), the same geriatrician screened the remaining other four wards (N = 43) from the same nursing home, of whom 19 were enrolled and 18 eventually participated in the SG.

The cognitive and physical assessments for all participants took place at baseline (T0) and after an intervention period of six weeks (T1). A trained research assistant, blinded for the intervention, administrated the cognitive and physical function tests at T0 and T1. The research assistant conducted the measurements at the same time of the day for a given patient.

Intervention

Exercise and social visit sessions were provided in an individually supervised format for a period of six weeks. An individually supervised format was chosen because dementia is related to behavioral problems, such as apathy and agitation and this may cause inactivating thoughts and difficulties in initiating movement [1]. For safety reasons, institutionalized patients who live in a closed ward are required to have personal guidance for activities outside the ward. Each participant received five, 30-minute-long sessions during each of the six weeks. Four allocated trained research assistants delivered the two intervention programs and kept a log on the indices of feasibility.

Exercise group. Each week, the EG participated in three walking sessions and two strength training sessions. Walking sessions took place in the corridors of the nursing home or on paved outdoor walking paths near the nursing home. In accordance with ACSM guidelines for aerobic activity, our aim was to offer walking sessions at a moderate to high intensity level [17]. If a participant requested rest, an appropriate rest period was included in the 30-minute-long session. As soon as patients recovered, walking was resumed. The trainer monitored the intensity-level of the walks by asking the patients rate of perceived exertion (RPE). RPE was measured at the end of each session. The goal was to reach RPE-scores between 12–15 (e.g. 'somewhat hard' - 'hard', maximum score 20) [17].

In accordance with ACSM guidelines for strength training, the EG participated in two strength training sessions per week. These

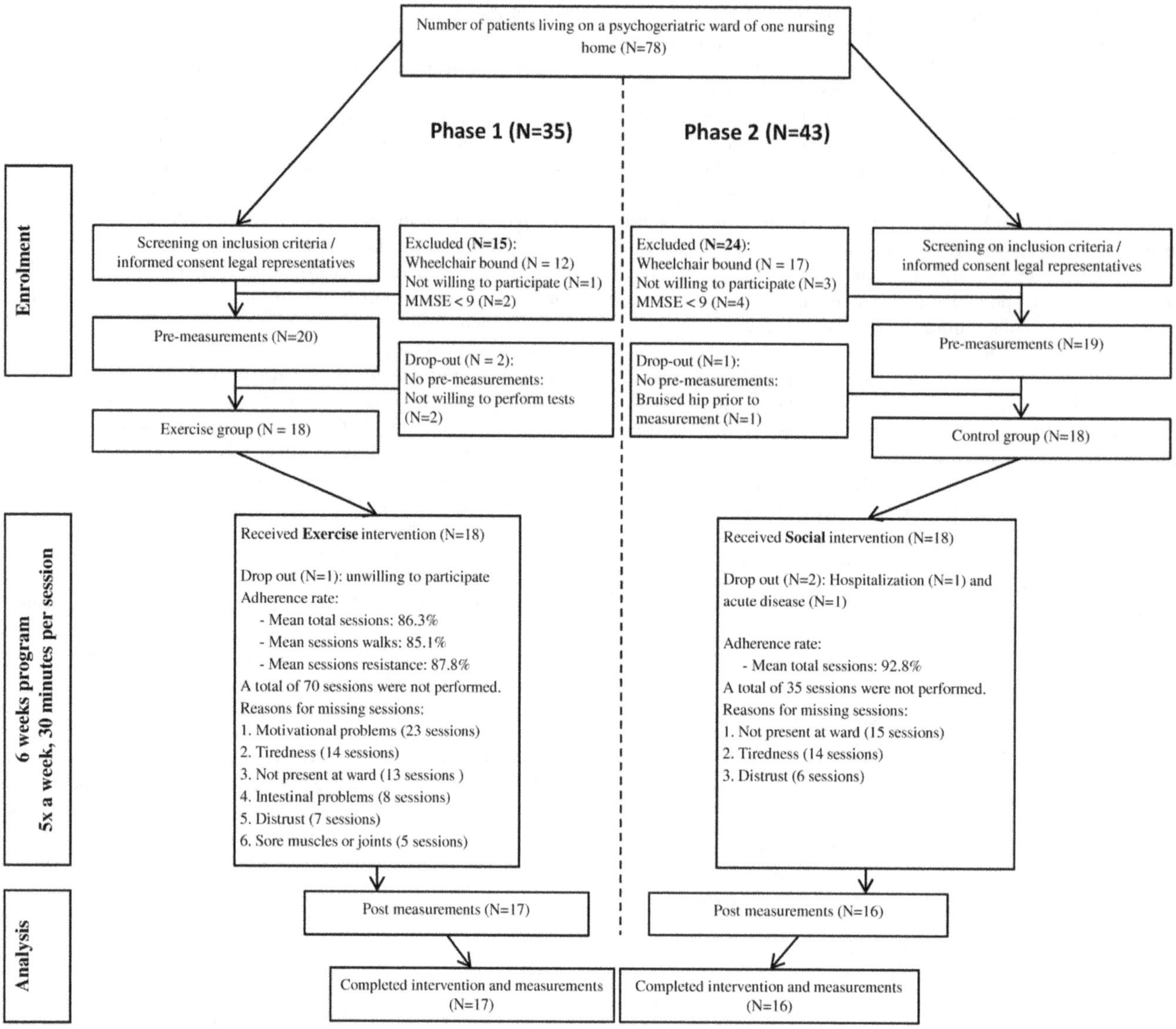

Figure 1. Flowchart of the study. Phase 1 (left side) determined feasibility by including a combined exercise group. Phase 2 (right side) explored the effects of the program by including a social visits group.

sessions were conducted in the patient's personal room on two non-consecutive days with at least 48 h between sessions [17]. Strength exercises focused on lower-limb strengthening to activate large muscle groups known to contribute to gait speed, balance, and mobility [11,18]. The exercises were as follows: (1) seated knee extension, (2) plantar flexion through toe raises, while holding both hands of the trainer, (3) hip abduction by moving the straight leg sideways, while standing behind and holding on to a chair, and (4) hip extension by moving the straight leg backwards, while standing behind and holding on to a chair. An exercise program targeting the same muscle groups was successful in improving mobility and leg strength in community dwelling older adults, recovering from a hip fracture [19]. Exercise intensity increased gradually by increasing the number of repetitions and by affixing small weights to the ankle. In accordance with ACSM guidelines for strength training, our aim was to offer a moderate to hard intensity strength exercise program at an RPE of 12–15 (e.g. 'somewhat hard' - 'hard') [17]. To minimize the chance for an injury, overload, and drop-out, all participants started with three sets of 8 repetitions for each leg without weights. When an exercise was performed with ease and according to protocol as judged by the trainer (RPE<12 e.g. fairly light), the number of repetitions was increased to 10 in the next session, and 12 thereafter. When a participant was able to correctly perform 12 repetitions without weights, at an RPE<12, 0.5 kg was attached to the ankle. After the weight was attached, patients performed eight repetitions and progressed as described before. The trainers increased the weights from 0 kg to a maximum of 1.5 kg in 0.5 kg increments to reach RPE 12–15. For plantar flexion, the number of repetitions increased in increments of 2 with each session, to a maximum of 30 repetitions.

Social group. The SG received individualized social visits for the same duration and frequency as the EG. Social engagement may have a positive effect on cognitive function in patients with dementia [20]. Therefore, to control for social engagement, activities during social visits were small talk while sitting in a chair.

Measurements

Feasibility. We obtained the recruitment rate at the psychogeriatric ward of one nursing home for participating in the combined exercise program. We defined an intervention feasible when the rate of program adherence is high (>75%), the number of drop-out low (<20%), no adverse events occur, and participants complete the program according to protocol.

Cognitive function. Cognitive function was measured with a neuropsychological test battery that covered the domains global cognitive function, verbal memory, visual attention, and executive function. Tests used in this study were based on a review [21] and a study-protocol [22].

Mini Mental State Examination (MMSE) measures the global level of cognitive function [23]. Scores range from 0–30.

Faces Recognition Test, as a subtest of the Rivermead Behavioral Memory Test (RBMT), measures visual long term memory/attention [24]. Version A was used. Five cards with faces were shown to the participant, each for five seconds. After ten minutes, ten cards were presented; five cards were shown before and five cards presented new faces. The participant had to recognize if a face was shown before or not. The total score is the number of correct answers minus the number of incorrect answers. Scores ranged between −10 and +10. A higher score represented a better performance.

Pictures Recognition Test, as a subtest of the RBMT, measures visual long term memory/attention [24]. The versions A + B were combined. Ten cards with objects were presented, each card for five seconds. After ten minutes, twenty cards were presented; ten were shown before and ten cards presented new objects. The participant had to recognize if an object was shown before or not. The total score was the number of correct answers minus the number of incorrect answers. Scores ranged between −20 and + 20. A higher score represented a better performance.

Visual Memory Span Forward and Backward, as a subtest of the Wechsler Memory Scale Revised (WMS-R), consisted of printed squares on a card [25]. Participants were instructed to repeat a number of tapping sequences that became longer with each trial. The test consisted of a forward and backward condition. The forward condition measured attention and immediate visual memory. The backward condition measured attention and visual working memory, an executive function. Scores of both sub-tests ranged between 0–14. A higher score represented better performance.

Digit Span Test Forward and Backward are subtests from the WMS-R [25]. The forward condition consists of increasingly long sequences of orally presented numbers at a rate of one digit per second. Participants were asked to repeat the exact same sequence of numbers immediately. In the backward condition participants were asked to repeat the sequence in reverse order. It is suggested that the forward condition taps more into the short-term memory and the backward condition more into working memory, an executive function. Each condition ends when a participant fails to recall two strings of the same length or repeated an eight-digit sequence correctly. The scores for both conditions range between 0–21.

8-Words Test Direct-Recall and Recognition is a list-learning test for people with memory problems [26]. Eight words were orally presented five times in a row. Every time, directly after presenting the words, participants were asked to repeat as many words as possible. The first outcome measure was the total number of correct words over five trials (Direct-Recall score 0–40). After 15 minutes the examiner orally presents 16 words among which eight words presented in the direct-recall phase and eight new words. The participant had to recognize if a word was presented before (Recognition score 0–16).

Verbal Fluency Test evaluated executive function [27,28]. Participants were asked to name as many examples of 'animals' as possible in one minute. After a few minutes, they were asked to name as many examples of 'professions' in one minute. The outcome measure was the total number of animals and professions.

Picture Completion Test, as a sub-test of the Groningen Intelligence Test, measures visual perception and alertness to detail (executive function). During the test, incomplete drawn figures were presented [29]. Participants were instructed to describe the picture as a whole. The pictures increased in difficulty as the test progressed. With five false answers in a row the test was stopped. Scores ranged from 0–20, with one point for each correct answer.

Stroop Task consisted of three subtasks [30]. Each task was performed as quickly as possible over a timed period of 45 seconds. Card 1 presented black-printed words 'red', 'green', 'blue', and 'yellow'. Participants were instructed to read as many words as possible in the right order (left to right, top to bottom). Card 2 presented solid colored patched blocks which were red, green, blue, and yellow. As many of these colors needed to be named in the right order. Finally, Card 3 presented colored words. That is, each word was printed in a different color (i.e. the word 'blue' printed in yellow ink). The ink-color needed to be named and the highly provocative word-reading response needed to be inhibited. The final score was Card 2 minus Card 3. A lower final score indicated a better performance of inhibition, an executive function.

Physical function. Physical function was measured with a test battery that covered the domains of walking endurance, lower limb strength, mobility, and balance as suggested previously [21,22]. Participants were allowed to use a walking aid.

Six-Minute Walk Test measures walking endurance [31,32]. Participants were instructed to walk as long a distance as they could in six minutes. Each pre-set round was 26.3 meters and the distance was measured until the nearest meter. Stops and rests were included in the test performance.

Sit-to-Stand Test measures lower body strength in older adults [33]. To increase feasibility, participants were allowed to use upper limbs to rise from the chair. Participants were asked to stand-up and sit-down as many times as possible in thirty seconds. Ending in a standing position was counted as 0.5 stand.

Quadriceps strength test measures strength of the quadriceps femoris muscle [34]. A participant was instructed to generate maximal isometric knee extension force of the left leg, then the right leg while resting the arms on the thighs. The test was performed three times with 30 seconds of rest between trials. During the measurements, the maximum knee extension force was not visible for the participant. The highest score was given in kilograms. At baseline the maximum knee extension force of both legs was recorded. The highest score of either the left or right leg was recorded as outcome score. Then, after the six-week-long intervention period, the strongest leg at baseline (e.g. left or right leg) was tested again for maximum knee extension force.

Timed Up & Go Test quantifies functional mobility [35]. Participants were asked to rise from a standard chair (0.47 m height, horizontal seat and armrests), walk three meter to an orange cone, walk around it, and return in their chair in fully seated position. The test was performed two times and the mean time in seconds was used as score.

Six-meter Timed Walk measures walking speed [36]. Participants were instructed to walk six meters at a comfortable pace in a straight line, actively passing a line set at six meters. The test was performed twice and the fastest time was noted. As an outcome measure, walking speed (meters per second) over the last five meters of the test was calculated to exclude start-up speed.

Frailty and Injuries Cooperative Studies of Intervention Techniques (FICSIT-4) measures static balance control [37,38]. Participants were asked to perform four different stances: (1) feet together, (2) semi-tandem, (3) tandem, and (4) single-leg without assistive device. Every stance had to hold for 10 seconds. The score on the FICSIT-4 scale ranged from 0 to 5 with a higher score indicating better performance.

Figure of Eight Test measures dynamic balance [39,40]. Participants walked two laps of a standard figure-eight trajectory, as quickly and accurately as possible. The fastest time of two trials was noted, and the results were converted into walking speed (meters per second). Furthermore, oversteps outside the Figure of Eight were noted.

Statistical analysis

SPSS Statistics 20 was used for data management and analyses. Possible group differences at baseline between EG and SG were analyzed for personal characteristics as well as cognitive and physical outcomes using Mann-Whitney or Fisher's tests. Difference scores between posttest (T1) and pretest (T0) for the EG and SG were calculated followed by Mann-Whitney U tests to compare the difference scores between EG and SG. The two-sided level of significance for global cognitive function was set at $p<.05$. To correct for alpha-inflation we used Bonferroni corrected alpha values for the cognitive domains verbal memory ($p<.05/3$ tests = .017), visual attention ($p<.05/3$ tests = .017), and executive function ($p<.05/5$ tests = .010). The level of significance for the physical domain walking endurance was set at $p<.05$, lower limb strength at $p=.025$ ($p<.05/2$ tests), mobility at $p=.025$ ($p<.05/2$ tests), and balance at $p=.012$ ($p<0.05/3$ tests). To explore the relation between cognitive change and physical change in the total study population, we used Spearman's correlations between the difference scores of the cognitive and physical tests. The magnitude of effects between the EG and SG were displayed as a Cohen's d Effect Size (ES). ESs were calculated with Cohen's d formula: $d = [(\text{post}_{EG} - \text{pre}_{EG}) - (\text{post}_{SG} - \text{pre}_{SG})] / Sqrt\,[([s^2 \text{pre}_{EG} (n_{EG}) + s^2 \text{pre}_{SG} (n_{SG})] / [n_{EG} + n_{SG}]) + ([s^2 \text{post}_{EG} (n_{EG}) + s^2 \text{post}_{SG} (n_{SG})] / [n_{EG} + n_{SG}]) / 2]$ [41].

To adjust for changes in SG, which may be initiated by natural course or social engagement, the formula as stated above included both values for the EG and SG. Cohen's benchmarks were used to indicate small ($d=0.20$), moderate ($d=0.50$), and large ($d=0.80$) ESs.

Results

Table 1 shows that patients in the two groups at baseline were not significantly different in age, gender, use of a walking aid, and global cognitive function measured with the MMSE.

Feasibility

We managed to recruit 33 (46%) of 78 patients in a Dutch nursing home. Figure 1 shows that the rates of adherence (EG = 86%/SG = 93%) were similar in the two groups and it also shows reasons for non-participation such as motivational problems and tiredness. Three dropouts occurred (e.g. 2 due to not willing to perform the pretests, 1 due to injury) but these dropouts were not related to the intervention. Adverse effects included sore leg muscles (6 participants EG; 0 SG) and a sense of exertion (12 participants EG; 0 SG) but resulted in no dropouts. In total, all of the participants in the EG completed the 30-minute walks according to protocol. Further, 15 of 17 participants completed all strength exercises according to protocol. Two participants were unable to perform the toe rises while standing with the trainer's assistance and these patients performed toe rises in the seated position when lifting the heels.

Changes in cognitive function

Table 2 presents the cognitive function data. The two intervention groups did not significantly differ at baseline in all cognitive tests. There were no changes in MMSE after either interventions (EG: 0%, SG: −3%). Performance in Faces Recognition Test, Pictures Recognition Test, and Visual Memory Span Forward was 6%, 22%, and 15% higher, respectively, in the EG, while the corresponding values in the SG were 2%, 13%, and 6% lower ($d=0.13$, $d=0.46$, $d=0.68$, respectively). There were no differences between the EG and SG in the verbal memory tests. Finally, the EG scored 12%, 19%, and 13% higher on the Digit Span Backward Test, GIT incomplete figures test, and STROOP test, respectively. In comparison, the SG scored 8%, 8%, and 6% higher on these tests, respectively ($d=0.21$, $d=0.27$, $d=0.23$, respectively). None of the between-group differences in cognitive test scores reached statistical significance.

Changes in physical function

Table 3 presents the physical function data. The EG and SG were similar at baseline in the physical function tests. Performance in the Six Minute Walk Test improved 17% in EG, and decreased 12% in SG ($d=0.70$). Walking Speed also improved 18% in the EG but decreased 11% in the SG ($d=0.91$). The EG improved 4% in knee extension strength while the SG lost 20% strength ($d=0.66$). The EG gained 15% on the FICSIT-4 and the SG lost 1% ($d=0.43$). No significant correlation larger than rho = .20 was found between any of the physical and cognitive change scores.

Table 1. Baseline characteristics of the Exercise group and the Social group.

Characteristic	Exercise group (N = 17)	Social group (N = 16)	p-value
Age, years (Mean ± SD)	86.1±3.8	84.1±5.7	.118[a]
Male (%)	23.5%	25.0%	.958[b]
Use of walking aid (%)	29.4%	37.5%	.709[b]
Mini Mental State Examination (Mean ± SD)	16.5±4.4	16.8±4.3	.822[a]

Note: [a], Mann-Whitney U Test, [b], Fisher's Exact Test: $p<.05$.

Table 2. Cognitive function data for the Exercise group and Social group at baseline (T0) and after 6 weeks (T1).

	Exercise group				Social group				Exercise vs. Social		
Cognitive function tests	**Pre-measure (T0) (Mean ± SD)**	**Post-measure (T1) (Mean ± SD)**	**T0 - T1 (%)**	**N**	**Pre-measure (T0) (Mean ± SD)**	**Post-measure (T1) (Mean ± SD)**	**T0 - T1 (%)**	**N**	***d***	**U**	**p***
Domain: Global cognition											
Mini Mental State Examination	16.5±4.4	16.5±4.6	0%	17	16.8±4.3	16.3±4.1	−3%	16	0.13	123.5	.657
Domain: Visual attention											
Faces Recognition Test	5.4±2.9	5.8±2.9	+6%	17	3.3±4.0	3.2±2.6	−2%	16	0.13	85.5	.114
Pictures Recognition Test	8.8±7.7	10.7±6.9	+22%	17	10.1±6.9	8.8±7.8	−13%	16	0.46^{S}	90.0	.165
Visual Memory Span Forward	4.6±1.7	5.3±1.5	+15%	17	4.6±1.3	4.3±1.6	−6%	16	0.68^{M}	67.5	.022
Domain: Verbal memory											
Digit Span Test Forward	8.9±3.2	9.8±2.1	+10%	17	8.4±2.8	8.9±2.4	+5%	16	0.17	118.5	.503
8-Words Test – Direct-Recall	14.5±7.3	15.1±6.7	+4%	17	12.8±8.1	13.2±7.4	+4%	16	0.01	126.0	.970
8-Words Test - Recognition	10.5±2.2	11.1±2.7	+5%	17	10.7±3.3	11.9±2.3	+12%	16	−0.27	126.0	.970
Domain: Executive function											
Verbal Fluency Test	13.6±8.1	13.9±7.7	+2%	17	11.9±6.2	12.2±7.1	+3%	16	0.00	135.0	.986
Digit Span Test Backward	5.7±2.1	6.4±1.9	+12%	17	4.3±2.2	4.6±1.6	+8%	15	0.21^{S}	112.5	.576
Picture Completion Test	4.9±2.3	5.9±2.0	+19%	17	3.9±2.4	4.2±2.8	+8%	16	0.27^{S}	122	.631
Stroop Task	28.9±12.7	24.9±12.5	+13%	15	23.8±11.8	22.4±8.6	+6%	11	0.23^{S}	75.5	.721
Visual Memory Span Backward	3.7±2.0	3.9±1.5	+5%	17	2.8±1.8	2.9±1.4	+4%	16	0.03	109.0	.502

Note: SD, Standard deviation; T0, Baseline; T1, 6-week posttest;
^{S}, small Cohen's *d* effect size;
^{M}, medium Cohen's *d* effect size;
*, Bonferroni corrected p-values were set at $p < 0.05$ for the domain global cognitive function, $p<.017$ for domain visual attention, $p<.017$ for domain verbal memory, and $p<.010$ for domain executive function.

Table 3. Physical function data for the Exercise group and Social group at baseline (T0) and after 6 weeks (T1).

	Exercise group				Social group				Exercise vs. Social		
Physical function tests	**Pre-measure (T0) (Mean ± SD)**	**Post-measure (T1) (Mean ± SD)**	**T0 - T1 (%)**	**N**	**Pre-measure (T0) (Mean ± SD)**	**Post-measure (T1) (Mean ± SD)**	**T0 - T1 (%)**	**N**	***d***	**U**	**p***
Domain: Walking endurance											
Six Minute Walk Test (m)	216.8±90.60	254.6±99.0	+17%	15	252.4±105.2	221.8±110.8	−12%	14	0.70[M]	51.00	.031*
Domain: Leg strength											
Sit to Stand test (no.)	7.9±3.3	8.7±3.3	+10%	16	8.8±3.0	8.3±3.2	−5%	16	0.41[S]	94.0	.210
Quadriceps strength test (kg)[a]	21.8±10.7	22.7±10.5	+4%	16	25.8±10.2	20.5±6.3	−20%	9	0.66[M]	28.0	.012*
Domain: Mobility											
Timed Up and Go Test (s)	18.5±8.7	16.6±6.2	+10%	16	17.6±7.4	18.4±8.9	+5%	16	0.35[S]	171.5	.102
Six-meter Timed Walk (m/s)	0.8±0.3	0.9±0.3	+18%	16	0.9±0.2	0.8±0.2	−11%	16	0.91[L]	51.0	.003*
Domain: Balance											
FICSIT-4	2.4±1.0	2.8±0.6	+15%	16	2.7±1.0	2.7±1.2	−1%	16	0.43[S]	92.0	.184
Figure of Eight speed (m/s)	0.4±0.2	0.5±0.2	+14%	16	0.5±0.3	0.5±0.2	−2%	16	0.32[S]	97.0	.254
Figure of Eight oversteps (no.)	6.7±6.2	5.8±6.6	+14%	16	5.9±8.1	7.8±9.3	−33%	16	0.39[S]	172.5	.093

Note: SD, Standard deviation; T0, Baseline; T1, 6-week posttest; FICSIT-4, Frailty and Injuries Cooperative Studies of Intervention Techniques;
[S], small Cohen's *d* effect size;
[M], medium Cohen's *d* effect size;
[L], large Cohen's *d* effect size;
[a], maximum knee extension force of the strongest leg (e.g. left or right) was measured at pretest and posttest; *, Bonferroni corrected p-values were set at $p < 0.05$ for domain walking endurance, $p < .025$ for domain leg strength, $p < .025$ for domain mobility, and $p < .017$ for domain balance.

Discussion

The purpose of the study was to determine the feasibility of a combined aerobic and strength training program and to perform an exploratory analysis concerning the effects of such an exercise program on cognitive and physical function in institutionalized patients with dementia. Because this was a pilot study using small sample sizes, the results should be considered preliminary and viewed with caution. Still, the current results could serve as a basis for future larger randomized clinical trials.

Feasibility

The individually supervised format of administering the intervention contributed to feasibility. We defined that an exercise program was feasible if the adherence rate was high (>75%), the number of drop outs low (<20%), no adverse events occurred, and the exercise program was performed according to protocol. We consider the mean adherence rate of 84% high and encouraging for future studies. Our rate was 31% higher than the mean adherence in a 12-month group-walking exercise program using patients with mild cognitive impairment [42] and 9% higher than a one-on-one 12-week home-based combined exercise program in a similar patient group [14]. The much shorter intervention period compared with the other studies could explain our substantially higher adherence rate. Therefore, a longer duration exercise program is needed to further study the adherence on a longer term.

All patients were able to perform the aerobic part of the training program according to protocol and 15 out of 17 patients performed the strength part of the training program according to protocol. A factor that contributed to the high program adherence was that all patients started the training program at a generally low-intensity, working their way up to higher intensity levels as the program progressed. The progressive training character, with a low baseline training intensity, may have contributed to higher adherence rates. As a result, no major adverse events other than sore leg muscles, a feeling of exertion, and no program related drop out occurred. Furthermore, progressive training is important because adherence rate in institutionalized patients with dementia is negatively affected by low self-efficacy and low external locus of control [43,44]. Progressive, individually supervised training in the current study may have resulted in a more personalized approach and one-on-one feedback may have led to better participation during the exercise programs and higher adherence rates compared to group interventions. While an individually supervised format of treating institutionalized patients with dementia can be effective in keeping adherence rates high as in the present study, it is also time intensive and potentially costly. However, we experienced that perhaps the most effective way to deliver exercise programs in dementia patients is in an individually supervised format. This is supported by knowledge that patients with dementia suffer from behavioral problems, such as apathy and agitation, which may cause inactivating thoughts and problems in the initiation of movement [1]. A possible practical solution to offer a personal individualized training regime is to involve volunteers and family members to offer such programs in a structured and frequent way.

In total, 46% of the patients with dementia who lived in an institutionalized setting met the inclusion criteria and were willing to participate. Therefore, the generalizability of this study is limited to patients who are able to walk independently, with or without a walking aid and were willing to exercise. The main reason why walking and leg-strength training was not possible was that 37% of the residents was wheelchair bound. Different training strategies are needed for this group, which should focus at both aerobic training and upper-extremity training to maintain or improve handgrip and arm strength because these are key contributors to functional ability and independency in activities of daily life [45]. A possible exercise program could consist of an arm-bike exercise combined with upper body strength training.

Cognitive function

A six-week exercise program did not significantly improve cognitive function. However, there was a medium effect size only for the Visual Memory Span Forward, a visuospatial attention and memory test. This finding is in line with other studies, demonstrating positive effects of exercise on visuospatial but not on verbal processes [46]. This selective effect on visuospatial memory was also found in a meta-analysis of Colcombe & Kramer [6] and suggested a mediating role for a specific part of the hippocampus. The involvement of the hippocampal area was shown by an aerobic exercise program, which led to increased anterior hippocampal volume, and had little effect on the posterior hippocampal part in healthy older adults [47]. Neurons found in the anterior part of the hippocampus were selectively associated with visuospatial memory [48], and are more prone to age related atrophy than the neurons in the posterior hippocampus [49]. So, the current study provides some evidence that these selective effects of exercise on visuospatial memory are also present in older adults with dementia who participated in our combined aerobic and strength training program. Again, these results need to be interpreted with caution and studied further in larger randomized clinical trials over a longer intervention period.

The present data failed to confirm previously reported improvements in executive function after an exercise intervention in frail sedentary cognitively-impaired older adults [4]. A possibility to achieve more change over time is to perform an exercise program over a longer intervention period (e.g. 12 weeks) [3,4]. Furthermore, measurements in cognitively impaired older adults may be less sensitive to change compared with measurements in cognitively non-impaired older adults due to large score variation [50]. We attempted to control for possible intraday variation by performing the measurements at the same time of the day (e.g. morning or afternoon). However, a small sample size, and therefore the use of non-parametric tests, led to the use of difference scores, resulting in lower test reliability. Therefore, future studies should replicate this study with a larger sample size to eliminate this problem.

Physical function

A combination of aerobic and strength exercise sessions led to improvements in tests that measured walking endurance, leg strength, and mobility. The current improvements of leg strength and functional mobility are also in line with results of a six-week, twice to three times per week strength exercise training program [51], emphasizing that a short-term six-week exercise program may already result in beneficial change of physical functions. These improvements should conceptually increase the ability to walk [10] and achieve higher VO_2-peak levels during aerobic activities [52]. In turn, this may promote cerebral blood flow, which is associated with higher level of cognitive function [12,53]. However, we found no association between physical function change scores and cognitive function change scores. We suggest this may relate to different rates of change over time between physical and cognitive function [54]. It remains to be seen if the motor improvements eventually result in correlated improvements in cognitive function in proportion to intervention duration or if the beneficial effects of exercise intervention reach a saturation point. Therefore, long-term intervention studies are needed.

Conclusions

The present pilot study showed that it is feasible to conduct a high-frequency combined aerobic and strength training program in institutionalized patients with dementia. The data also show selective visual attention improvements in cognitive function and more robust changes in motor function in favor of the exercise compared with the social visit intervention. These initial positive results are encouraging and warrant the execution of randomized clinical trials involving higher patient numbers and longer duration.

Acknowledgments

The staff of healthcare institution De Dilgt (ZINN), The Netherlands and all participants and their families are greatly acknowledged. We thank Freek Nieuwhof, Alyt Oppewal, and Annemiek Bielderman for their contribution to the data collection. Finally, we thank the colleagues of the Technical Department of the Center for Human Movement Sciences, University Medical Center Groningen for their technical support during this study.

Author Contributions

Conceived and designed the experiments: WJRB EJAS MJGVH. Performed the experiments: WJRB. Analyzed the data: WJRB EJAS FB TH LVDW MJGVH. Wrote the paper: WJRB EJAS FB TH LVDW MJGVH.

References

1. Perri R, Monaco M, Fadda L, Caltagirone C, Carlesimo GA (2013) Neuropsychological correlates of behavioral symptoms in Alzheimer's disease, frontal variant of frontotemporal, subcortical vascular, and lewy body dementias: A comparative study. J Alzheimers Dis 39: 669–677.
2. Luppa M, Luck T, Weyerer S, Konig HH, Brahler E, et al. (2010) Prediction of institutionalization in the elderly. A systematic review. Age Ageing 39: 31–38.
3. Blankevoort CG, van Heuvelen MJ, Boersma F, Luning H, de Jong J, et al. (2010) Review of effects of physical activity on strength, balance, mobility and ADL performance in elderly subjects with dementia. Dement Geriatr Cogn Disord 30: 392–402.
4. Heyn P, Abreu BC, Ottenbacher KJ (2004) The effects of exercise training on elderly persons with cognitive impairment and dementia: A meta-analysis. Arch Phys Med Rehabil 85: 1694–1704.
5. Forbes D, Thiessen EJ, Blake CM, Forbes SC, Forbes S (2013) Exercise programs for people with dementia. Cochrane Database Syst Rev 12: CD006489.
6. Colcombe S, Kramer AF (2003) Fitness effects on the cognitive function of older adults: A meta-analytic study. Psychol Sci 14: 125–130.
7. Liu-Ambrose T, Donaldson MG (2009) Exercise and cognition in older adults: Is there a role for resistance training programmes? Br J Sports Med 43: 25–27.
8. Huang T, Larsen KT, Ried-Larsen M, Moller NC, Andersen LB (2014) The effects of physical activity and exercise on brain-derived neurotrophic factor in healthy humans: A review. Scand J Med Sci Sports 24: 1–10.
9. Schafer JH, Glass TA, Bolla KI, Mintz M, Jedlicka AE, et al. (2005) Homocysteine and cognitive function in a population-based study of older adults. J Am Geriatr Soc 53: 381–388.
10. LaRoche DP, Millett ED, Kralian RJ (2011) Low strength is related to diminished ground reaction forces and walking performance in older women. Gait Posture 33: 668–672.
11. Krist L, Dimeo F, Keil T (2013) Can progressive resistance training twice a week improve mobility, muscle strength, and quality of life in very elderly nursing-home residents with impaired mobility? A pilot study. Clin Interv Aging 8: 443–448.
12. Nation DA, Hong S, Jak AJ, Delano-Wood L, Mills PJ, et al. (2011) Stress, exercise, and Alzheimer's disease: A neurovascular pathway. Med Hypotheses 76: 847–854.
13. Wiesmann M, Kiliaan AJ, Claassen JA (2013) Vascular aspects of cognitive impairment and dementia. J Cereb Blood Flow Metab 33: 1696–1706.
14. Steinberg M, Leoutsakos JM, Podewils LJ, Lyketsos CG (2009) Evaluation of a home-based exercise program in the treatment of Alzheimer's disease: The maximizing independence in dementia (MIND) study. Int J Geriatr Psychiatry 24: 680–685.
15. Vreugdenhil A, Cannell J, Davies A, Razay G (2012) A community-based exercise programme to improve functional ability in people with Alzheimer's disease: A randomized controlled trial. Scand J Caring Sci 26: 12–19.
16. Hinrichsen GA, Niederehe G (1994) Dementia management strategies and adjustment of family members of older patients. Gerontologist 34: 95–102.
17. Nelson ME, Rejeski WJ, Blair SN, Duncan PW, Judge JO, et al. (2007) Physical activity and public health in older adults: Recommendation from the American College of Sports Medicine and the American Heart Association. Med Sci Sports Exerc 39: 1435–1445.
18. Chandler JM, Duncan PW, Kochersberger G, Studenski S (1998) Is lower extremity strength gain associated with improvement in physical performance and disability in frail, community-dwelling elders? Arch Phys Med Rehabil 79: 24–30.
19. Mangione KK, Craik RL, Palombaro KM, Tomlinson SS, Hofmann MT (2010) Home-based leg-strengthening exercise improves function 1 year after hip fracture: A randomized controlled study. J Am Geriatr Soc 58: 1911–1917.
20. Bassuk SS, Glass TA, Berkman LF (1999) Social disengagement and incident cognitive decline in community-dwelling elderly persons. Ann Intern Med 131: 165–173.
21. Bossers WJ, van der Woude LH, Boersma F, Scherder EJ, van Heuvelen MJ (2012) Recommended measures for the assessment of cognitive and physical performance in older patients with dementia: A systematic review. Dement Geriatr Cogn Dis Extra 2: 589–609.
22. Volkers KM, Scherder EJ (2011) The effect of regular walks on various health aspects in older people with dementia: Protocol of a randomized-controlled trial. BMC Geriatr 11: 38-2318-11-38.
23. Folstein MF, Folstein SE, McHugh PR (1975) "Mini-mental state". A practical method for grading the cognitive state of patients for the clinician. J Psychiatr Res 12: 189–198.
24. Wilson B, Cockburn J, Baddely A (1987) The Rivermead Behavioural Memory Test. London: Thames Valley Test Company.
25. Wechsler D (1987) Wechsler memory scale - revised. New York, NY: The Psychological Corporation.
26. Lindeboom J, Jonker C (1989) Amsterdam dementia screening test, manual. Lisse: Swets and Zeitlinger.
27. Brucki SM, Rocha MS (2004) Category fluency test: Effects of age, gender and education on total scores, clustering and switching in Brazilian Portuguese-speaking subjects. Braz J Med Biol Res 37: 1771–1777.
28. Rosen VM, Engle RW (1997) The role of working memory capacity in retrieval. J Exp Psychol Gen 126: 211–227.
29. Luteijn F, Van der Ploeg FA (1983) Manual Groningen intelligence test (in Dutch: Handleiding Groninger intelligentie test). Swets and Zeitlinger.
30. Hammes J (1973) The STROOP color-word test: Manual (in Dutch: De STROOP kleur-woord test: Handleiding). Amsterdam: Swets and Zeitlinger.
31. Enright PL (2003) The six-minute walk test. Respir Care 48: 783–785.
32. Tappen RM, Roach KE, Buchner D, Barry C, Edelstein J (1997) Reliability of physical performance measures in nursing home residents with Alzheimer's disease. J Gerontol A Biol Sci Med Sci 52: M52–5.
33. Jones CJ, Rikli RE, Beam WC (1999) A 30-s chair-stand test as a measure of lower body strength in community-residing older adults. Res Q Exerc Sport 70: 113–119.
34. Verkerke GJ, Lemmink KA, Slagers AJ, Westhoff MH, van Riet GA, et al. (2003) Precision, comfort and mechanical performance of the quadriso-tester, a quadriceps force measuring device. Med Biol Eng Comput 41: 283–289.
35. Podsiadlo D, Richardson S (1991) The timed "up & go": A test of basic functional mobility for frail elderly persons. J Am Geriatr Soc 39: 142–148.
36. Guralnik JM, Seeman TE, Tinetti ME, Nevitt MC, Berkman LF (1994) Validation and use of performance measures of functioning in a non-disabled older population: MacArthur studies of successful aging. Aging (Milano) 6: 410–419.
37. Ory MG, Schechtman KB, Miller JP, Hadley EC, Fiatarone MA, et al. (1993) Frailty and injuries in later life: The FICSIT trials. J Am Geriatr Soc 41: 283–296.
38. Rossiter-Fornoff JE, Wolf SL, Wolfson LI, Buchner DM (1995) A cross-sectional validation study of the FICSIT common data base static balance measures. frailty and injuries: Cooperative studies of intervention techniques. J Gerontol A Biol Sci Med Sci 50: M291–7.

39. Frandin K, Sonn U, Svantesson U, Grimby G (1995) Functional balance tests in 76-year-olds in relation to performance, activities of daily living and platform tests. Scand J Rehabil Med 27: 231–241.
40. Jarnlo G, Nordell E (2003) Reliability of the modified figure of eight - a balance performance test for elderly women. Physiother Theory Pract 19: 35–43.
41. Cohen J (1988) Statistical power analysis for the behavioral sciences (2nd ed.). Hillsdale New Jersey: Lawrence Erlbaum.
42. Tak EC, van Uffelen JG, Paw MJ, van Mechelen W, Hopman-Rock M (2012) Adherence to exercise programs and determinants of maintenance in older adults with mild cognitive impairment. J Aging Phys Act 20: 32–46.
43. Rhodes RE, Martin AD, Taunton JE, Rhodes EC, Donnelly M, et al. (1999) Factors associated with exercise adherence among older adults. an individual perspective. Sports Med 28: 397–411.
44. Schutzer KA, Graves BS (2004) Barriers and motivations to exercise in older adults. Prev Med 39: 1056–1061.
45. Rogers SD, Jarrot SE (2008) Cognitive impairment and effects on upper body strength of adults with dementia. J Aging Phys Act 16: 61–68.
46. Yaguez L, Shaw KN, Morris R, Matthews D (2011) The effects on cognitive functions of a movement-based intervention in patients with Alzheimer's type dementia: A pilot study. Int J Geriatr Psychiatry 26: 173–181.
47. Erickson KI, Voss MW, Prakash RS, Basak C, Szabo A, et al. (2011) Exercise training increases size of hippocampus and improves memory. Proc Natl Acad Sci U S A 108: 3017–3022.
48. Broadbent NJ, Squire LR, Clark RE (2004) Spatial memory, recognition memory, and the hippocampus. Proc Natl Acad Sci U S A 101: 14515–14520.
49. Raji CA, Lopez OL, Kuller LH, Carmichael OT, Becker JT (2009) Age, Alzheimer disease, and brain structure. Neurology 73: 1899–1905.
50. Blankevoort CG, van Heuvelen MJ, Scherder EJ (2013) Reliability of six physical performance tests in older people with dementia. Phys Ther 93: 69–78.
51. Thomas VS, Hageman PA (2003) Can neuromuscular strength and function in people with dementia be rehabilitated using resistance-exercise training? Results from a preliminary intervention study. J Gerontol A Biol Sci Med Sci 58: 746–751.
52. Fiser WM, Hays NP, Rogers SC, Kajkenova O, Williams AE, et al. (2010) Energetics of walking in elderly people: Factors related to gait speed. J Gerontol A Biol Sci Med Sci 65: 1332–1337.
53. Brown AD, McMorris CA, Longman RS, Leigh R, Hill MD, et al. (2010) Effects of cardiorespiratory fitness and cerebral blood flow on cognitive outcomes in older women. Neurobiol Aging 31: 2047–2057.
54. Etnier JL, Nowell PM, Landers DM, Sibley BA (2006) A meta-regression to examine the relationship between aerobic fitness and cognitive performance. Brain Res Rev 52: 119–130.

5

The Effects of Exercise on Synaptic Stripping Require Androgen Receptor Signaling

Caiyue Liu[1], Patricia J. Ward[2], Arthur W. English[2]*

1 Department of Plastic and Reconstructive Surgery, Changzheng Hospital, Second Military Medical University, Shanghai, China, 2 Department of Cell Biology, Emory University School of Medicine, Atlanta, Georgia, United States of America

Abstract

Following peripheral nerve injury, synapses are withdrawn from axotomized motoneurons. Moderate daily treadmill exercise, which promotes axon regeneration of cut peripheral nerves, also influences this synaptic stripping. Different exercise protocols are required to promote axon regeneration in male and female animals, but the sex requirements for an effect of exercise on synaptic stripping are unknown. In male and female C57BL/6 mice, the sciatic nerve was transected in the mid-thigh. Mice were then exercised five days per week for two weeks, beginning on the third post-transection day. Half of the exercised mice were trained by walking slowly (10 M/min) on a level treadmill for one hour per day (continuous training). Other mice were interval trained; four short (two min) sprints at 20 M/min separated by five minute rest periods. A third group was untrained. The extent of synaptic contacts made by structures immunoreactive to vesicular glutamate transporter 1 and glutamic acid decarboxylase 67 onto axotomized motoneurons was studied in confocal images of retrogradely labeled cells. Both types of presumed synaptic contacts were reduced markedly in unexercised mice following nerve transection, relative to intact mice. No significant reduction was found in continuous trained males or interval trained females. Reductions in these contacts in interval trained males and continuous trained females were identical to that observed in untrained mice. Treatments with the anti-androgen, flutamide, blocked the effect of sex-appropriate exercise on synaptic contacts in both males and females. Moderate daily exercise has a potent effect on synaptic inputs to axotomized motoneurons. Successful effects of exercise have different requirements in males and females, but require androgen receptor signaling in both sexes.

Editor: Alan R. Harvey, The University of Western Australia, Australia

Funding: This work was funded by NIH Grants NS057190 and HD032571 from the USPHS. The funders had no role in study design, data collection and analysis, decision to publish, or preparation of the manuscript.

Competing Interests: The authors have declared that no competing interests exist.

* E-mail: medae@emory.edu

Introduction

Axons in injured peripheral nerves have the capacity for regeneration, but functional recovery after peripheral nerve injury is poor [1,2]. Following transection of a peripheral nerve, a withdrawal of nearly half of the synaptic inputs onto the somata and proximal dendrites of the axotomized motoneurons is found (reviewed in [3]). Both excitatory and inhibitory inputs are withdrawn. Over time, many of these inputs are restored, but those containing vesicular glutamate transporter 1 (VGLUT1), and arising mainly from primary afferent neurons [4,5] remain withdrawn [3]. The irreversible withdrawal of synapses arising from these stretch-sensitive afferents is thought to be an important factor contributing to the loss of the stretch reflex in self-reinnervated muscles [6] and may contribute significantly to the poor functional recovery found clinically after recovery from peripheral nerve injury.

We have shown that moderate exercise in the form of daily treadmill training after peripheral nerve injury produced a substantial enhancement of axon regeneration [7]. We also found a profound sex difference in the requirements for exercise to promote axon regeneration in cut peripheral nerves [8]. Continuous training (an hour of daily slow walking) enhances axon regeneration in male mice, but not in female mice while interval training (a series of interrupted short sprints) is effective in female and not male mice. Following sciatic nerve transection, we also showed that the expected loss of contacts onto motoneurons by synaptic structures was not observed in interval trained female mice [9]. One goal of this study was to examine whether a similar sex difference in the requirements for the effects of exercise on synaptic withdrawal was found.

Androgens are well known to play important roles in recovery following peripheral nerve injury. Treatments with testosterone induced acceleration of functional recovery from lower limb paralysis following sciatic nerve crush in the rat [10,11]. Such treatments are thought to promote elongation of regenerating axons, as they decrease time to recovery after both facial nerve crush injury [12,13] and recurrent laryngeal nerve injury [14]. In the central nervous system (CNS), testosterone propionate treatment significantly attenuated the amount of synaptic withdrawal and the decrease in average length of the remaining synapses in an adult male hamster model of facial nerve transection [15]. A similar reduction of synapse loss was found after testosterone treatment in male rats exposed to chronic stress [16]. All of these effects of androgens require signaling through the androgen receptor. Exposure to flutamide, a potent non-steroidal anti-androgen, completely abolished the testosterone-induced enhancing effects on facial nerve regeneration [17].

Castration eliminates the effect of continuous training on enhancement of axon regeneration in male mice. Treatments of unexercised female mice with an inhibitor of aromatase, an enzyme that converts androgens or their precursors into estradiol, enhanced axon regeneration significantly [8]. Treatments of both male and female mice with flutamide blocked the enhancing effect of exercise on axon regeneration in peripheral nerves completely [18]. Based on these results, we hypothesized that androgens also would be required for the effects of exercise in restoring withdrawn synapses from axotomized motoneurons in both males and females.

To test this hypothesis, we used flutamide to block signaling through the androgen receptor and then evaluated the extent of contacts made by excitatory (VGLUT1) and inhibitory (glutamic acid decarboxylase, GAD67) immunoreactive terminals on the somata and proximal-most dendrites of both intact and axotomized motoneurons in exercised and unexercised female and male mice. We report here that exercise has similar effects on synaptic contacts to axotomized motoneurons in male and female mice, that the requirements for exercise to produce these effects are different in male and female mice, and that this effect of exercise is blocked completely by flutamide treatments in both males and females.

Materials and Methods

Ethical Statements

All experimental procedures conformed to the Guidelines for the Use of Animals in Research of the Society for Neuroscience and were approved by the Institutional Animal Care and Use Committee of Emory University (Protocol #2002017).

Animals

Experiments were conducted on 64 wild type (C57BL/6J) adult (>2 months old) mice weighing 18 g–32 g. Mice were randomly divided into six groups for both females and males as follows: (1): sciatic nerve intact; (2): right sciatic nerve transection without treadmill exercise; (3): right sciatic nerve transection plus treadmill exercise; (4): sciatic nerve intact plus flutamide treated; (5): right sciatic nerve transection plus flutamide treated; (6): right sciatic nerve transection plus treadmill exercise and flutamide treated. For the exercised and untreated animals (group 3), two different exercise protocols, continuous and interval (see below) were applied to males and females. The numbers of mice studied were based on a power sample size estimate [19] using a power of 0.8, alpha = 0.05 and the inter-animal standard deviations (0.5–0.8%) and changes in synaptic coverage reported in the literature [3,20] as a reasonable expectation of anticipated differences between groups. For N = 4, as in most of the groups studied, a true difference in means of 1.66% was estimated. The numbers of mice in each group are shown in Table 1.

Surgical procedures

All mice were subjected to two survival surgeries while anesthetized with isoflurane. Three days prior to sciatic nerve transection surgery, the motoneuron cell bodies were labeled bilaterally by injecting the retrograde tracer, cholera toxin beta subunit (CTB) conjugated with Alexafluor 555 (Invitrogen) (1 µg/µl in distilled water), into the right and left gastrocnemius and tibialis anterior muscles respectively (1 µl each) of isoflurane anesthetized mice [21]. After the tracer had been taken up and transported to motoneuron cell bodies, the animals were again anesthetized and the right sciatic nerve was cut in the mid-thigh. The left sciatic nerve remained intact. To rule out any effect of trophic molecules in the distal segment of the cut nerve [22,23] or from the muscle targets of motoneurons, we chose not to repair the cut nerves.

To assess the requirement for androgen receptor signaling on the effect of exercise on synaptic withdrawal after injury, flutamide, an androgen receptor antagonist, was applied systemically in a sustained release dosage form [24]. Capsules composed of 15 mm long Silastic tubing (1.57 mm i.d.; 3.18 mm o.d.; Dow Corning Corp., Midland, MI) were packed with 5 mm of flutamide powder (2-methyl-*N*-[4-nitro-3-(trifluoromethyl)phenyl]-propanamide; Sigma Aldrich, Seelze, Germany) and flanked on each side by 5 mm wooden stint segments. The ends of the capsules were then covered externally by Medical Adhesive A (Dow Corning). Capsules were soaked in normal saline solution at 37°C for 24 hours prior to implantation to prime the flutamide powder for release. Using this approach, the flutamide was released gradually, by diffusing through the tubing, the rate of release being roughly proportional to the capsule surface area [25]. Two flutamide capsules (ca. 16.8 mg of flutamide) were implanted subcutaneously in each animal three days prior to the onset of treadmill training. We have shown previously that this approach is effective in blocking androgen receptors [18].

Treadmill training

Beginning on the third day post-nerve transection, mice were treadmill trained for five days a week for two weeks, using either an interval or continuous paradigm [7]. We have previously reported a sex difference in the effect of treadmill training in promoting axon regeneration from cut peripheral nerves [8]. To evaluate whether the same difference in the effect of treadmill training on synaptic withdrawal was found, different groups of male and female mice were trained either continuously for one hour at a slow treadmill speed of 10 m/min (continuous training) or as four repetitions at a faster speed of 20 m/min for two minutes with a five-minute rest periods interspersed (interval training).

Tissue harvesting and preparation

Two weeks after nerve transection, mice were euthanized with an overdose of pentobarbital (150 mg/kg) and perfused through the heart with saline, followed by periodate-lysate-paraformaldehyde fixative [26]. The L3-L5 segments of spinal cord were removed and stored overnight in 20% sucrose solution at 4°C for cryoprotection. Serial transverse sections were cut at 20 µm on a cryostat and mounted directly onto subbed slides. Standard immunohistological procedures were performed to detect the synaptic vesicle proteins glutamic acid decarboxylase protein 67 (GAD67) (Millipore #MAB5406, USA) or vesicular glutamate transporter 1 (VGLUT1) (Synaptic Systems GmbH #TO30326, Germany). Glutamic acid decarboxylase (GAD), the rate-limiting enzyme in the synthesis of gamma amino butyric acid (GABA), the main inhibitory neurotransmitter in the central nervous system, is found as two isoforms, known by their molecular weights as GAD67 and GAD65. The majority of GABAergic boutons in the ventral horn of the spinal cord are strongly immunoreactive for GAD67 and originate from interneurons in the spinal cord [27]. Synaptic terminals onto motoneurons that are immunoreactive for VGLUT1 have been shown to originate mainly from primary afferent neurons [4,5]. We assumed that because the proportions of inputs immunoreactive for VGLUT1 arising from other sources is quite small, any contributions that they might make to the findings presented below were not considered. Sections were incubated in primary antibodies, diluted in 1:2000 for rabbit anti-VGLUT1, 1:200 for mouse anti-GAD67, for 24 hours at room

Table 1. Summary of Animals Studied by Treatment Condition.

	Exercise				
Sciatic n. Transection	Continuous	Interval	Flutamide	Sex	N
No	No	No	No	M	8
No	No	No	No	F	8
No	No	No	Yes	M	4
No	No	No	Yes	F	4
Yes	No	No	No	M	4
Yes	No	No	No	F	4
Yes	Yes	No	No	M	4
Yes	No	Yes	No	M	4
Yes	Yes	No	No	F	4
Yes	No	Yes	No	F	4
Yes	No	No	Yes	M	4
Yes	No	No	Yes	F	4
Yes	Yes	No	Yes	M	4
Yes	No	Yes	Yes	F	4
TOTAL					64

temp. After washing in 0.1 M PBS for 3 times, the sections were incubated with secondary antibodies (Alexafluor 488, goat anti-rabbit IgG or goat anti-mouse IgG) for 2 hours at room temp to detect immunofluorescence. All the incubations and reactions were separated by 3×10 min washes in 0.1 M PBS.

Microscopy and imaging analysis

All analyses of tissue sections in this study were performed in such a way that the person collecting images and taking measurements from the collected images was unaware, while performing these tasks, of the experimental conditions applied to the tissues. Histological sections of L3–L5 spinal cord were viewed with a laser scanning confocal microscope (Zeiss LSM510). Labeled motoneurons were selected for study only if they contained labeling that filled the somata and extended into the proximal dendrites and their cell borders could be recognized. Twenty to 40 high magnification (40x) RGB images of individual labeled motoneuron cell bodies were obtained, at a confocal Z-dimension thickness of 1 μm, from each side of each spinal cord studied.

All measurements from these images were made using ImageJ software, using a method analogous to that of Wang et al, [28]. A region of interest (ROI) was created around the perimeter of each motoneuron studied (Fig. 1, top), and used to study contacts made by structures immunoreactive to synapse-specific proteins. Because we considered that the identification of this ROI was critical to all subsequent analyses, we tried to make the determination of cell outline as objective as possible. We used the thresholding function of ImageJ while viewing only the red channel of the RGB images; the one containing images of the retrograde label in the motoneuron, because the contrast between the border of the cells studied and the neuropil is so substantial. Cells in which such contrast in the red channel was not entirely clear were not studied. Once a ROI was established, a plot profile (Fig. 1, bottom) was then created to measure the fluorescence intensity, along the region of interest, in the green channel of the RGB image in which immunoreactivity for different synaptic vesicle proteins was displayed. Then, the mean fluorescence intensity (plus the 95% confidence interval) in this latter channel was measured *within* the ROI and used to establish the background fluorescence intensity threshold for that cell. We assumed that any fluorescence within the ROI on this channel was non-specific. We assumed that any fluorescence intensity values in the profile plot for each cell studied that were greater than this threshold represented contact of the motoneuron by structures immunoreactive for the synaptic vesicle protein studied. In Figure 1 (Top) the locations of three (among several) such locations along the ROI are shown. The percentage of the perimeter of the cell profile in which contact by such VGLUT1+ or GAD67+ immunoreactive structures was found was calculated and expressed as percent synaptic coverage. Mean values of percent synaptic coverage by VGLUT1+ and GAD67+ structures were determined for each mouse studied.

We assume that these structures immunoreactive for synapse-specific proteins that are in very close proximity to the outline of the labeled motoneurons represent synaptic contacts made on the motoneurons. This assumption has been supported by others. Immunoreactive structures identified using the same antibodies as used here have been shown to contain synaptic active zones and, after extensive high magnification reconstruction, to be in very close contact to the somata of intracellularly filled motoneurons [29]. However, without higher resolution images available through electron microscopy, we acknowledge that we cannot rule out that at least some of the contacts we have studied might be separated from the motoneuron soma by ultra-fine processes of glial cells.

Statistical analysis

All data are expressed as means ± SEM. Significance of differences in mean percent synaptic coverage between groups and between cohorts within groups was evaluated using analysis of variance (ANOVA) (Statistica, StatSoft, Tulsa, OK). When the omnibus test for significance was met ($p<0.05$), paired post-hoc testing (Tukey's honest significant differences (HSD)) was applied.

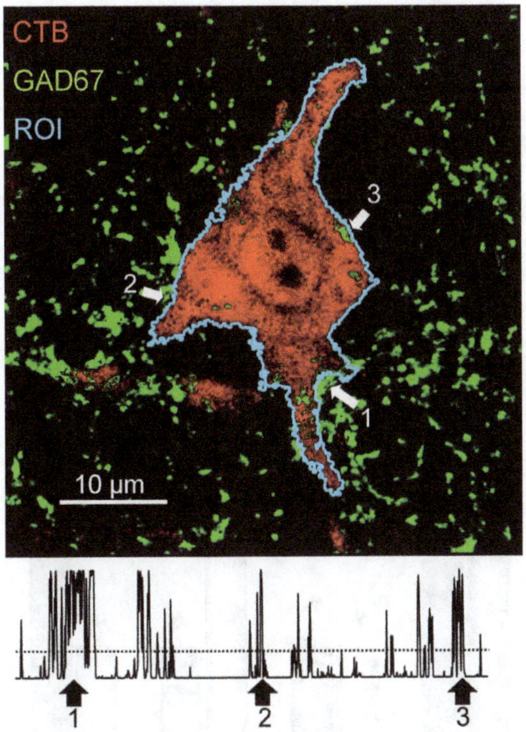

Figure 1. A single retrogradely labeled motoneuron (red) is shown to demonstrate the measurements made throughout this study. This image is from a histological section reacted with an antibody to glutamic acid decarboxylase 67 (GAD67, green). A region of interest (ROI) around the perimeter of this profile of the motoneuron visible in this confocal image was created (cyan line) and the green fluorescence intensity was measured beneath the ROI. In the resulting plot profile (bottom), a threshold intensity (horizontal dashed line) was established, based on the red intensity within the ROI. Intensity values above this threshold were assumed to represent contacts of the motoneuron soma and structures immunoreactive for synapse-specific antigens. Arrows are placed at three examples of the several clusters of contacts in the image and the corresponding position of the plot profile.

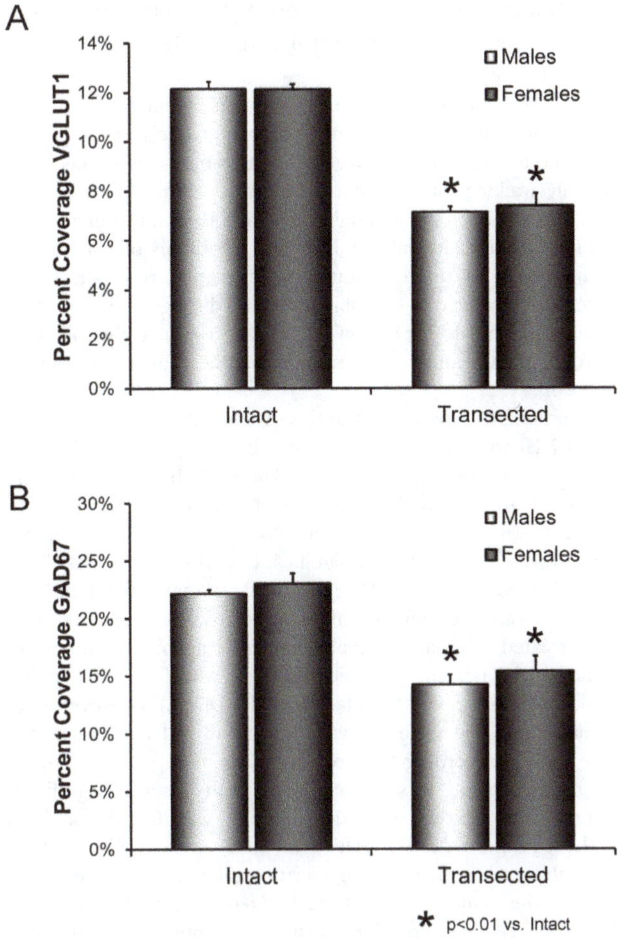

Figure 2. A. Mean (±SEM) percent coverage of motoneuron somata by structures immunoreactive for VGLUT1 in intact male and female mice and male and female mice two weeks following sciatic nerve transection. B. Mean (±SEM) percent coverage of motoneuron somata by structures immunoreactive for GAD67 in intact male and female mice and male and female mice two weeks following sciatic nerve transection.

Results

We studied the effect of moderate daily exercise on changes in synaptic contacts made by terminals of afferent neurons immunoreactive for the synapse-specific proteins VGLUT1 and GAD67 onto motoneurons following peripheral nerve injury. Structures containing VGLUT1 are assumed to be excitatory terminals arising from primary afferent neurons [4,5]. Most of them are permanently withdrawn following peripheral nerve transection [3]. Terminals containing GAD67 arise from inhibitory interneurons in the spinal cord. They are withdrawn transiently following peripheral nerve transection [3]. Although these are not all of the different types of synapses that make contact with spinal motoneurons, we studied them as different models of synapses that are withdrawn following nerve injury.

Sciatic nerve transection results in synaptic withdrawal in both male and female mice

The extent of contacts made by structures immunoreactive for the synapse-specific proteins VGLUT1 and GAD67 onto the somata and proximal-most dendrites of retrogradely labeled motoneurons were studied in intact male and female mice and in male and female mice two weeks after transection of the sciatic nerve. The resulting measurements are expressed as percent synaptic coverage. Following transection of the sciatic nerve, synapses are withdrawn from the somata of the axotomized motoneurons. The extent of this reduction in percent synaptic coverage is shown quantitatively, as means (± SEM) in Figure 2. The results of ANOVA for the effects of sex and transection were significant, both for VGLUT1 ($F_{3,20} = 38.77$, $p<0.01$) and GAD67 ($F_{3,20} = 32.92$, $p<0.01$). Statistically significant reductions in percent synaptic coverage by VGLUT1 immunoreactive (IR) structures following sciatic nerve transection were found in both males and females (HSD, $p<0.01$ for both) (Fig. 2A). No significant sex difference was found. Coverage by GAD67- IR structures was reduced after transection (HSD, $p<0.01$ in both males and females) (Fig 2B) and no significant sex difference was encountered.

Sex-appropriate exercise influences the withdrawal of synaptic terminals from motoneurons after peripheral nerve injury

We have shown that enhancing axon regeneration in cut peripheral nerves requires quite different exercise protocols in male and female mice [8]. Regeneration is enhanced in male mice by daily walking for one hour at a slow treadmill speed (10 M/min), termed continuous training. Females respond similarly only to more intense interval training (four repetitions of two minute sprints at 20 M/min, separated by 5 minute rest periods), a pattern of exercise that resembles that used during voluntary wheel running in mice [30]. Thus we wanted to evaluate the effects of exercising male and female mice using these different training protocols.

Mean (±SEM) percent synaptic coverage by VGLUT1-IR and GAD67-IR structures is shown for the different groups in Figure 3. Data for intact and untrained mice, described above and shown in Figure 2, are included to make comparisons easier. For both VGLUT1-IR and GAD67-IR contacts, the results of the omnibus test from the ANOVA were significant (VGLUT1, $F_{7,33} = 49.58$, $p<0.01$; GAD67, $F_{7,33} = 24.78$, $p<0.01$). In male mice that were exercised with a continuous training protocol and female mice that were treated with an interval training protocol, no significant reduction in percent synaptic coverage was found for either marker, relative to that for intact mice (HSD, n.s.). However, both in male mice that were interval trained and in female mice that were trained according to a continuous training protocol, a quite different outcome was observed. In both cases a significant reduction in percent synaptic coverage was found for both VGLUT1 and GAD67, relative to intact mice (HSD, $p<0.01$ for both), and neither was significantly different from untrained mice of the same sex (HSD, n.s.). Exercise has the same sex-dependent requirements for effects on synaptic inputs to spinal motoneurons as found for the effects of exercise in promoting axon regeneration in the periphery.

Treatments with flutamide block the effects of exercise on synaptic withdrawal after peripheral nerve injury in both male and female mice

We measured the effects of sex-appropriate exercise on the extent of contacts onto the somata of retrogradely labeled motoneurons two weeks after sciatic nerve transection in male and female mice that were treated with the non-steroidal anti-androgen, flutamide. As controls, we performed the same flutamide treatments in intact mice and unexercised mice whose sciatic nerves had been transected. The mean (± SEM) *percent change* in synaptic coverage by VGLUT1- IR and GAD67-IR structures in these animals, relative to that found in intact and untreated mice, is shown in Figure 4. Based on the results of ANOVA, significant differences were found for both VGLUT1 ($F_{9,30} = 27.21$, $p<0.01$) and GAD67 ($F_{9,30} = 21.89$, $p<0.01$). In intact male and female flutamide-treated mice, no significant reduction in synaptic coverage, was found relative to intact untreated mice, for either VGLUT1 or GAD67 (HSD, n.s, for both). The percent change in synaptic coverage is not significantly different from zero. Following sciatic nerve transection, a significant reduction (HSD, $p<0.01$) in contacts by VGLUT1+ synaptic structures or GAD67+ synaptic structures, relative to intact mice, was found in untreated mice and in flutamide-treated mice, whether or not the mice were exercised appropriately (continuous for males, interval for females). Flutamide treatment blocked the effect of exercise in both males and females.

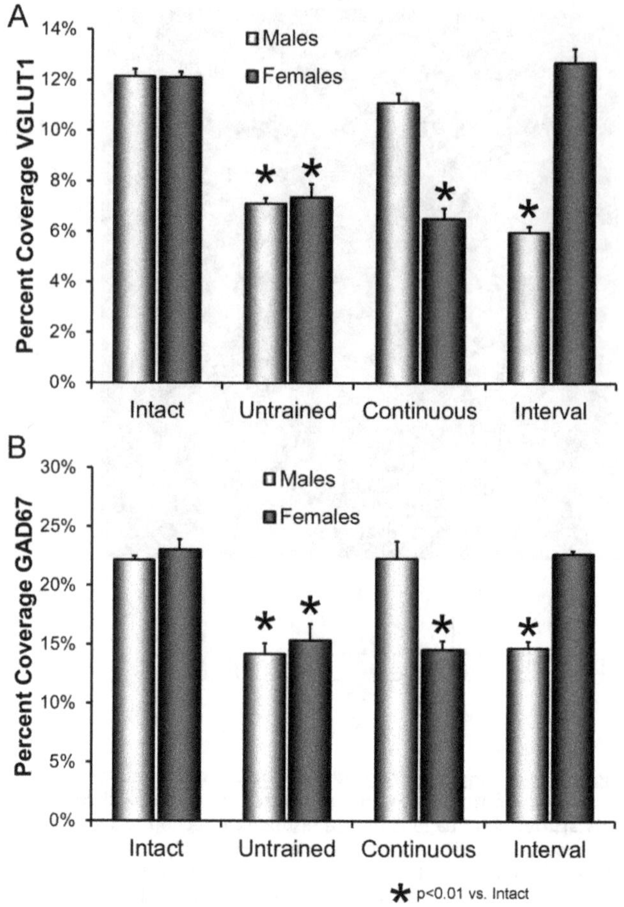

Figure 3. Effects of treadmill exercise on synaptic withdrawal from axotomized motoneurons. A. The mean (±SEM) proportions of motoneuron somata in contact with structures immunoreactive for VGLUT1 are shown for intact mice and in mice two weeks after sciatic nerve transection that were either untrained or exercised using a continuous or interval training protocol. Separate bars are shown for data from males and females. B. As in A, except for contacts immunoreactive to GAD67. In both panels, the data for intact and untrained animals are the same as shown in Figure 2.

In addition, in flutamide-treated male mice, the reduction in percent synaptic coverage by GAD67-IR structures following sciatic nerve transection was significantly (HSD, $p<0.01$) greater (i.e. larger negative percent change in synaptic coverage) than in flutamide-treated females, whether or not the animals were exercised. This proportional decrease in synaptic coverage in injured, flutamide treated males is also significantly greater than found in untreated and unexercised males. No significant sex differences were found in the contacts made by VGLUT1-IR structures.

Discussion

Despite the capacity for regeneration by axons in cut peripheral nerves, poor functional outcomes after peripheral nerve injury are common [1,2]. Slow and inefficient axon regeneration are often cited as a reason for this poor clinical outcome [31]. Changes in the circuitry of the central nervous system are considered far less often. When peripheral nerves are injured, a withdrawal of nearly half of the synaptic inputs from the somata and proximal dendrites of the axotomized motoneurons is found as well [3]. Many of these

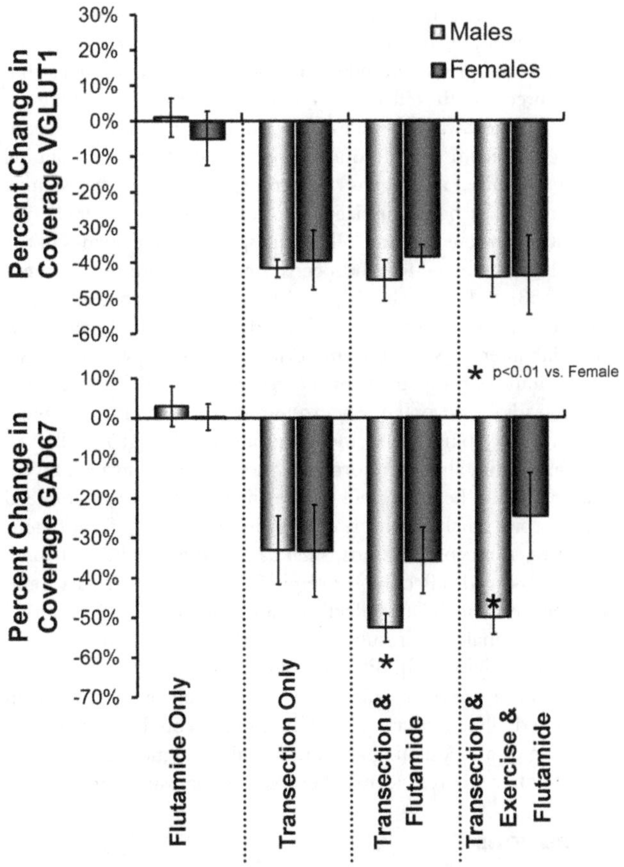

Figure 4. Mean (+SEM) percent change in synaptic coverage, relative to intact mice, in intact mice treated only with flutamide, mice two weeks following sciatic nerve transection that were untreated and unexercised, mice two weeks following sciatic nerve transection that were treated with flutamide only, and mice two weeks following sciatic nerve transection that were both exercised and treated with flutamide. Data are shown for males and females separately. Males were exercised with a continuous training protocol. Females were exercised with interval training. Data for VGLUT1 are in the top panel. Data for GAD67 are in the bottom panel.

synaptic inputs are restored over time, but those arising from primary afferent neurons and expressing VGLUT1 in their terminals are not [3].

We [7], and others (e.g.[32]) have shown that moderate exercise in the form of daily treadmill training, if applied shortly after peripheral nerve injury, will promote axon regeneration. Male and female mice respond to different exercise protocols in very different ways [8]. Slow continuous walking for one hour per day is effective in enhancing axon regeneration only in males, while interval training, a series of short sprints separated by rest periods, is effective in females but not in males. Pharmacologic blocking of the androgen receptor eliminated the effectiveness of exercise in promoting axon regeneration in both sexes [18].

We studied immunoreactive contacts made by two different types of synapses onto motoneurons. Excitatory (VGLUT1+) contacts made mainly by primary afferent neurons and inhibitory (GAD67+) contacts arising from within the central nervous system were studied as models of synapses that are withdrawn from the somata of motoneurons following peripheral nerve transection. One important finding of this study is that if both male and female mice are appropriately exercised following peripheral nerve injury, the anticipated reduction in synaptic coverage on the axotomized motoneurons by both of these types of synapses is not found. The requirements for exercise to produce this effect differ dramatically between males and females. In interval trained males and continuous trained females, the coverage of the somata of axotomized motoneurons by structures immunoreactive for VGLUT1 and GAD67 is reduced to the same extent as in unexercised mice. In contrast, no significant reduction in percent synaptic coverage was found in continuous trained males and interval trained females. Thus the very same sex-dependent difference in the requirement for the effect of exercise to promote axon regeneration in the periphery also is a requirement for the effect of exercise on the withdrawal of these synaptic inputs onto axotomized motoneurons.

The cellular mechanism by which synapses are withdrawn from motoneurons following peripheral nerve transection is not well known. Initial observations [33,34,35,36] were used to suggest that processes of reactive astrocytes and/or microglia, which proliferate and surround axotomized motoneurons, might play an important role, but based on the results of more recent studies [37], a shift in attention to axotomy induced changes in the motoneurons has occurred. In particular, the decline in production of cell adhesion molecules by axotomized motoneurons has been shown to precede the actual withdrawal of synapses [20,36,38,39], suggesting that, in intact animals, these molecules are part of an active, retrograde signaling mechanism that promotes synapse retention. In addition, immune system-related molecules, such as the major histocompatibility complex (MHC) class I molecules [39] and members of the complement family [40] have been associated with synaptic withdrawal. In mice null for MHC class I (MHC class Ia), greater synaptic withdrawal was found after peripheral nerve transection than in wild type controls, while markedly less synaptic stripping was found after nerve injury in mice lacking complement protein C3. These findings were used to suggest that immune molecules might regulate both the shedding and retention of synapses [41]. Of considerable interest is the finding that MHC class Ia has been found in both motoneurons and microglia following peripheral nerve transection [41]. Whether our finding that no synaptic withdrawal is observed following peripheral nerve transection if mice are appropriately exercised is the result of decreased expression of complement protein C3 expression or even increased expression of MHC class I is not known at this time, but seems a fruitful avenue for future studies.

A second, and not mutually exclusive mechanism has emerged from the results of manipulation of the retrograde signaling molecule nitric oxide (NO) [42]. Peripheral axotomy results in the production of NO in somatic motoneurons, and associated reactive astrocytes, cells that do not normally produce it. Diffused NO acts directly on presynaptic terminals, activating a signaling pathway eventually leading to microtubule disruption and withdrawal. The NO also acts indirectly on the synaptic inputs. Within the axotomized motoneurons it blocks the secretion of brain derived neurotrophic factor (BDNF) at synaptic sites [43], which eventually leads to effects on cytoskeletal actin in the afferent neural terminals and mechanical destabilization of synaptic inputs. Blocking either NO production with neuronal nitric oxide synthase (nNOS) inhibitors [44] or the effects of direct downstream signaling components [45] blocks nerve crush-induced synaptic stripping. Inducing nNOS activity in motoneurons using viral constructs induces synaptic stripping in intact animals [46].

The effects of our exercise protocols on NO production following peripheral axotomy are not known, but we have shown that the effect of exercise, *both* in enhancing axon regeneration in the periphery [47] and in restoring withdrawn synaptic inputs from motoneurons [48] following peripheral nerve injury, is lost in motoneuron-specific BDNF knockout mice. Based on these observations, we suggest that one role of neuronal BDNF is to promote stabilization of synaptic inputs onto motoneurons. Consistent with this postulate, the expression of BDNF is increased transiently in motoneurons following transection of their axons and then decreases rapidly at about the time that synapses begin to be withdrawn [49]. Application of BDNF to the proximal segment of a cut eye muscle nerve restored synaptic inputs stripped from the axotomized oculomotor motoneurons [50]. It is known that treadmill training results in an increased expression of neurotrophins, especially BDNF, in spinal motoneurons [51], with a time course that is appropriate to impact synaptic withdrawal following peripheral nerve injury.

The nature of the stimulus provided by exercise that triggers this increase in BDNF expression is not clear. One means of regulation of the BDNF gene in neurons is activity [52] and the anticipated increase in activity of motoneurons found with exercise has been suggested as an explanation for the increased BDNF expression [53]. However, the finding presented above and elsewhere [18] that signaling through the androgen receptor is required for the effects of exercise on axon regeneration and synaptic stripping are consistent with a role of androgens as a stimulus to motoneuron expression of BDNF. Indeed, androgen treatments of castrated animals produced a substantial and prolonged increase in BDNF expression in facial motoneurons [54] and attenuated the amount of synaptic withdrawal after facial nerve transection [15], as well as accelerated peripheral motor axon regeneration [55]. Precisely how this combination of activity and androgens might contribute to increased expression and secretion of motoneuron BDNF is not known, nor is the relationship between BDNF signaling through the trkB receptor and the expression of cell adhesion molecules implicated in synaptic stabilization. We do not know why different exercise protocols are required in males and females. We interpret our finding that interval training in male mice and continuous treadmill training in female mice promotes *neither* enhanced axon regeneration *nor* an effect on synaptic inputs to motoneurons to mean that these forms of exercise in the different sexes do not result in sufficient combinations of increased activity and androgen availability to influence these processes. However, until we can examine the effects of a greater diversity of exercise protocols on the expression of signaling molecules such as BDNF and trkB in identified populations of motoneurons, this interpretation must remain entirely speculative.

The source of the androgens may differ in males and females. The testes are the primary source of androgens in males, and because castrating male mice blocked the effects of exercise on axon regeneration in cut nerves [8], gonadal androgens must be considered the prime candidate for the source of androgens that are required for the effects of continuous treadmill training on synaptic withdrawal in males. In females, since no significant increase in serum testosterone was noted after interval training [48], the required androgens must come from some other source. Sex steroids can be synthesized in a number of tissues, including the central nervous system [56]. In the spinal cord, enzymes in the biosynthetic pathway for androgens are found both in motoneurons [57,58] and glial cells [59,60,61,62], indicating that these cells could be a source of localized production of androgens. Of particular interest is the enzyme cytochrome C P450 aromatase, which catalyzes the conversion of testosterone and its precursors into estradiol, a potent neurosteroid. If exercise inhibited aromatase in spinal cord motoneurons and/or glial cells, an increased availability of androgens and decreased availability of estradiol might be expected in the vicinity of the axotomized motoneurons. Such localized change in expression of androgens and estrogen receptor ligands, such as estradiol, could contribute to the observed effects of exercise on synaptic inputs onto motoneurons. Such an effect is not unprecedented. Interval training in female rats resulted in a marked depression of muscle aromatase activity [63]. Pharmacologic inhibition of aromatase resulted in a marked enhancement of axon regeneration in unexercised female mice [8]. This notion could be tested by measuring or manipulating aromatase activity in motoneurons and glial cells after different forms of exercise in male and female mice.

Conclusions

Moderate daily treadmill training following peripheral nerve transection can affect the extent of contacts made by excitatory and inhibitory synaptic inputs with the somata motoneurons. The requirements for effective exercise treatments are different for males and females. Cellular signaling through the androgen receptor is required for the effects of exercise in both sexes. Exercise could be a potent and low-technology treatment to help maintain circuitry in the central nervous system, but the requirements for its effect will require careful consideration.

Author Contributions

Conceived and designed the experiments: CL PJW AE. Performed the experiments: CL PJW AE. Analyzed the data: CL PJW AE. Contributed reagents/materials/analysis tools: CL PJW AE. Wrote the paper: CL PJW AE.

References

1. Frostick SP, Yin Q, Kemp GJ (1998) Schwann cells, neurotrophic factors, and peripheral nerve regeneration. Microsurgery 18: 397–405.
2. Scholz T, Krichevsky A, Sumarto A, Jaffurs D, Wirth GA, et al. (2009) Peripheral nerve injuries: an international survey of current treatments and future perspectives. J Reconstr Microsurg 25: 339–344.
3. Alvarez FJ, Titus-Mitchell HE, Bullinger KL, Kraszpulski M, Nardelli P, et al. (2011) Permanent central synaptic disconnection of proprioceptors after nerve injury and regeneration. I. Loss of VGLUT1/IA synapses on motoneurons. J Neurophysiol 106: 2450–2470.
4. Todd AJ, Hughes DI, Polgar E, Nagy GG, Mackie M, et al. (2003) The expression of vesicular glutamate transporters VGLUT1 and VGLUT2 in neurochemically defined axonal populations in the rat spinal cord with emphasis on the dorsal horn. Eur J Neurosci 17: 13–27.
5. Alvarez FJ, Villalba RM, Zerda R, Schneider SP (2004) Vesicular glutamate transporters in the spinal cord, with special reference to sensory primary afferent synapses. J Comp Neurol 472: 257–280.
6. Cope TC, Clark BD (1993) Motor-unit recruitment in self-reinnervated muscle. J Neurophysiol 70: 1787–1796.
7. Sabatier MJ, Redmon N, Schwartz G, English AW (2008) Treadmill training promotes axon regeneration in injured peripheral nerves. Exp Neurol 211: 489–493.
8. Wood K, Wilhelm JC, Sabatier MJ, English AW (2012) Sex differences in the effects of treadmill training on axon regeneration in cut peripheral nerves. Dev Neurobiol 72: 688–698.
9. English AW, Wilhelm JC, Sabatier MJ (2011) Enhancing recovery from peripheral nerve injury using treadmill training. Ann Anat 193: 354–361.
10. Brown T, Khan T, Jones K (1999) Androgen induced acceleration of functional recovery after rat sciatic nerve injury. Restor Neurol Neurosci 15: 289–295.
11. Brown T, Storer P, Oblinger M, Jones K (2001) Androgenic enhancement of betaII-tubulin mRNA in spinal motoneurons following sciatic nerve injury. Restor Neurol Neurosci 18: 191–198.
12. Jones K, Storer P, Drengler S, Oblinger M (1999) Differential regulation of cytoskeletal gene expression in hamster facial motoneurons: effects of axotomy and testosterone treatment. J Neurosci Res 57: 817–823.

13. Fargo KN, Alexander TD, Tanzer L, Poletti A, Jones KJ (2008) Androgen regulates neuritin mRNA levels in an in vivo model of steroid-enhanced peripheral nerve regeneration. J Neurotrauma 25: 561–566.
14. Brown TJ, Pittman AL, Monaco GN, Benscoter BJ, Mantravadi AV, et al. (2013) Androgen treatment and recovery of function following recurrent laryngeal nerve injury in the rat. Restor Neurol Neurosci 31: 169–176.
15. Jones KJ, Durica TE, Jacob SK (1997) Gonadal steroid preservation of central synaptic input to hamster facial motoneurons following peripheral axotomy. J Neurocytol 26: 257–266.
16. Matsumoto A (2005) Testosterone prevents synaptic loss in the perineal motoneuron pool in the spinal cord in male rats exposed to chronic stress. Stress 8: 133–140.
17. Kujawa KA, Tanzer L, Jones KJ (1995) Inhibition of the accelerative effects of testosterone on hamster facial nerve regeneration by the antiandrogen flutamide. Exp Neurol 133: 138–143.
18. Thompson NJ, Sengelaub DR, English AW (2014) Enhancement of peripheral nerve regeneration due to treadmill training and electrical stimulation is dependent on androgen receptor signaling. Dev Neurobiol 74: 531–540.
19. Lenth RV (2006) Java Applets for Power and Sample Size [Computer software]. Retrieved 01/10/2013, from http://www.stat.uiowa.edu/~rlenth/Power.
20. Oliveira A, Thams S, Lidman O, Piehl F, Hökfelt T, et al. (2008) A role for MHC class I molecules in synaptic plasticity and regeneration of neurons after axotomy. Proc Natl Acad Sci U S A 101: 17843–17848.
21. Al-Majed AA, Neumann CM, Brushart TM, Gordon T (2000) Brief electrical stimulation promotes the speed and accuracy of motor axonal regeneration. J Neurosci 20: 2602–2608.
22. Funakoshi H, Frisen J, Barbany G, Timmusk T, Zachrisson O, et al. (1993) Differential expression of mRNAs for neurotrophins and their receptors after axotomy of the sciatic nerve. J Cell Biol 123: 455–465.
23. Griesbeck O, Parsadanian AS, Sendtner M, Thoenen H (1995) Expression of neurotrophins in skeletal muscle: quantitative comparison and significance for motoneuron survival and maintenance of function. J Neurosci Res 42: 21–33.
24. Jones SL, Ismail N, King L, Pfaus JG (2012) The effects of chronic administration of testosterone propionate with or without estradiol on the sexual behavior and plasma steroid levels of aged female rats. Endocrinology 153: 5928–5939.
25. Smith E, Damassa D, Davidson J (1977) Hormone Administration: Peripheral and Intracranial Implants. In: RD M, editor. Methods Psychobiol. New York: Academic Press. pp. 259–279.
26. McLean IW, Nakane PK (1974) Periodate-lysate-paraformaldehyde fixative. A new fixative for immunoelectron microscopy. J Histochem Cytochem 22: 1077–1083.
27. Hughes DI, Mackie M, Nagy GG, Riddell JS, Maxwell DJ, et al. (2005) P boutons in lamina IX of the rodent spinal cord express high levels of glutamic acid decarboxylase-65 and originate from cells in deep medial dorsal horn. Proc Natl Acad Sci U S A 102: 9038–9043.
28. Wang Y, Pillai S, Wolpaw JR, Chen XY (2006) Motor learning changes GABAergic terminals on spinal motoneurons in normal rats. Eur J Neurosci 23: 141–150.
29. Rotterman TM, Nardelli P, Cope TC, Alvarez FJ (2014) Normal distribution of VGLUT1 synapses on spinal motoneuron dendrites and their reorganization after nerve injury. J Neurosci 34: 3475–3492.
30. De Bono JP, Adlam D, Paterson DJ, Channon KM (2006) Novel quantitative phenotypes of exercise training in mouse models. Am J Physiol Regul Integr Comp Physiol 290: R926–934.
31. Hoke A (2013) Experimental neurology and state of preclinical research. Exp Neurol 239: A1.
32. Udina E, Puigdemasa A, Navarro X (2011) Passive and active exercise improve regeneration and muscle reinnervation after peripheral nerve injury in the rat. Muscle & Nerve 43: 500–509.
33. Blinzinger K, Kreutzberg G (1968) Displacement of synaptic terminals from regenerating motoneurons by microglial cells. Z Zellforsch 85: 145–157.
34. Graeber M, Kreutzberg G (1986) Astrocytes increase in glial fibrillary acidic protein during retrograde changes of facial motor neurons. J Neurocytol 15: 363–373.
35. Aldskogius H, Liu L, Svensson M (1999) Glial responses to synaptic damage and plasticity. J Neurosci Res 58: 33–41.
36. Zelano J, Berg A, Thams S, Hailer NP, Cullheim S (2009) SynCAM1 expression correlates with restoration of central synapses on spinal motoneurons after two different models of peripheral nerve injury. J Comp Neurol 517: 670–682.
37. Perry VH, O'Connor V (2010) The role of microglia in synaptic stripping and synaptic degeneration: a revised perspective. ASN Neuro 2: e00047.
38. Berg A, Zelano J, Thams S, Cullheim S (2013) The extent of synaptic stripping of motoneurons after axotomy is not correlated to activation of surrounding glia or downregulation of postsynaptic adhesion molecules. PLoS ONE 8: e59647.
39. Oliveira AL, Thams S, Lidman O, Piehl F, Hokfelt T, et al. (2004) A role for MHC class I molecules in synaptic plasticity and regeneration of neurons after axotomy. Proc Natl Acad Sci U S A 101: 17843–17848.
40. Berg A, Zelano J, Stephan A, Thams S, Barres BA, et al. (2012) Reduced removal of synaptic terminals from axotomized spinal motoneurons in the absence of complement C3. Exp Neurol 237: 8–17.
41. Thams S, Oliveira A, Cullheim S (2008) MHC class I expression and synaptic plasticity after nerve lesion. Brain Res Rev 57: 265–269.
42. Moreno-Lopez B, Sunico CR, Gonzalez-Forero D (2011) NO orchestrates the loss of synaptic boutons from adult "sick" motoneurons: modeling a molecular mechanism. Mol Neurobiol 43: 41–66.
43. Jovanovic JN, Benfenati F, Siow YL, Sihra TS, Sanghera JS, et al. (1996) Neurotrophins stimulate phosphorylation of synapsin I by MAP kinase and regulate synapsin I-actin interactions. Proc Natl Acad Sci U S A 93: 3679–3683.
44. Sunico CR, Portillo F, Gonzalez-Forero D, Moreno-Lopez B (2005) Nitric-oxide-directed synaptic remodeling in the adult mammal CNS. J Neurosci 25: 1448–1458.
45. Sunico CR, Gonzalez-Forero D, Dominguez G, Garcia-Verdugo JM, Moreno-Lopez B (2010) Nitric oxide induces pathological synapse loss by a protein kinase G-, Rho kinase-dependent mechanism preceded by myosin light chain phosphorylation. J Neurosci 30: 973–984.
46. Montero F, Sunico CR, Liu B, Paton JF, Kasparov S, et al. (2010) Transgenic neuronal nitric oxide synthase expression induces axotomy-like changes in adult motoneurons. J Physiol 588: 3425–3443.
47. Wilhelm JC, Cucoranu D, Xu M, Chmielewski S, Holmes T, et al. (2012) Cooperative roles of BDNF expression in neurons and Schwann cells are modulated by exercise to facilitate nerve regeneration. J Neurosci 32: 5002–5009.
48. Krakowiak JR, Wilhelm JC, English AW (2010) Effect of treadmill training on synaptic stripping of axotomized mouse motoneurons. Abstr Soc Neurosci.
49. Gordon T (2009) The role of neurotrophic factors in nerve regeneration. Neurosurg Focus 26: E3.
50. Davis-Lopez de Carrizosa M, Morado-Diaz C, Tena J, Benitez-Temino B, Pecero M, et al. (2009) Complimentary actions of BDNF and Neurotrophin-3 on the firing patterns and synaptic composition of motoneurons. J Neurosci 29: 575–587.
51. Gomez-Pinilla F, Ying Z, Opazo P, Roy RR, Edgerton VR (2001) Differential regulation by exercise of BDNF and NT-3 in rat spinal cord and skeletal muscle. Eur J Neurosci 13: 1078–1084.
52. Hong EJ, McCord AE, Greenberg ME (2008) A biological function for the neuronal activity-dependent component of Bdnf transcription in the development of cortical inhibition. Neuron 60: 610–624.
53. Gomez-Pinilla F, Ying Z, Roy RR, Molteni R, Edgerton VR (2002) Voluntary exercise induces a BDNF-mediated mechanism that promotes neuroplasticity. J Neurophysiol 88: 2187–2195.
54. Sharma N, Marzo SJ, Jones KJ, Foecking EM (2010) Electrical stimulation and testosterone differentially enhance expression of regeneration-associated genes. Exp Neurol 223: 183–191.
55. Kujawa KA, Kinderman NB, Jones KJ (1989) Testosterone-induced acceleration of recovery from facial paralysis following crush axotomy of the facial nerve in male hamsters. Exp Neurol 105: 80–85.
56. Turgeon JL, Carr MC, Maki PM, Mendelsohn ME, Wise PM (2006) Complex actions of sex steroids in adipose tissue, the cardiovascular system, and brain: Insights from basic science and clinical studies. Endocrine Rev 27: 575–605.
57. Coirini H, Gouezou M, Liere P, Delespierre B, Pianos A, et al. (2002) 3 Beta-hydroxysteroid dehydrogenase expression in rat spinal cord. Neuroscience 113: 883–891.
58. Rakotoarivelo C, Petite D, Lambard S, Fabre C, Rouleau C, et al. (2004) Receptors to steroid hormones and aromatase are expressed by cultured motoneurons but not by glial cells derived from rat embryo spinal cord. Neuroendocrinology 80: 284–297.
59. Gottfried-Blackmore A, Sierra A, Jellinck PH, McEwen BS, Bulloch K (2008) Brain microglia express steroid-converting enzymes in the mouse. J Steroid Biochem 109: 96–107.
60. Garcia-Ovejero D, Azcoitia I, Doncarlos LL, Melcangi RC, Garcia-Segura LM (2005) Glia-neuron crosstalk in the neuroprotective mechanisms of sex steroid hormones. Brain Res Brain Res Rev 48: 273–286.
61. Saldanha CJ, Duncan KA, Walters BJ (2009) Neuroprotective actions of brain aromatase. Front Neuroendocrin 30: 106–118.
62. Patte-Mensah C, Penning TM, Mensah-Nyagan AG (2004) Anatomical and cellular localization of neuroactive 5 alpha/3 alpha-reduced steroid-synthesizing enzymes in the spinal cord. J Comp Neurol 477: 286–299.
63. Aizawa K, Iemitsu M, Otsuki T, Maeda S, Miyauchi T, et al. (2008) Sex differences in steroidogenesis in skeletal muscle following a single bout of exercise in rats. J Appl Physiol 104: 67–74.

6

Differences in Supraspinal and Spinal Excitability during Various Force Outputs of the Biceps Brachii in Chronic- and Non-Resistance Trained Individuals

Gregory E. P. Pearcey[1], Kevin E. Power[1], Duane C. Button[1,2]*

1 School of Human Kinetics and Recreation, Memorial University of Newfoundland, St. John's, NL, Canada, 2 Faculty of Medicine, Memorial University of Newfoundland, St. John's, NL, Canada

Abstract

Motor evoked potentials (MEP) and cervicomedullary evoked potentials (CMEP) may help determine the corticospinal adaptations underlying chronic resistance training-induced increases in voluntary force production. The purpose of the study was to determine the effect of chronic resistance training on corticospinal excitability (CE) of the biceps brachii during elbow flexion contractions at various intensities and the CNS site (i.e. supraspinal or spinal) predominantly responsible for any training-induced differences in CE. Fifteen male subjects were divided into two groups: 1) chronic resistance-trained (RT), (n = 8) and 2) non-RT, (n = 7). Each group performed four sets of ~5 s elbow flexion contractions of the dominant arm at 10 target forces (from 10%–100% MVC). During each contraction, subjects received 1) transcranial magnetic stimulation, 2) transmastoid electrical stimulation and 3) brachial plexus electrical stimulation, to determine MEP, CMEP and compound muscle action potential (M_{max}) amplitudes, respectively, of the biceps brachii. All MEP and CMEP amplitudes were normalized to M_{max}. MEP amplitudes were similar in both groups up to 50% MVC, however, beyond 50% MVC, MEP amplitudes were lower in the chronic RT group ($p<0.05$). CMEP amplitudes recorded from 10–100% MVC were similar for both groups. The ratio of MEP amplitude/absolute force and CMEP amplitude/absolute force were reduced ($p<0.012$) at all contraction intensities from 10–100% MVC in the chronic-RT compared to the non-RT group. In conclusion, chronic resistance training alters supraspinal and spinal excitability. However, adaptations in the spinal cord (i.e. motoneurone) seem to have a greater influence on the altered CE.

Editor: Alessio Avenanti, University of Bologna, Italy

Funding: This research was supported by a Memorial University start-up grant 208604. The funders had no role in study design, data collection and analysis, decision to publish, or preparation of the manuscript.

Competing Interests: The authors have declared that no competing interests exist.

* E-mail: dbutton@mun.ca

Introduction

Neural adaptations account for a large portion of the initial increase in strength following the commencement of a resistance training program [1–4]. Various stimulation techniques including transcranial magnetic stimulation (TMS), transcranial electrical stimulation (TES), transmastoid electrical stimulation (TMES), and peripheral nerve stimulation (i.e. Hoffman-reflex, H-reflex) have been used to examine these 'neural adaptations,' each with their own strengths and weaknesses. The results have determined that acute resistance training alters the corticospinal excitability (CE) of both upper- and lower-limb muscles, including the first dorsal interosseous (FDI) [5,6], extensor carpi radialis brevis [7], biceps brachii [8,9], rectus femoris [10,11] tibialis anterior [12] and soleus [13,14].

While it is generally accepted that initial strength gains during a resistance-training program are due to changes in CE, it is presently unclear whether the predominant site of those adaptations is of supraspinal or spinal origin, though it is likely that both are involved. TMS is often employed to assess CE. The difficulty of using TMS alone for determining changes in CE is that the amplitude of a TMS-induced motor evoked potential (MEP) could be affected anywhere along the corticospinal pathway (i.e. from corticoneurones in the brain to the motoneurones in the spinal cord). A relatively new and underutilized technique, TMES, which stimulates the corticospinal tracts independent of the corticoneurones, can be used in combination with TMS to identify whether or not changes in CE are of supraspinal or spinal origin [7,15,16].

As a resistance training program progresses, further increases in strength are thought to be mainly influenced by morphological adaptations of the muscle [1]. However, very few studies have examined how long-term (*chronic*) resistance training affects the manner in which the central nervous system (CNS) generates force output. Studies that have examined the tibialis anterior [17] and biceps brachii [18] suggest that there are no differences in CE between chronic resistance trained (RT) (2–3 years) and non-RT individuals. This apparent lack of change in CE may be due to the muscle group and protocols utilized. The tibialis anterior examined by Tallent and colleagues (2013) is not a muscle that individuals typically resistance train on a consistent basis and the TMS protocol used by del Olmo et al. (2006) could not differentiate between supraspinal and spinal excitability or whether the lack of change in MEP amplitude occurred due to a masking effect from increased spinal excitability. Research on a muscle that is extensively activated during resistance training (i.e.

biceps brachii) combined with a stimulation protocol capable of examining both supraspinal and spinal excitability may allow further insight into the neural adaptations induced via *chronic* resistance training.

In *non-training* studies examining elbow flexion and index finger abduction, MEPs and CMEPs recorded from the biceps brachii and brachioradialis increase similarly from weak to strong contractions and then decrease at the strongest contractions (i.e. ~>60 MVC); a response that also occurred in MEPs recorded from the FDI [19]. Oya at al. [20] also found similar MEP and CMEP responses in the soleus and medial gastrocnemius muscles. Both studies concluded that the decrease in both MEPs and CMEPs at the higher contraction intensities were due to spinal mechanisms. Only two studies have used stimulation techniques (TMS, TES and TMES) that produce MEPs and CMEPs to determine the effects of *acute* resistance training on CE and involved the FDI and extensor carpi radialis brevis [5,7]. Both studies concluded that enhanced force production following training was probably due to changes at the spinal, not supraspinal level. It remains to be determined how CE in chronic-RT individuals is modulated over various contraction intensities, and if so, whether or not the modulation is predominantly supraspinal or spinal in origin.

The objectives of the current study were to determine: 1) the effect of *chronic* resistance training on CE of the biceps brachii during isometric elbow flexion contractions at various intensities and 2) if there was an effect, the CNS site (i.e. supraspinal or spinal) predominantly responsible for any training-induced differences in CE. Based on the work by Carroll et al. (2002, 2009), we hypothesized that CE would be altered in the biceps brachii of chronic-RT individuals during strong, but not weak elbow flexion contractions, mainly due to increased spinal excitability. A portion of the current results have been reported elsewhere in abstract form [21].

Methods

Subjects

Fifteen apparently healthy subjects without history of neurological disease volunteered for the study. The 15 subjects were divided into two groups consisting of 8 chronic-RT males (height 180.6±5.23 cm, weight 87.9±9.28 kg, age 24.3±2.03 years) and 7 non-RT males (height 177.7±4.34 cm, weight 72.4±10.93 kg, age 22.5±5.99 years) who were all recreationally active. All subjects were recruited from the university population. Subjects in the chronic-RT group had at least 2 continuous years (≥3 times per week) of resistance training experience. The chronic-RT group routinely performed a variety of compound, multi-jointed exercises. The subjects in the non-RT group had no resistance training experience. Subjects were verbally informed of all procedures, and if willing to participate, read and signed a written consent form. Subjects also completed a magnetic stimulation safety checklist designed [22] to screen for potential contraindications with magnetic stimulation procedures prior to the start of the experiment. The Memorial University of Newfoundland Interdisciplinary Committee on Ethics in Human Research approved the study (20131456-HK) and was accordance with the Tri-Council guideline in Canada with full disclosure of potential risks to subjects.

Experimental Set-up

To determine elbow flexor forces, subjects sat in an upright position with hips, knees and elbows flexed at 90° with forearms supinated and resting on padded support. The upper torso rested against the backrest and was secured with straps around the waist and shoulders. The wrist of the dominant arm was inserted into a padded strap, attached by a high-tension wire that measured force using a load cell (Omegadyne Inc., Sunbury, OHIO). The subjects performed 5s isometric contractions with all forces detected by the load cell, which were amplified (x1000) (CED 1902) and displayed on a computer screen (Fig. 1A).

Electromyography (EMG) activity was recorded from the biceps brachii and triceps brachii muscles. Surface EMG recording electrodes (MediTrace Pellet Ag/AgCl electrodes, disc shape, and 10 mm in diameter, Graphic Controls Ltd., Buffalo, NY) were placed 2 cm apart (centre to centre) over the mid-muscle belly of the subject's biceps brachii. Since the EMG activity recorded from the three triceps brachii muscles is similar during an MVC of the elbow extensors (elbow flexed at 90 and shoulder at 0 of flexion, as performed in the current study) [23], we chose to record EMG from the lateral head of the triceps brachii muscle. A ground electrode was secured on the lateral epicondyle. Thorough skin preparation for all electrodes included shaving hair off the desired area, removal of dead epithelial cells from the desired area with abrasive sand paper, followed by cleansing with an isopropyl alcohol swab. An inter-electrode impedance of <5 kOhms was obtained prior to recording to ensure an adequate signal-to-noise ratio. EMG signals were amplified (x1000) (CED 1902) and filtered using a 3-pole Butterworth with cutoff frequencies of 10–1000 Hz. All signals were analog-digitally converted at a sampling rate of 5 KHz using a CED 1401 interface and Signal 4 software (Cambridge Electronic Design Ltd., Cambridge, UK). Recordings were made from the dominant arm for each subject.

Stimulation conditions. Motor responses from the biceps brachii were elicited via 1) transcranial magnetic stimulation (TMS), 2) transmastoid electrical stimulation (TMES)and 3) brachial plexus electrical stimulation at Erb's point. Stimulation intensities used for TMS and TMES were adjusted so that the evoked potentials produced by each, MEPs and CMEPs, respectively, were of similar amplitude and normalized to a maximal M-wave (M_{max}). Stimulation intensities were set during an isometric elbow flexion contraction equal to 5% of MVC.

Transcranial magnetic stimulation. MEP responses of the biceps brachii were elicited via TMS over the motor cortex in the left or right hemisphere (depending on arm dominance) using a circular coil (13.5 cm outside diameter) attached to a Magstim 200 stimulator (Magstim, Dyfed, UK). The coil was placed horizontally over the vertex with the direction of the current flow to specifically activate the left or right cortex. To locate vertex, the distances from nasion to inion and from tragus to tragus were measured and marks were placed halfway directly on the scalp for both measurements. The intersection of both halfway marks was defined as vertex. During a 5% MVC, the stimulation intensity was altered to elicit a MEP amplitude that was between 10–20% of the M_{max} amplitude. The stimulator setting used to evoke MEP amplitude that was between 10–20% of the M_{max} amplitude was then used for the remainder of the experiment.

Transmastoid electrical stimulation. CMEP responses of the biceps brachii were elicited via electrical stimulation of the corticospinal tracts. Stimulation was elicited via adhesive Ag-AgCl electrodes fixed to the skin over the mastoid processes and current was passed between them (100 μs duration, 150–350 mA; model DS7AH, Digitimer Ltd, Welwyn Garden City, UK) with the anode on the right side and cathode on the left side and vice versa depending on hand dominance [24,25]. During a 5% MVC, the stimulation intensity was altered to elicit a CMEP amplitude that matched the MEP amplitude. This stimulation intensity was used to evoke a CMEP for all contractions in the experimental protocol.

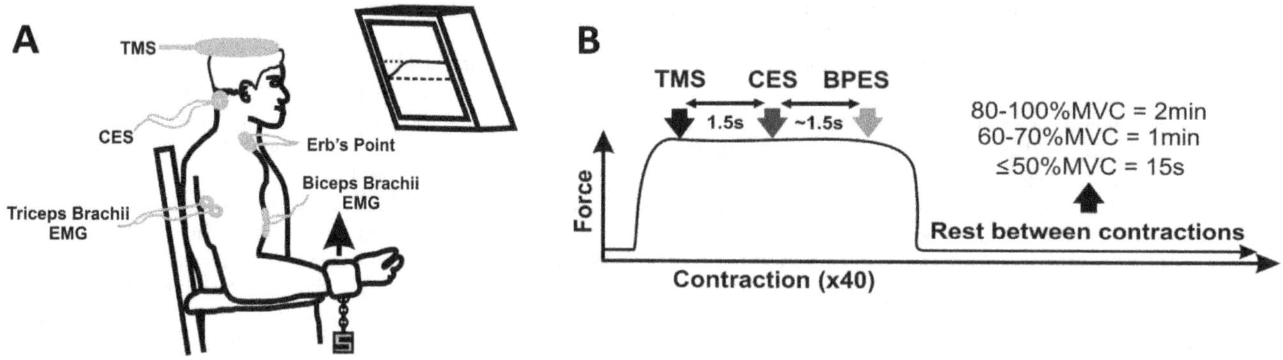

Figure 1. Experimental protocol. (A) Schematic diagram of experimental apparatus for elbow flexion from 10–100% MVC and stimulation location. (B) Subjects performed 4 sets of 10–100% MVCs (40 contractions in total) and received transcranial magnetic stimulation of the motor cortex (black arrow, at 1.0 s), cervicomedullary electrical stimulation of the corticospinal tracts (white arrow, at 2.5 s) and brachial plexus electrical stimulation (Erb's point) of the peripheral nerve (grey arrow, at 4.0 s) following the onset of muscle contraction. The amount of rest given between contractions depended on the contraction intensity (i.e. percentage of MVC) and is illustrated at the far right.

TMS and TMES evoked potentials were matched in amplitude to ensure that a similar portion of the motoneurone pool was activated by each stimulus. For example, if MEPs were much larger than CMEPs, then one could suggest that the TMS response would be examining the excitability of different portions of the motoneurone pool. Close attention to the latency of the CMEPs was monitored because evoked stimulation to the mastoid processes can activate axons near the ventral roots which subsequently decreases the onset latency of the CMEP by ~2 ms [26]. Since the onset latency of the CMEP was ~3 ms shorter than the MEP and ~3 ms longer than M_{max} we are confident that we were stimulating the descending corticospinal tracts.

Brachial plexus electrical stimulation (referred to as Erb's point hereafter). To evoke a M_{max} in the biceps brachii, electrical stimulation was applied to Erb's point during a 5% MVC. Erb's point was electrically stimulated via adhesive Ag-AgCl electrodes (diameter 10 mm) fixed to the skin over the supraclavicular fossa (cathode) and the acromion process (anode). Current pulses (200 μs duration, 100–300 mA) were delivered via a constant current stimulator (DS7AH, Digitimer Ltd, Welwyn Garden City, UK). The electrical current was gradually increased until the M-wave of the biceps brachii no longer increased. The stimulator setting used to evoke M_{max} at 5% MVC was then used for the remainder of the experiment.

Experimental Protocol

In a single experimental session (~1.5 hrs) subjects first performed isometric contractions for 5 s at various low intensities to get accustomed to producing varying contraction intensities. The subjects then performed an elbow flexor MVC. Following the MVC, subjects were exposed to the 3 stimulation conditions 1) Erb's point, 2) TMS and 3) TMES while performing a 5% MVC to determine the stimulation intensities to be used throughout the experiment. Once the stimulation intensities were determined, the subjects began the experimental protocol. Subjects performed a voluntary isometric contraction protocol which included four sets of 5 s contractions of the dominant elbow flexors at 10 target forces (i.e. 10, 20, 30, 40, 50, 60, 70, 80, 90, and 100% of MVC) for a total of 40 contractions (i.e. 4 contractions at each target force). For each contraction the target force and the force exerted by the subjects were displayed on a computer screen. Subjects were required to match the target force with their exerted force and maintain it for 5 s. Once the subject reached the prescribed force they received triggered TMS and TMES and a manual Erb's point stimulation at 1, 2.5, and ~4 s, respectively (Fig. 1B). Due to the experimental set-up it was only possible to trigger 2 stimulators. At the start of each set, subjects performed a MVC and all subsequent target forces within that set were made relative to it. The order of contractions was randomized for intensities between 10 and 90% of MVC. Fig. 2 shows the raw data from one subject for all of the contraction intensities in one set (Fig. 2A) and the MEP, CMEP and M-wave responses of the bicep brachii recorded during those contractions (Fig. 2B).

Due to the high volume of contractions and potential fatigue effects, the protocol was pseudo-randomized as stated above. To further minimize the effect of fatigue there was 2 minutes of rest following 90 and 100% MVCs, 1 minute of rest following 60, 70, and 80% MVCs and at least 10 s of rest following all forces at and below 50% MVC (Fig. 1B) [20]. Immediately following the completion of the contraction protocol subjects performed one additional MVC to determine whether or not the contraction protocol induced fatigue. Verbal encouragement to match the target forces was given during all contraction intensities.

Data Analysis and Statistics

Average biceps brachii force and average biceps and triceps brachii root mean square EMG (rmsEMG) were measured at each contraction intensity for a 1 s period between TMS and TMES stimulations. Biceps brachii rmsEMG activity recorded from 10–90% MVC was normalized to 100% MVC. Muscle co-activation was quantified by computing the ratio between the triceps/biceps rmsEMG at all contraction intensities from 10–100% MVC.

Biceps brachii MEP, CMEP and M-wave peak-to-peak amplitudes (see Table 1 for all average chronic-RT and non-RT amplitude values at each contraction intensity) and onset latencies were measured from all %MVC forces in each set. In total there were four MEP, CMEP and M-wave responses recorded and averaged for each contraction intensity. MEPs and CMEPs peak-to-peak amplitudes were normalized to M-wave amplitude at each %MVC force. Since amplitudes and areas give similar results we chose to measure the amplitudes for comparison [27,28]. Onset latencies for MEP, CMEP and M-waves were defined as the time between the stimulus artifact and the onset of the evoked potential. Force and rmsEMG averages were also measured for 50 ms prior

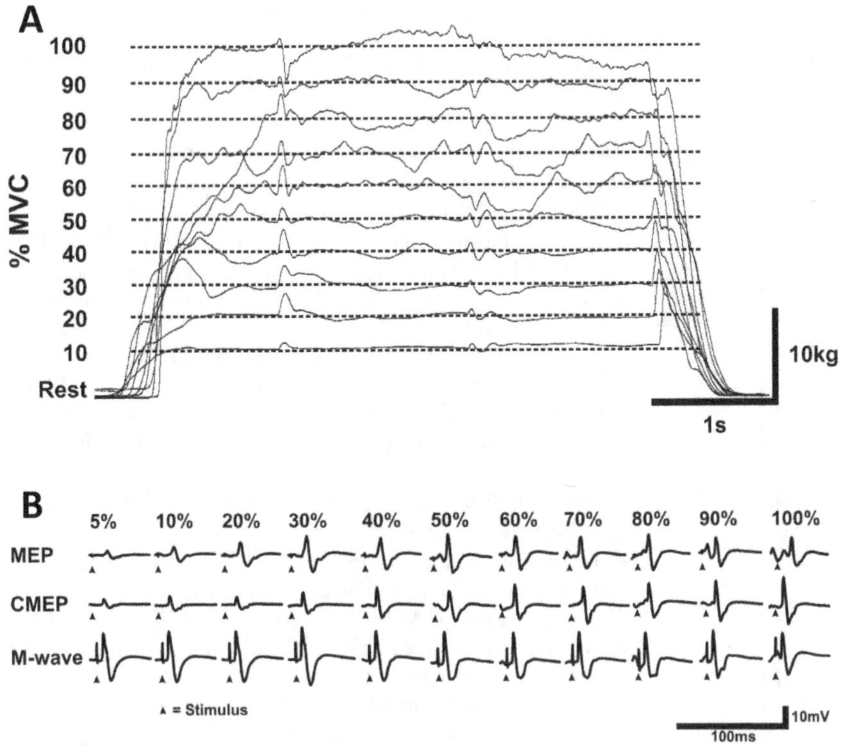

Figure 2. Force output from 10–100% MVC and corticospinal responses of the biceps brachii recorded from a chronic-RT subject. (A) Individual raw data traces from a single subject of one set of contractions from 10–100% MVC with the three stimuli: transcranial magnetic (MEP), cervicomedullary (CMEP) and brachial plexus stimulation (M-wave). Additional force is superimposed on the actual force following each stimulus at each contraction intensity. (B) Individual raw data traces from the same subject showing EMG responses (MEP-top, CMEP-middle, and M-wave-bottom) of the biceps brachii following each stimulus. Arrows indicate the time of stimulation.

to each stimulus for each %MVC force. All data were analyzed off-line using Signal 4.0 software (CED, UK).

A series of one-way ANOVAs were performed to compare between group (chronic-RT vs. non-RT) differences from 10–100% MVC for all dependent variables using SPSS (SPSS 18.0 for Macintosh, IBM Corporation, Armonk, New York, USA). *F*-ratios were considered statistically significant at $p<0.05$. Descriptive statistics in text, table and figures include means ± SE.

Results

Control measures at 5% MVC

In the present study, stimulation intensities were determined to induce MEP and CMEP amplitudes in the biceps brachii that were ~10–20% of M_{max} during an active contraction performed at 5% MVC. The average TMS, TMES and Erb's point stimulation intensities required to evoke MEP, CMEP and M_{max} at 5% MVC in chronic-RT and non-RT groups were 60.0±5.69% MSO and 58.8±2.35% MSO, 202.0±16.61 mA and 204.5±22.48 mA and 164.7±10.43 mA and 162.5±24.00 mA, respectively. There were no between group differences in stimulation intensities to induce, MEP (p = 0.86), CMEP (p = 0.80) and M_{max} (p = 0.95) responses in the biceps brachii.

At 5% MVC the average MEP, CMEP and M_{max}, amplitudes in chronic-RT and non-RT groups were, 1.9±0.48 mV and 2.3±0.22 mV, 1.9±0.43 mV and 2.3±0.17 mV and 12.0±2.80 mV and 12.4±0.97 mV, respectively. Average MEP and CMEP amplitudes in chronic-RT and non-RT groups were ~15.8% and 18.5% of M_{max}, respectively. There were no between group differences for, MEP (p = 0.84), CMEP (p = 0.92) or M_{max} (p = 0.60) amplitudes.

There were no between group differences (p-values ranging from p = 0.31 to p = 0.71) for M_{max} amplitudes from 10–100% MVC.

The latencies from the stimulus artefact to the onset of the MEP, CMEP and M_{max} responses of the biceps brachii were measured to ensure that the supraspinal, spinal and nerve sites, respectively were being activated. MEP, CMEP and M_{max} average latencies for all subjects were 11.8±0.11 ms, 8.6±0.08 ms and 5.02±0.03 ms, respectively.

During all contraction intensities, elbow flexion force and biceps brachii rmsEMG were measured for 50 ms prior to each stimulation type (TMS, TMES, and Erb's point) to ensure that force and background neuromuscular activity was similar within each contraction intensity and across the same relative contraction intensities (i.e. 40% MVC in sets 1–4, see Fig. 3) throughout the contraction protocol. The average pre-stimulus (pre-TMS, -TMES and -Erb's point) elbow flexion force and biceps brachii rmsEMG values were similar (p≥0.14) within and across all contraction intensities (10–100% MVC) throughout the contraction protocol.

Elbow flexor force output in chronic-RT and non-RT

Overall, the chronic-RT group was able to exert 30% more force at 100% MVC than the non-RT group (p<0.001). Also, the absolute elbow flexor forces at all percentages of MVC were greater (p<0.001) in the chronic-RT group. The slopes of the absolute-relative target force relationship were 0.425 (r = 0.99) and

Table 1. Raw data for amplitudes of motor evoked potentials (MEPs), cervicomedullary motor evoked potentials (CMEPs) and muscle compound action potentials (M-wave) in chronic-RT and non-RT groups from 10–100% maximum voluntary contraction (MVC).

Chronic-RT										
%MVC	**10**	**20**	**30**	**40**	**50**	**60**	**70**	**80**	**90**	**100**
MEP Amplitude (mV)	3.3±0.75	5.0±1.02	7.3±1.31	8.0±1.57	8.1±1.71	7.6±1.57	7.4±1.45	7.0±1.41	6.8±1.44	6.4±1.49
CMEP Amplitude (mV)	2.3±0.82	2.9±0.85	4.3±1.18	5.1±1.48	5.2±1.65	5.3±1.47	5.3±1.64	5.6±1.94	6.2±1.84	6.0±1.74
M-wave Amplitude (mV)	13.0±2.51	12.3±2.33	12.3±2.50	12.1±2.32	11.5±2.20	11.5±2.12	11.7±2.21	10.9±2.26	11.5±2.47	10.6±2.39
Non-RT										
Target %MVC	**10**	**20**	**30**	**40**	**50**	**60**	**70**	**80**	**90**	**100**
MEP Amplitude (mV)	3.0±0.54	4.9±0.83	7.3±0.71	7.3±0.75	7.1±0.77	7.6±0.89	7.2±0.83	6.9±0.83	6.7±0.83	6.4±0.73
CMEP Amplitude (mV)	2.7±0.44	3.0±0.53	4.2±1.09	4.9±1.11	5.4±1.27	5.9±1.51	5.2±1.13	5.5±1.24	5.1±1.09	4.9±1.06
M-wave Amplitude (mV)	11.2±0.77	10.9±0.87	10.9±1.04	10.0±1.29	10.2±1.33	10.5±1.48	10.0±1.49	9.7±1.37	9.9±1.42	9.3±1.34

Data are reported as means±SE.

0.293 (r = 0.99) in the chronic-RT and non-RT groups, respectively (Fig. 4). As the relative target force increased the difference in absolute forces between the chronic-RT and non-RT groups became greater.

Corticospinal excitability of the biceps brachii during relative force outputs

MEP amplitudes recorded from the chronic-RT group were 14.5% ($p = 0.043$), 15% ($p = 0.022$), 14.3% ($p = 0.041$), 16% ($p = 0.023$) less than the non-RT group at 60, 70, 90 and 100% MVC, respectively (Fig. 5A). CMEP amplitudes recorded from chronic-RT and non-RT groups were not different ($p \leq 0.22$) (Fig. 5B). There were no between group differences for MEP (chronic-RT, 11.9±0.10 ms and non-RT, 11.6±0.18 ms, $p = 0.15$) and CMEP (chronic-RT, 8.7±0.09 ms and non-RT, 8.6±0.15 ms, $p = 0.69$) onset latencies at any contraction intensity.

Corticospinal excitability of the biceps brachii during absolute force outputs

To determine the change in MEP and CMEP responses between chronic-RT and non-RT over each absolute force output we made a ratio of MEP and CMEP to the average absolute background force 50 ms prior to each stimulus at every target force, as per Carroll et al. [5].

The ratio of MEP amplitude to absolute force recorded from the chronic-RT group was reduced, by 26 to 42% (p-values ranging from $p < 0.007$ to $p < 0.001$) from 10–100% MVC compared to the non-RT group (Fig. 6A). The ratio of CMEP amplitude to absolute force recorded from the chronic-RT group was also reduced by 25 to 46% (p-values ranging from $p = 0.011$ to $p < 0.001$) from 10–100% MVC compared to the non-RT group (Fig. 6B).

Biceps brachii activation and triceps:biceps coactivation ratios in chronic-RT and non-RT

To determine the change in normalized biceps brachii rmsEMG between chronic-RT and non-RT over each absolute force output we made a ratio of normalized rmsEMG to the average absolute force recorded during each target force. The normalized rmsEMG to the absolute force ratio was higher (ranging from 12 to 45%) in the non-RT than chronic-RT from 10–100% MVC, but only statistically higher by 29.7% ($p = 0.016$), 31.9% ($p = 0.041$), 42.9% ($p = 0.019$ and 44.9% ($p = 0.001$) at 10, 80, 90, and 100% MVC, respectively. There was also a trend ($p = 0.077$ and 0.071) for it to be higher at 20 and 70% MVC, respectively (Fig. 7A).

The chronic-RT group had lower tricep:bicep coactivation ratios by 45–60% (p-values ranging from $p = 0.003$ to 0.032) over all contraction intensities compared to the non-RT group (Fig. 7B).

Discussion

This is the first study to clearly demonstrate that the increased force generating capabilities of *chronically* resistance-trained individuals is accompanied by corticospinal plasticity. MEP amplitudes were smaller in the chronic-RT group during elbow flexion forces >50% of MVC when compared to the non-RT group, whereas CMEP amplitudes did not differ between groups. This implies that at higher contraction intensities supraspinal excitability is lower in chronic-RT individuals while spinal excitability is similar when compared to non-RT individuals. However, even with the techniques utilized it is difficult to determine whether the observed difference in MEP amplitude following *chronic*

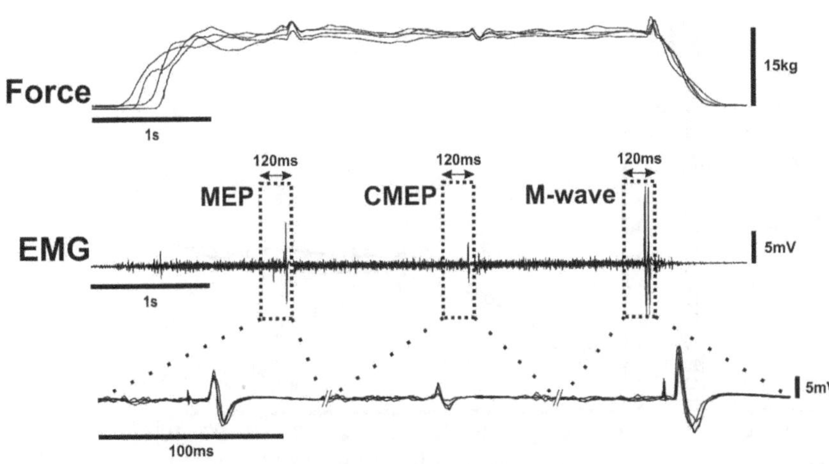

Figure 3. Consistency of the elbow flexion force tracing procedure and corticospinal responses in the biceps brachii within and between set contractions recorded from a chronic-RT subject. Individual raw data traces from a single subject for 4 contractions across four sets at 40% MVC (TOP). Individual raw data traces from the same subject showing EMG responses of the biceps brachii following each stimulus (transcranial magnetic - MEP, cervicomedullary - CMEP and brachial plexus - M-wave) for the 4 contractions (middle). Boxes were placed around the MEP, CMEP and M-wave and magnified for clearer illustration (bottom). MEPs, CMEPs and M-waves were very consistent within each contraction and between set contractions at the same relative intensity. Since TMS and TMES were triggered at 1 s and 2.5 s, respectively during all contraction intensities, MEPs and CMEPs overlap in the EMG Waveform. Erb's point stimulation was manually triggered at ~4 s thus M-waves do not overlap. In the magnified M-wave waveform, M-waves from each contraction were matched by the onset of stimulus artifact.

resistance training is due to predominantly supraspinal or spinal mechanisms.

In the present study it is possible that: 1) supraspinal excitability was similar between groups and spinal excitability was higher in chronic-RT individuals. MEP amplitudes were decreased in chronic-RT individuals because increased firing frequencies of the spinal motoneurones masked, to a small extent, the actual size of the MEP; 2) supraspinal and spinal excitability were increased in chronic-RT individuals. MEP amplitudes were decreased in chronic-RT individuals because increased firing frequencies of the spinal motoneurones masked, to a great extent, the actual size of

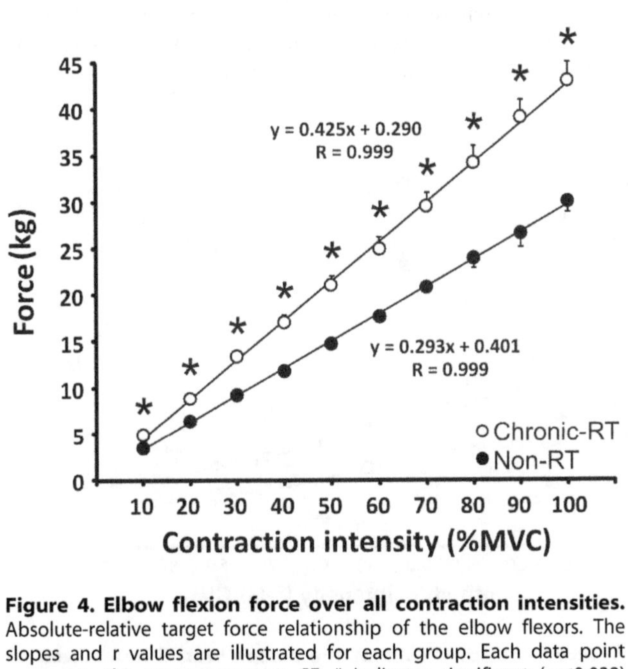

Figure 4. Elbow flexion force over all contraction intensities. Absolute-relative target force relationship of the elbow flexors. The slopes and r values are illustrated for each group. Each data point represents the group means ± SE. * Indicates significant ($p \leq 0.032$) differences between groups.

the MEP; 3) supraspinal excitability was decreased in chronic-RT individuals but compensated for by an increased firing frequency of the spinal motoneurones which may allow for a reduction in supraspinal drive required for force production and movement. We suggest that the commonality between all three scenarios is an increase in the firing rate of the spinal motoneurone following *chronic* resistance training.

It is currently unknown whether the neural adaptations that accompany the commencement of a resistance training program are the same, maintained and (or) amplified in chronic-RT individuals. There are two research studies on *acute* resistance training, however, that support the current findings. Carroll et al. [5] found that a 4-week resistance training program of the index finger abductor increases strength while significantly reducing FDI MEP amplitudes (via TMS and TES) when assessed between 40–60% of MVC. Since all motor units in the FDI muscle are recruited by ~50% of MVC [29,30] they did not assess MEPs and CMEPs beyond 60% MVC. Carroll et al. (2009) subsequently showed a reduction in MEP and CMEP amplitudes at 50 and 75% of MVC in the extensor carpi radialis brevis following 4 weeks of resistance training. They suggest that the decreased MEP amplitude following training is most likely due to training-induced spinal motoneurone adaptations such as an increased firing rate and (or) modulation of motoneurone intrinsic properties. Changes in the after-hyperpolarization potential (AHP) (i.e. increased duration and (or) amplitude) [31] and (or) higher firing rates of the spinal motoneurone [32,33] may reduce the probability of a motoneurone to respond to TMS, subsequently "masking" the MEP response.

Though it is not known if or how the AHP changes in response to resistance training, increased motoneurone AHP amplitude has been shown in animals following endurance training [34] and motor training [35]. In humans, increased strength following dynamic resistance training has been shown to be due to production of extra doublets and increased maximal firing rate [36,37] leading to temporal summation of force output. Other biophysical properties of the spinal motoneurone can also be modified. Following an endurance training program, spinal

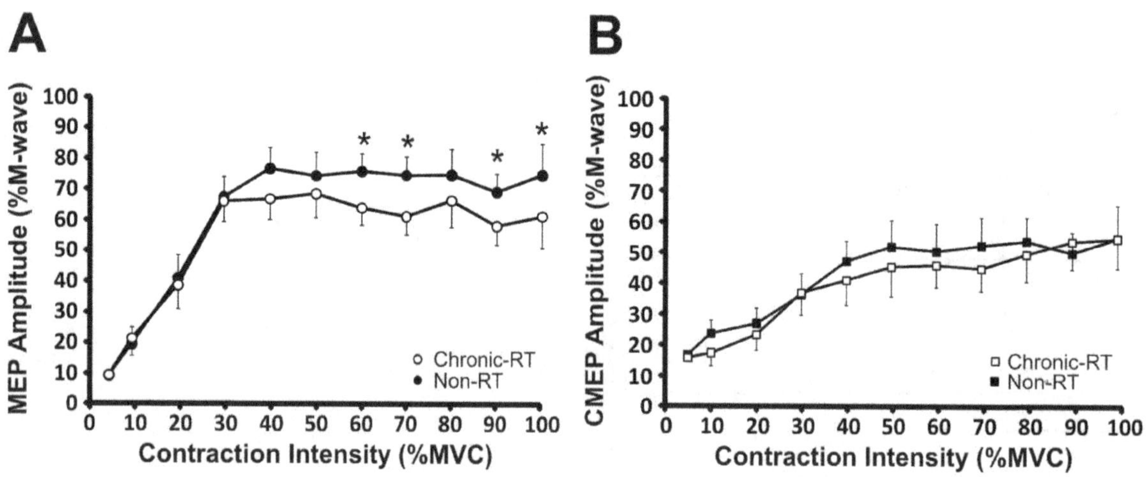

Figure 5. Between group differences in corticospinal responses (A) MEPs and (B) CMEPs of the biceps brachii during elbow flexion from 10-100% MVC. Each data point represents group means ± SE. * Indicates a significant ($p \leq 0.043$) difference between groups.

motoneurones are characterized by a lowering of the voltage threshold for action potential initiation and a decreased spike rise time [38], both of which could increase firing frequency. Activation of persistent inward currents can also significantly increase and maintain motoneurone firing frequency in the presence of lower synaptic input in animals and humans [39–42]. Although it is not known how training affects persistent inward currents, it is thought that these currents will be strongly modulated via the monoaminergic system during exercise [43,44], subsequently increasing motoneurone firing frequency and enhancing force. If motoneurone properties were altered following resistance training in a similar manner to the aforementioned putative mechanisms, the result would be a reduction in the effort required for their activation and enhanced firing frequencies. This could lead to increased force output. On the other hand, recent research has shown activity-dependent depressions of F-waves (following various duration maximal effort contractions in the tibialis anterior and abductor digiti minimi illustrating decreases in the excitability of the initial segment and (or) soma-dendritic membrane [45,46] which would lead to a decreased force output. However, the effect of *chronic* resistance training on these depressions and the excitability of the initial segment or soma-dendritic membrane is unknown.

Based on our findings and those of others, there is a strong argument for an increased motoneurone firing frequency at high force output (i.e. >50% MVC) in the chronic-RT group. It is inconclusive if *chronic* resistance training affected spinal motoneurone recruitment patterns during force production because CMEPs did not differ between groups. CMEP amplitudes were recorded from the biceps brachii from 10–100% MVC as a measure of motoneurone recruitment because motor units of the biceps brachii are recruited up to and beyond 90% MVC [29]. The effects of resistance training on motor unit recruitment are relatively unknown. In animals, endurance training decreased the current required to discharge a motoneurone to fire but not the amount of current required to elicit an action potential 50% of the time (i.e. rheobase current) [47]. In humans, Van Cutsem et al. [36] showed a shift in tibialis anterior motor unit recruitment

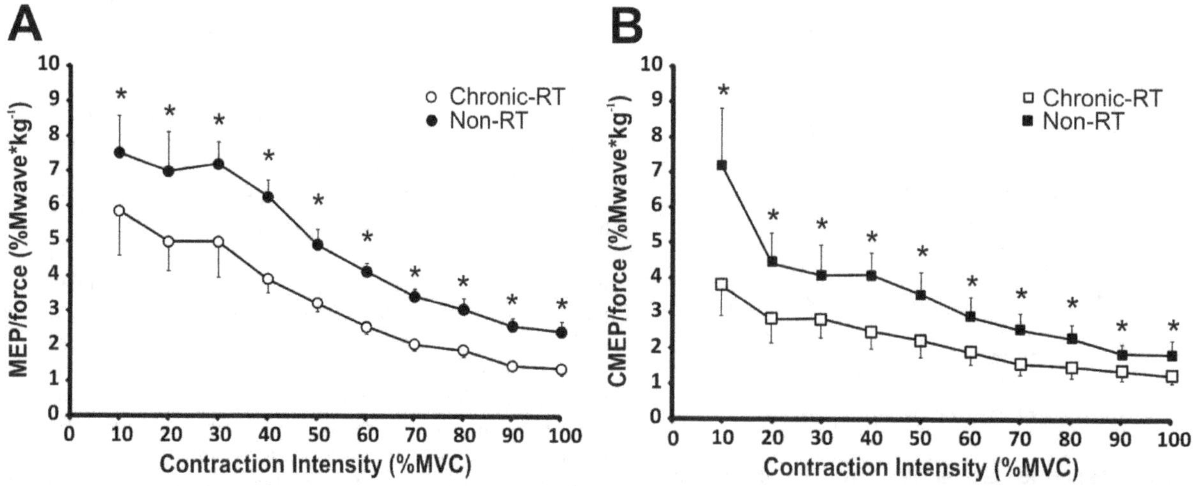

Figure 6. Between group differences in corticospinal responses (A) MEPs and (B) CMEPs of the biceps brachii normalized to absolute elbow flexion forces from 10–100% MVC. Each data point represents group means ± SE. * Indicates a significant ($p \leq 0.015$) difference between groups.

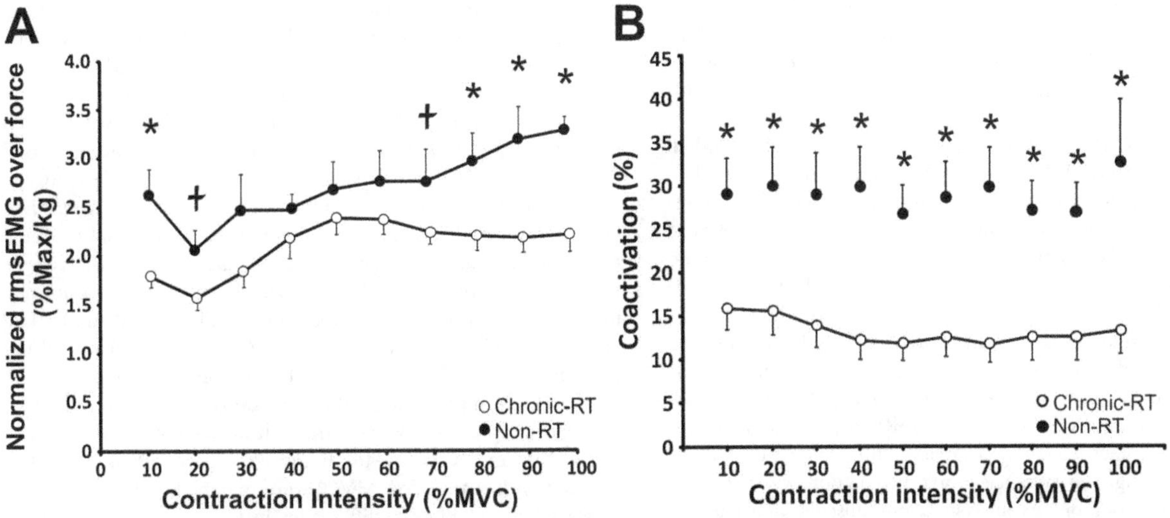

Figure 7. Biceps brachii activation during muscle contraction from 10–100% MVC. (A) Normalized rmsEMG to absolute elbow flexion forces recorded from 10–100%MVC. (B) Muscle coactivation (EMG of triceps:biceps brachii) 10–100% MVC. Each data point represents group means ± SE. * Indicates a significant ($p \leq 0.041$ and $p < 0.001$ for activation and coactivation, respectively) difference between groups. Ł Indicates a trend ($p \leq 0.075$) for between group differences.

thresholds (i.e. earlier activation) via needle electrodes following resistance training. Adam et al., (1998) demonstrated that the FDI of the dominant hand had lower motor unit recruitment thresholds compared to the FDI of the non-dominant hand. Thus, the voltage threshold or recruitment threshold of spinal motoneurones can be altered. If similar mechanisms were at play in the present study one would have expected the CMEP amplitudes to have been higher in the chronic-RT group at lower contraction intensities when compared to the non-RT group, perhaps due the clustering of motoneurone thresholds. This did not occur but might be a result of the TMES protocol used, which may not have been sensitive enough to detect this type of adaptation. The TMES current used was not set to find CMEP threshold, rather it was set to induce a CMEP amplitude that was ~15–20% of M_{max}. A higher TMES current could have recruited motoneurones that would have not been recruited at a threshold current giving similar CMEP amplitudes in both groups over all relative contraction intensities. Nonetheless, altered motoneurone properties following resistance training can account for some of the increased strength that occurs with resistance training.

Following resistance training, supraspinal excitability has been shown to increase, not change, or decrease, with concomitant increases in strength. Increased supraspinal excitability following an *acute* resistance training program has been demonstrated in the tibialis anterior [12], soleus [14], rectus femoris [10,11] and biceps brachii [8] muscles, possibly due to reduced intracortical inhibition [10,11]. Other studies have shown no difference in supraspinal excitability following *chronic* resistance training of the tibialis anterior [17] or *acute* resistance training of the FDI [6] and biceps brachii [18] muscles. In fact, Jensen et al. (2005) actually showed decreased supraspinal excitability of the biceps brachii muscle following *acute* resistance training. A decrease in supraspinal excitability could potentially occur since resistance training attenuates movement-related cortical potentials [48] thereby enhancing the neural economy within the connections between the neurons in the cortex. These contradictory results may be a result of differences in the 1) muscles examined, 2) contraction protocols, 3) type and combination of stimulation techniques used (see review by McNeil et al. [49] for details), 4) stimulation protocol and 5) complexity of the resistance training movements [3]. Unfortunately, none of these aforementioned studies used TMES (i.e. CMEPs) to determine the impact that training induced changes in spinal motoneurones would have on CE. It has been suggested that TMS and TMES combined have advantages over other stimulation techniques in determining the CNS sites for changes in CE (see reviews by Martin et al. [16], McNeil et al. [49] and Carroll et al. [3] for more detail). There are now three studies (the present study, and Carroll et al, 2002 and 2009) that employed both TMS and TMES to determine whether CE is altered predominantly at the supraspinal or spinal level following resistance training. All three studies showed similar results (increased strength and similar MEP and CMEP responses) using different stimulation protocols on different muscles following very different training programs. Essentially the three studies illustrate that at higher relative contraction intensities (i.e. >50% MVC) altered CE appears to be predominately influenced by spinal mechanisms.

Irrespective of training status there appears to be a shift from supraspinal to spinal control of force output at relative contraction intensities >50% of MVC. In both groups, the MEP (Fig. 5A) amplitude increases to a greater degree than the CMEP (Fig. 5B) amplitude from 5–40% MVC and then plateaus. The greater increase in MEP amplitude compared to CMEP amplitude from 10–40% MVC would indicate that CE was predominantly supraspinally mediated. Following 50% MVC both MEP and CMEP amplitudes plateaued indicating that at higher contraction intensities any change in CE was predominantly spinally mediated. In non-training studies, increased CE at the supraspinal level during weak contractions (<50%MVC) has also been reported [50–53]. Martin et al. [19] also demonstrated that MEPs and CMEPs of the biceps brachii during strong contractions (>50% MVC) changed similarly, suggesting that spinal mechanisms (i.e. the motoneurone) are responsible for changes in the evoked potentials. Interestingly, the biceps MEP amplitude-force curve (Figure 5A) shown here (increase in MEP amplitude up to 30–40% MVC) is not similar to that found previously (increase in MEP amplitude up to 80% MVC [54] rather it was similar to that found in a rate coding muscle such as the abductor digiti minimi [54]. It is possible that the stimulation intensity used by Gelli et al. (2007), was lower, thus allowing a more sensitive measure for MEPs (smaller increments in MEP amplitude without a 'ceiling effect'). However, this is speculative and cannot be concluded with certainty.

MEPs and CMEPs were decreased in the chronic-RT compared to the non-RT group at all absolute forces from 10–100% MVC indicating that both supraspinal and spinal excitability were lower with chronic resistance training per given amount of force generated. Carroll et al, (2002) and (2009) showed the same results after only four weeks of resistance training. In the chronic-RT group the increase in absolute force at all contraction intensities was due to neural and (or) muscle adaptations (see review by Folland and Williams [1], for details). Although we did not assess muscle girth or fat-free body mass, the chronic-RT group was ~15 kg heavier than the non-RT group, likely due, at least in part, to increased muscle mass. Thus, following chronic resistance training, the enhanced force production was probably due to a combination of nervous system and muscular adaptations.

The chronic-RT group also had a lower absolute force-agonist EMG relationship. Biceps brachii EMG activity normalized to force was lower at every (although not statistically, see Fig. 7A) contraction intensity from 10–100% MVC in the chronic-RT group. Other studies have found a shift in the force–agonist EMG relationship (i.e., greater force for the same level of activation) following chronic resistance training (2–6 months) [55–57]. In the present study, the chronic-RT group also had decreased triceps brachii:biceps brachii coactivation ratios from 10–100% MVC compared to the non-RT group. On average, triceps activation was ~15% of biceps activation in the chronic-RT group whereas it was ~30% in the non-RT group (Fig. 7B) and these percentages were similar across all contraction intensities. Decreased co-activation has been shown to occur as a result of resistance training [37,58–60] which may be due to increased sensitivity to descending motor commands at the spinal level or a decrease in reciprocal inhibition [61]. A shift in the force-agonist EMG relationship and decreased muscle coactivation would make the agonist muscle more efficient during a given contraction intensity and potentially reduce the amount of CE required to produce force.

The current study has several potential limitations. Based on our findings and others we suggest that there is an enhanced motoneurone firing frequency as a result of chronic resistance training. However, the stimulation techniques employed here cannot decipher whether this enhanced firing frequency is due to intrinsic properties of the motoneurone or changes to pre-motoneuronal sites (i.e. cortico-motoneuronal synapse). Indeed, the H-reflex is potentiated by resistance training, illustrating a pre-motoneuronal and/or motoneuronal adaptation [13]. The methodological protocol employed in the current study may have influenced the results, though we don't think this is the case. The order of stimulation techniques (i.e. MEP, CMEP, M-wave) was not randomized from contraction to contraction. Since the force and EMG prior to each stimulus were not different within each contraction the stimuli should not have affected the amplitude of the MEP or CMEP. Furthermore, M-wave did not differ between groups at any contraction intensity, thus MEP and CMEP amplitudes were likely due to changes at the supraspinal or spinal level and not due to differences in excitation across the muscle fibres. Fatigue related to the number of contractions performed throughout the protocol probably did not affect MEP and CMEP amplitudes either since the MEP and CMEP amplitudes did not differ from set to set at the same contraction intensity (see Fig. 3) and perhaps most telling, there was no significant difference between the pre- and post-contraction protocol MVCs ($p = 0.28$). All MEP and CMEP amplitudes recorded at a very low contraction intensity (5% MVC) were matched and did not differ between groups. Finally, differences in CE between groups were probably not due to changes in conduction speed or synaptic transmission along the corticospinal pathway because there were no differences between MEP and CMEP onset-latencies between groups at any contraction intensity.

In conclusion, enhanced strength resulting from chronic resistance training is in part due to altered CE. The predominant site for the altered CE is probably at the motoneurone. This was evidenced by a decreased MEP amplitude in chronic-RT compared to non-RT individuals at relative forces >50% MVC. Both MEP and CMEP amplitudes normalized to absolute force were lower in the chronic-RT group at all contraction intensities from 10–100% MVC. Thus, any training-induced enhancement in force production will allow for reduced corticospinal drive. A shift in the force-agoinst EMG relationship and decreased coactivation also occurred in the chronic-RT group and may contribute to the reduction in CE. *Chronic* resistance training substantially increases force output in part due to altered CE supraspinally and especially spinally (i.e. the spinal motoneurone).

Acknowledgments

The authors would like to thank Dr. Timar Alkanani at Memorial University for technical assistance and Michael Monks and David Bradbury-Squires for assistance in data collection and analysis.

Author Contributions

Conceived and designed the experiments: GP KP DB. Performed the experiments: GP KP DB. Analyzed the data: GP KP DB. Contributed reagents/materials/analysis tools: GP KP DB. Wrote the paper: GP KP DB.

References

1. Folland JP, Williams AG (2007) The adaptations to strength training: morphological and neurological contributions to increased strength. Sports Med 37: 145–168.
2. Del Balso C, Cafarelli E (2007) Adaptations in the activation of human skeletal muscle induced by short-term isometric resistance training. J Appl Physiol (1985) 103: 402–411.
3. Carroll TJ, Selvanayagam VS, Riek S, Semmler JG (2011) Neural adaptations to strength training: moving beyond transcranial magnetic stimulation and reflex studies. Acta physiologica 202: 119–140.
4. Carroll TJ, Riek S, Carson RG (2001) Neural adaptations to resistance training: implications for movement control. Sports medicine 31: 829–840.
5. Carroll TJ, Riek S, Carson RG (2002) The sites of neural adaptation induced by resistance training in humans. The Journal of physiology 544: 641–652.
6. Kidgell DJ, Pearce AJ (2010) Corticospinal properties following short-term strength training of an intrinsic hand muscle. Human movement science 29: 631–641.
7. Carroll TJ, Barton J, Hsu M, Lee M (2009) The effect of strength training on the force of twitches evoked by corticospinal stimulation in humans. Acta physiologica 197: 161–173.
8. Kidgell DJ, Stokes MA, Castricum TJ, Pearce AJ (2010) Neurophysiological responses after short-term strength training of the biceps brachii muscle. Journal of strength and conditioning research/National Strength & Conditioning Association 24: 3123–3132.
9. Jensen JL, Marstrand PC, Nielsen JB (2005) Motor skill training and strength training are associated with different plastic changes in the central nervous system. J Appl Physiol (1985) 99: 1558–1568.
10. Weier AT, Pearce AJ, Kidgell DJ (2012) Strength training reduces intracortical inhibition. Acta Physiol (Oxf) 206: 109–119.
11. Goodwill AM, Pearce AJ, Kidgell DJ (2012) Corticomotor plasticity following unilateral strength training. Muscle & nerve 46: 384–393.
12. Griffin L, Cafarelli E (2007) Transcranial magnetic stimulation during resistance training of the tibialis anterior muscle. J Electromyogr Kinesiol 17: 446–452.

13. Aagaard P, Simonsen EB, Andersen JL, Magnusson P, Dyhre-Poulsen P (2002) Neural adaptation to resistance training: changes in evoked V-wave and H-reflex responses. J Appl Physiol (1985) 92: 2309–2318.
14. Beck S, Taube W, Gruber M, Amtage F, Gollhofer A, et al. (2007) Task-specific changes in motor evoked potentials of lower limb muscles after different training interventions. Brain Res 1179: 51–60.
15. McNeil CJ, Giesebrecht S, Gandevia SC, Taylor JL (2011) Behaviour of the motoneurone pool in a fatiguing submaximal contraction. The Journal of physiology 589: 3533–3544.
16. Martin PG, Hudson AL, Gandevia SC, Taylor JL (2009) Reproducible measurement of human motoneuron excitability with magnetic stimulation of the corticospinal tract. Journal of neurophysiology 102: 606–613.
17. Tallent J, Goodall S, Hortobagyi T, St Clair Gibson A, Howatson G (2013) Corticospinal responses of resistance-trained and un-trained males during dynamic muscle contractions. J Electromyogr Kinesiol 23: 1075–1081.
18. del Olmo MF, Reimunde P, Viana O, Acero RM, Cudeiro J (2006) Chronic neural adaptation induced by long-term resistance training in humans. European journal of applied physiology 96: 722–728.
19. Martin PG, Gandevia SC, Taylor JL (2006) Output of human motoneuron pools to corticospinal inputs during voluntary contractions. Journal of neurophysiology 95: 3512–3518.
20. Oya T, Hoffman BW, Cresswell AG (2008) Corticospinal-evoked responses in lower limb muscles during voluntary contractions at varying strengths. Journal of applied physiology 105: 1527–1532.
21. Pearcey GEP, Bradbury-Squires DJ, Monks M, Power KE, Button DC (2013) Does Corticospinal excitability differ in trained and untrained individuals during various contraction intensities? Applied Physiology, Nutrition, and Metabolism 38: 1069.
22. Rossi S, Hallett M, Rossini PM, Pascual-Leone A (2011) Screening questionnaire before TMS: an update. Clin Neurophysiol 122: 1686.
23. Davidson AW, Rice CL (2010) Effect of shoulder angle on the activation pattern of the elbow extensors during a submaximal isometric fatiguing contraction. Muscle Nerve 42: 514–521.
24. Gandevia SC, Petersen N, Butler JE, Taylor JL (1999) Impaired response of human motoneurones to corticospinal stimulation after voluntary exercise. J Physiol 521 Pt 3: 749–759.
25. Ugawa Y, Rothwell JC, Day BL, Thompson PD, Marsden CD (1991) Percutaneous electrical stimulation of corticospinal pathways at the level of the pyramidal decussation in humans. Ann Neurol 29: 418–427.
26. Taylor JL (2006) Stimulation at the cervicomedullary junction in human subjects. Journal of electromyography and kinesiology: official journal of the International Society of Electrophysiological Kinesiology 16: 215–223.
27. Martin PG, Weerakkody N, Gandevia SC, Taylor JL (2008) Group III and IV muscle afferents differentially affect the motor cortex and motoneurones in humans. The Journal of physiology 586: 1277–1289.
28. Levenez M, Garland SJ, Klass M, Duchateau J (2008) Cortical and spinal modulation of antagonist coactivation during a submaximal fatiguing contraction in humans. J Neurophysiol 99: 554–563.
29. De Luca CJ, LeFever RS, McCue MP, Xenakis AP (1982) Behaviour of human motor units in different muscles during linearly varying contractions. J Physiol 329: 113–128.
30. de Luca CJ, Foley PJ, Erim Z (1996) Motor unit control properties in constant-force isometric contractions. J Neurophysiol 76: 1503–1516.
31. Jones KE, Bawa P (1997) Computer simulation of the responses of human motoneurons to composite 1A EPSPS: effects of background firing rate. J Neurophysiol 77: 405–420.
32. Matthews PB (1999) The effect of firing on the excitability of a model motoneurone and its implications for cortical stimulation. J Physiol 518 (Pt 3): 867–882.
33. Olivier E, Bawa P, Lemon RN (1995) Excitability of human upper limb motoneurones during rhythmic discharge tested with transcranial magnetic stimulation. The Journal of physiology 485 (Pt 1): 257–269.
34. Beaumont E, Gardiner P (2002) Effects of daily spontaneous running on the electrophysiological properties of hindlimb motoneurones in rats. J Physiol 540: 129–138.
35. Carp JS, Wolpaw JR (1994) Motoneuron plasticity underlying operantly conditioned decrease in primate H-reflex. J Neurophysiol 72: 431–442.
36. Van Cutsem M, Duchateau J, Hainaut K (1998) Changes in single motor unit behaviour contribute to the increase in contraction speed after dynamic training in humans. J Physiol 513 (Pt 1): 295–305.
37. Vila-Cha C, Falla D, Farina D (2010) Motor unit behavior during submaximal contractions following six weeks of either endurance or strength training. J Appl Physiol (1985) 109: 1455–1466.
38. Beaumont E, Gardiner PF (2003) Endurance training alters the biophysical properties of hindlimb motoneurons in rats. Muscle Nerve 27: 228–236.
39. Lee RH, Heckman CJ (1998) Bistability in spinal motoneurons in vivo: systematic variations in rhythmic firing patterns. J Neurophysiol 80: 572–582.
40. Lee RH, Heckman CJ (1998) Bistability in spinal motoneurons in vivo: systematic variations in persistent inward currents. J Neurophysiol 80: 583–593.
41. Heckman CJ, Johnson M, Mottram C, Schuster J (2008) Persistent Inward Currents in Spinal Motoneurons and Their Influence on Human Motoneuron Firing Patterns. Neuroscientist.
42. Button DC, Gardiner K, Marqueste T, Gardiner PF (2006) Frequency-current relationships of rat hindlimb {alpha}-motoneurones. J Physiol 573: 663–677.
43. Gardiner P, Dai Y, Heckman CJ (2006) Effects of exercise training on alpha-motoneurons. J Appl Physiol 101: 1228–1236.
44. Heckman CJ (2003) Active conductances in motoneuron dendrites enhance movement capabilities. Exerc Sport Sci Rev 31: 96–101.
45. Khan SI, Giesebrecht S, Gandevia SC, Taylor JL (2012) Activity-dependent depression of the recurrent discharge of human motoneurones after maximal voluntary contractions. J Physiol 590: 4957–4969.
46. Rossi A, Rossi S, Ginanneschi F (2012) Activity-dependent changes in intrinsic excitability of human spinal motoneurones produced by natural activity. J Neurophysiol 108: 2473–2480.
47. MacDonell CW, Button DC, Beaumont E, Cormery B, Gardiner PF (2012) Plasticity of rat motoneuron rhythmic firing properties with varying levels of afferent and descending inputs. Journal of neurophysiology 107: 265–272.
48. Falvo MJ, Sirevaag EJ, Rohrbaugh JW, Earhart GM (2010) Resistance training induces supraspinal adaptations: evidence from movement-related cortical potentials. Eur J Appl Physiol 109: 923–933.
49. McNeil CJ, Butler JE, Taylor JL, Gandevia SC (2013) Testing the excitability of human motoneurons. Frontiers in human neuroscience 7: 152.
50. Di Lazzaro V, Restuccia D, Oliviero A, Profice P, Ferrara L, et al. (1998) Effects of voluntary contraction on descending volleys evoked by transcranial stimulation in conscious humans. The Journal of physiology 508 (Pt 2): 625–633.
51. Taylor JL, Petersen NT, Butler JE, Gandevia SC (2002) Interaction of transcranial magnetic stimulation and electrical transmastoid stimulation in human subjects. J Physiol 541: 949–958.
52. Mazzocchio R, Rothwell JC, Day BL, Thompson PD (1994) Effect of tonic voluntary activity on the excitability of human motor cortex. J Physiol 474: 261–267.
53. Ugawa Y, Terao Y, Hanajima R, Sakai K, Kanazawa I (1995) Facilitatory effect of tonic voluntary contraction on responses to motor cortex stimulation. Electroencephalogr Clin Neurophysiol 97: 451–454.
54. Gelli F, Del Santo F, Popa T, Mazzocchio R, Rossi A (2007) Factors influencing the relation between corticospinal output and muscle force during voluntary contractions. Eur J Neurosci 25: 3469–3475.
55. Garfinkel S, Cafarelli E (1992) Relative changes in maximal force, EMG, and muscle cross-sectional area after isometric training. Med Sci Sports Exerc 24: 1220–1227.
56. Narici MV, Hoppeler H, Kayser B, Landoni L, Claassen H, et al. (1996) Human quadriceps cross-sectional area, torque and neural activation during 6 months strength training. Acta Physiol Scand 157: 175–186.
57. Hakkinen K, Komi PV (1983) Electromyographic changes during strength training and detraining. Med Sci Sports Exerc 15: 455–460.
58. Enoka RM (1997) Neural adaptations with chronic physical activity. J Biomech 30: 447–455.
59. Carolan B, Cafarelli E (1992) Adaptations in coactivation after isometric resistance training. J Appl Physiol (1985) 73: 911–917.
60. Tillin NA, Pain MT, Folland JP (2011) Short-term unilateral resistance training affects the agonist-antagonist but not the force-agonist activation relationship. Muscle Nerve 43: 375–384.
61. Dragert K, Zehr EP (2013) High-intensity unilateral dorsiflexor resistance training results in bilateral neuromuscular plasticity after stroke. Exp Brain Res 225: 93–104.

7

Fibre-Specific Responses to Endurance and Low Volume High Intensity Interval Training: Striking Similarities in Acute and Chronic Adaptation

Trisha D. Scribbans[1], Brittany A. Edgett[1], Kira Vorobej[2], Andrew S. Mitchell[2], Sophie D. Joanisse[3], Jennifer B. L. Matusiak[1], Gianni Parise[3], Joe Quadrilatero[2], Brendon J. Gurd[1]*

1 School of Kinesiology and Health Studies, Queen's University, Kingston, Ontario, Canada, **2** Department of Kinesiology, University of Waterloo, Waterloo, Ontario, Canada, **3** Department of Kinesiology, McMaster University, Hamilton, Ontario, Canada

Abstract

The current study involved the completion of two distinct experiments. Experiment 1 compared fibre specific and whole muscle responses to acute bouts of either low-volume high-intensity interval training (LV-HIT) or moderate-intensity continuous endurance exercise (END) in a randomized crossover design. Experiment 2 examined the impact of a six-week training intervention (END or LV-HIT; 4 days/week), on whole body and skeletal muscle fibre specific markers of aerobic and anaerobic capacity. Six recreationally active men (Age: 20.7±3.8 yrs; VO_2peak: 51.9±5.1 mL/kg/min) reported to the lab on two separate occasions for experiment 1. Following a muscle biopsy taken in a fasted state, participants completed an acute bout of each exercise protocol (LV-HIT: 8, 20-second intervals at ~170% of VO_2peak separated by 10 seconds of rest; END: 30 minutes at ~65% of VO_2peak), immediately followed by a muscle biopsy. Glycogen content of type I and IIA fibres was significantly ($p<0.05$) reduced, while p-ACC was significantly increased ($p<0.05$) following both protocols. Nineteen recreationally active males (n = 16) and females (n = 3) were VO_2peak-matched and assigned to either the LV-HIT (n = 10; 21±2 yrs) or END (n = 9; 20.7±3.8 yrs) group for experiment 2. After 6 weeks, both training protocols induced comparable increases in aerobic capacity (END: Pre: 48.3±6.0, Mid: 51.8±6.0, Post: 55.0±6.3 mL/kg/min LV-HIT: Pre: 47.9±8.1, Mid: 50.4±7.4, Post: 54.7±7.6 mL/kg/min), fibre-type specific oxidative and glycolytic capacity, glycogen and IMTG stores, and whole-muscle capillary density. Interestingly, only LV-HIT induced greater improvements in anaerobic performance and estimated whole-muscle glycolytic capacity. These results suggest that 30 minutes of END exercise at ~65% VO_2peak or 4 minutes of LV-HIT at ~170% VO_2peak induce comparable changes in the intra-myocellular environment (glycogen content and signaling activation); correspondingly, training-induced adaptations resulting for these protocols, and other HIT and END protocols are strikingly similar.

Editor: Stephen E. Alway, West Virginia University School of Medicine, United States of America

Funding: Funding was provided by the Natural Sciences and Engineering Research Council of Canada (NSERC) and the Canada Foundation for Innovation (CFI). The funders had no role in study design, data collection and analysis, decision to publish, or preparation of the manuscript.

Competing Interests: The authors have declared that no competing interests exist.

* E-mail: gurdb@queensu.ca

Introduction

Endurance (END) training and interval training, consisting of either sprint interval training (SIT; repeated bouts of 'all out' exercise [e.g. Repeated Wingates]) or high-intensity interval training (HIT; repeated bouts of exercise below an all out intensity) result in comparable adaptations in both performance and skeletal muscle metabolism. These include: improvements in maximal oxygen uptake (VO_2peak) [1–7] and aerobic exercise performance [7–9], increases in markers of mitochondrial content, oxidative capacity [1–3,8,10], intramuscular glycogen [8] and triglyceride stores [3], capillary density [4,6,11], lipid oxidation [1,3,10], and reductions in substrate level (phosphocreatine and glycogen) phosphorylation [1]. Given the markedly reduced training dose (exercise energy expenditure and training time) associated with many high-intensity protocols, these data demonstrate the ability of high intensity exercise to induce physiological adaptations without the requirement for large training volumes.

The potency of HIT high-intensity exercise has recently been demonstrated by several studies employing a low volume- (LV) high-intensity interval training (HIT) protocol requiring a fraction of the training dose (total training time of ~4 min/day) necessary for END and many other HIT protocols. Similar to other larger dose HIT protocols, studies utilizing LV-HIT have demonstrated improvements in VO_2peak [9,12,13], anaerobic exercise capacity [12,13], and increased mitochondrial protein content (cytochrome *c* oxidase (COX) subunit I and COX IV)[13] that are equivalent to those induced by END [9,12]. While there is an abundance of literature demonstrating the efficacy of HIT at inducing adaptations, the mechanisms by which substantially lower doses of high intensity exercise induce adaptations typically associated with high dose END are not completely understood, specifically, similarities/differences in fibre-type specific adaptations induced by HIT and END have not been completely described.

Table 1. Experiment 1 participant characteristics (N = 6), mean (SD) unless otherwise indicated.

Age (yrs)	20.7(3.8)
Height (cm)	183.7(9.3)
Body mass (kg)	77.8(2.8)
Absolute VO_2 (mL/min)	4025(306)
Relative VO_2 (mL/kg/min)	51.9(5.1)
HRpeak (BPM)	196(7)
WRpeak (W)	264.1(41.6)
Mean power (W) LV-HIT (actual)	481.4(60.1)
Mean power (W) LV-HIT (prescribed)	448.0(70.5)
Mean power (W) endurance (actual)	173.7(29.8)
Mean power (W) endurance (prescribed)	172.0(27.1)

Note: LV-HIT mean power represents the average power output during the 8 intervals not including rest periods. BPM, beats per minute; cm, centimeters; kg, kilograms; min, minute; RER, respiratory exchange ratio; s, seconds; W, watts; yrs, years.

For example, several recent reports suggest that improvements in aerobic exercise capacity and performance following HIT result primarily from peripheral adaptations [14,15]. These adaptations, specifically the induction of mitochondrial biogenesis, result from the activation of signaling cascades which increase transcription of mitochondrial genes via the activation [16,17] and/or increased expression of peroxisome proliferator-activated receptor gamma co-activator 1 alpha (PGC-1α) [18]. Given that END and HIT result in similar increases in whole-muscle markers of mitochondrial content and oxidative capacity [1–3,8,10], it is not surprising that acute activation of signaling pathways, measured in whole-muscle homogenates, following a single bout of END and HIT are also comparable [19–21]. However, it is not clear if these whole-muscle measures reflect similar adaptations across distinct fibre populations within a trained muscle, or whether HIT induces adaptations in different populations of fibres. More specifically, whether the well characterized recruitment of type II fibres associated with higher intensities of exercise, including continuous supramaximal [22–24] and intermittent maximal [25] exercise result in different fibre recruitment patterns between LV-HIT and END is unknown. Further, whether variations in acute fibre recruitment result in distinctive fibre adaptations following chronic LV-HIT and END is also not known; however, it is possible that different recruitment patterns and fibre-type specific adaptations may partially explain the potency of high intensity exercise and more specifically, LV-HIT.

To examine these issues we performed 2 distinct experiments. The purpose of experiment 1 was to examine: 1) fibre recruitment patterns, as reflected by reductions in glycogen content of each fibre-type population, and 2) whole-muscle and fibre-type specific signalling pathway activation following an acute bout of LV-HIT and END exercise. The purpose of experiment 2 was to examine: 1) changes in aerobic and anaerobic exercise performance, and 2) fibre-type specific adaptations in oxidative and glycolytic capacities, substrate storage and whole-muscle capillary density resulting from 6 weeks of LV-HIT and END training. We hypothesized that an acute bout of LV-HIT would result in the activation of a greater number of type II muscle fibres than END exercise, and that resulting fibre-specific metabolic adaptations following training would reflect these differences in acute fibre recruitment.

Materials and Methods

Ethics Statement

All experimental procedures performed on human participants were approved by the Health Sciences Human Research Ethics Board at Queen's University and conformed to the Declaration of Helsinki. Verbal and written explanation of the experimental protocol and associated risks was provided to all participants prior to obtaining written informed consent.

Experimental Design

The current study involved the completion of two distinct experiments. Experiment 1 compared fibre specific and whole muscle responses to acute bouts of either low-volume high-intensity interval training (LV-HIT) or moderate-intensity continuous cycle exercise (END) in a randomized crossover design. Experiment 2 examined the impact of a six-week training intervention (END or LV-HIT 4 days/week), on whole body and skeletal muscle fibre specific markers of aerobic and anaerobic capacity. All physiological testing and training for both experiments was performed on a Monark Ergomedic 874 E stationary ergometer (Vansbro, Sweden). Participants were asked to refrain from alcohol and exercise 24 hours before, and caffeine 12 hours before all experimental days in experiment 1 and pre- and post-training testing days in experiment 2.

Experiment 1

Participants. Six recreationally active males volunteered to participate in the study (participant characteristics are presented in Table 1). No participants were involved in more than 3 hours of aerobic exercise (running, jogging, etc.) per week.

Physiological testing. On their first visit to the lab participants completed a VO_2peak incremental ramp test to exhaustion as described previously [26], and height and weight were recorded. Gas exchange was measured throughout the test with a metabolic cart (Moxus AEI Technologies, Pittsburgh, PA), with VO_2peak and heart rate (HR) peak calculated as the highest value of continuous 30 second averages for each measure during the protocol. Peak O_2 pulse was calculated by dividing absolute VO_2peak by HRpeak from the incremental ramp protocol. Work rate (WR) was collected continuously throughout the test and peak aerobic power (WRpeak) was calculated using the average WR from the last 30 seconds of the test.

Exercise interventions. Participants reported to the lab in the morning following an overnight fast (≥12 h) after consuming a standardized dinner the night before [Stouffer's Sauté Sensations Country Beef Pot Roast (540 kcal; 56 g carbohydrate (CHO), 20 g fat, 14 g protein) and 500 mL of 2% milk (260 kcal; 12 g CHO, 5 g fat, 9 g protein)]. A fasted, resting muscle biopsy (Rest) was taken from the vastus lateralis under superficial local anaesthesia (2% lidocaine, with epinephrine) using the Bergstrom needle biopsy technique [27] adapted with suction. An additional incision was made, and covered with sterile gauze, approximately 1 cm from the resting biopsy site to allow for immediate removal of the post-exercise muscle sample. Participants then rested in the lab for 30 minutes or 55 minutes before completing a bout of END or LV-HIT, respectively. Immediately following each exercise bout a second muscle biopsy was taken (Ex). The LV-HIT exercise protocol was performed as described previously [12,13]. Briefly, participants completed eight 20-second intervals at 170% of VO_2peak separated by 10 seconds of rest eight times, for a total of four-minutes. During rest periods participants cycled against no load at a cadence of their choice. The END exercise protocol consisted of 30 minutes of continuous cycling at 65% of VO_2peak. Each exercise bout was performed at the same time of day for all subjects and were performed one week apart (7 days).

Experiment 2

Participants. Nineteen recreationally active males (n = 16) and females (n = 3) volunteered to participate in this study (participant characteristics are presented in Table 1). No participants were involved in more than 3 hours of aerobic exercise (running, jogging, etc.) per week or involved in any structured training program within the past six months. Participants were VO_2peak-matched and assigned to either the LV-HIT (n = 10) or endurance (n = 9) group.

Training interventions. All participants completed training four days a week for six weeks (week 4 only had 3 training sessions due to the mid-training VO_2peak test for a total of 23 sessions). Both the LV-HIT and END training protocols were the same as those utilized in experiment 1 (see above for descriptions). Participants descended and ascended 4 flights of stairs as a warm-up prior to all training sessions. Revolutions per minute (RPM) data was collected for each training session in order to confirm training intensity.

Physiological testing. During baseline testing (Pre) participants reported to the lab in the morning following an overnight fast (≥8 h). Participants were fed a standardized breakfast [plain bagel (190 kcal; 1 g fat, 36 g CHO, 7 g protein) with 15 g of peanut butter (90 kcal; 8 g fat, 4 g CHO, 3 g protein) and 200 mL of apple juice (90 kcal; 0 g fat, 22 g CHO, 0 g protein)] and rested for 1 hour before a muscle biopsy was taken from their vastus lateralis under superficial local anaesthesia (2% lidocaine, with epinephrine) using the Bergstrom needle biopsy technique (1) adapted with suction.

Forty-eight hours following the muscle biopsy participants returned to the lab to complete a VO_2peak incremental ramp test to exhaustion as described previously [26]. Following completion of the VO_2peak test, participants rested for 30 minutes before completing a repeated Wingate protocol consisting of 2 minutes of load-less cycling followed by four 30 second Wingates (7.5% body weight), separated by 4.5 minutes of load-less cycling. RPM was collected continuously and peak (first 5 second average) and mean power (average for total 30 seconds) were determined for the first Wingate. Total work performed during all 4 Wingate bouts was also calculated. Twenty-four hours after the VO_2peak and Wingate tests, participants reported to the lab and completed a 500 kcal time to completion (TTC) trial at a self-selected cadence as quickly as possible as described previously [28,29].

A VO_2peak incremental ramp test to exhaustion was performed half way through training (Mid) on the first day of week 4 in order to adjust training loads. As a result participants only completed 3 training sessions in week 4. Post-training (Post) testing began 72 hours following the last training session of week 6 and was conducted in an identical manner as the baseline testing. (See above for details).

Immunofluorescent and Histochemical Analysis

Immunofluorescent analysis of myosin heavy chain isoforms was performed as previously described [30] using primary antibodies against myosin heavy chain (MHC) I (BA-F8), MHCIIa (SC-71), and MHCIIx (6H1) (Developmental Studies Hybridoma Bank, Iowa City, IA, USA), followed by isotype-specific fluorescent secondary antibodies. This allowed for the identification of type I (blue), type IIA (green), type IIX (red), as well as hybrid fibre types (IIAX). For all analyses type IIX and type IIAX fibres were analyzed together (type IIAX/IIX) given their relatively low percentage. Fibre type composition was determined by counting all fibres within a muscle cross-section.

Quantification of capillary density [31] and fibre-type specific phosphorylated-AMP-activated protein kinase alpha (p-AMPKα) [32] was adapted from previous work. Briefly, sections were fixed in 4% paraformaldehyde for 10 minutes, followed by permeabilization with 0.5% TritonX-100 for 30 minutes, and then blocked in 10% goat serum for 30 minutes. Sections were incubated overnight in 5% goat serum with the appropriate primary antibodies specific for the endothelium (PECAM) and sarcolemma (dystrophin) (Developmental Studies Hybridoma Bank, Iowa City, IA, USA) or p-AMPKα (Thr^{172}) (Cell Signaling Technology, Danvers, MA, USA). After 3×5 minute washes in PBS, sections were incubated for 1 hour in 5% goat serum with the appropriate fluorescent secondary antibodies (Life Technologies, Burlington, ON, CA).

For all immunofluorescent procedures, sections were mounted with Prolong Gold Antifade Reagent (Life Technologies, Burlington, ON, CA) and imaged the following day. All sections were visualized with an Axio Observer Z1 microscope (Carl Zeiss, Jena, TH, DE). Individual images were taken across the entire muscle cross-section and assembled into a composite panoramic image using AxioVision software (Carl Zeiss). Compiled images were matched to fibre-type images and ~30 of each fibre type were randomly selected and analyzed. Data were expressed relative to the values obtained in type I fibers, which were assigned a reference value of 1.0, and reported as mean optical density in arbitrary units (AU). This method was utilized for all immunofluorescent and histochemical analyses except for the determination of capillary density where 3 separate areas per sample were analyzed for number of capillaries. Fibre-specific p-AMPKα fluorescence was performed in ImageJ (National Institutes of Health, Bethesda, MD, USA) and was determined by subtracting the average fluorescence of the slide background (>5 per slide) from each individual fibre's fluorescence.

As a general indicator of oxidative and glycolytic potential, histochemical staining for succinate dehydrogenase (SDH) [33] and α-glycerophosphate dehydrogenase (GPD) [34] activity was performed [30]. Intramuscular triglyceride (IMTG) content was determined with Oil Red O (ORO) staining [35], whereas glycogen content was determined using the Periodic Acid Schiff (PAS) [36]. Images were acquired with a bright field Nikon microscope linked to a PixelLink digital camera. Individual images were taken across the entire muscle cross-section and assembled

Table 2. Quantitative RT-PCR primer sequences.

	Forward Primer	Reverse Primer
PGC-1α	Cacttacaagccaaaccaacaact	caatagtcttgttctcaaatgggga
SIRT1	Agaacatagacacgctggaaca	caagatgctgttgcaaaggaacc
GCN5	Aaggaccccgaccagctcta	gggaagcggatgacctcgta
RIP140	Gttccactcagcccagcagt	agaccctgcacagcccaagt
GAPDH	cctcctgcaccaccaactgctt	gaggggccatccacagtcttct

Note: GAPDH, glyceraldehyde 3-phosphate dehydrogenase; GCN5, general control non-derepressible 5; PGC-1α, peroxisome proliferator-activated receptor gamma coactivator 1 alpha; RIP140, receptor-interacting protein 140; SIRT1, silent mating type information regulation 2 homolog 1.

into a composite panoramic image using Microsoft Image Composite Editor (ICE) (Microsoft, Redmond, WA, USA). Image analysis was performed in ImageJ by converting color images to 8-bit, and calculated by subtracting background staining from the mean grey value of individual fibres. Estimated oxidative and glycolytic capacities were calculated by summing the calculated capacities of each fibre type together. Capacities for each fibre type were calculated by multiplying the mean SDH (oxidative) or GPD (glycolytic) activity for each fibre-type by the percent of that fibre present within each participant's sample.

Western Blotting

Samples were homogenized, total protein was determined, and sample loading, separation and transfer were performed as described previously [29]. All phosphorylated protein contents are expressed relative to total protein content at rest. Samples were run in duplicate and equal protein loading was confirmed with GAPDH analysis. For protein detection, commercially available antibodies were used for GAPDH (Millipore, Billerica, MA, USA), p-p38 MAPK (Thr^{180}/Tyr^{182}), p-38 MAPK, p-AMPKα (Thr^{172}), AMPKα, p-ACC (Ser^{79}), and ACC (Cell Signaling Technologies, Danvers, MA, USA). Membranes were blocked with 5% bovine serum albumin (BSA) in Tris-buffered saline with Tween-20 (TBS-T) (0.1%) and were immunoblotted with primary antibodies (1:1000). Proteins were visualized by chemiluminescence detection, according to the manufacturer's instructions (Millipore, Billerica, MA, USA). Blots were quantified using the Fluorochem HD2 System (Cell Biosciences, Santa Clara, CA, USA).

RNA Extraction

RNA was extracted using the TRIzol/RNeasy method (Qiagen Sciences, Valencia, CA, USA). Briefly, approximately 20 mg of frozen muscle was added to Lysing Matrix D tubes (MP Biomedicals, Solon, OH, USA), containing 1 mL of TRIzol Reagent (Life Technologies, Burlington, ON, Canada). Muscle samples were homogenized using the FastPrep-24 Tissue and Cell Homogenizer (MP Biomedicals, Solon, OH, USA) for 40 sec at a setting of 6 m/sec. 200 µl of chloroform reagent was added to homogenized samples (Sigma-Aldrich, Oakville, ON, CA), mixed for 15 sec, incubated at room temperature for 5 minutes and centrifuged for 10 minutes at 12000 g at 4°C. The aqueous phase was transferred to a new tube and equal amounts of 70% ethanol was added and mixed. The mixture was transferred into an RNeasy mini-spin column and RNA was purified following the commercially available E.Z.N.A. Total RNA Kit 1 (Omega Bio-Tek, Norcross, GA, USA) as per manufacturer's instructions. The RNA concentration and purity was quantified using the Nano-Drop 1000 spectrophotometer (Thermo Fisher Scientific, Rockville, MD, USA). RNA integrity was assessed using a bioanalyzer (Agilent 2100 Bioanalyzer; Agilent Technologies). Average RNA Integrity Number (RIN) values were 6.4.

Quantitative Real-time PCR

Individual samples were reverse transcribed using the commercially available high capacity cDNA reverse transcription kit (Applied Biosystems, Foster City, CA, USA), according to the manufacturer's instructions, using an Eppendorf Mastercycler epgradient thermal cycler (Eppendorf, Mississauga, ON, CA). Reactions were run using RT^2 real-time SYBR Green qPCR master mix (SABioscience; Qiagen Sciences, Germantown, MD, USA), prepared using the epMotion 5075 Eppendorf automated pipetting system (Eppendorf, Mississauga, ON, CA) and carried out in duplicate with an Eppendorf $realplex^2$ Master Cycler epgradientS (Eppendorf, Mississauga, ON, CA). Primer sequences are shown in Table 2. Relative mRNA expression was calculated using the ΔCt method and fold changes from PRE was calculated using the ΔΔCt method [37]. Gene expression was normalized to the housekeeping gene GAPDH.

Statistical Analysis

For both experiments, a two-way, repeated measures ANOVA was used to compare the effect of condition (END and LV-HIT) and time (Rest/Ex and Pre/Post) for all muscle derived data and pre- to post-training physiological testing data from experiment 2. All fibre-type specific analyses were performed within a particular fibre-type. Differences in fibre-type specific expression of p-AMPKα were determined using paired students t-tests comparing mean fluorescence between fibre-types at that time point (Rest and Ex). For estimated glycolytic capacity, where no interaction effect or main effects of training were observed, paired student t-tests were utilized to examine within group changes. All statistical analysis was performed using GraphPad Prism v 5.01 (GraphPad Software Inc., La Jolla, CA, USA). Statistical significance was accepted at $p<0.05$ and all data are presented as means ± SD.

Results

Experiment 1

Exercise bout characteristics. All participants completed each exercise protocol at a work rate corresponding to 65.7±3.8% and 183.2±9.5% VO_2peak for the END and LV-HIT exercise bouts, respectively. Mean prescribed and actual WR for both protocols are presented in Table 1.

Immunofluorescent and histochemical analysis. Representative images are presented in Figure 1A. While no interaction effect was observed for either type I or type IIA fibres, a significant ($p<0.05$) main effect of exercise for muscle glycogen content was present for type I (END–42%, LV-HIT–55%; Fig. 1B) and IIA (END–72%,

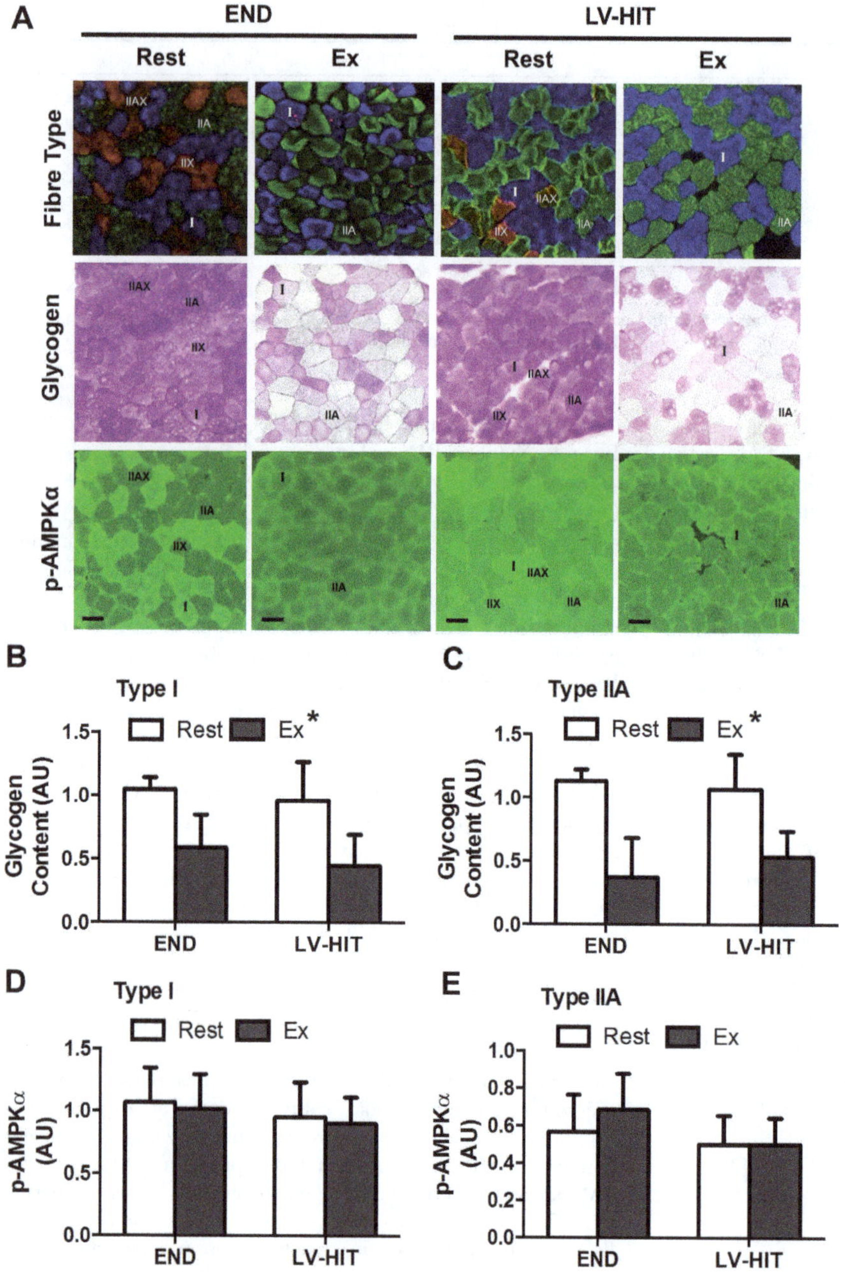

Figure 1. Effects of acute exercise on fibre-type specific glycogen depletion and phosphorylation of AMPKα. A: Representative slides of immunofluorescent fibre-type analysis (blue fibres are type I, green are type IIA, red/green are type IIAX/IIX) with serial sections of glycogen (periodic acid-Schiff staining) and p-AMPKα Thr^{172} content before (Rest) and immediately after (Ex) an acute bout of END or LV-HIT. B–C: Fold change in glycogen content from Rest and Ex in type I and IIA fibres. D–E: Fold change in p-AMPKα content from Rest and Ex in type I and IIA fibres. Bars represent 100 µm. AU, arbitrary units; µm, micrometre. *Significant ($p<0.05$) main effect of exercise.

LV-HIT–49%; Fig. 1C) fibres. As a result of type IIAX/IIX (END, n = 3; LV-HIT, n = 4) fibres not being present in all samples, they were excluded from analysis.

There was no interaction effect, or effect of exercise for p-AMPKα content in type I (Fig. 1D) or type IIA (Fig. 1E) fibres (see representative slides Fig. 1A). A similar lack of effect of exercise on p-AMPKα content was observed with whole muscle Western Blot analysis (see below). Type I fibres expressed significantly ($p<0.05$) greater levels of p-AMPKα than both type IIA and IIAX/IIX fibres at rest and post-exercise.

Western blotting. There was no effect (Fig. 2A and C) of exercise on p-AMPKα Thr^{172} or p-p38MAPK Thr^{180}/Tyr^{182} (see representative blots, Fig. 2D). However a main effect ($p<0.05$) of exercise was observed for p-ACC Ser^{79} (Fig. 2B).

Experiment 2

Aerobic exercise performance and oxidative capacity. A main effect of training ($p<0.05$) on relative VO_2peak (Fig. 3A) was observed at both Mid and Post testing (Percent change from pre: END: +15.5%, LV-HIT: +13.9%). A significant ($p<0.05$) main effect of training on absolute VO_2peak and peak HR was also

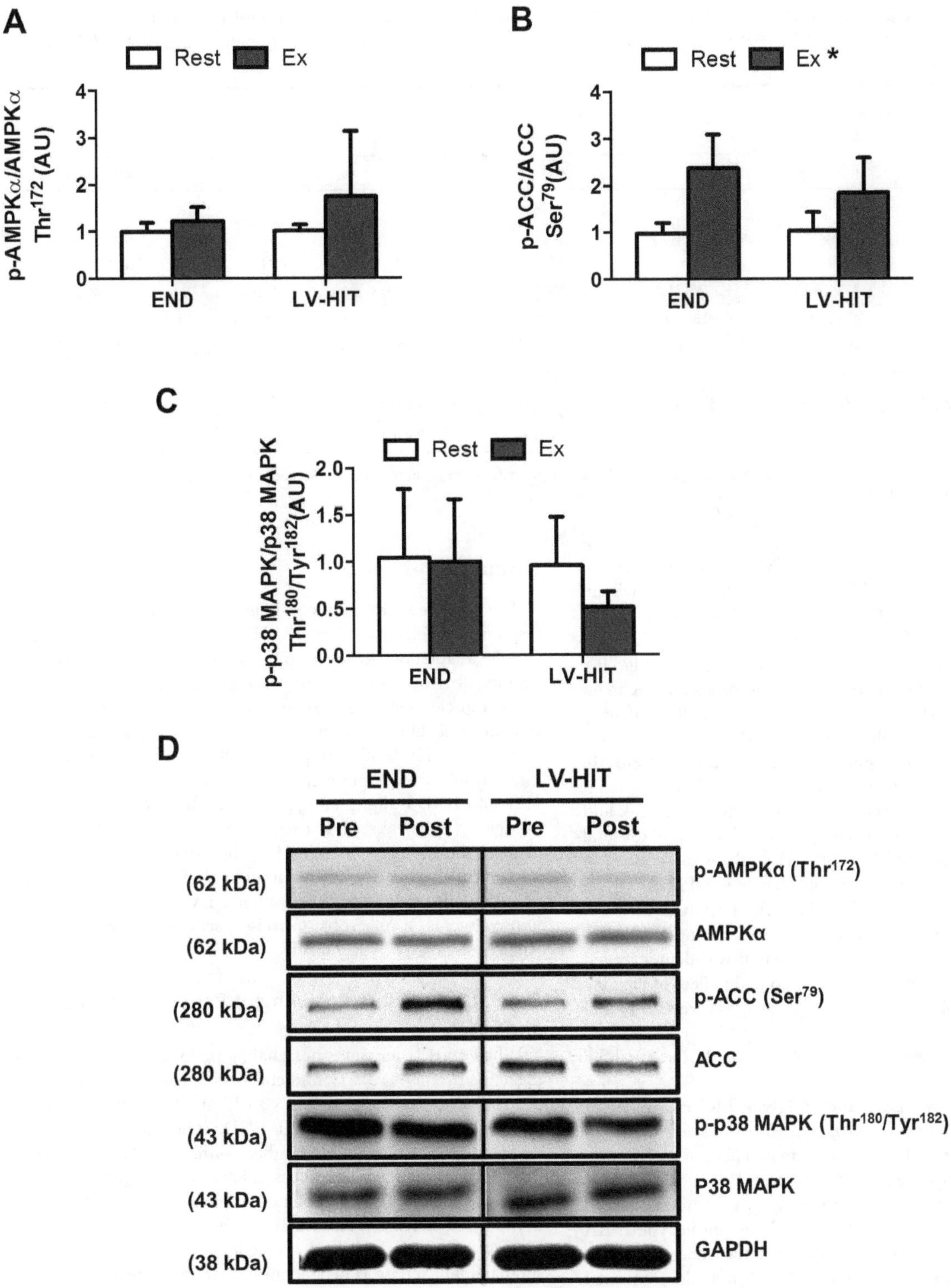

Figure 2. Effects of an acute bout of endurance (END) and low-volume high-intensity interval training (LV-HIT) on whole-muscle signaling. A–D: Fold change in p-AMPKα Thr^{172} (A), p-ACC Ser^{79} (B) and p38 MAPK Thr^{180}/Tyr^{182} (C) content from Rest and Ex. D: Representative western blots, including loading control are also shown. AU, arbitrary units. *Significant ($p<0.05$) main effect of exercise.

demonstrated, while no effect of training was observed for WRpeak (Table 3). A significant ($p<0.05$) main effect of training was also observed for the time to complete the 500 kcal test (Percent change from pre: END: +20.4%, LV-HIT: +15.3%; Fig. 3B).

A main effect of training ($p<0.05$) was demonstrated for fibre distribution of type I and type IIAX/IIX fibres, with the percentage of type I fibres increasing and type IIAX/IIX fibres decreasing following training (Fig. 3D). No effect of training was demonstrated for the percentage fibre distribution for type IIA

Table 3. Experiment 2 participant characteristics (N = 19) for low volume high-intensity interval (LV-HIT) training (n = 10) and endurance (END) training (n = 9) at baseline (pre), mid-training (mid) and following 6 weeks of training (post); mean (SD) unless otherwise indicated.

	END			LV- HIT		
	Pre	Mid	Post	Pre	Mid	Post
Age (yrs)	21(4)	-	-	21(2)	-	-
Height (cm)	180(7)	-	-	175(10)	-	-
Body mass (kg)	74(9)	74(8)	74(9)	71(17)	71(17)	71(17)
Absolute VO_2 (mL/min)*	3534(768)	3743(715)	4050(760)	3440(913)	3703(1007)	3910(1094)
Relative VO_2 (mL/kg/min)*	47.6(8.3)	50.6(7.4)	54.6(7.6)	48.3(6.1)	51.8(6.0)	54.9(6.2)
HRpeak (bpm)*	194(11)	190(9)	191(9)	195(7)	192(6)	193(3)
WRpeak (W)	255(62)	285(56)	281(58)	250(58)	262(53)	258(63)
Wingate peak power (W)*†	718(142)	-	704(147)	654(146)	-	718(184)
Wingate mean power (W)*†	570(119)	-	594(122)	498(141)	-	580(131)

Note: *Main effect of training, $p<0.05$; †significant interaction, $p<0.05$. BPM, beats per minute; cm, centimeters; kg, kilograms; min, minute; mL, milliliter; RER, respiratory exchange ratio; s, seconds; W, watts; yrs, years.

(Fig. 3D) fibres (see representative slides Fig. 3C). A main effect of training ($p<0.05$) was observed for fold change in SDH activity in type I (n = 9), type IIA (n = 9) and type IIAX/IIX (n = 6)(Fig. 3E, see representative slides Fig. 3C). A main effect of training ($p<0.05$) was also observed for estimated oxidative capacity (Fig. 3F).

Cardiovascular capacity and capillary density. A main effect of training ($p<0.05$) was observed for capillary density (Fig. 4B) (see representative slides Fig. 4A) and O_2 pulse (Fig. 4C).

Anaerobic exercise performance and glycolytic capacity. A significant interaction effect ($p<0.05$) and a main effect of training ($p<0.05$) were demonstrated for both peak and mean power in the first Wingate completed (Table 3), and for total work completed across all 4 Wingates (Fig. 5B). A main effect of training ($p<0.05$) was observed for fold change in GPD activity in type I fibres (see representative slides Fig. 5A). There was no effect of training observed for GPD activity in type IIA and IIAX/IIX fibres, while a significant ($p<0.05$) interaction was demonstrated for type IIA fibres (Fig. 5C). There was no main effect of training for estimated glycolytic capacity (Fig. 5D); however, paired students t-tests demonstrated a significant ($p<0.05$) increase in estimated glycolytic capacity post-training (Post) in the LV-HIT group only.

Intramuscular glycogen and triglyceride content. A main effect of training ($p<0.05$) was observed for glycogen content in type I fibres. There was no main effect of training for percent change of glycogen content in type IIA and IIAX/IIX fibres (Fig. 6B, see representative slides Fig. 6A). A main effect of training ($p<0.05$) was observed for IMTG content in type I, IIA and IIAX/IIX fibres (Fig. 6C, see representative slides Fig. 6A).

mRNA expression. Unpaired students t-tests demonstrated no difference in fold change of PGC-1α (END [n = 9]: 1.46±1.10 AU; HIT: 0.87±0.40 AU), general control non-derepressible (GCN) 5 (END [n = 9]: 1.04±0.74 AU; HIT: 0.81±0.45 AU) and receptor-interacting protein (RIP) 140 mRNA (END [n = 9]: 0.98±0.42 AU; HIT: 0.81±0.37 AU) expression between groups, and a significantly ($p<0.05$) higher fold change of silent mating type information regulation 2 homolog 1 (SIRT1) mRNA expression in the END group only (END [n = 9]: 1.19±0.57 AU; HIT: 0.74±0.23 AU) following training.

Discussion

The present study examined both fibre recruitment patterns in response to acute bouts of LV-HIT and END, and fibre-type specific adaptations following 6 weeks of either LV-HIT or END training. In experiment 1, we observed comparable changes in whole-muscle cellular signaling and glycogen depletion derived estimates of fibre recruitment following LV-HIT and END. Consistent with similar responses following the acute exercise bouts, results from experiment 2 demonstrate that 6 weeks of LV-HIT and END training induced comparable increases in aerobic capacity (VO_2peak) and exercise performance (TTC trial), changes in fibre-type distribution, fibre-type specific oxidative and glycolytic capacity, glycogen and IMTG storage, and whole-muscle capillary density. Interestingly, LV-HIT induced greater improvements in anaerobic exercise performance and estimated whole-muscle glycolytic capacity than END.

Experiment 1: Fibre Recruitment Patterns during LV-HIT and END

Whole-muscle measures of signaling pathway activation following acute exercise [19–21], and chronic increases in mitochondrial protein/oxidative capacity [1–3,8,10] are typically comparable following interval training and END. The current study was designed to investigate whether these similarities in whole-muscle measures are masking differences in fibre-type specific adaptations that may help explain the potency of high-intensity exercise and, more specifically, LV-HIT. Fibre recruitment, as indicated by fibre-type specific glycogen depletion, following steady state submaximal exercise is dependent on exercise intensity with type I fibres being preferentially recruited during low intensity exercise and type II fibres being progressively recruited with increasing exercise intensity [24,38,39]. Based on this relationship, we hypothesized that LV-HIT (~170% VO_2peak WR) would result in a greater number of recruited fibres (both type I and II) than END (~65% VO_2peak WR) which would recruit primarily type I fibres.

Contrary to our hypothesis, we observed equivalent reductions ($p<0.05$) in glycogen content in type I and IIA fibres following both protocols (Fig. 1B and C), suggesting that fibre recruitment during LV-HIT and END is comparable. While these data are

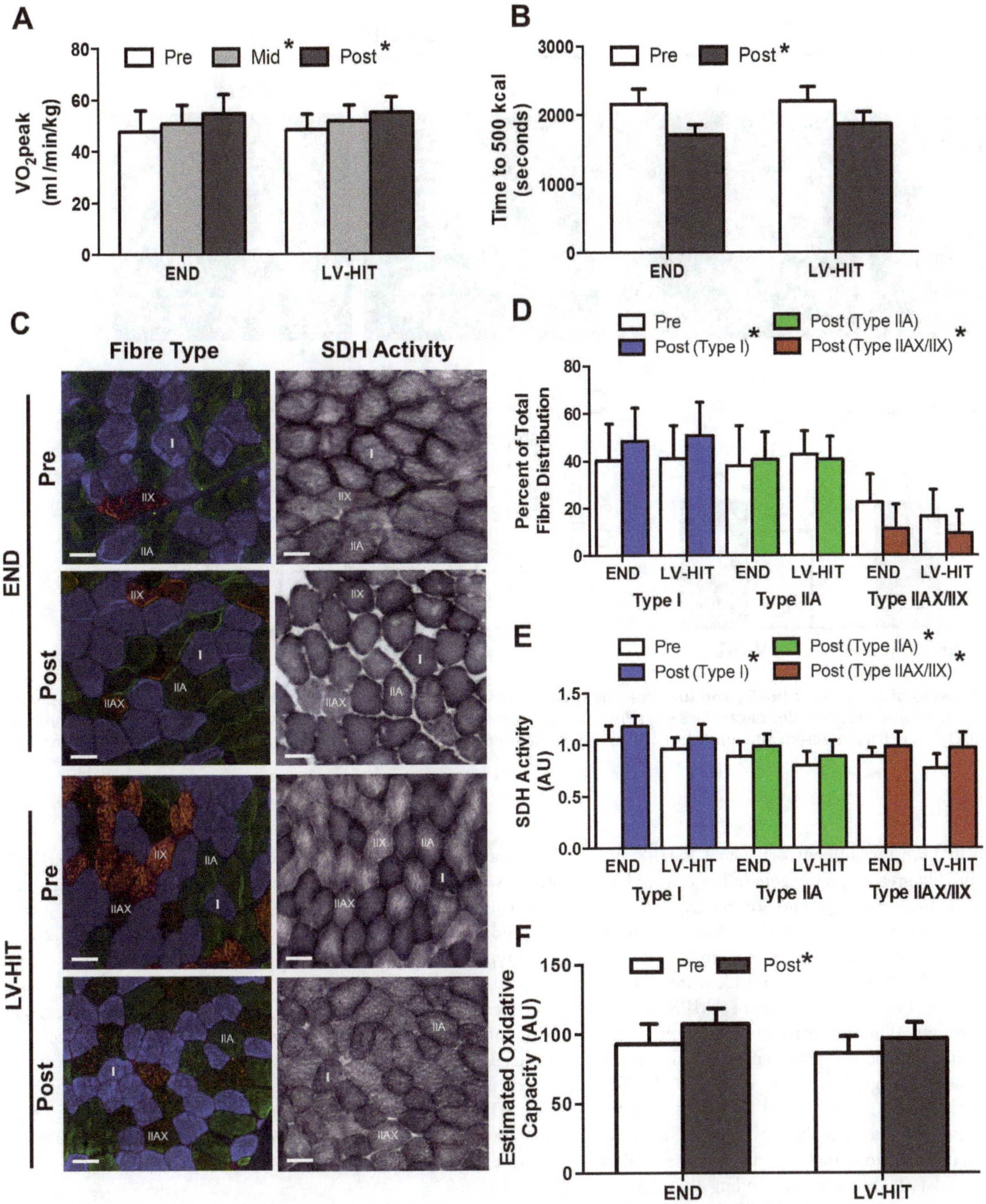

Figure 3. Effects of training (LV-HIT) on aerobic exercise performance, fibre-type distribution and fibre specific oxidative capacity. Relative VO_2peak (A) and time to 500 kcal (B) at Pre, Mid, and Post for both END and LV-HIT groups are shown. C: Representative slides of immunofluorescent fibre-type analysis (blue fibres are type I, green are type IIA, red/green are type IIAX/IIX) with serial sections of succinate dehydrogenase (SDH) activity Pre and Post END or LV-HIT. D: Percentage of total fibre distribution of type I, IIA and IIAX/IIX fibres Pre and Post END or LV-HIT. E: Fibre-type specific fold change in SDH activity post-training compared to pre-training in type I, IIA and IIAX/IIX fibres. F: Absolute change in estimated oxidative capacity. Bars represent 100 μm. AU, arbitrary units; μm, micrometre. *Significant ($p<0.05$) main effect of exercise.

consistent with both type I and IIA fibres being recruited during supramaximal exercise [22–25], the observed glycogen depletion in both fibre types following END is somewhat surprising [24,25,38]. Regardless, in combination with previous demonstrations of type IIA fibre glycogen depletion during submaximal exercise [38,39] our results suggest that there is a threshold intensity associated with the recruitment of a significant percentage of type IIA fibres and that this threshold is below ~65% of VO_2peak. Thus, it would appear that similarities in whole-muscle measures of signaling pathway activation between interval training and END observed previously [19–21], and between LV-HIT and END observed in the current study (Fig. 2), likely result from similar fibre recruitment patterns.

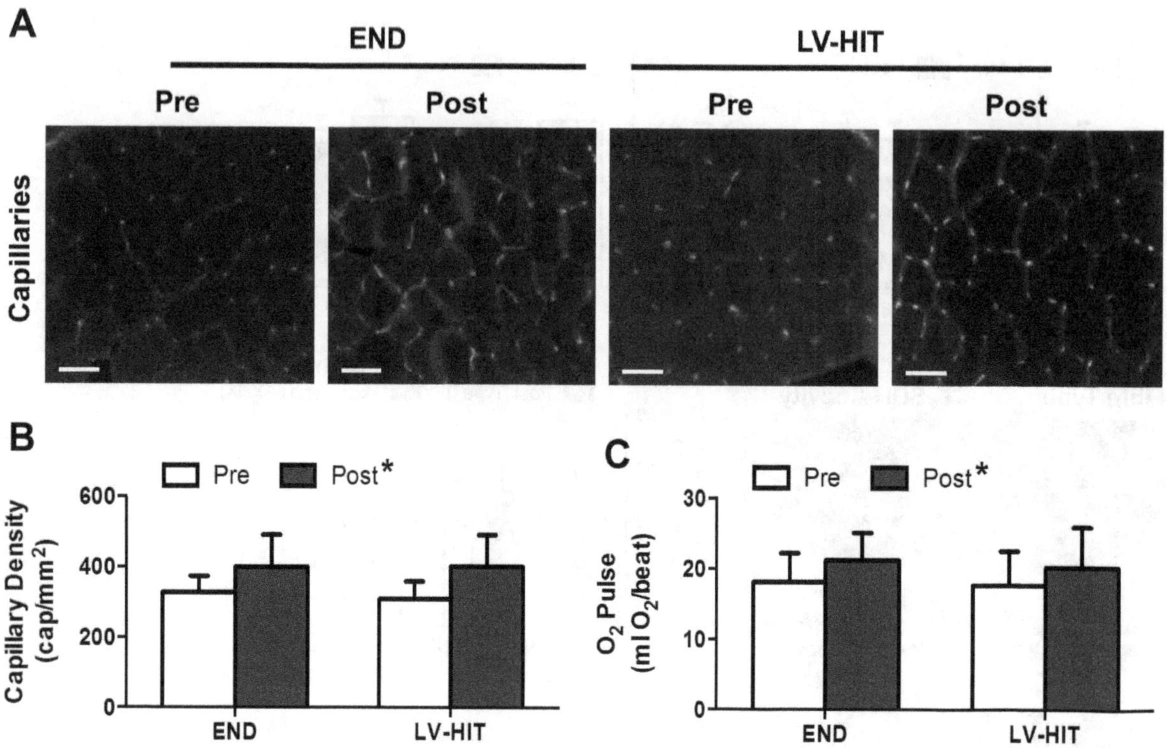

Figure 4. Effects of 6 weeks of endurance (END) and low-volume high-intensity interval training (LV-HIT) on cardiovascular capacity and capillary density. A: Representative slides of capillarisation Pre and Post training. B: Absolute change in capillary density (capillaries/mm^2). C: Change in O_2 pulse (mL O_2/beat). Bars represent 100 µm. mL, milliliter; mm, millimeter; O_2, oxygen; µm, micrometre. *Significant ($p<0.05$) main effect of exercise.

Given the equivalent fibre recruitment between LV-HIT and END, and the substantially greater power generation during LV-HIT, it seems reasonable to assume that a greater relative intensity of signal activation would be experienced within individual fibres during LV-HIT. It is therefore somewhat surprising that fibre-type specific phosphorylation of AMPK (Fig. 1D and E), whole-muscle phosphorylation of ACC (a downstream target of AMPK; Fig. 2) and p38 MAPK were not different between conditions. This finding is consistent with a previous report demonstrating similar activation of intramuscular signaling between END (~70% VO_2max) and submaximal (~90% VO_2max) HIT [19], but not with the recent observation that signaling events are intensity dependent when continuous submaximal exercise (~40 vs. ~80% VO_2peak) was compared [40]. Further, the finding that AMPK and p38 phosphorylation were not increased following LV-HIT is in contrast to observation made following SIT [18]. The reasons for this discrepancy in intramuscular signalling are unclear, however the brevity of the LV-HIT protocol utilized in the current study, compared to the longer duration of SIT protocols utilized previously, suggests that the duration of exercise may be an important factor underlying the activation of these pathways. Collectively, these results suggest that END exercise at an intensity >65% VO_2peak results in both similar fibre recruitment and activation of intramuscular signaling pathways as more intense, lower dose HIT. Additionally, it appears that the intensity/duration threshold required to activate intracellular signaling events associated with the induction of mitochondrial biogenesis within an individual muscle fibre is achieved by both LV-HIT and END exercise at intensities equal to, or greater than 65% VO_2peak and a duration of at least 30 minutes [19,40]. This assertion is supported by the presence of similar levels of PGC-1α mRNA and other genes related to mitochondrial biogenesis following 90 minutes of continuous submaximal (~65% VO_2peak) and supramaximal (~120% VO_2peak) interval exercise [20,21] in both type I and IIA fibres [21].

In summary, experiment 1 of the current study demonstrated that recruitment of muscle fibres (type I and IIA) during a single bout of LV-HIT or END are similar, as is activation of intracellular signaling pathways. Given that type I and IIA fibres represent ~90% of the total fibre population of the vastus lateralis (Fig. 3D) [30], the assumption that changes in both type I and type IIA fibres are accurately reflected in whole-muscle measures of intracellular signaling appears to be appropriate.

Experiment 2: Fibre Specific Adaptations to LV-HIT and END Training

Exercise training increases the maximal activity and content of mitochondrial enzymes involved in oxidative metabolism, capillary density, and intramuscular triglyceride and glycogen stores [1–4,6,8,10,11]. Collectively, these adaptations contribute to improved skeletal muscle oxidative potential, fatty acid oxidative capacity, and improve aerobic capacity and exercise performance (VO_2peak, time to fatigue trials, etc.). Based on the recent argument that improvements in aerobic capacity and performance following interval training are driven primarily by peripheral adaptations [14,15], and the previously discussed hypothesis that LV-HIT would recruit additional different muscle fibres than END, we examined fibre-type specific adaptations to both LV-HIT and END training.

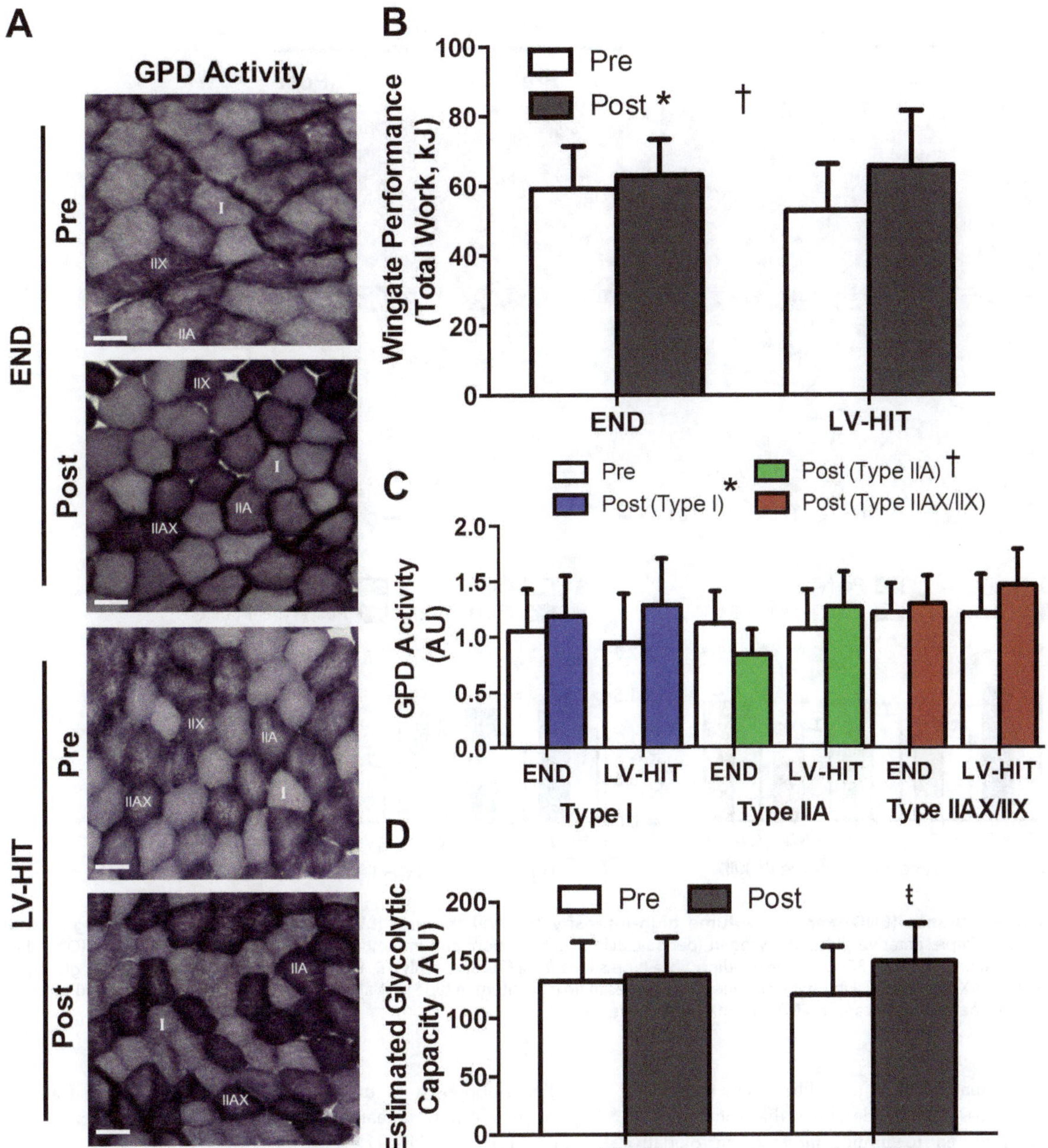

Figure 5. Effects of endurance (END) and low-volume high-intensity interval training (LV-HIT) on anaerobic exercise performance and glycolytic capacity. A: Representative slides of α-glycerophosphate dehydrogenase (GPD) activity Pre and Post training (see Fig. 3C for corresponding fibre-type slides). B: Total work performed during all 4 Wingate bouts. C: Fibre-type specific fold change in GPD activity post-training compared to pre-training in type I, IIA and IIAX/IIX fibres. D: Absolute change in estimated glycolytic capacity. Bars represent 100 μm. AU, arbitrary units; μm, micrometre. †Significant ($p<0.05$) group by time interaction, *Significant ($p<0.05$) main effect of exercise, ǂSignificant ($p<0.05$) within group difference (derived from paired t-test).

Aerobic Exercise Performance and Oxidative Capacity

As has been previously observed [9,12], we demonstrated similar improvements in VO_2peak and aerobic exercise performance (Fig. 3A and B) following 6 weeks of LV-HIT and END. Consistent with these whole body adaptations, comparable increases in SDH activity, a mitochondrial protein correlated with mitochondrial content [41], were observed across all fibre-types following both LV-HIT and END (Fig. 3E). Additionally, changes in whole muscle gene expression of proteins associated with mitochondrial biogenesis were similar following both training protocols. While others have reported comparable increases in fibre specific cytochorome c oxidase (COX) protein content following SIT and END [3], COX is not highly correlated with mitochondrial content ($r = 0.55$) [41]. Our results supports these assumptions but are derived from SDH activity, a protein which correlates much more highly with mitochondrial content ($r = 0.73$) [41]. These adaptations are also consistent with the muscle fibre activation patterns observed during a single bout of LV-HIT and END in experiment 1 suggesting that recruitment of fibres during repeated acute bouts of LV-HIT and END (i.e. training) results in

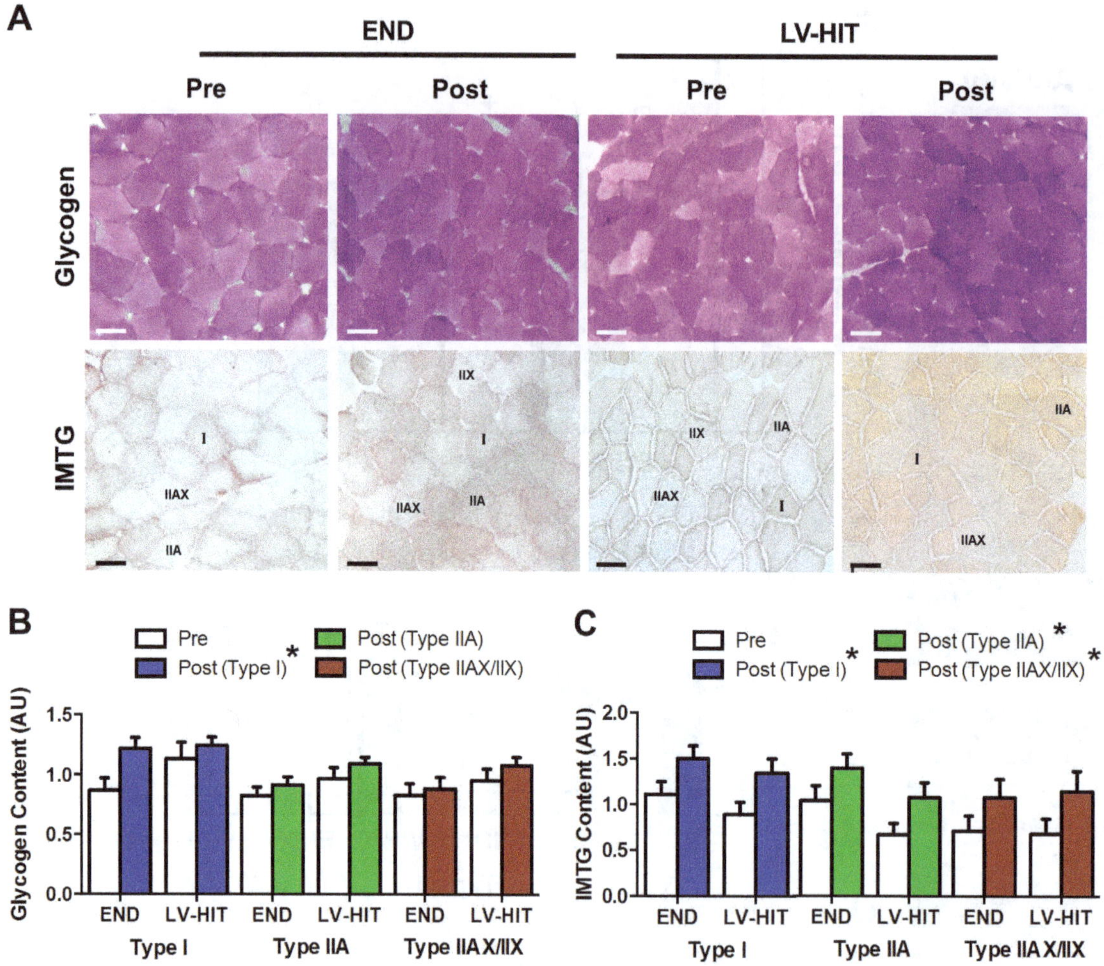

Figure 6. Effects of endurance (END) and low-volume high-intensity interval training (LV-HIT) on intramuscular glycogen and triglyceride storage. A: Representative slides of glycogen (periodic acid-Schiff reaction) and intramuscular triglyceride (IMTG) content (Oil red O staining) Pre and Post training (see Fig. 3C for corresponding fibre-type slides for IMTG stain only). B. Fibre-type specific fold changes in glycogen content in type I, IIA and IIAX/IIX fibres. C. Fibre-type specific fold changes in IMTG content in type I, IIA and IIAX/IIX fibres. Bars represent 100 µm. AU, arbitrary units; µm, micrometre. *Significant ($p<0.05$) main effect of exercise.

increases in oxidative capacity within those fibres. The results also further strengthen the assertion made above that the intensity/duration threshold required to induce increases in oxidative capacity within a given fibre are reached by both the LV-HIT and END protocols utilized in the present study.

Further, both groups demonstrated an increased proportion of type I fibres concomitant with a reduction in type IIAX/IIX fibres (Fig. 3D). While several studies have demonstrated myofiber transitions resulting in a greater percentage of oxidative fibres (type I) following HIT and END training [42,43], our results are not consistent with several reports demonstrating increases in type IIA fibres with concurrent reductions in type I fibres following several weeks of SIT [44–47]. While the exact mechanism(s) responsible for contraction-induced changes in myofiber composition remain to be completely described, contraction frequency has been demonstrated to influence fibre-type synthesis [48] with high-frequency activation inducing the synthesis of fast twitch myosin. Importantly, our END and LV-HIT protocols required participants to cycle at the same speed (80 RPM), while the load was changed in order to manipulate training intensity. This may explain why we observed increases in type I fibres and reductions in type IIAX/IIX fibres following 6 weeks of both LV-HIT and END, as opposed to those studies employing SIT, a training protocol typically demanding maximal pedaling frequency and contraction rates [44–47].

Combined, the increases in fibre-type specific SDH activity and the increase proportion of type I fibres resulted in an increase in estimated whole-muscle oxidative capacity (Fig. 3F) following both training protocols. These results support prior observations of comparable increases in whole-muscle markers of oxidative capacity and enzymes associated with oxidative metabolism [1,3,18,49,50] following HIT or SIT and END training. We also observed similar increases in capillary density (Fig. 4B), data which are consistent with previous studies reporting comparable increases in capillary density following SIT and END [4,6,11]. While these results are in agreement with improvements in aerobic capacity and performance following interval training being mediated by peripheral adaptations, the similar changes in estimated oxidative capacity, capillary density and O_2 pulse in both groups (Fig. 4C) are not consistent with suggestions that increases in VO_2peak are supported by different mechanisms following LV-HIT and END [14].

Anaerobic Exercise Performance and Glycolytic Capacity

Six weeks of LV-HIT and END resulted in improved anaerobic exercise performance (total work; Fig. 5B) and anaerobic capacity (peak and mean power; Table 3). Importantly, improvements for all indices of anaerobic performance/capacity were greater for LV-HIT than END. Consistent with these results, changes in GPD activity were similar in type I fibres (Fig. 5C) while a significant interaction effect was observed in type IIA fibres such that an increased GPD activity was only observed in this fibre population following LV-HIT. Additionally, our estimate of whole-muscle glycolytic capacity demonstrated a trend towards an increase following LV-HIT only (no main effect of training; paired t-test significant within LV-HIT only; Fig. 5D). These results are consistent with previous demonstrations that HIT and SIT improve anaerobic exercise performance [1,49], while changes in glycolytic enzyme activity have been observed following SIT but not END [5,50–52]. While the exact mechanisms responsible for our observed differences in anaerobic exercise capacity and performance between groups are unknown, it appears that they may be attributable to factors beyond the peripheral skeletal muscle adaptations examined in the present study. One such peripheral factor could be an improved skeletal muscle lactic acid buffering capacity, which has been observed following SIT [8], but not HIT [53]. Another potential mechanism may be differences in adaptations of central origin, such as rate of fibre recruitment, firing rate and motor unit synchronization. SIT in conjunction with END training results in increased motor unit recruitment and total work performed during a repeated Wingate test compared to END training alone [54], which suggests that improvements in neuromuscular characteristics may partially explain the greater improvements in Wingate performance and anaerobic capacity following LV-HIT.

Limitations and Future Directions

The sample size of experiment 1 ($n = 6$) was relatively small and it is therefore possible that a larger sample size may have yielded different results. However, while an increased sample size might have allowed for subtle differences between LV-HIT and END to be detected (for both glycogen depletion and intramuscular signalling), we do not believe that the limited statistical power associated with the small sample studies impaired our ability to conclude that both type I and IIA fibres are recruited during both of exercise protocols examined in the current study. Additionally, we have observed a dissociation between phosphorylation of AMPK and phosphorylation of ACC, an interesting result that reflects previously published results [18,40,55]. While we are unable to comment with certainty regarding why this dissociation exists, it is possible that differential phosphorylation of $\alpha 1$ and $\alpha 2$ AMPK sub-units [56,57] may impair the ability to estimate changes in AMPK activity based on changes in global AMPK phosphorytion. Thus, while we were unable to conduct this analysis on samples from the present study, the potential that phosphorylation of ACC is a more sensitive measure of AMPK activity than phosphorylation of AMPK itself raises the possibility the fibre specific differences in ACC phosphorylation may be present following exercise. This represents an important area for future research. It would also be of interest to investigate whether similar acute activation of intramuscular signalling pathways following LV-HIT and END result similar activation and expression of PGC-1α and other genes associated with the induction of mitochondrial biogenesis in the hours following exercise.

Perspectives/Conclusions

Numerous recent investigations have attempted to elucidate the mechanisms by which interval training and END training induce similar improvements in aerobic capacity and exercise performance (VO_2peak, time to fatigue trails, etc.) [18,19,40,55,58]. Collectively, these studies suggest that the intramuscular signaling required to elicit these adaptations are equivalently stimulated by both low intensity exercise of long duration and high-intensity exercise of short duration. While the minimum duration of low intensity exercise required to elicit adaptation remains unknown, very brief bouts of high-intensity exercise appear to be sufficient [9,12,13]. From an exercise prescription perspective, exercise resulting in the largest degree of intramuscular signaling activation in the greatest amount of muscle fibres would presumably result in the greatest degree of adaptation. What remains largely unknown, however, is whether differences in fibre recruitment and the magnitude of signal activation within individual fibre-types between interval training and END exercise are obscured by whole muscle analyses. Our results demonstrate that LV-HIT and END produce similar: a) glycogen depletion across fibre types (indicative of similar fibre recruitment), b) changes in intramuscular signaling, and c) fibre-type specific increases in oxidative capacity, intramuscular glycogen and triglyceride content, whole-muscle capillary density and O_2pulse. Remarkably, these results suggest that 30 minutes of END exercise at $\sim$65% VO_2peak or 4 minutes of LV-HIT at $\sim$170% VO_2peak induce comparable deviations of the intra-myocellular environment (glycogen content and signaling activation); correspondingly, training-induced adaptations resulting for these protocols, and other interval training and END protocols [1,8], appear comparable. The one exception to this equivocality is the capacity of LV-HIT to induce greater improvements in anaerobic adaptations than END. Thus, our results suggest that the mechanisms responsible for adaptation following chronic LV-HIT and END are the same, with the supramaximal exercise intensity inherent with LV-HIT permitting their manifestation in significantly less exercise time.

Collectively, results from this study suggest that the potency of high-intensity exercise resides is its ability to activate the mechanisms that trigger the induction of exercise-induced adaptation in a drastically reduced exercise time compared to traditional END training. However, while END exercise at intensities greater than $\sim$65% VO_2peak are of adequate intensity to elicit "maximal" fibre recruitment (i.e. type I and IIA fibres) and the manifestation of chronic adaptations, at present the minimal duration of exercise at these relatively low intensities required for comparable adaptations is not known. Our results, and others [9], suggest that 30 minutes is adequate; however, given that our assumptions regarding the minimal dose of exercise required for adaptations having been recently challenged [59,60], the minimal duration of moderate intensity END required to induce adaptation is an interesting area for future research.

Acknowledgments

We would like to thank a very dedicated group of volunteers without whom this study would not have been possible.

Author Contributions

Conceived and designed the experiments: TDS BJG. Performed the experiments: TDS BAE KV ASM. Analyzed the data: TDS BAE KV ASM JBM SDJ GP JQ BJG. Contributed reagents/materials/analysis tools: GP JQ BJG. Wrote the paper: TDS BJG.

References

1. Burgomaster KA, Howarth KR, Phillips SM, Rakobowchuk M, MacDonald MJ, et al. (2008) Similar metabolic adaptations during exercise after low volume sprint interval and traditional endurance training in humans. J Physiol 586: 151–160. doi:10.1113/jphysiol.2007.142109.
2. Saltin B, Nazar K, Costill DL, Stein E, Jansson E, et al. (1976) The Nature of the Training Response; Peripheral and Central Adaptations to One-Legged Exercise. Acta Physiol Scand 96: 289–305.
3. Shepherd SO, Cocks M, Tipton KD, Ranasinghe AM, Barker TA, et al. (2013) Sprint interval and traditional endurance training increase net intramuscular triglyceride breakdown and expression of perilipin 2 and 5. J Physiol 591: 657–675. doi:10.1113/jphysiol.2012.240952.
4. Cocks M, Shaw CS, Shepherd SO, Fisher JP, Ranasinghe AM, et al. (2013) Sprint interval and endurance training are equally effective in increasing muscle microvascular density and eNOS content in sedentary males. J Physiol 591: 641–656. doi:10.1113/jphysiol.2012.239566.
5. Fournier M, Ricci J, Taylor AW, Ferguson RJ, Montpetit RR, et al. (1982) Skeletal muscle adaptation in adolescent boys: sprint and endurance training and detraining. Med Sci Sports Exerc 14: 453–456.
6. Daussin FN, Zoll J, Dufour SP, Ponsot E, Lonsdorfer-Wolf E, et al. (2008) Effect of interval versus continuous training on cardiorespiratory and mitochondrial functions: relationship to aerobic performance improvements in sedentary subjects. Am J Physiol Regul Integr Comp Physiol 295: R264–R272. doi:10.1152/ajpregu.00875.2007.
7. Eddy DO, Sparks KL, Adelizi DA (1977) The effects of continuous and interval training in women and men. Eur J Appl Physiol Occup Physiol 37: 83–92.
8. Gibala MJ, Little JP, van Essen M, Wilkin GP, Burgomaster KA, et al. (2006) Short-term sprint interval versus traditional endurance training: similar initial adaptations in human skeletal muscle and exercise performance. J Physiol 575: 901–911. doi:10.1113/jphysiol.2006.112094.
9. McRae G, Payne A, Zelt JGE, Scribbans TD, Jung ME, et al. (2012) Extremely low volume, whole-body aerobic-resistance training improves aerobic fitness and muscular endurance in females. Appl Physiol Nutr Metab. 37: 1124–1131. doi:10.1139/h2012-093.
10. Terada S, Tabata I, Higuchi M (2004) Effect of high-intensity intermittent swimming training on fatty acid oxidation enzyme activity in rat skeletal muscle. Jpn J Physiol 54: 47–52.
11. Vogiatzis I, Terzis G, Nanas S, Stratakos G, Simoes DCM, et al. (2005) Skeletal muscle adaptations to interval training in patients with advanced COPD. Chest 128: 3838–3845. doi:10.1378/chest.128.6.3838.
12. Tabata I, Nishimura K, Kouzaki M, Hirai Y, Ogita F, et al. (1996) Effects of moderate-intensity endurance and high-intensity intermittent training on anaerobic capacity and VO2max. Med Sci Sports Exerc 28: 1327–1330.
13. Ma JK, Scribbans TD, Edgett BA, Colin Boyd J, Simpson CA, et al. (2013) Extremely low-volume, high-intensity interval training improves exercise capacity and increases mitochondrial protein content in human skeletal muscle. OJMIP 03: 202–210. doi:10.4236/ojmip.2013.34027.
14. MacPherson REK, Hazell TJ, Olver TD, Paterson DH, Lemon PWR (2011) Run Sprint Interval Training Improves Aerobic Performance but Not Maximal Cardiac Output. Med Sci Sports Exerc 43: 115–122. doi:10.1249/MSS.0b013e3181e5eacd.
15. Jacobs RA, Lundby C (2013) Mitochondria express enhanced quality as well as quantity in association with aerobic fitness across recreationally active individuals up to elite athletes. J Appl Physiol 114: 344–350. doi:10.1152/japplphysiol.01081.2012.
16. Pilegaard H, Saltin B, Neufer PD (2003) Exercise induces transient transcriptional activation of the PGC-1 gene in human skeletal muscle. J Physiol 546: 851–858. doi:10.1113/jphysiol.2002.034850.
17. Wright DC, Han D-H, Garcia-Roves PM, Geiger PC, Jones TE, et al. (2007) Exercise-induced Mitochondrial Biogenesis Begins before the Increase in Muscle PGC-1 Expression. J Biol Chem 282: 194–199.
18. Gibala MJ, McGee SL, Garnham AP, Howlett KF, Snow RJ, et al. (2009) Brief intense interval exercise activates AMPK and p38 MAPK signaling and increases the expression of PGC-1 in human skeletal muscle. J Appl Physiol 106: 929–934. doi:10.1152/japplphysiol.90880.2008.
19. Bartlett JD, Hwa Joo C, Jeong TS, Louhelainen J, Cochran AJ, et al. (2012) Matched work high-intensity interval and continuous running induce similar increases in PGC-1 mRNA, AMPK, p38, and p53 phosphorylation in human skeletal muscle. J Appl Physiol 112: 1135–1143. doi:10.1152/japplphysiol.01040.2011.
20. Wang L, Psilander N, Tonkonogi M, Ding S, Sahlin K (2009) Similar Expression of Oxidative Genes after Interval and Continuous Exercise. Med Sci Sports Exerc 41: 2136–2144. doi:10.1249/MSS.0b013e3181abc1ec.
21. Wang L, Sahlin K (2011) The effect of continuous and interval exercise on PGC-1α and PDK4 mRNA in type I and type II fibres of human skeletal muscle. Acta Physiologica 204: 525–532. doi:10.1111/j.1748-1716.2011.02354.x.
22. Greenhaff PLP, Nevill MEM, Soderlund KK, Bodin KK, Boobis LHL, et al. (1994) The metabolic responses of human type I and II muscle fibres during maximal treadmill sprinting. J Physiol 478 (Pt 1): 149–155.
23. Vøllestad NK, Tabata I, Medbø JI (1992) Glycogen breakdown in different human muscle fibre types during exhaustive exercise of short duration. Acta Physiol Scand 144: 135–141.
24. Gollnick PD, Piehl K, Saltin B (1974) Selective glycogen depletion pattern in human muscle fibres after exercise of varying intensity and at varying pedalling rates. J Physiol 241: 45–57.
25. Essén B (1978) Glycogen depletion of different fibre types in human skeletal muscle during intermittent and continuous exercise. Acta Physiol Scand 103: 446–455. doi:10.1111/j.1748-1716.1978.tb06239.x.
26. Edgett BA, Foster WS, Hankinson PB, Simpson CA, Little JP, et al. (2013) Dissociation of Increases in PGC-1α and Its Regulators from Exercise Intensity and Muscle Activation Following Acute Exercise. PLoS One 8: e71623. doi:10.1371/journal.pone.0071623.t003.
27. Bergstrom J (1975) Percutaneous needle biopsy of skeletal muscle in physiological and clinical research. Scand J Clin Lab Invest 35: 609–616.
28. Jeukendrup A, Saris WH, Brouns F, Kester AD (1996) A new validated endurance performance test. Med Sci Sports Exerc 28: 266–270.
29. Boyd JC, Simpson CA, Jung ME, Gurd BJ (2013) Reducing the Intensity and Volume of Interval Training Diminishes Cardiovascular Adaptation but Not Mitochondrial Biogenesis in Overweight/Obese Men. PLoS One 8: e68091. doi:10.1371/journal.pone.0068091.t002.
30. Bloemberg D, Quadrilatero J (2012) Rapid Determination of Myosin Heavy Chain Expression in Rat, Mouse, and Human Skeletal Muscle Using Multicolor Immunofluorescence Analysis. PLoS One 7: e35273. doi:10.1371/journal.pone.0035273.t005.
31. Cebasek V, Kubínová L, Ribaric S, Erzen I (2004) A novel staining method for quantification and 3D visualisation of capillaries and muscle fibres. Eur J Histochem 48: 151–158.
32. Lee-Young RS, Canny BJ, Myers DE, McConell GK (2009) AMPK activation is fiber type specific in human skeletal muscle: effects of exercise and short-term exercise training. J Appl Physiol 107: 283–289. doi:10.1152/japplphysiol.91208.2008.
33. Blanco CE, Sieck GC, Edgerton VR (1988) Quantitative histochemical determination of succinic dehydrogenase activity in skeletal muscle fibres. Histochem J 20: 230–243.
34. Halkjaer-Kristensen JJ, Ingemann-Hansen TT (1979) Microphotometric analysis of NADH-tetrazolium reductase and alpha-glycerophosphate dehydrogenase in human quadriceps muscle. Histochem J 11: 127–136.
35. Koopman RR, Schaart GG, Hesselink MKM (2001) Optimisation of oil red O staining permits combination with immunofluorescence and automated quantification of lipids. Histochem Cell Biol 116: 63–68. doi:10.1007/s004180100297.
36. Quadrilatero J, Bombardier E, Norris SM, Talanian JL, Palmer MS, et al. (2010) Prolonged moderate-intensity aerobic exercise does not alter apoptotic signaling and DNA fragmentation in human skeletal muscle. Am J Physiol Endocrinol Metab 298: E534–E547. doi:10.1152/ajpendo.00678.2009.
37. Livak KJ, Schmittgen TD (2001) Analysis of relative gene expression data using real-time quantitative PCR and the 2(-Delta Delta C(T)) Method. Methods 25: 402–408. doi:10.1006/meth.2001.1262.
38. Vøllestad NKN, Blom PCP (1985) Effect of varying exercise intensity on glycogen depletion in human muscle fibres. Acta Physiol Scand 125: 395–405.
39. Vøllestad NK, Vaage O, Hermansen L (1984) Muscle glycogen depletion patterns in type I and subgroups of type II fibres during prolonged severe exercise in man. Acta Physiol Scand 122: 433–441. doi:10.1111/j.1748-1716.1984.tb07531.x.
40. Egan B, Carson BP, Garcia-Roves PM, Chibalin AV, Sarsfield FM, et al. (2010) Exercise intensity-dependent regulation of peroxisome proliferator-activated receptor γ coactivator-1α mRNA abundance is associated with differential activation of upstream signalling kinases in human skeletal muscle. J Physiol 588: 1779–1790. doi:10.1113/jphysiol.2010.188011.
41. Larsen S, Nielsen J, Hansen CN, Nielsen LB, Wibrand F, et al. (2012) Biomarkers of mitochondrial content in skeletal muscle of healthy young human subjects. J Physiol 590: 3349–3360. doi:10.1113/jphysiol.2012.230185.
42. Russell AP, Feilchenfeldt J, Schreiber S, Praz M, Crettenand A, et al. (2003) Endurance training in humans leads to fiber type-specific increases in levels of peroxisome proliferator-activated receptor-γ coactivator-1 and peroxisome proliferator-activated receptor-α in skeletal muscle. Diabetes 52: 2874–2881.
43. Simoneau JA, Lortie G, Boulay MR, Marcotte M, Thibault MC, et al. (1985) Human skeletal muscle fiber type alteration with high-intensity intermittent training. Eur J Appl Physiol Occup Physiol 54: 250–253.
44. Jansson E, Esbjörnsson M, Holm I, Jacobs I (1990) Increase in the proportion of fast-twitch muscle fibres by sprint training in males. Acta Physiol Scand 140: 359–363.
45. Allemeier CA, Fry AC, Johnson P, Hikida RS, Hagerman FC, et al. (1994) Effects of sprint cycle training on human skeletal muscle. J Appl Physiol 77: 2385–2390.
46. Esbjörnsson MM, Hellsten-Westing YY, Balsom PDP, Sjödin BB, Jansson EE (1993) Muscle fibre type changes with sprint training: effect of training pattern. Acta Physiol Scand 149: 245–246.
47. Dawson B, Fitzsimons M, Green S, Goodman C, Carey M, et al. (1998) Changes in performance, muscle metabolites, enzymes and fibre types after short sprint training. Eur J Appl Physiol Occup Physiol 78: 163–169.
48. Pette D, Vrbová G (1985) Invited review: neural control of phenotypic expression in mammalian muscle fibers. Muscle Nerve 8: 676–689.

49. Burgomaster KA, Hughes SC, Heigenhauser GJF, Bradwell SN, Gibala MJ (2005) Six sessions of sprint interval training increases muscle oxidative potential and cycle endurance capacity in humans. J Appl Physiol 98: 1985–1990. doi:10.1152/japplphysiol.01095.2004.
50. Rodas G, Ventura JL, Cadefau JA, Cussó R, Parra J (2000) A short training programme for the rapid improvement of both aerobic and anaerobic metabolism. Eur J Appl Physiol 82: 480–486. doi:10.1007/s004210000223.
51. MacDougall JD, Hicks AL, MacDonald JR, McKelvie RS, Green HJ, et al. (1998) Muscle performance and enzymatic adaptations to sprint interval training. J Appl Physiol 84: 2138–2142.
52. Phillips SM, Green HJ, Tarnopolsky MA, Heigenhauser GJ, Grant SM (1996) Progressive effect of endurance training on metabolic adaptations in working skeletal muscle. Am J Physiol 270: E265–E272.
53. Bishop D, Edge J, Thomas C, Mercier J (2008) Effects of high-intensity training on muscle lactate transporters and postexercise recovery of muscle lactate and hydrogen ions in women. Am J Physiol Regul Integr Comp Physiol 295: R1991–R1998. doi:10.1152/ajpregu.00863.2007.
54. Creer AR, Ricard MD, Conlee RK, Hoyt GL, Parcell AC (2004) Neural, metabolic, and performance adaptations to four weeks of high intensity sprint-interval training in trained cyclists. Int J Sports Med 25: 92–98. doi:10.1055/s-2004-819945.
55. Little JP, Safdar A, Cermak N, Tarnopolsky MA, Gibala MJ (2010) Acute endurance exercise increases the nuclear abundance of PGC-1 in trained human skeletal muscle. Am J Physiol Regul Integr Comp Physiol 298: R912–R917. doi:10.1152/ajpregu.00409.2009.
56. Treebak JT, Birk JB, Rose AJ, Kiens B, Richter EA, et al. (2007) AS160 phosphorylation is associated with activation of alpha2beta2gamma1- but not alpha2beta2gamma3-AMPK trimeric complex in skeletal muscle during exercise in humans. Am J Physiol Endocrinol Metab 292: E715–E722. doi:10.1152/ajpendo.00380.2006.
57. Birk JB, Wojtaszewski JFP (2006) Predominant α2/β2/3 AMPK activation during exercise in human skeletal muscle. J Physiol 577: 1021–1032. doi:10.1113/jphysiol.2006.120972.
58. Little JP, Safdar A, Bishop D, Tarnopolsky MA, Gibala MJ (2011) An acute bout of high-intensity interval training increases the nuclear abundance of PGC-1 and activates mitochondrial biogenesis in human skeletal muscle. Am J Physiol Regul Integr Comp Physiol 300: R1303–R1310. doi:10.1152/ajpregu.00538.2010.
59. Tjønna AE, Leinan IM, Bartnes AT, Jenssen BM, Gibala MJ, et al. (2013) Low- and High-Volume of Intensive Endurance Training Significantly Improves Maximal Oxygen Uptake after 10-Weeks of Training in Healthy Men. PLoS One 8: e65382. doi:10.1371/journal.pone.0065382.s002.
60. Hazell TJ, MacPherson REK, Gravelle BMR, Lemon PWR (2010) 10 or 30-s sprint interval training bouts enhance both aerobic and anaerobic performance. Eur J Appl Physiol 110: 153–160. doi:10.1007/s00421-010-1474-y.

8

Prevalence of Metabolic Syndrome in COPD Patients and Its Consequences

Marie-Kathrin Breyer[1,2,3]*, Martijn A. Spruit[2], Corrine K. Hanson[4], Frits M. E. Franssen[2], Lowie E. G. W. Vanfleteren[2], Miriam T. J. Groenen[2], Piet L. B. Bruijnzeel[5], Emiel F. M. Wouters[1,2], Erica P. A. Rutten[2]

1 Department of Respiratory Medicine, Maastricht University Medical Center + (MUMC+), Maastricht, the Netherlands, **2** Program Development Center (CIRO), Center of expertise for chronic organ failure, Horn, the Netherlands, **3** Department of Respiratory and Critical Care Medicine and Ludwig Boltzmann Institute for COPD and Pulmonary Epidemiology, Otto Wagner Hospital, Vienna, Austria, **4** Division of Medical Nutrition Education, School of Allied Health Professions, University of Nebraska Medical Center, Ohmaha, Nebraska, United States of America, **5** Inflammation Neuroscience and Respiratory, AstraZeneca, Molndal, Sweden

Abstract

Background: The prevalence of metabolic syndrome in COPD patients and its impact on patient related outcomes has been little studied. We evaluated the prevalence of metabolic syndrome and clinical and functional characteristics in patients with COPD and healthy subjects.

Methods: 228 COPD patients and 156 healthy subjects were included. Metabolic syndrome was defined using criteria of the IDF. In all patients spirometry, body composition, functional exercise performance, and mood and health status were assessed. Groups were stratified for BMI and gender.

Results: Metabolic syndrome was present in 57% of the COPD patients and 40% of the healthy subjects. After stratification for BMI, presence of metabolic syndrome in patients with a BMI ≥25 kg/m^2 was higher than in healthy peers. Patients with metabolic syndrome and a BMI <25 kg/m^2 had higher BMI, fat free mass index and bone mineral density, and a lower 6MWD than the BMI matched patients without metabolic syndrome. Spirometry, maximal ergometry, mood and health status, and blood gases were not different between those groups. In COPD patients with metabolic syndrome self-reported co-morbidities and medication use were higher than in those without.

Conclusion: Metabolic syndrome is more prevalent in overweight or obese COPD patients than in BMI matched healthy subjects. Metabolic syndrome did not additionally impact patients' functional outcomes, but did impact the prevalence of co-morbidities.

Editor: Joseph Devaney, Children's National Medical Center, Washington, United States of America

Funding: MKB was funded by the Ludwig Boltzmann Institute for COPD and Respiratory Epidemiology, Vienna, Austria. AstraZeneca provided support in the form of a salary for author PLBB, but did not have any additional role in the study design, data collection and analysis, decision to publish, or preparation of the manuscript. The specific roles of the authors are articulated in the author contributions section.

Competing Interests: PLBB is an employee of AstraZeneca. EFMW is a member of the scientific advisory boards for GSK, Nycomed and Novartis and received lecture fees from GSK, AstraZeneca, Nycomed, Numico and Novartis. There are no patents, products in development or marketed products to declare.

* Email: marie.breyer@gmx.at

Introduction

Chronic obstructive pulmonary disease (COPD) is characterized by persistent airflow limitation that is usually progressive. Additionally, exacerbations and co-existing morbidities contribute to the overall severity in the individual patient [1]. Indeed, cardiovascular co-morbidities are common in COPD [2] and are associated with an increased mortality risk [3,4]. So far, the underlying mechanisms are only partially understood. In addition to smoking, other factors may contribute including advanced age, medications, systemic inflammation and metabolic disturbances.

Metabolic syndrome is a common metabolic disorder defined as a complex of interrelated cardiovascular risk factors [5]. Metabolic syndrome is age dependent [6] and has been related to several other health conditions [7] and an increased mortality risk [8]. In addition, metabolic syndrome has clinically relevant negative effects on subjects exercise capacity [9], as well as on health status [10], while protective effects are described on bone mineral density (BMD) [11].

To date, the prevalence of metabolic syndrome in COPD patients compared to healthy subjects has been studied scarcely [12]. Marquis and colleagues reported an increased prevalence in 38 COPD patients compared to 34 healthy subjects (47% vs. 21%, respectively) [13]. A comparable prevalence of metabolic syndrome in COPD was reported by Watz and colleagues [14], but no healthy control group was included in this study.

COPD patients with metabolic syndrome are physically less active and have increased levels of systemic inflammation

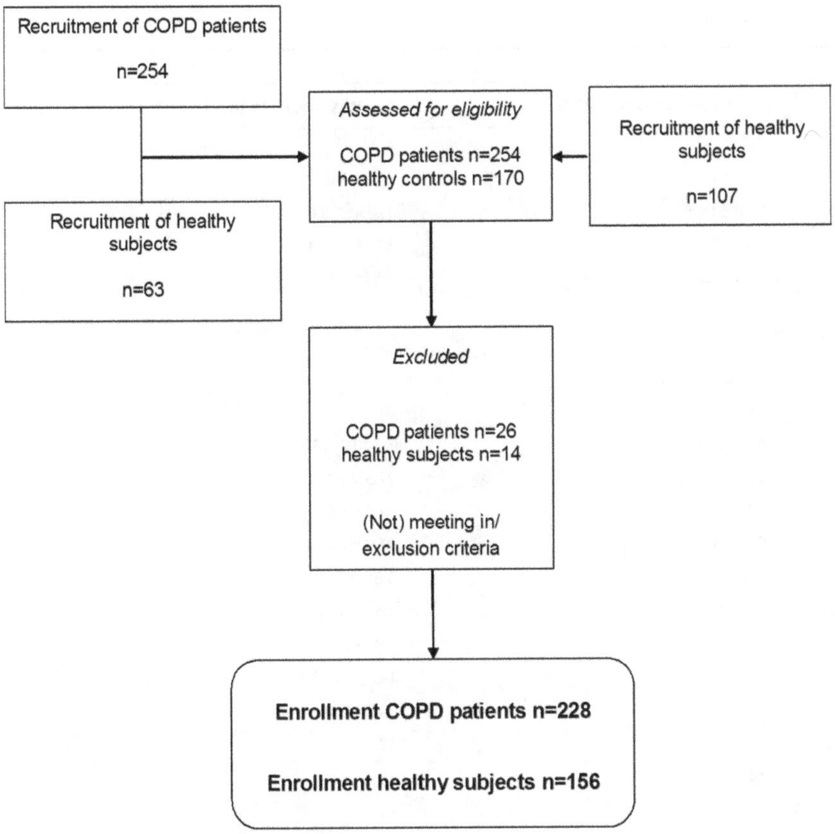

Figure 1. Patient flow diagram.

compared to COPD patients without metabolic syndrome [14]. To date it remains largely unknown whether and to what extent other clinical outcomes, like spirometry, functional exercise performance, mood and health status, and the prevalence of cardiovascular co-morbidity might differ between COPD patients with and without metabolic syndrome. Therefore, we think it is of great interest to get more insight of the impact of metabolic syndrome on COPD patients' clinical outcomes in order to better characterise this subgroup of COPD patients.

In the present study we evaluated the prevalence of metabolic syndrome in COPD patients compared to healthy subjects. We hypothesize that the prevalence of metabolic syndrome is higher in the patients. In addition, clinical and functional characteristics of COPD patients with and without metabolic syndrome were studied.

Methods

Study population

Data were prospectively collected in 228 clinically stable COPD patients and 156 healthy subjects from 2007–2012. All patients and 55 healthy subjects were recruited as part of the CIROCO study and 101 control subjects were recruited from another observational prospective study. For both studies, inclusion criteria for the COPD patients were: diagnosis of COPD, GOLD I–IV [15] and no respiratory tract infection or exacerbation at least 4 weeks prior to the study. Exclusion criteria for both groups were any kind of oncologic pathology less than 5 years prior to the study.

Ethics statement

Study 1 (CIROCO study): Ethical approval number: 10-3-067. Medical ethical committee of the Maastricht University Medical Centre. Study 2 ethical approval number: 10-3-033, Medical ethical committee of the Maastricht University Medical Centre, www.controlled-trials.com, ISRCTN86049077. All participants gave written informed consent.

International Diabetes Federation (IDF) definition of metabolic syndrome [5]

Waist circumference (WC ≥94 cm in European men or ≥80 cm in European women)

Plus two of the following:

- glucose >100 mg/dL (5.6 mmol/L) or previously diagnosed type II diabetes;
- triglyceride ≥150 mg/dL (1.7 mmol/L) or specific treatment for this lipid abnormality;
- high density lipoprotein (HDL) <40 mg/dL (1.03 mmol/L) in men or <50 mg/dL (1.29 mmol/L) in women or specific treatment for this lipid abnormality;
- systolic blood pressure ≥130 mmHg and/or diastolic blood pressure ≥85 mmHg or treatment of previously diagnosed hypertension;

Lung function and arterial blood gases

Lung function parameters were collected using standardized spirometry (Masterlab, Viasys, Germany). The degree of severity

Table 1. Baseline characteristics of the total study population.

	COPD patients (n = 228)	healthy subjects (n = 156)
Gender, %male	59	45*
age, years	63.7±7.1	60.1±7.4*
FEV_1, %pred	52.8±18.6	120.4±15.8*
FVC, %pred	96.1±19.1	122.8±21.3*
FEV_1/FVC	40.9±12.2	78.1±6.5*
smoking status		
never smoker, %	0	77*
former smoker, %	73	23*
current smoker, %	27	0*
Pack years, n#	43.0 (29.4–58.5)	3.5 (0.0–15.3)*
BMI, kg/m^2	26.2±5.1	27.3±4.2†
FFMI, kg/m^2	17.0±2.4	17.9±3.6*
Waist circumference, cm	98.5±14.3	93.9±10.7*
Plasma glucose level, mmol/L	5.8±1.2	5.6±0.7
Plasma triglyceride level, mmol/L	1.5±0.9	1.5±1.1
Plasma HDL level, mmol/L	1.7±0.5	1.8±0.5†
Systolic blood pressure, mmHg	138.6±21.4	142.7±20.3
Diastolic blood pressure, mmHg	82.2±9.7	84.3±9.1†
High waist circumference$, %	79	79
High glucose level$, %	49	45
High triglyceride level$, %	31	22
High HDL level$, %	10	8
High systolic blood pressure$, %	61	75*
High diastolic blood pressure$, %	33	46*
Metabolic syndrome$, %	57	40*

Data are presented: mean ± SD, percentages or #median (interquartile range) if data were not normal distributed.
FEV_1, forced expiratory volume in the first second; FVC, forced vital capacity; BMI, body mass index; FFMI, fat free mass index; HDL, high density lipoprotein.
$according to the IDF.
Other symbols:
*p<0.01,
†p<0.05 compared with COPD patients.

of airflow limitation was classified according to the GOLD guidelines [15]. Arterial oxygen tensions (PaO2) and arterial carbon dioxide tension (PaCO2) have been analyzed in the patients only.

Anthropometric parameters

Fat free mass index (FFMI) and bone mineral density (BMD) have been assessed using a dual x-ray absorptiometry (DEXA) scan (Lunar Prodigy; GE Healthcare, Madison, WI, USA). FFMI was calculated as: FFM in kilogram divided by squared height in meters. Low FFM was defined as FFMI $\leq$15 (females) or $\leq$16 (males) kg/m^2. BMD has been defined by a T-score (hip and lumbar spine) >-1, Osteopenia -2.5 and -1, and osteoporosis by a T-score ≤ -2.5.

Exercise capacity and mood status

In patients peak cycling load has been assessed by incremental ergometry cycling test and functional exercise capacity by six-minute walking distance test (6MWD). The St. George Respiratory Questionnaire (SGRQ) has been used to assess disease-specific health status [16]. Assessment of mood status has been done using the Hospital Anxiety and Depression Scale (HADS) [17].

Additional parameters

The Modified Medical Research Council (MRC) dyspnoea scale, subjects' smoking status, number of pack years, the use of long-term oxygen therapy (LTOT), the Charlson Co-morbidity Index (CCI) [18] and current pharmacological treatment were recorded.

Statistical analyses

Besides whole group comparison, both the patient and healthy subject groups were stratified for BMI (cut-off of 25 kg/m^2) and for gender to evaluate the prevalence of the metabolic syndrome. Categorical variables are described as frequencies, while continuous variables were checked for normality and described as mean ± SD or median (inter-quartile range; for pack years). Evaluation of group differences (patients vs. healthy subjects, patients with vs. without metabolic syndrome) in means for continuous variables was done using the Unpaired Student's t-test, and for categorical variables the chi-square test. Logistic regression was performed to

Table 2. Body composition and criteria of metabolic syndrome of the study population by BMI.

	BMI <25 kg/m²		BMI ≥25 kg/m²	
	COPD patients (n = 97)	**healthy subjects (n = 47)**	**COPD patients (n = 131)**	**healthy subjects (n = 109)**
BMI, kg/m²	21.7±2.4	23.0±1.5*	29.4±3.9	29.1±3.5
FFMI, kg/m²	15.3±1.5	15.8±1.9†	18.3±2.1	18.8±3.7
Waist circumference, cm	87.4±10.6	83.3±7.7†	107±10.7	98.5±8.2*
Plasma glucose level, mmol/L	5.5±0.9	5.4±0.6	6.0±1.3	5.7±0.7†
Plasma triglyceride level, mmol/L	1.3±0.6	1.2±0.6	1.7±1.0	1.6±1.3
Plasma HDL level, mmol/L	1.8±0.5	2.0±0.5†	1.4±0.4	1.7±0.4
Systolic blood pressure, mmHg	136.5±19.9	135.1±18.5	140±22.3	146±20.2†
Diastolic blood pressure, mmHg	82.3±9.5	80.2±8.9	82.2±9.9	86.1±8.6*
High waist circumference$, %	49	57	100	88*
High glucose level$, %	41	36	55	49
High triglyceride level$, %	20	17	40	25†
High HDL level$, %	5	6	13	8
High systolic blood pressure$, %	55	55	66	83*
High diastolic blood pressure$, %	33	23	33	56†
Metabolic syndrome$, %	29	17	77	50*

Data are presented: mean ± SD or percentages. BMI, body mass index; FFMI, fat free mass index; HDL, high density lipoprotein.
$according to the IDF.
Other symbols:
*p<0.01,
†p<0.05 compared with COPD patients.

test whether COPD patients had a higher risk of having metabolic syndrome after correction for age, gender and BMI. All analyses were performed using the Statistical Package for the Social Sciences (SPSS) version 20 for Windows. A *p*-value of ≤0.05 was considered significant.

Results

Prevalence of metabolic syndrome and its components

A diagram of participant flow is shown in **Figure 1**. The COPD patients were characterised by moderate to severe airflow limitation (**Table 1**). Compared to healthy, patients were slightly older, had a higher number of pack years and male gender was predominant. While BMI and FFMI were lower, WC was higher in the patients. Plasma HDL concentration and diastolic BP were lower in the patients. Prevalence of a high systolic and diastolic BP, one of the criteria of metabolic syndrome, was more prevalent in healthy than in the patients, but metabolic syndrome was more prevalent in the patients than in healthy subjects. After stratification for BMI: the subgroup of patients with a BMI ≥25 kg/m² were matched for BMI with their healthy peers, but BMI was lower in the subgroup of patients with BMI <25 kg/m² compared to their healthy peers (**Table 2**). Further, in the subgroups of subjects with BMI <25 kg/m², WC was higher and plasma HDL concentration was lower in patients than in healthy, but the prevalence of the metabolic syndrome was comparable. In the logistic regression on metabolic syndrome, COPD patients had a 60% more chance of having metabolic syndrome than control subjects after correction for age, gender and BMI (**Table 3**).

Figure 2 and 3 provide an overview of the prevalence of metabolic syndrome and its components in patients and healthy subjects after stratification for gender and BMI. No differences were found between men and women with BMI <25 kg/m² (**Figure 2, A and B**). In the subjects with BMI ≥25 kg/m² (**Figure 3, A and B**), WC, systolic and diastolic BP, and the prevalence of the metabolic syndrome were different between men and women.

Table 3. Logistic regression with metabolic syndrome as dependent variable.

	OR	CI	P-value
Age	1.03	0.99–1.06	0.11
Gender (male = 1)	0.58	0.37–0.92	0.02
BMI (BMI<25 kg/m² = 1)	6.85	4.13–11.36	<0.01
Group (COPD = 1)	0.39	0.24–0.64	<0.01

The interaction term group*BMI was not significant, so it was excluded from the model. Abbreviations: OR: odds ratio; CI: 95th percentile confident interval.

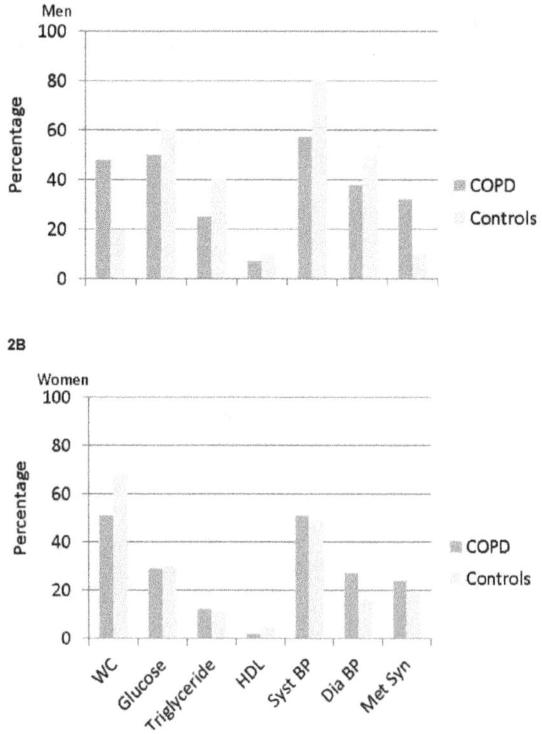

Figure 2. A and B. Prevalence of metabolic syndrome and its components in male and female COPD and healthy subjects with BMI <25 kg/m^2. WC, waist circumference; HDL, high density lipoprotein; Syst BP, systolic blood pressure; Dia BP, diastolic blood pressure; Met Syn, metabolic syndrome.

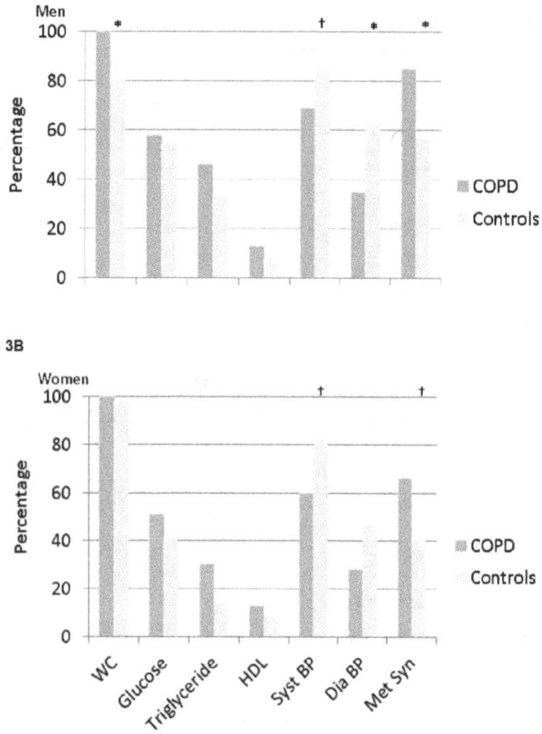

Figure 3. A and B. Prevalence of metabolic syndrome and its components in male and female COPD and healthy subjects by BMI >25 kg/m^2. WC, waist circumference; HDL, high density lipoprotein; Syst BP, systolic blood pressure; Dia BP, diastolic blood pressure; Met Syn, metabolic syndrome. *$p<0.01$, †$p<0.05$ compared to COPD patients.

Characteristics of patients with and without metabolic syndrome

Even after stratification for BMI, the markers of body composition, BMI and FFMI were higher in patients with compared to those without metabolic syndrome (**Table 4**). Further, in the patients with BMI <25 kg/m^2, patients with metabolic syndrome had a lower prevalence of low muscle mass and a lower 6MWD compared to patients without metabolic syndrome. In addition, the proportion of patients using statins and BP lowering drugs was higher when having metabolic syndrome. In the patients with BMI ≥ 25 kg/m^2, male gender was predominant and BMD of the lumbar spine was higher in the patients with compared to those without metabolic syndrome. Also the proportion of patients with co-morbidities, and the proportion of patients using statins, β-blockers and BP lowering drugs was higher in the patients with compared to those without metabolic syndrome. Other characteristics like spirometry, GOLD stages and combined COPD assessment, peak cycling load, prevalence of osteopenia/osteoporosis, use of LTOT, arterial blood gases, dyspnea, symptoms of anxiety and depression, and health status were similar between COPD patients with and without metabolic syndrome.

Discussion

The present study reports on two important findings: first, metabolic syndrome is more prevalent in overweight to obese patients with COPD compared to BMI matched healthy subjects. In the present cohort, no difference in the frequency of metabolic syndrome was observed in low to normal weight patients and healthy subjects. Second, the presence of metabolic syndrome in COPD patients had no functional consequences, but it coincided with more cardiovascular co-morbidity and type II diabetes.

Fifty seven percent of the COPD patients were diagnosed with metabolic syndrome, a prevalence comparable with previous studies [13,14]. However, this percentage was significantly higher compared to the healthy subjects, despite the presence of a lower BMI. Indeed, after stratification for BMI, the prevalence of metabolic syndrome was not significantly different in the subjects with BMI <25 kg/m^2, but the prevalence of metabolic syndrome was significantly higher in the patients compared to the healthy subjects in the group with BMI ≥ 25 kg/m^2. According to the IDF, the prevalence of metabolic syndrome is largely driven by abdominal obesity. In fact, it was recently shown that patients with obstructive lung disease have more visceral fat mass compared to healthy subjects [19]. Here, these findings are indirectly confirmed by the observation that even after stratification for BMI patients in both BMI sub-groups have higher WC than their matched healthy peers. It is uncertain why abdominal obesity is more prevalent in COPD patients compared to healthy subjects, but various factors including poor nutrition and an inactive lifestyle may play an important role [19]. It is remarkable that the prevalence of metabolic syndrome is only higher in the patients with BMI ≥ 25 kg/m^2. Furthermore, cardiovascular co-morbidity was more prevalent in the patients with metabolic syndrome and BMI ≥ 25 kg/m^2. These data imply that BMI contribute to the cardiovascular co-morbidity in COPD on top of metabolic syndrome.

Table 4. Clinical and functional characteristics of the COPD patients by metabolic syndrome.

	BMI <25 kg/m²		BMI ≥25 kg/m²	
	Metabolic syndrome		Metabolic syndrome	
	with (n = 28)	without (n = 69)	with (n = 101)	without (n = 30)
age, years	64.3±6.6	62.9±7.2	64.1±7.2	63.7±7.3
male, %	64	55	65	40†
FEV_1, % pred.	45.2±18.9	49.4±20.5	57.5±17.0	52.1±15.9
FVC, % pred.	92.8±23.3	97.5±17.7	95.8±19.4	97.1±16.9
FEV_1/FVC, % pred.	35.6±9.9	37.8±13.4	44.6±11.6	40.2±9.3
GOLD I, II, III, IV, %	0, 43, 36, 21	7, 36, 41, 16	8, 59, 27, 6	7, 50, 40, 3
Combined COPD assessment A, B, C, D, %	32, 11, 4, 54	18, 23, 17, 42	23, 43, 2, 32	27, 30, 10, 33
BMI, kg/m²	23.2±1.3	21.1±2.5*	30.1±4.1	27.3±2.2*
FFMI, kg/m²	15.9±1.3	15.0±1.5*	18.6±2.2	17.1±1.5*
Low muscle mass, %	32	72*	4	7
BMD hip, g/cm²	0.80±0.10	0.80±0.15	0.89±0.13	0.89±0.23
BMD lumbar spine, g/cm²	1.04±0.16	1.01±0.20	1.14±0.18	1.05±0.16†
osteopenia , %	46	41	56	60
osteoporosis, %	50	49	19	20
6MWD, m	438.0±122.1	491.9±97.3†	460.4±95.5	474.6±125.3
6MWD, %pred	73.7±21.3	80.5±14.7	82.4±16.6	81.6±19.9
peak load, watts	68.0±19.4	68.2±23.8	81.7±28.6	78.2±38.4
peak load, %pred	56.6±31.5	55.1±23.8	61.9±25.8	65.9±26.9
smoking status				
never smoker, %	0	0	0	3
former smoker, %	64	64	79	73
current smoker, %	36	36	21	23
pack years, n#	38.5 (27.3–56.2)	43.8 (28.5–59.7)	43.8 (31.5–58.8)	38.3 (30.6–56.1)
LTOT, %	14	20	13	23
pH	7.44±0.03	7.43±0.03	7.43±0.02	7.44±0.09
$PaCO_2$, kPa	5.3±0.7	5.3±0.6	5.3±0.6	5.5±0.6
PaO_2, kPa	9.3±1.1	9.6±1.1	9.5±1.0	9.3±1.2
MRC	2.3±1.3	1.9±1.0	2.2±1.1	2.0±1.2
HADS, anxiety	6.0±3.8	6.5±4.3	6.0±3.8	7.2±4.2
depression	5.4±3.6	5.6±3.4	5.8±3.7	5.7±3.6
SGRQ, total score	52.2±16.2	49.8±18.1	52.7±16.9	50.3±19.7
symptom score	54.8±18.8	57.7±21.4	55.2±19.9	53.4±23.0
activity score	65.6±20.8	65.6±23.2	71.0±21.0	66.7±21.6
impact score	39.3±21.4	38.9±21.6	41.2±18.0	40.0±21.8
Charlson Co-morbidity Index				
CVD, %	32	22	39	27
Myocardial infarct, %	4	6	18	0†
Peripheral vascular disease, %	14	13	22	13†
Type II diabetes, %	7	3	8	3†
Medication use				
Inhaled CS, %	14	12	13	13
Oral CS, %	14	7	8	10
Statins, %	46	7*	47	3*
Beta-blockers, %	21	9	26	7†
Anti-diabetics, %	7	3	6	3

Table 4. Cont.

	BMI <25 kg/m^2		BMI ≥25 kg/m^2	
	Metabolic syndrome		Metabolic syndrome	
	with (n = 28)	without (n = 69)	with (n = 101)	without (n = 30)
Insulin, %	0	0	3	3
Blood pressure lowering drugs, %	54	28†	61	17*

Data are mean ± SD or percentages or #median (interquartile range) if data were not normal distributed.
FEV_1, forced expiratory volume in the first second; FVC, forced vital capacity; BMI, body mass index; FFMI, fat free mass index; BMD, bone mineral density; 6MWD, six minute walking distance; LTOT, long term oxygen therapy; $PaCO_2$, arterial carbon dioxide tension; PaO_2, arterial oxygen tension; CVD, cardiovascular disease; inhaled and oral CS, inhaled and oral corticosteroids; MRC, modified Medical Research Council; HADS, Hospital Anxiety and Depression Scale; SGRQ, St. George Respiratory Questionnaire.
*$p<0.01$,
$^†p<0.05$ compared to patients without the metabolic syndrome.

The presence of metabolic syndrome was independent of the degree of airflow limitation. One other manuscript reported a slightly higher prevalence of metabolic syndrome in mild to moderate COPD patients [14]. In the present study most patients had COPD GOLD stage II or III, but no difference in the prevalence of metabolic syndrome within the various GOLD stages of COPD could be identified. Indeed, in the general population metabolic syndrome is associated with restrictive ventilatory patterns but not with obstructive lung function impairments [20]. This association is mainly driven by abdominal obesity, which is particularly present in patients with moderate airflow obstruction.

In patients with BMI <25 kg/m^2, patients with metabolic syndrome had lower 6MWD compared to the patients without metabolic syndrome. This is a surprising finding as the prevalence of low muscle mass, which is associated with decreased exercise tolerance [21], was lower in the patients with metabolic syndrome. On the other hand, metabolic syndrome contributes to a lower exercise capacity assessed by treadmill test in healthy subjects [9,22] and lower physical activity levels have been found in COPD patients with compared to those without metabolic syndrome [14]. However, differences in body composition were not taken into account as possible confounder. Interestingly, in the patients with BMI ≥25 kg/m^2 metabolic syndrome did not affect functional exercise performance.

In the present study the prevalence of osteoporosis in COPD patients ranges from 20% up to 50% depending on BMI. To date no data are available on levels of BMD in COPD patients with metabolic syndrome. In the present study we did not find an association between the prevalence of metabolic syndrome and the prevalence of osteoporosis, but we did find a higher BMD of the lumbar spine in the patients with BMI ≥25 kg/m^2 and metabolic syndrome. In the NHANES study, performed in the general population it was shown that subjects with metabolic syndrome have higher BMD compared to subjects without metabolic syndrome (after correcting for multiple confounders) and these results were mainly driven by an increased abdominal obesity [11]. Indeed, even a protective effect of criteria of metabolic syndrome against non-vertebral fractures has been described in patients with type II diabetes [23]. This effect could be partly explained by an increased mechanical load on the cortical skeleton [24] and increased insulin levels promoting bone formation due to an increased fat mass [25]. There aside, in COPD it is already shown that circulating leptin, a cytokine produced and secreted by adipocytes, appears to act as a mediator between fat mass and bone mass [26]. More studies should be performed to investigate whether metabolic syndrome in COPD could have a protective effect on osteoporosis.

COPD is known to have a negative impact on the disease-specific health status and the effect increases even more with increased disease severity [27]. Identifying factors related to a decreased health status in COPD are, besides lung function impairment [27], exercise intolerance [28], dyspnoea, anxiety [29], and body composition [30]. In general chronic conditions, such as type II diabetes, hypertension as well as dyslipidaemia are well known to affect patients' health status. Thus, it can be expected that subjects having metabolic syndrome also suffer from an impaired health status [31,32]. In COPD co-morbid conditions might lead to a further decrease in health status. However, results from our study show that COPD patients having metabolic syndrome are not additionally affected in their disease-specific health status.

Finally the latest global strategy for the diagnosis, management and prevention of COPD (GOLD) highlighted the importance of co-morbidities in COPD. In particular, cardiovascular diseases, lung cancer, osteoporosis, depression, and metabolic disorders, such as type II diabetes, as they have a significant impact on prognosis and some of them even have been found to be the most frequent cause of death in mild COPD [1]. The here presented results indicate that having metabolic syndrome increases the co-morbidity index, particularly in those patients with an overweight or obese BMI. Therefore metabolic syndrome has to be identified and treated appropriately in patients with COPD.

The following methodological considerations have to be taken into account: firstly, healthy subjects were slightly younger than the COPD patients. However, it is unlikely that a mean age difference of about 3 years explains the difference in the prevalence of the metabolic syndrome. Secondly, blood pressure of the healthy was relatively high. Indeed, hypertension was the most mentioned co-morbidity among the healthy. Further, subjects were not allowed to take their blood lowering drugs before the tests. Thirdly, no metabolic effects of metabolic syndrome are taken into account in the present study. Nevertheless, there is evidence that metabolic syndrome is associated with disturbed adipokine metabolism, insulin resistance [33], and with increased systemic inflammation [14]. These studies did however not include healthy subjects and future research has to unravel whether this is a COPD specific effect. Fourth, the present study had a cross-sectional study design and longitudinal studies are warranted to investigate the long term effects of metabolic syndrome on cardiovascular and other morbidities in patients with COPD.

In conclusion, in contrast to normal weight patients, metabolic syndrome is more prevalent in overweight and obese patients with COPD compared to BMI matched healthy subjects. Both, lung function impairment and functional parameters did not differ between COPD patients with and those without metabolic syndrome. Additionally, the prevalence of osteoporosis and disease-specific health status were not altered by the presence of metabolic syndrome, while metabolic syndrome has shown to contribute to an increased co-morbidity index.

Acknowledgments

AstraZeneca provided support in the form of a salary for author PLBB, but did not have any additional role in the study design, data collection and analysis, decision to publish, or preparation of the manuscript. The specific roles of the authors are articulated in the 'author contributions' section.

Author Contributions

Conceived and designed the experiments: EFMW EPAR MAS. Performed the experiments: MTJG. Analyzed the data: MKB FMEF LEGWV EPAR CKH. Contributed reagents/materials/analysis tools: PLBB EFMW. Wrote the paper: MKB.

References

1. Barnes PJ, Celli BR (2009) Systemic manifestations and comorbidities of COPD. Eur Respir J 33: 1165–1185.
2. Curkendall SM, DeLuise C, Jones JK, Lanes S, Stang MR, et al. (2006) Cardiovascular disease in patients with chronic obstructive pulmonary disease, Saskatchewan Canada cardiovascular disease in COPD patients. Ann Epidemiol 16: 63–70.
3. Mannino DM, Thorn D, Swensen A, Holguin F (2008) Prevalence and outcomes of diabetes, hypertension and cardiovascular disease in COPD. Eur Respir J 32: 962–969.
4. Divo M, Cote C, de Torres JP, Casanova C, Marin JM, et al. (2012) Comorbidities and risk of mortality in patients with chronic obstructive pulmonary disease. Am J Respir Crit Care Med 186: 155–161.
5. Alberti KG, Zimmet P, Shaw J (2006) Metabolic syndrome–a new world-wide definition. A Consensus Statement from the International Diabetes Federation. Diabet Med 23: 469–480.
6. Eckel RH, Grundy SM, Zimmet PZ (2005) The metabolic syndrome. Lancet 365: 1415–1428.
7. Isomaa B, Almgren P, Tuomi T, Forsen B, Lahti K, et al. (2001) Cardiovascular morbidity and mortality associated with the metabolic syndrome. Diabetes Care 24: 683–689.
8. Lakka HM, Laaksonen DE, Lakka TA, Niskanen LK, Kumpusalo E, et al. (2002) The metabolic syndrome and total and cardiovascular disease mortality in middle-aged men. Jama 288: 2709–2716.
9. Ribisl PM, Lang W, Jaramillo SA, Jakicic JM, Stewart KJ, et al. (2007) Exercise capacity and cardiovascular/metabolic characteristics of overweight and obese individuals with type 2 diabetes: the Look AHEAD clinical trial. Diabetes Care 30: 2679–2684.
10. Ford ES, Li C (2006) Physical activity or fitness and the metabolic syndrome. Expert Rev Cardiovasc Ther 4: 897–915.
11. Kinjo M, Setoguchi S, Solomon DH (2007) Bone mineral density in adults with the metabolic syndrome: analysis in a population-based U.S. sample. J Clin Endocrinol Metab 92: 4161–4164.
12. Wells G (2013) Metabolic syndrome and diabetes mellitus in COPD: European Respiratory Monograph.
13. Marquis K, Maltais F, Duguay V, Bezeau AM, LeBlanc P, et al. (2005) The metabolic syndrome in patients with chronic obstructive pulmonary disease. J Cardiopulm Rehabil 25: 226–232; discussion 233–224.
14. Watz H, Waschki B, Kirsten A, Muller KC, Kretschmar G, et al. (2009) The metabolic syndrome in patients with chronic bronchitis and COPD: frequency and associated consequences for systemic inflammation and physical inactivity. Chest 136: 1039–1046.
15. Vestbo J, Hurd SS, Agusti AG, Jones PW, Vogelmeier C, et al. (2013) Global Strategy for the Diagnosis, Management, and Prevention of Chronic Obstructive Pulmonary Disease: GOLD Executive Summary. Am J Respir Crit Care Med 187: 347–365.
16. Jones PW, Quirk FH, Baveystock CM, Littlejohns P (1992) A self-complete measure of health status for chronic airflow limitation. The St. George's Respiratory Questionnaire. Am Rev Respir Dis 145: 1321–1327.
17. Zigmond AS, Snaith RP (1983) The hospital anxiety and depression scale. Acta Psychiatr Scand 67: 361–370.
18. Charlson ME, Pompei P, Ales KL, MacKenzie CR (1987) A new method of classifying prognostic comorbidity in longitudinal studies: development and validation. J Chronic Dis 40: 373–383.
19. van den Borst B, Gosker HR, Koster A, Yu B, Kritchevsky SB, et al. (2012) The influence of abdominal visceral fat on inflammatory pathways and mortality risk in obstructive lung disease. Am J Clin Nutr 96: 516–526.
20. Leone N, Courbon D, Thomas F, Bean K, Jego B, et al. (2009) Lung function impairment and metabolic syndrome: the critical role of abdominal obesity. Am J Respir Crit Care Med 179: 509–516.
21. Schols AM, Mostert R, Soeters PB, Wouters EF (1991) Body composition and exercise performance in patients with chronic obstructive pulmonary disease. Thorax 46: 695–699.
22. Wong CY, O'Moore-Sullivan T, Fang ZY, Haluska B, Leano R, et al. (2005) Myocardial and vascular dysfunction and exercise capacity in the metabolic syndrome. Am J Cardiol 96: 1686–1691.
23. Yamaguchi T, Kanazawa I, Yamamoto M, Kurioka S, Yamauchi M, et al. (2009) Associations between components of the metabolic syndrome versus bone mineral density and vertebral fractures in patients with type 2 diabetes. Bone 45: 174–179.
24. Reid IR (2006) Obesity and osteoporosis. Ann Endocrinol (Paris) 67: 125–129.
25. Reid IR (2010) Fat and bone. Arch Biochem Biophys 503: 20–27.
26. Pobeha P, Ukropec J, Skyba P, Ukropcova B, Joppa P, et al. (2011) Relationship between osteoporosis and adipose tissue leptin and osteoprotegerin in patients with chronic obstructive pulmonary disease. Bone 48: 1008–1014.
27. Ferrer M, Alonso J, Morera J, Marrades RM, Khalaf A, et al. (1997) Chronic obstructive pulmonary disease stage and health-related quality of life. The Quality of Life of Chronic Obstructive Pulmonary Disease Study Group. Ann Intern Med 127: 1072–1079.
28. Ketelaars CA, Schlosser MA, Mostert R, Huyer Abu-Saad H, Halfens RJ, et al. (1996) Determinants of health-related quality of life in patients with chronic obstructive pulmonary disease. Thorax 51: 39–43.
29. Hajiro T, Nishimura K, Tsukino M, Ikeda A, Koyama H, et al. (1998) Comparison of discriminative properties among disease-specific questionnaires for measuring health-related quality of life in patients with chronic obstructive pulmonary disease. Am J Respir Crit Care Med 157: 785–790.
30. Shoup R, Dalsky G, Warner S, Davies M, Connors M, et al. (1997) Body composition and health-related quality of life in patients with obstructive airways disease. Eur Respir J 10: 1576–1580.
31. Roriz-Cruz M, Rosset I, Wada T, Sakagami T, Ishine M, et al. (2007) Stroke-independent association between metabolic syndrome and functional dependence, depression, and low quality of life in elderly community-dwelling Brazilian people. J Am Geriatr Soc 55: 374–382.
32. Tsai AG, Wadden TA, Sarwer DB, Berkowitz RI, Womble LG, et al. (2008) Metabolic syndrome and health-related quality of life in obese individuals seeking weight reduction. Obesity (Silver Spring) 16: 59–63.
33. Minas M, Kostikas K, Papaioannou AI, Mystridou P, Karetsi E, et al. (2011) The association of metabolic syndrome with adipose tissue hormones and insulin resistance in patients with COPD without co-morbidities. COPD 8: 414–420.

9

Exercise Training during Normobaric Hypoxic Confinement Does Not Alter Hormonal Appetite Regulation

Tadej Debevec[1]*, Elizabeth J. Simpson[2], Ian A. Macdonald[2], Ola Eiken[3], Igor B. Mekjavic[1]

1 Department of Automation, Biocybernetics and Robotics, Jozef Stefan Institute, Ljubljana, Slovenia, **2** MRC/Arthritis Research UK Centre for Musculoskeletal Ageing Research, University of Nottingham Medical School, School of Life Sciences, Queen's Medical Centre, Nottingham, United Kingdom, **3** Department of Environmental Physiology, Swedish Aerospace Physiology Centre, Royal Institute of Technology, Stockholm, Sweden

Abstract

Background: Both exposure to hypoxia and exercise training have the potential to modulate appetite and induce beneficial metabolic adaptations. The purpose of this study was to determine whether daily moderate exercise training performed during a 10-day exposure to normobaric hypoxia alters hormonal appetite regulation and augments metabolic health.

Methods: Fourteen healthy, male participants underwent a 10-day hypoxic confinement at ~4000 m simulated altitude ($F_iO_2 = 0.139 \pm 0.003\%$) either combined with daily moderate intensity exercise (Exercise group; $N = 8$, Age $= 25.8 \pm 2.4$ yrs, BMI $= 22.9 \pm 1.2$ kg·m^{-2}) or without any exercise (Sedentary group; $N = 6$ Age $= 24.8 \pm 3.1$ yrs, BMI $= 22.3 \pm 2.5$ kg·m^{-2}). A meal tolerance test was performed before (Pre) and after the confinement (Post) to quantify fasting and postprandial concentrations of selected appetite-related hormones and metabolic risk markers. ^{13}C-Glucose was dissolved in the test meal and $^{13}CO_2$ determined in breath samples. Perceived appetite ratings were obtained throughout the meal tolerance tests.

Results: While body mass decreased in both groups (-1.4 kg; $p = 0.01$) following the confinement, whole body fat mass was only reduced in the Exercise group (-1.5 kg; $p = 0.01$). At Post, postprandial serum insulin was reduced in the Sedentary group (-49%; $p = 0.01$) and postprandial plasma glucose in the Exercise group (-19%; $p = 0.03$). Fasting serum total cholesterol levels were reduced (-12%; $p = 0.01$) at Post in the Exercise group only, secondary to low-density lipoprotein cholesterol reduction (-16%; $p = 0.01$). No differences between groups or testing periods were noted in fasting and/or postprandial concentrations of total ghrelin, peptide YY, and glucagon-like peptide-1, leptin, adiponectin, expired $^{13}CO_2$ as well as perceived appetite ratings ($p > 0.05$).

Conclusion: These findings suggest that performing daily moderate intensity exercise training during continuous hypoxic exposure does not alter hormonal appetite regulation but can improve the lipid profile in healthy young males.

Editor: Manlio Vinciguerra, University College London, United Kingdom

Funding: The study was supported, in part, by the European union funding programme FP7 (PlanHab project; Grant no. 284438), the European Space Agency (ESA) Programme for European Cooperating States (ESTEC/Contract No. 40001043721/11/NL/KML: Planetary Habitat Simulation), and by the Slovene Research Agency (Contract no. L3-3654: Zero and reduced gravity simulation: The effect on the cardiovascular and musculoskeletal systems). The funders had no role in study design, data collection and analysis, decision to publish, or preparation of the manuscript.

Competing Interests: The authors have declared that no competing interests exist.

* E-mail: tadej.debevec@ijs.si

Introduction

High altitude sojourns are often associated with significant weight loss [1]. While several factors appear to be involved in this phenomenon, growing evidence suggest that appetite reduction plays an important role [2]. Indeed, decreased appetite and energy intake, collectively termed "altitude anorexia" is frequently reported during high altitude exposures and can induce negative energy balance, especially when coupled with increased levels of physical activity [3,4].

Altitude-related appetite modulation is not entirely understood. Initially, the observed appetite reduction was only linked to acute mountain sickness [5]. However, the reported reductions in appetite, as well as energy intake, after altitude sickness symptoms subside imply other underlying mechanisms [1]. Among these, hormonal regulation might potentially play a role since several appetite-related gut hormones, and adipokines are affected by acute and/or prolonged hypoxic exposure [2,6].

Acute hypoxia has been shown to reduce circulating levels of the appetite-stimulating hormone, ghrelin, both in the fasted [7] and fed state [6,8], although the fasting ghrelin concentration reportedly returns to baseline levels after 7 and 49 days of continuous exposure [7,9]. On the other hand, hypoxia has been shown to increase serum levels of the satiety-signaling hormone leptin, both acutely [7,10,11] and after 7 days at altitude [7]. Reports in the literature present contradictory findings with regard to both ghrelin and leptin responses to hypoxia [9,12], presumably attributable to different experimental paradigms (hypobaric vs. normobaric hypoxia, rest vs. exercise and different hypoxic doses). Another potential explanation for the discrepancies between the outcomes is the fact that some studies measured total ghrelin [6,7] while others measured the acylated ghrelin [8] known to be essential for ghrelin appetite-stimulating effects [13]. To date, the contribution of other potential anorexigenic hormonal modulators that can be altered by hypoxic exposures such as peptide YY (PYY) [8] and glucagon-like peptide-1 (GLP-1) [10], has received less attention. Hence, their role and contribution to altitude-related appetite reduction is currently unclear.

Similarly to hypoxia, acute or chronic exercise significantly modulates hormonal appetite regulation [14]. Acute exercise transiently suppresses appetite, while chronic exercise training typically results in an augmented appetite leading to a restoration of the exercise-induced energy imbalance [15]. Although the exact mechanisms of these exercise-induced acute appetite alterations are unclear, reductions in ghrelin and increases in PYY and GLP-1 have been proposed as the key underlying factors [15,16]. Long-term studies have also indicated that chronic exercise training can improve appetite control system sensitivity [17] and augment fasting and postprandial satiety sensations [18]. While combining hypoxia and exercise is mostly used by athletes aiming to improve performance [19], it is gaining popularity as a novel modality for treatment of obesity with related comorbidities [2,20,21]. It has been suggested that hypoxia and exercise synergistically enhance metabolic health, since both individually up-regulate glucose, glycolysis and satiety related genes through hypoxia-inducible factor-1 stabilization [22–24]. Training under hypoxic condition has already been shown capable of improving metabolic status and glycemic control in healthy individuals [25,26] and clinical populations [27]. However, the potential additive effects of exercise during prolonged hypoxic exposure on hormonal appetite regulation and metabolic risk factors have, to our knowledge, not yet been investigated. Only one study to date investigated the effects of rest and exercise in acute (7-hrs) hypoxia on specific appetite regulating markers, and noted that both hypoxia and exercise reduce hunger and ghrelin concentrations [8]. Given the potential application of hypoxia and exercise for improving metabolic health and fighting the escalating obesity pandemic, their combined effects on appetite regulation should be further elucidated. Moreover, the potential contribution of physical exertion to hormonal appetite modulations observed during prolonged high altitude sojourns is currently unresolved.

Accordingly, this study sought to determine the acute and prolonged effects of continuous normobaric hypoxic exposure and exercise training on hormonal appetite regulation and select metabolic risk factors. The participants underwent 10 days of normobaric hypoxic confinement, either with daily moderate-intensity exercise training, or without any exercise. It was hypothesized that the addition of exercise training to continuous hypoxia would result in further reduction of appetite, through a synergistic effect of hypoxia and exercise. We additionally hypothesized that performing exercise training during continuous hypoxia would further augment select indices of metabolic health.

Materials and Methods

Ethics statement

The present study was approved by the National Committee for Medical Ethics at the Ministry of Health of the Republic of Slovenia and conformed to the guidelines of the Declaration of Helsinki. The participants were informed in detail about the experimental procedures as well as the potential risks involved, and signed a written informed consent prior to the start of the study.

Participants

Potential participants were invited to take part in this study through local advertisement. Exclusion criteria included chronic diseases, smoking, hematological, pulmonary and kidney disorders, use of any hormonal, metabolic or orexigenic/anorexigenic medications as well as any dietary manipulations within the last year. Applicants who had recently ($\leq$1 month) been exposed to normobaric or hypobaric hypoxia (above 2000 m) were also ineligible to participate. Following initial laboratory screening and medical examination, 16 healthy males, all recreationally active low altitude residents (<500 m), were selected and equally assigned, in a randomized manner, to either the Exercise or the Sedentary group. As a result of medical issues during the confinement period (appendicitis, adaptation problems), two participants from the Sedentary group had to be withdrawn from the study. Consequently, eight participants in the Exercise (age $=25.8\pm2.4$ yrs, height $=179.1\pm3.1$ cm; BMI $=22.9\pm1.2$ kg·m^{-2}, % body fat $=22.8\pm6.2$, peak O_2 uptake in normoxia (VO_{2peak}) $=42.6\pm6.1$ mL·kg^{-1}·min^{-1}) and six participants in the Sedentary group (age $=24.8\pm3.1$ yrs, height $=177.7\pm3.5$ cm; BMI $=22.3\pm2.5$ kg·m^{-2}, % body fat $=21.9\pm4.7$, VO_{2peak} $=42.2\pm5.0$ mL·kg^{-1}·min^{-1}) finished the study and only their data is reported in this paper.

Experimental design

This randomized, prospective trial was performed in the normobaric hypoxic facility of the Olympic Sports Center Planica in Rateče, Slovenia, situated 900 m above sea level. The study protocol, outlined in Figure 1, consisted of an initial testing period (Pre), a 10-day normobaric hypoxic confinement, combined either with daily moderate-intensity exercise training (Exercise group), or without any training (Sedentary group), and of an after testing period (Post). The participants were requested to arrive at the facility three days prior to the start of the protocol in order to familiarize them to the environment and to standardize their diet. They were accommodated in the hypoxic facility for the whole duration of the study protocol. A meal tolerance test (MTT) was performed at Pre and Post to determine the participants fasting metabolic status and postprandial metabolic responses. During the Pre testing period, the participants also performed graded exercise tests both under normoxic and hypoxic conditions to determine their VO_{2peak} and enable appropriate training intensity calculations.

Experimental procedures

Normobaric hypoxic confinement. The participants were confined for 10 consecutive days to the hypoxic facility comprising ten double bedrooms, living area, dining area and connecting hallway. The confinement began on the morning of Day 1 and finished on the morning of Day +1 (Post), following the MTT, such that the cumulative individual hypoxic exposure time was exactly 240 hours. The normobaric hypoxic gas was generated and maintained using a Vacuum Pressure Swing Adsorption system (VPSA, b-Cat, Tiel, The Netherlands), that continuously delivered the oxygen depleted air into the confinement area to simulate an altitude of ~4000 m (Fraction of inspired O_2 (F_IO_2) $=0.139\pm0.003$; Partial pressure of inspired O_2 (P_IO_2) $=88.2\pm0.6$ mmHg). Air samples were automatically drawn from each bedroom at 15-min intervals and analyzed by the VPSA system for O_2 and CO_2 fraction. The accumulated carbon dioxide

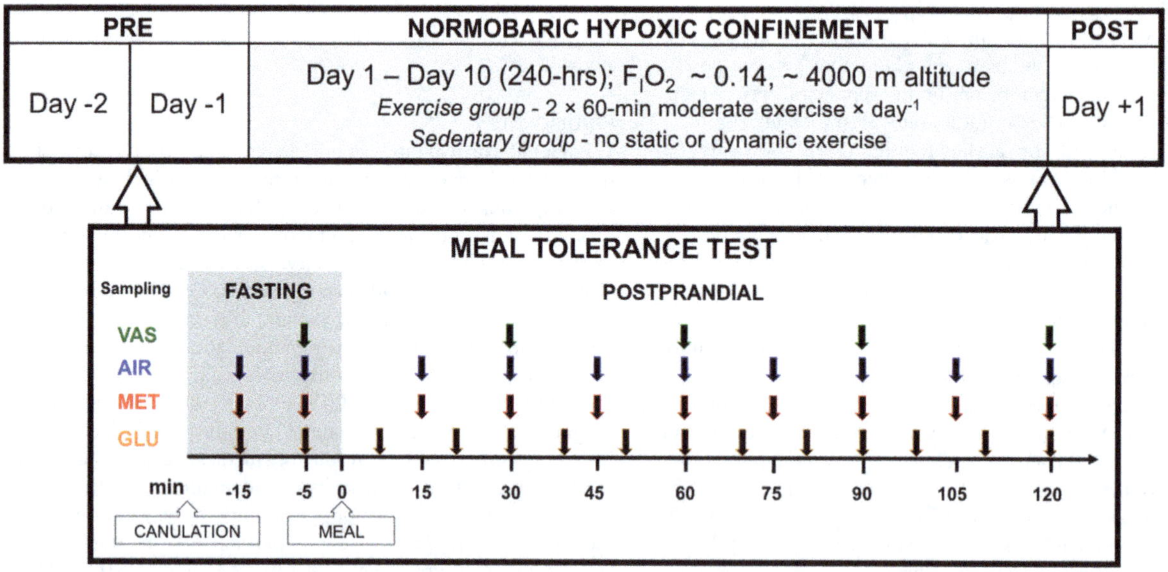

Figure 1. Study protocol and meal tolerance test outline. The meal tolerance test (MTT) was performed in the morning, one day before (Day -1) and just prior to exiting the 10-day confinement (morning of Day +1). F_IO_2, Fraction of inspired oxygen; VAS, Visual analogue scale for perceived appetite rating; AIR, Exhaled air sampling for determination of ^{13}C isotope; MET, Blood sampling for determination of metabolic markers: total ghrelin, peptide YY, Glucagon-like peptide-1 and insulin at all samplings and leptin, adiponectin, free fatty acids, triacylglycerols, cholesterol, and catecholamines during fasting samplings only; GLU, Blood sampling for plasma glucose concentration determination.

level within the confinement area did not exceed 0.5% at any time. The environmental conditions on the whole floor were stable throughout the protocol (temperature $=23.1\pm1.0°C$; relative humidity $=56\pm8\%$ and ambient pressure $=682\pm4$ mmHg). The participants wore portable, ambient O_2 analyzers with audible alarm (Rae PGM-1100, California, U.S.) at all times. Systolic and diastolic blood pressure (BP), heart rate (HR) and capillary oxyhaemoglobin saturation (SpO_2) were measured each morning using an automated blood pressure cuff (Withings BP monitor; Withings, Les Moulineaux, France) and a finger oximetry device (3100 WristOx, Nonin Medicals, Minnesota, U.S.), respectively. Additionally, acute mountain sickness (AMS) symptoms and severity (Lake Louise score (LLS; 0–15)) were quantified daily using the self-assessment portion of the Lake Louise mountain sickness questionnaire [28]. AMS was defined as presence of headache and concomitant LLS of 3 or more.

Diet and fluid intake. The diet was individually adjusted, with the same macronutrient composition (expressed as percentage macronutrient contribution to total energy intake) used for all participants. The basal energy requirement of each participant was calculated using the Mifflin equation [29]. To account for the different energy expenditure requirements of the interventions, the values were subsequently multiplied by a physical activity level factor of 1.8 and 1.4 for the Exercise and Sedentary group, respectively. The targeted daily energy intakes were 3166 ± 219 kcal for the Exercise and 2380 ± 80 kcal for the Sedentary group. The menus were prepared using the web-based application Open Platform for Clinical Nutrition (OPKP (www.opkp.si), Jozef Stefan Institute, Ljubljana, Slovenia). The OPKP enables individual planning and monitoring of dietary intakes based on food tables. Five meals (breakfast, morning snack, lunch, afternoon snack and dinner) were served per day, with portion size adjusted according to the OPKP calculations to achieve the required energy intake for each individual. All meals were prepared in the facility kitchen by the staff of the Olympic Sport Centre. To provide each individual with the exact targeted intakes all food items were weighed on a precision (±0.1 g) scale (TPT 6C, Libela ELSI, Celje, Slovenia) prior to each meal. In case of any leftovers, the unconsumed food items were re-weighed and the outcome deducted from the initial weight to provide the actual food intake. The actual intakes were then used in final dietary analysis performed individually using the OPKP system (Table 1). The participants were encouraged to consume the meals provided in their entirety. They were allowed to drink water and unsweetened tea *ad libitum*, and were advised to drink at least 2 liters of fluid per day [30].

Baseline exercise testing. Details of the exercise testing and training protocol are presented elsewhere [31]. Briefly, all participants performed an incremental test to task failure on an electronically braked cycle-ergometer (Ergo Bike Premium, Daum electronics, Fürth, Germany) prior to the start of the confinement, to assess their baseline aerobic capacity. After an initial 2-min warm up at 60 W, the workload was increased by 25 $W\cdot min^{-1}$ until task failure (cycling cadence below 60 rpm). A calibrated metabolic cart (Quark CPET, Cosmed, Rome, Italy) was used for breath-by-breath gas exchange measurement. The average O_2 uptake during the last minute of the test was calculated and reported as VO_{2peak}.

Additionally, participants in the Exercise group performed a graded exercise test to task failure (cadence <60 rpm) under normobaric hypoxic condition ($F_IO_2=0.14$) to determine the altitude specific peak power output that was used to calculate exercise training intensity. During the test, the participants breathed the humidified hypoxic gas mixture through a facemask, using a low resistance two-way valve (2700 NRBV, Hans Rudolph Inc., Shawnee, U.S.).

Exercise training. The exercise group participants performed two 60-min training sessions daily on a bicycle fitted to a mechanically braked indoor cycle trainer (Elite SuperChrono Forte, Fontaniva, Italy). Exercise sessions were performed during the morning and afternoon hours under the same environmental conditions ($F_IO_2=0.140\pm0.004$; $P_IO_2=88.8\pm0.6$ mmHg). The

Table 1. Average daily nutritional intakes in the Exercise and Sedentary group during the 10-Day normobaric hypoxic confinement.

	Exercise group	Sedentary group
Energy intake (kcal)	2601±383 ##	2213±192 **
Carbohydrate (g)	344±106	286±60 *
Protein (g)	113±30	94±19 *
Fat (g)	84±23	76±20
Carbohydrate (% daily intake)	63±19	62±13
Protein (% daily intake)	21±5	22±4
Fat (% daily intake)	16±4	16±4
H_2O (mL)	4872±1465	3283±1342 **
Fe (mg)	15.4±2.4	13.6±1.2 *
Na (mg)	4069±481	3428±477 *
Ca (mg)	1098±145	896±67 **

Values are means ± SD. * indicates significant differences compared to the Exercise group (* $p<0.05$, ** $p<0.01$); # indicates significant differences compared to pre-calculated intake (## $p<0.01$); H_2O, Water; Fe, Iron; Na, Sodium; Ca, Calcium.

targeted training HR was 140±8 beats·min^{-1} corresponding to the HR measured at 50% of the altitude specific peak power output attained during the baseline hypoxic test. HR and SpO_2 exercise responses were recorded using a short-range telemetry system (iBody, Wahoo Fitness, Atlanta, U.S.) and a finger oximetery device (3100 WristOx, Nonin Medicals, Minnesota, U.S.), respectively. The Sedentary group participants were not allowed to perform any static or dynamic exercise throughout the confinement period.

Body mass and composition. Body mass, whole-body composition and regional body composition and (% body fat, fat mass and fat-free mass (FFM)) were assessed at Pre and Post using a fan-beam dual-energy X-ray absorptiometry scanner ((DXA) Discovery W - QDR series, Hologic, Bedford U.S.). To optimize the reproducibility of the DXA measures the participants were always scanned in the morning, fasted and well rested. Both leg and android (abdomen) regions of interest used for the regional analysis were defined as detailed previously [32]. The precision of DXA for *in vivo* body composition measurements has previously been demonstrated [33]. The scans were subsequently analyzed by the same experienced researcher using the Hologic APEX System Software (version 3.1.2).

Meal tolerance test (MTT). The MTT protocol is outlined in Figure 1. The MTT was performed in a quiet, thermally comfortable laboratory (temperature =22.6±0.9°C; relative humidity =48.3±6.8%), with participants in a semi-supine position. The first MTT was performed in the morning of the Day -1 (Pre) and the second commenced following exactly 240-hrs of confinement on the morning of Day +1, prior to exiting hypoxic environment (Post). The participants refrained from exhaustive exercise, and from alcohol and coffee consumption and were placed on a standardized, prescribed diet for two days prior to the first MTT. The last meal before both tests was a standardized dinner served exactly 12-hrs before the start of the MTT. The MTT comprised fasting sample collection, standardized meal ingestion at time 0, and subsequent postprandial sample collection for two hrs. Breath samples for determination of ^{13}C isotope in expired CO_2, used as an indicator of the glucose uptake and the rate of gastric emptying, were obtained at 15-min intervals throughout the MTT. Perceived appetite ratings were obtained at 30-min intervals during the MTT. A standardized liquid meal (Ensure Plus vanilla flavor, Abbott nutrition laboratories Ltd., Maidenhead, U.K.) with an energy value of 1.5 kcal·mL^{-1} was used. Both, the meal volume (5 mL·kg^{-1}) and the amount of diluted ^{13}C isotope-labeled glucose (9.2 mg·kg^{-1}) were calculated according to each individual's body weight on the day of the MTT. The average volume and energy content of the liquid meal were 366.8±40.5 mL and 550±61 kcal, respectively. The average liquid meal comprised 73.9±8.1 g of carbohydrate, 22.8±2.5 g of protein and 18.0±1.9 g of fat. The participants were requested to consume the liquid meal in its entirety.

Blood sampling. Arterialized venous blood samples were obtained from a 20-gauge cannula (Venflon, Becton Dickinson Infusion Therapy, Helsingborg, Sweden) inserted retrograde into a vein on the dorsum of the wrist or the forearm. A 7-cm extension catheter (Connecta, Becton Dickinson Infusion Therapy, Helsingborg, Sweden) was attached to allow blood to be sampled away from the hand. The catheterized arm was placed in a hot box (Handwarmer, MEU University of Nottingham, Nottingham, U.K.) at least 15 minutes before the first blood sampling to provide a constantly high hand temperature throughout the MTT (air temperature within the heated box ~55°C). The cannula was flushed with saline solution (0.9% Sodium Chloride, Baxter Healthcare, Norfolk U.K.) after each sampling. To account for the cannula dead space and saline blood dilution, two mL of blood was drawn and discarded before each sampling. The first two fasting samples (8 mL) were obtained before the ingestion of the meal (−15 & −5 min) with additional samples (6 mL) collected at 15-min intervals throughout the MTT (15, 30, 45, 60, 75, 90, 105 & 120 min). The plasma concentration of total ghrelin, PYY, GLP-1, insulin and plasma glucose were determined at all sampling points, while the concentrations of serum leptin, adiponectin, high-density lipoprotein cholesterol (HDL-C), low-density lipoprotein cholesterol (LDL-C), total cholesterol, plasma free-fatty acids (FFA), triacylglycerols (TAG), and catecholamines (adrenaline & noradrenaline) were only determined from the two fasting samples. A 0.5 mL blood sample was also obtained every 10 min to monitor the plasma glucose concentration throughout the MTT. To determine any acute changes in the measured markers an additional fasting venous blood sample (6 mL) was obtained following the first 24-hrs of confinement (morning of Day 2), by venepuncture from the antecubital vein.

The sampled blood for determination of total ghrelin and PYY was collected into a precooled EDTA tube (Vacutainer K2E, Becton Dickinson, Plymouth, U.K.) containing 50 μl of Trasylol, whereas a pre-cooled EDTA tube containing 50 μl of Dipeptidyl peptidase-4 was used for GLP-1 determination. For fasting TAG and catecholamine assessment, the blood was collected into a continuously ice-cooled Lithium Heparin tube (Vacutainer LH, Becton Dickinson, Plymouth, U.K.) containing 50 μl of ethylene glycol tetraacetic acid (EGTA) and 10 μl of the lipase inhibitor, tetrahydrolipostatin. 50 μl of EGTA was added to a precooled Lithium Heparin tube (Vacutainer LH, Becton Dickinson, Plymouth, U.K.) used to collect the fasting sample for FFA determination. These samples were immediately centrifuged (3500 rpm; 10-min @ 4°C) using a laboratory centrifuge (Centric 200R, Tehtnica Železniki, Železniki, Slovenia). The remaining sample was collected into a separate tube (Vacutainer SST II Advance tube, Becton Dickinson, Plymouth, U.K.) for serum insulin, leptin, adiponectin and cholesterol determination, and centrifuged, as detailed above, after standing at room temperature for 15 minutes to allow clotting to occur. Blood samples for glucose concentration determination were collected in a safe-seal fluoride oxalate tube (Microtube FH, Sarstedt, Nümbrecht, Deutschland) and immediately centrifuged (13500 rpm; 1-min @ ~22°C) in a micro centrifuge (Mini, Labogene, Lynge, Denmark). The plasma was transferred into a microtube (Microtube Cap, Sarstedt, Nümbrecht, Deutschland) and frozen at −80°C immediately after the MTT for subsequent analysis performed less than 6 months after the study.

Biochemistry. The analysis of all plasma and serum samples was performed in duplicate using the methods outlined below. Appropriate radioimmunoassays (EMD Millipore, Billerica, U.S.) were used to determine the concentration of total ghrelin, PYY, insulin, leptin, and adiponectin. GLP-1 concentration was determined using sandwich ELISA (EMD Millipore, Billerica, U.S.), comprising amide acid GLP-1 7-36 and 7-37. The glucose concentration was assessed using the glucose oxidase enzymatic method (YSI Inc., Yellow Springs, Ohio, USA).

The concentration of FFA, TAG, HDL-C, LDL-C and total cholesterol was determined using spectrophotometry (ABX Pentra 400, Horiba Medical, Montpellier, France). Adrenaline and noradrenaline concentrations were determined by extraction of both from the plasma (HPLC – ECD; Glutathione preservative E4378, Sigma-Aldrich Company Ltd., Dosert, U.K.), followed by high performance liquid chromatography with electrochemical detection [34]. The intra-assay coefficient of variation (CV) for leptin, FFA, TAG, HDL-C, LDL-C and total cholesterol (analyzed in a single run) were 1.0%, 1.5%, 2.9%, 1.3%, 1.0% and 4.6%, respectively. The inter-assay CV for total ghrelin, PYY, GLP-1, insulin, plasma glucose, adiponectin, adrenaline and noradrenaline (analyzed in multiple runs) were 9.1%, 6.7%, 4.9%, 7.4%, 2.3%, 8.6%, 11.8% and 17.2%, respectively.

Isotope ^{13}C tracer protocol. Ubiquitously labeled ^{13}C glucose, tested for pyrogenicity and sterility (Cambridge Isotope Laboratories, Inc., Andover, U.S.) was dissolved in the individual's liquid meal immediately prior to the MTT. The breath sampling protocol is based on the principle that the ingested substrate is absorbed, metabolized, and a measurable metabolite subsequently expelled through the respiratory system. The rate of appearance of ^{13}C isotope in exhaled breath CO_2 is a product of the rate of gastric emptying, absorption from the gut, uptake by metabolizing tissues and oxidation of the liquid meal. Exhaled breath samples were collected into a 500 mL breath-sampling bag using a one-way valve, before the meal ingestion (−15 & −5 min) and at 15-min intervals postprandially (15, 30, 45, 60, 75, 90, 105 & 120 min). At each sampling point, duplicate 12-mL breath vials (Exetainer, Labco Limited, Lampeter, U.K.) were filled from the breath-sampling bag using a catheter (Vacutainer adapter, Becton Dickinson, Plymouth, U.K.). All $^{13}CO_2$ samples were analyzed in triplicate using continuous flow isotope ratio mass spectrometry (VG Isochrom, VG Analytical, Manchester, U.K.) less than six months after the study.

Perceived appetite ratings. Visual analogue scores (VAS) were obtained before and during the MTT using a custom-designed application on an iPad tablet (Apple, Cupertino, USA) to assess perception of hunger, fullness, desire to eat, and prospective food consumption (PFC) [35]. The VAS scale was a 100 mm digital line, anchored to the left with 'sensation not felt at all' and to the right with 'sensation felt the greatest'. A similar VAS collection method using a handheld electronic device has been validated previously [36]. The participants were instructed to place a vertical line according to their perceived feeling at that particular point in time for all included questions. VAS were filled by the participants 5 min before the liquid meal ingestion and 30 min, 60 min, 90 min and 120 min thereafter. The Composite Satiety Score (CSS) was subsequently calculated from the obtained scores using the following formula (higher the score, higher the level of subjective satiety): CSS = (Fullness + (100 − Desire) + (100 − Hunger) + (100 – PFC))/4. CSS scores were also obtained throughout the confinement period before and after breakfast, lunch and dinner.

Statistical analysis and calculations. All data were coded and analyzed using Statistica 12.0 for Windows (StatSoft, Tulsa, USA). Prior to analysis the data were tested for normality of distribution using a modified Kolmogorov-Smirnov test. Student's independent-samples t-test was used to compare participants' baseline characteristics and average daily energy and macronutrient intakes between groups. Area under the curve (AUC) was calculated for total ghrelin, PYY, GLP-1, insulin, plasma glucose and CSS changes during the MTT, using the conventional trapezoid rule. Due to blood clotting and resulting inability to obtain the last two blood samples during one of the Post MTT tests the AUC values were calculated over 90-min for total ghrelin, PYY, GLP-1 and insulin and over 100-min for glucose. The Pre data obtained at 105 and 120-min from this individual were omitted from the analysis. A 1-way repeated measures unbalanced ANOVA analysis was used to define the effect of the 10-day confinement on BP, HR, SpO_2, LLS [group (Exercise & Sedentary) × Time (Day1–Day10)] and fasting metabolic markers (leptin, adiponectin, FFA, TAG, cholesterol and catecholamines), calculated AUC values and body-composition changes [group (Exercise & Sedentary) × testing period (Pre & Post)]. A 2-way repeated measures unbalanced ANOVA [group (Exercise & Sedentary) × testing period (Pre & Post) × time (MTT Pre & Post prandial responses)] was used to define the effect of the 10-day confinement on the CSS and metabolic markers, measured throughout the MTT (total ghrelin, PYY, GLP-1, insulin, glucose). Tukey's HSD *post hoc* test was employed to define the specific differences when ANOVA analysis revealed a significant F-ratio for the main effect or an interaction. Pearson's correlation coefficient was used to define bivariate correlations between changes in whole body fat and fat free mass (Pre-Post) and changes in fasting levels of total ghrelin, PYY, GLP-1, insulin, glucose and leptin. Values are represented as mean ± SD in the text and tables and as mean ± SEM in the figures. Statistical significance was set a priori at $\alpha = 0.05$.

The ^{13}C glucose results are expressed as a change of ^{13}C using the $^{13}CO_2$ enrichment equations. The differences between the measured ^{13}C enrichment in the expired CO_2 and the international standard for ^{13}C abundance (0.010767) were calculated and expressed as atoms %. The values were normalized and define the total amount of units for delta change after a standardized meal (total amount of the substrate metabolized). Insulin resistance was quantified before (Pre) and after (Post) the confinement by the homeostatic model assessment (HOMA IR) method [37] using the following formula: HOMA IR = (fasting insulin (mU·l^{-1})) × (fasting glucose (mmol·l^{-1}))/22.5.

For metabolic parameters with significant main effects or interactions, ANOVA revealed the following observed statistical analysis power: 0.98 for total ghrelin (time effect), 0.96 for PYY (time effect), 0.98 for GLP-1 (time effect), 0.87 for insulin (time × testing period effect), 0.78 for glucose (time × testing period effect), 0.93 for leptin (time effect), 0.89 for adiponectin (time effect), 0.64 for TAG (time effect), 0.82 for noradrenalin (time effect), 0.67 for LDL-C (time × group effect), 0.85 for total cholesterol (time effect) and 0.84 for CSS (time effect).

Results

Participants

Except for one participant with acute appendicitis, and one with general adaptation problems, all others underwent the confinement without any significant adverse effects. AMS was present in 4 participants in the Exercise group, and 3 in the Sedentary group on Day 1. The average LLS values were comparable between groups throughout the confinement (Exercise = 1.5 [0–6]; Sedentary = 1.4 [0–7]; mean [range]).

The participants in the Exercise group performed all 20 training sessions. The average training HR responses (142±11 beats·min^{-1}) were within the targeted levels and the average SpO_2 values were 85% [76–89%] (mean [range]). Average daily systolic, but not diastolic BP was higher in the Exercise group than in the Sedentary group (125±9 mmHg vs 119±12 mmHg; p = 0.01). A significant decrease in resting daily HR over the confinement period was only noted in the Exercise group (p<0.01), with HR decreasing from 100±12 beats·min^{-1} at Day 1 to 80±12 beats·min^{-1} on Day 10. The SpO_2 was higher on Day 10 (87 [83–92%]) than on Day 1 (81 [77–84%]; p<0.01) in the Exercise group, and tended to be lower compared to Sedentary group on Day 3 (Exercise = 83 [78–88%]; Sedentary = 88 [86–91%]; p = 0.09 (mean [range])).

Diet and fluid intake

The average daily energy, macronutrient, water, and selected micronutrient intakes of both groups are presented in Table 1. Compared to the pre-calculated levels the actual average energy intake was significantly lower only in the Exercise group (2601±383 kcal; p<0.01), while the Sedentary group intake only tended to be lower (2213±192 kcal; p>0.05). Average daily total water intake, was significantly higher in the Exercise (4.87±1.46 L; p<0.01) compared to the Sedentary (3.28±1.34 L) group. As a consequence of greater food consumption, the iron, sodium, and calcium intakes were significantly higher in the Exercise compared to the Sedentary group (p<0.05) (Table 1).

Body mass and composition

Body mass, whole body fat mass, whole body FFM as well as leg FFM were significantly lower in the Sedentary than the Exercise group prior to the study. Body mass was significantly reduced in both groups following the 10-day confinement period (Exercise = −1.4 kg; Sedentary = −1.4 kg; p<0.05). As noted in Table 2, whole body fat mass was significantly reduced after the confinement in the Exercise group whereas no changes were observed in whole body % body fat and FFM (p>0.05) in either group. After the confinement, the leg fat mass significantly decreased (p = 0.03) and the leg FFM significantly increased (p = 0.01) in the Exercise group only. No differences significant differences were observed in the regional android fat or FFM (Table 2).

Hormonal appetite markers

Fasting levels and postprandial levels of total ghrelin, PYY and GLP-1 were not significantly different between groups (p>0.05), or between Pre and Post MTT tests within groups (p>0.05; Figure 2, 3). As noted in Table 3, fasting morning values of total ghrelin, PYY and GLP-1 were similar on Day 2 compared to Pre (p>0.05). The AUC values for total ghrelin, PYY and GLP-1 was also comparable between groups at Pre and did not significantly change at Post (p>0.05; Table 4). No significant differences were noted in fasting leptin and adiponectin levels (p>0.05) between Pre and Post values and between the groups (Table 3).

Changes (Pre-Post) in fasting leptin concentration were significantly correlated to changes in whole body fat mass following the confinement (Pre-Post; r = −0.70, p = 0.01). No correlation was found between changes in whole body fat mass and whole body FFM and changes in fasting levels of total ghrelin (r = 0.33, r = 0.02, p>0.05), PYY (r = −0.32, r = 0.38, p>0.05), GLP-1 (r = 0.05, r = −0.01, p>0.05).

Perceived appetite ratings

The CSS values during the MTT are presented in Figure 4. No significant differences were noted either between groups (p>0.05), or between Pre and Post testing (p>0.05). No significant differences in CSS were observed throughout the MTT in the Exercise group (p>0.05). Also, CSS AUC was not significantly different between groups and testing periods (p>0.05; Table 4). Morning fasting daily CSS values were comparable between groups throughout the whole confinement period except on Day 2 with significantly lower values in the Exercise (44±6 mm), than the Sedentary group (56±7 mm; p<0.05) as well as compared to Pre fasting values (53±5 mm; p<0.05). The average aggregate daily CSS values obtained throughout the confinement period were comparable between groups (Exercise group = 63±2 mm, Sedentary group = 62±3 mm; p>0.05)

Insulin sensitivity

Insulin resistance, quantified by HOMA IR was similar between groups at Pre and only significantly decreased following the confinement in the Sedentary group (Exercise group: Pre = 2.23±0.47, Post = 1.85±0.43, p>0.05; Sedentary group: Pre = 2.27±0.38; Post = 1.71±0.25, p = 0.03).

No differences were noted between groups in fasting and postprandial insulin kinetics (p>0.05) at both study days. Compared to Pre, the insulin levels were significantly reduced at 40-min postprandial sampling during the Post MTT (p = 0.01; Figure 3) in the Sedentary group. The insulin AUC was significantly reduced in both groups following the confinement (p = 0.04; Table 4). Fasting glucose was comparable between groups and did not change following the confinement (Exercise group: Pre = 5.03±0.16, Post = 4.76±0.30; Sedentary group: Pre = 4.89±0.27; Post = 4.74±0.18; p>0.05). Postprandial glucose concentration was significantly lower at 50–70 min sampling at Post compared to Pre in the Exercise group only (p = 0.03; Figure 5). Postprandial glucose was significantly increased between 20–90 min sampling points during the Pre (p = 0.04) and at 20–40 min and 100–110 min samplings during the Post (p = 0.01) in the Exercise group (Figure 5). In the

Table 2. Body mass, whole body (WB) composition and regional leg and android (abdomen) composition analysis (DXA) in both Exercise and Sedentary group before (Pre) and after (Post) the 10-Day normobaric hypoxic confinement.

	Exercise group		Sedentary group	
	Pre	**Post**	**Pre**	**Post**
Body mass (kg)	75.2±6.4	73.8±6.1#	68.8±10.1**	67.4±9.8#**
WB fat mass (kg)	17.4±5.9	15.9±5.4##	15.6±4.8**	14.7±5.1
WB fat free mass (kg)	57.8±3.9	57.9±3.7	53.2±5.4**	52.7±4.9
% Body fat (%)	22.8±6.2	21.2±5.8	21.6±4.4	21.3±4.8
Leg fat mass (kg)	6.3±0.6	5.6±0.6#	5.9±0.5	5.6±0.5
Leg fat free mass (kg)	17.5±0.5	18.0±0.4##	16.4±0.6**	16.1±0.4
Android fat mass (kg)	1.2±0.4	1.1±0.4	1.1±0.5	1.1±0.4
Android fat free mass (kg)	3.8±0.3	4.0±0.3	3.7±0.5	3.6±0.5

Values are means ± SD. ** indicates significant differences compared to the Exercise group ($p<0.01$);
# indicates significant differences compared to Pre (# $p<0.05$, ## $p<0.01$).

Sedentary group, glucose was elevated postprandially between 20–90 min sampling during the Pre and between 20–120 min during the Post MTT ($p = 0.01$). A trend for a reduction in glucose AUC following the confinement was observed in the Exercise group only ($p = 0.07$; Table 4).

Isotope ^{13}C

As illustrated in Figure 5, no significant differences ($p>0.05$) were observed between the Exercise and Sedentary group or between Pre and Post testing periods in atom percent excess of expired CO_2 isotopic enrichment kinetics following the standardized meal ingestion.

Lipid profile and catecholamines

Compared to Pre the TAG concentration was significantly increased in the Sedentary group ($p = 0.03$) on Day 2 (Table 3). No significant differences were observed in fasting levels of FFA ($p>0.05$) and TAG ($p>0.05$) between Pre and Post values and between the groups (Table 3). Total cholesterol was significantly increased in the Sedentary group on Day 2 ($p = 0.02$) and reduced

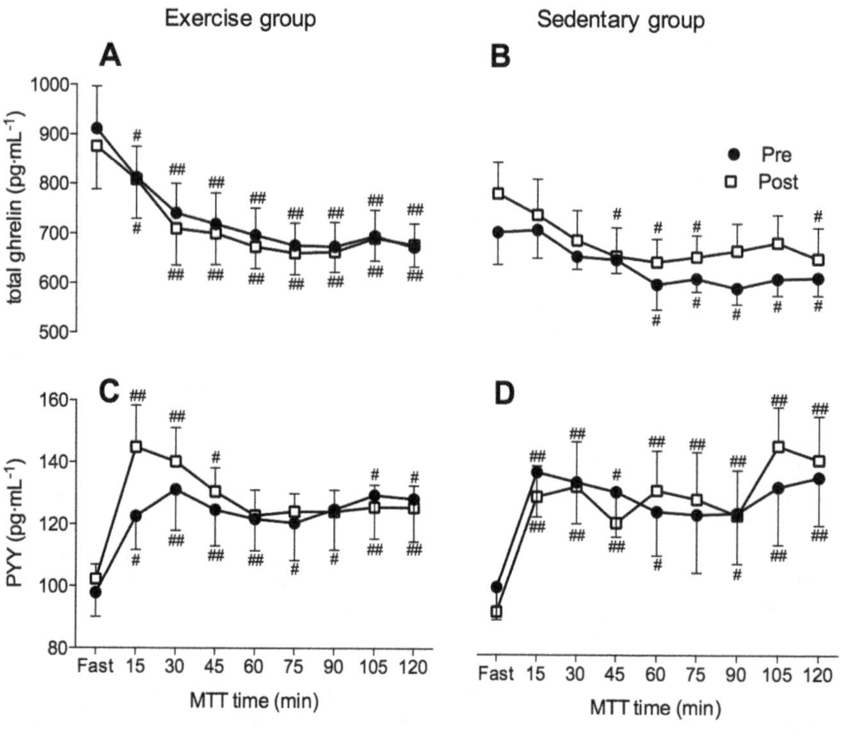

Figure 2. Total ghrelin and peptide YY (PYY) kinetics during the meal tolerance test in both Exercise (A, C) and Sedentary (B, D) group, respectively. The meal tolerance test (MTT) was performed before (Pre; closed circles) and after (Post; open squares) the confinement. Two-way repeated measures ANOVA analysis, followed by a Tukey's HSD *post hoc* test; # indicates significant differences compared to fasting values (# $p<0.05$; ## $p<0.01$). Values are mean ± SEM.

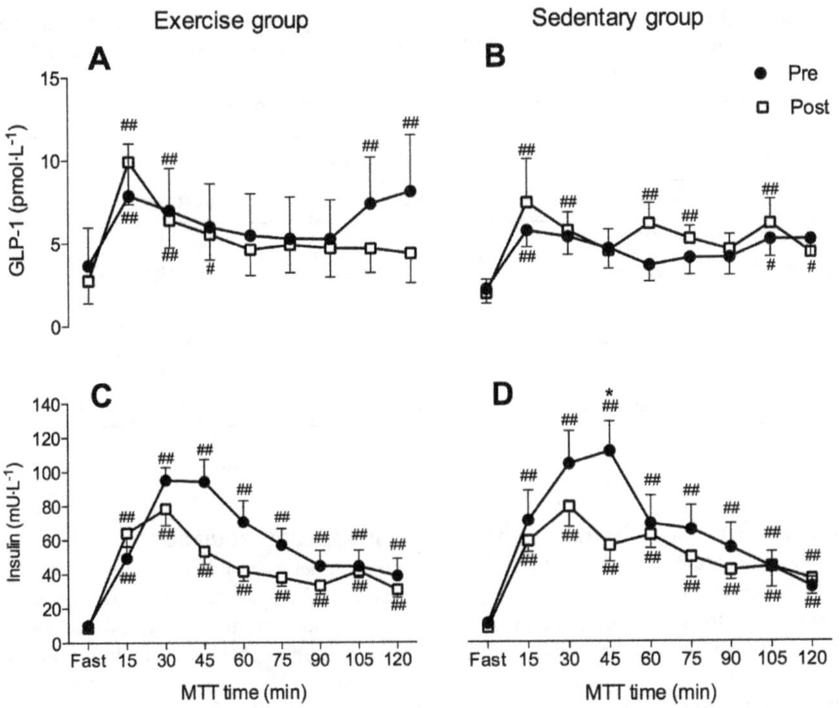

Figure 3. Glucagon-like peptide-1 (GLP-1) and insulin kinetics during the meal tolerance test in Exercise (A, C) and Sedentary (B, D) group, respectively. The meal tolerance test (MTT) was performed before (Pre; closed circles) and after (Post; open squares) the confinement. Two-way repeated measures ANOVA analysis, followed by a Tukey's HSD *post hoc* test; # indicates significant differences compared to fasting values (# $p<0.05$; ## $p<0.01$). * indicates significant differences compared to Pre values ($p<0.05$). Values are mean ± SEM.

at Post in the Exercise group only ($p=0.01$; Figure 6). As noted in Figure 6, LDL-C was significantly reduced in the Exercise group at Post ($p=0.01$). The LDL-C values at Post were lower in the Exercise compared to the Sedentary group ($p=0.04$). No differences were observed in the Sedentary group or in HDL-C values between groups or testing periods ($p>0.05$).

Noradrenaline levels were significantly increased on Day 2 in the Exercise group only ($p=0.01$) (Table 3). No significant differences were observed in fasting adrenaline ($p>0.05$) or noradrenaline ($p>0.05$) levels between Pre and Post values or between the two groups (Table 3).

Discussion

Main findings

This study investigated the effects of prolonged hypoxic exposure combined with, or without exercise training on hormonal

Table 3. Fasting levels of total ghrelin, peptide YY (PYY), glucagon-like peptide-1 (GLP-1), insulin, leptin, adiponectin, free fatty acids (FFA), triacylglycerols (TAG), adrenaline and noradrenaline in both Exercise and Sedentary group before (Pre), following the first 24-hrs of confinement (Day 2) and immediately after the 10-day confinement (Post).

	Exercise group			Sedentary group		
	Pre	Day 2	Post	Pre	Day 2	Post
Total ghrelin (pg·mL⁻¹)	911±239	817±162	876±247	705±160	743±145	782±155
PYY (pg·mL⁻¹)	97.8±21.8	93.8±13.3	102.2±13.6	101.7±25.6	96.8±31.2	93.8±20.7
GLP-1 (pmol·L⁻¹)	3.65±6.6	3.75±5.84	2.75±3.82	1.92±2.12	2.62±2.35	1.67±2.04
Insulin (mU·L⁻¹)	10.6±2.0	10.9±1.9	8.7±1.9	10.4±1.5	12.1±1.9	8.1±1.1##
Leptin (μg·L⁻¹)	4.91±3.53	6.92±4.22	3.65±2.02##	3.60±1.22	5.03±2.14	3.49±1.36
Adiponectin (μg·mL⁻¹)	7.41±3.26	7.97±3.63	6.12±3.43#	8.03±2.23	8.09±1.68	7.05±0.51
FFA (mmol·L⁻¹)	0.44±0.23	0.56±0.24	0.44±0.15	0.52±0.22	0.45±0.20	0.52±0.14
TAG (mmol·L⁻¹)	0.52±0.16	0.55±0.17	0.56±0.20	0.46±0.25	0.73±0.35*	0.55±0.28
Adrenaline (nmol·L⁻¹)	0.27±0.05	0.24±0.14	0.23±0.06	0.19±0.08	0.19±0.13	0.24±0.07
Noradrenaline (nmol·L⁻¹)	0.86±0.35	1.52±0.51*	1.16±0.26	0.95±0.67	1.29±0.49	1.28±0.39

Values are means ± SD. * indicates significant differences compared to Pre ($p<0.05$); # indicates significant differences compared to Day 2 (# $p<0.05$, ## $p<0.01$).

Table 4. Area under the curve calculated from total ghrelin, peptide YY (PYY), Glucagon-like peptide-1 (GLP-1), insulin, glucose and Composite satiety score (CSS) kinetics in both Exercise and Sedentary group during the meal tolerance test performed before (Pre) and after (Post) the 10-Day normobaric hypoxic confinement.

	Exercise group		Sedentary group	
	Pre	Post	Pre	Post
Total ghrelin (pg·mL^{-1}·90 min^{-1})	44379±9721	43220±10043	37808±5582	41157±8030
PYY (pg·mL^{-1}·90 min^{-1})	7318±1854	7755±1416	7714±2119	7597±1767
GLP^{-}1 (pmol·L^{-}1·90 min^{-1})	360±437	351±285	247±136	305±159
Insulin (mU·L^{-1}·90 min^{-1})	3941±1138	2965±561##	4348±2006	3170±849##
Glucose (mmol·L^{-1}·100 min^{-1})	664±63	605±44	662±78	631±59
CSS (mm·120 min^{-1})	2061±286	2391±288	2240±172	2092±154

Values are means ± SD. ## indicates significant differences compared to Pre ($p<0.01$).

appetite regulation and select metabolic markers. Contrary to our initial hypothesis, adding exercise to a 10-day hypoxic confinement did not significantly affect hormonal appetite regulation in fasted and postprandial states. Similarly, based on the ^{13}C tracer results, the passage of glucose from ingestion to breakdown and CO_2 excretion was also unaffected. The potentially beneficial effects of adding exercise to hypoxia observed in this study were the reduction in postprandial glucose response, a significant decrease in fasting total cholesterol, secondary to LDL-C reduction and a reduction of whole body fat mass.

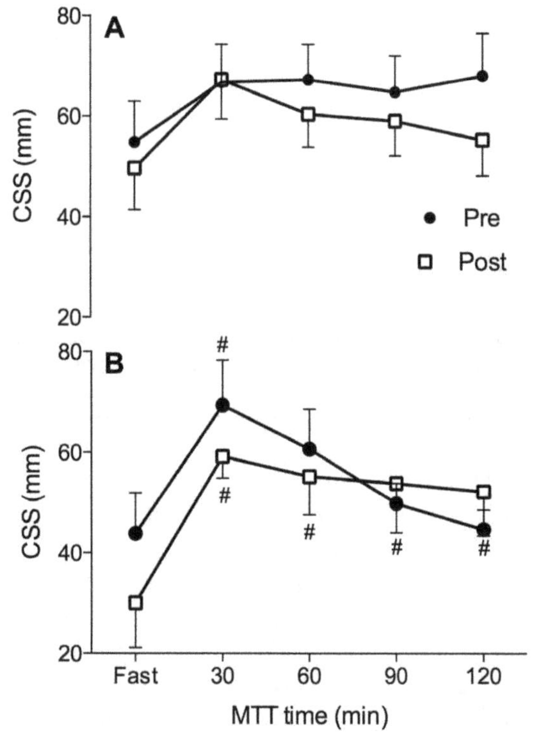

Figure 4. Composite satiety scores before (Fast) and at 30-min intervals throughout the meal tolerance test for both Exercise (A) and Sedentary group (B). One-way repeated measures ANOVA followed by Tukey's HSD *post hoc* test; # indicates significant differences compared to fasting values ($p<0.05$). Values are mean ± SEM.

Hypoxia and hormonal appetite regulation

Ghrelin is the only known appetite stimulating gut peptide, and it has been suggested to play a role in the altitude-related appetite modulation. Acute [6–8], but not chronic [7] hypoxic exposure has been shown to reduce circulating ghrelin levels. Interestingly, the fasting ghrelin levels in our study were unchanged both upon acute exposure (24-hrs), and after the 10-day exposure to a simulated altitude of 4000 m. Furthermore, postprandial ghrelin kinetics and the ghrelin AUC were also unaffected by hypoxic confinement *per se.* As the degree of hypoxia (~3500–4200 m altitude) and AMS responses were similar in the present and aforementioned studies [6–8], factors underlying the different outcomes are not obvious. These might include the diet and mode of hypoxia (i.e normobaric vs. hypobaric). It has to be noted however, that the lack of change in ghrelin concentration was also previously observed following chronic high-altitude altitude exposure [9].

The measured anorexigenic modulators leptin, GLP-1 and PYY were also unaffected by prolonged hypoxic exposure in our study. This seems contrary to the majority of other studies indicating that the levels of the satiety-inducing adipokine leptin increase as a result of acute hypoxic exposure [7,10,11]. However, the response of leptin to hypoxia has been widely debated and collective results from the reported studies are equivocal. Leptin has also been related to GLP-1 production in a rodent model, and subsequently a leptin appetite suppression through a GLP-1 mediated pathway was proposed [38]. To date only one study examined the response of GLP-1 to acute hypoxia and showed a tendency for increased GLP-1 postprandially with no changes in the fasting state [10]. The dependent relation between leptin and GLP-1 could therefore play a role in the lack of appetite regulation changes observed in this study. Similarly to GLP-1, only one study to date examined the effects of hypoxic exposure on PYY concentration and observed a tendency for lower PYY values in response to acute hypoxia than to normoxia [8]. Thus, implying that PYY might not be involved in hypoxia-induced appetite modulation. Our data also lend support to this notion as no significant changes in PYY after acute or prolonged hypoxic exposure were observed. The lack of changes in the measured hormonal appetite regulation markers following hypoxic confinement without concomitant exercise is also corroborated by the unchanged fasting and postprandial ratings of perceived appetite throughout the 10-day confinement. Collectively, the responses of the Sedentary group participants indicate that acute or prolonged exposure to simulated altitude of 4000 m does not seem to alter fasting and

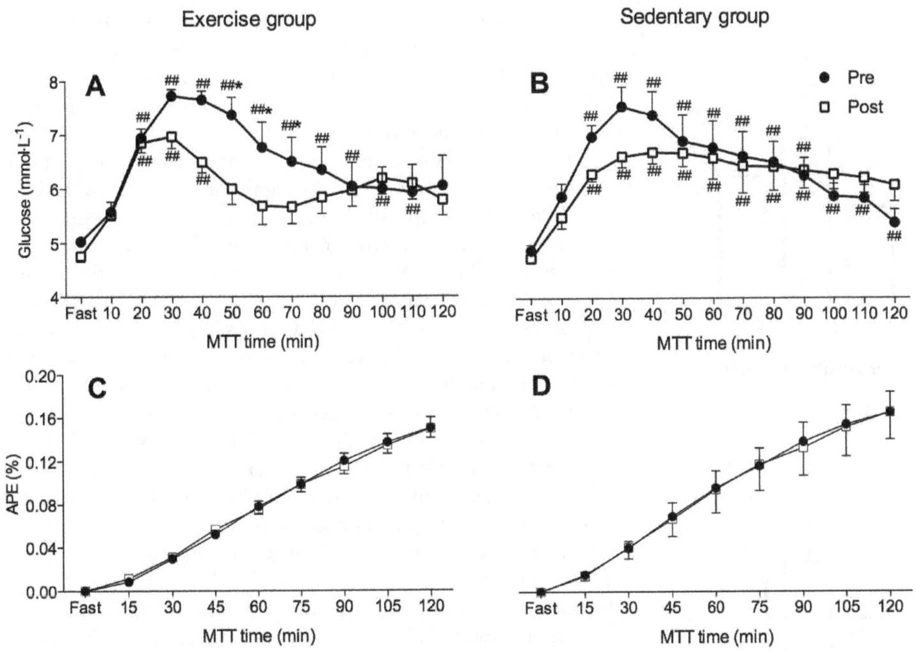

Figure 5. Plasma glucose kinetics and atom percent excess (APE) of expired CO_2 isotopic enrichment changes during the meal tolerance test in Exercise (A, C) and Sedentary group (B, D), respectively. The meal tolerance test (MTT) was performed before (Pre; closed circles) and after (Post; open squares) the confinement. Two-way repeated measures ANOVA followed by Tukey's HSD *post hoc* test; ## indicates significant differences compared to fasting values ($p<0.01$). * indicates significant differences compared to Pre values ($p<0.05$). Values are mean ± SEM.

postprandial (2-hrs) concentrations of ghrelin, leptin, GLP-1 and PYY plasma.

Hypoxia, exercise and hormonal appetite regulation

While many studies investigating concomitant hypoxia and exercise aimed to determine the potential beneficial effects on performance in athletes [19], very few scrutinized the combined effects on appetite regulation and metabolic health [8]. Moreover, no long-term study to date attempted to discern the separate effects of exercise, often associated with high altitude sojourns, and prolonged hypoxia on hormonal appetite regulation.

The hypothesis that combination of hypoxia and exercise might down-regulate appetite through modulation of orexigenic and anorexigenic hormones was recently tested in healthy sedentary men [26]. The participants in this study performed 12 training sessions over a four-week period (3 training sessions per week) under either hypoxia (~4000 m) or normoxia. Similarly to the current study they did not find any changes in fasting ghrelin, leptin and GLP-1 following hypoxic training although postprandial levels of leptin were increased in both the hypoxic and normoxic group. Interestingly, GLP-1 levels were only increased after the normoxic training. This is in line with previous studies demonstrating elevated GLP-1 levels following exercise training in normoxia [39], and suggests that GLP-1 might not play a role in combined exercise and hypoxia related appetite reduction. Wasse et al. [8] recently investigated ghrelin and PYY responses to acute hypoxic exposure, in combination with exercise and showed that there is a significant effect of both hypoxia and exercise on postprandial acylated ghrelin concentration. This was not confirmed in our study where total ghrelin was unchanged after the first 24-hrs of hypoxia as well as following 10 days of chronic hypoxia combined with exercise. This is in line with previous reports showing that ghrelin concentration can return to baseline upon prolonged exposure to hypoxia [7,9]. However, it has to be noted that we also did not observe any acute changes in total ghrelin levels. No changes in PYY concentration after combined hypoxia and exercise were observed in this study, which support the notion that PYY might not play a role in hypoxia induced hormonal appetite regulation [8]. This notion is further reinforced by reports suggesting that the addition of hypoxia to exercise might even suppress PYY compared to identical exercise performed in normoxic conditions [40].

No change in the perceived appetite ratings was also noted in the Exercise group during or after the 10-day confinement in spite of the fact that the actual intakes were lower then targeted. Both observations together could be suggestive of a reduced motivation to eat during combined hypoxia and exercise training. Collectively, this corroborates the unchanged hormonal appetite measures and also, importantly, indicates that the physical activity factors used for dietary intake calculations (1.4 Sedentary; 1.8 Exercise) were appropriate for both conditions.

Hypoxia, exercise and metabolic risk factors

Training in hypoxia has been shown to be superior to normoxic training for reducing fasting and postprandial insulin levels, insulin resistance [25] and improving glucose tolerance [41]. Based on these reports, and the fact that both hypoxia and exercise exert strong effects on the metabolic system, we reasoned that the addition of exercise to continuous hypoxic exposure would result in enhanced insulin sensitivity and lipid profiles. Especially, since hypoxia and exercise have been shown to up-regulate hypoxia-inducible factor 1α target genes [23] involved in glucose, oxygen uptake and lipid metabolism through increases in peroxisome proliferator activated receptor γ co-activator-1α [42]. However

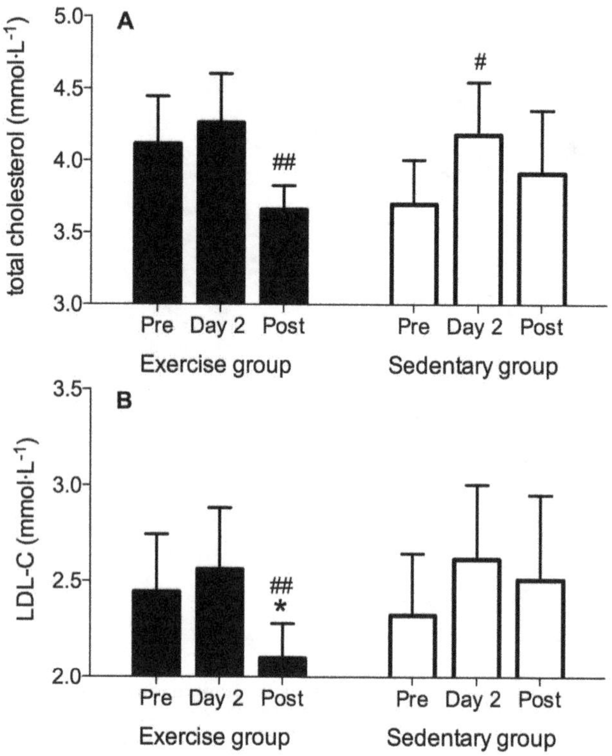

Figure 6. Fasting total cholesterol (A) and low-density lipoprotein cholesterol (LDL-C) levels in both Exercise and Sedentary group before (Pre), following the first 24-hrs of confinement (Day 2) and immediately after the confinement (Post). One-way repeated measures ANOVA followed by Tukey's HSD *post hoc* test; # indicates significant differences compared to Pre (# $p < 0.05$; ## $p < 0.01$). * indicates significant differences compared to the Sedentary group ($p < 0.05$). Values are mean ± SEM.

contrary to our hypothesis we did not observe any changes to measured metabolic variables as a result of exercise during prolonged hypoxia. Indeed the glycemic responses to feeding were similar in both groups, with significantly reduced insulin AUC at Post compared to Pre and no significant changes in glucose AUC in both groups. This finding supports the notion that hypoxia *per se* beneficially affects insulin postprandial kinetics [25,41]. While the glucose AUC was unchanged following the confinement in the Sendentary group, a tendency for a decreased glucose AUC was observed in the Exercise group. This observation could be explained by the increased glucose turnover previously documented following prolonged acclimatization to high altitudes [43]. Taken together, the glucose AUC and significant postprandial glucose concentration reductions, suggest that performing exercise training during hypoxic confinement might also results in improved postprandial insulin sensitivity although this was not observed in the present study. This hypothesis is in line with recent studies showing that the use of hypoxia during exercise training additively improves insulin sensitivity in sedentary individuals [26] and glycemic control in individuals with type 2 diabetes [27].

It has to be noted however that the postprandial insulin levels were only significantly reduced following the confinement in the Sedentary group. No significant changes in postprandial insulin kinetics were observed in the Exercise group in spite of the fact that glucose was reduced. Furthermore, the postprandial values of both glucose and insulin were, albeit not significantly, lower at Post compared to Pre following the confinement in both groups. The fact that these reductions were predominantly not significant could be explained by the relatively small sample size, potentially limiting the statistical significance of the outcomes.

Although beneficial effects of combining hypoxia and exercise training on TAG have been reported previously [25], we did not observe any additional effect of exercise during continuous hypoxia. Interestingly, we noted a significant increase in TAG in the Sedentary group after the first 24-hrs of confinement. Moreover, we did not observe any significant changes in FFA concentration during and after the confinement in either group although FFA reductions were previously reported following exercise performed at moderate altitudes due to their increased metabolic utilization during exercise and recovery [24]. The substrate metabolism responses could also be altered by the exercise-induced changes in catecholamine levels. Indeed, hypoxic training has been shown to potentiate the exercise-induced sympathetic activation [44]. This is in line with our findings indicating a significant increase in noradrenaline after the first 24-hrs of hypoxia in the Exercise group only.

Another potentially beneficial metabolic response of exercise in the present study, besides a tendency for a reduced postprandial glucose profile was a significant reduction in LDL-C and a concomitant total cholesterol reduction. Athough this has previously been reported to occur following hypoxic training [45], other studies did not find any changes in either total cholesterol or LDL-C following combined hypoxia and exercise [25,26].

In addition to select appetite and metabolic risk measures, the ^{13}C glucose tracer protocol was implemented in this study to indirectly assess postprandial glucose uptake and related gastric emptying. Even though it has been speculated that changes in gastro-intestinal flow/permeability might be involved in "altitude anorexia" [46], no changes in postprandial expired CO_2 isotopic enrichment kinetics were observed in this study. This is in line with other recent data [47] suggesting that both, glucose uptake and the rate of gastric emptying are unaffected by hypoxia.

Methodological considerations

To our knowledge, this is the first controlled study that explored the effects of long-term continuous exposure to hypoxia in combination with exercise training on hormonal appetite regulation and selected metabolic responses. The hypoxic nature of our intervention is clearly demonstrated by significant reductions in SpO_2 throughout the confinement period. While the SpO_2 values gradually increased during the ten-day confinement, as a result of the well-established hypoxic ventilatory acclimatization, the average values did not exceed 89% at any time.

The main strengths of the present study are standardized diet (i.e. macronutrient diet composition) as well as general living conditions (i.e. sleep, activity, environmental conditions) throughout the 10-day confinement period. Other studies investigating prolonged effects of training in hypoxia did not precisely control both the dietary composition and intake levels and that might have significantly affected the metabolic measures [20,21,25,26,41]. It has to be noted that although the dietary intakes were matched between groups in terms of macronutrient intake percentages the intakes were significantly lower in the Sedentary than in the Exercise group. Moreover, the fact that the participants in the Exercise group did not attain the targeted intakes resulted in a negative energy balance, also documented by the reductions in whole body fat mass. We can only speculate whether the reductions in fat mass observed in the Exercise group were a result of hypoxia and exercise or a consequence of insufficient energy intakes. The observed reductions in whole body fat mass are in line with the study by Haufe et al. [25] reporting similar reductions following a four-week hypoxic exercise training intervention. Nevertheless, the observed energy deficit and body composition changes might have influenced our metabolic outcomes since a negative energy balance resulting from reduced dietary intake has previously been shown to influence hormonal appetite regulation in healthy individuals [48]. An increase in basal metabolic rate as a result of exposure to hypoxia is also a factor that might have contributed to the negative energy balance and body mass reductions observed in both groups. While we did not perform the metabolic rate measurements, previous reports suggest that energy intake requirements at high altitudes may be higher as a consequence of increased basal metabolic rate [49].

While the results of this study extend our understanding of hormonal appetite regulation during combined exercise and hypoxia a few limitations of this study need to be addressed. First, the present study investigated the effects of normobaric rather than hypobaric hypoxia. Even though there are no known effects of pressure *per se* on hormonal appetite regulation, recent reports suggest that, for certain physiological functions, normobaric and hypobaric hypoxia do in fact induce somewhat different responses [50]. Second, due to the relatively small sample size the results should be interpreted with caution and it is warranted that the hypothesis of a synergistic effect of hypoxia and exercise is tested using higher number of participants. Third, to determine the potential orexigenic effects of combined hypoxia and exercise we measured resting and postprandial responses of total ghrelin rather than its acylated (active) form, suggested to mainly underlie the appetite inducing effects of ghrelin [13]. Finally, the dose of both, hypoxia and exercise should be taken into account when interpreting the findings of the present study. Based on previous reports indicating profound reductions in appetite as a result of exposures to extreme altitudes (>5000 m) [3], more severe hypoxia would probably exert larger effects on the measured appetite markers than those observed in the present study.

Conclusion

While some minor metabolic benefits of exercise training during normobaric hypoxic confinement were noted (i.e. decreased postprandial glucose response and reduced cholesterol levels), the findings of this study do not support the hypothesis that adding exercise training to hypoxic exposure significantly alters appetite regulation or improves metabolic outcomes. In addition, our findings indirectly indicate that glucose uptake and gut permeability are unaltered following prolonged hypoxia with or without exercise. Based on the current inconsistencies in the literature and given the escalating prevalence of obesity and metabolic dysfunctions, future well-controlled and powered dose-response trials are warranted to ultimately determine the potential of combining hypoxia and exercise for reducing appetite and improving cardiometabolic risk factors in both clinical populations and healthy humans.

Acknowledgments

We are grateful to the devoted participants who made this study possible. We would also like to thank Miss Iva Kumprej for her excellent laboratory assistance and Dr. Shawnda A. Morrison, Adam C. Mcdonnell and Miro Vrhovec for their invaluable contribution to the study. Last but not least we would like to acknowledge Mrs. Sally Cordon and Mrs. Karen Swift for their excellent work on sample biochemical analysis.

Author Contributions

Conceived and designed the experiments: TD EJS IAM OE IBM. Performed the experiments: TD EJS IBM. Analyzed the data: TD EJS. Contributed reagents/materials/analysis tools: EJS IAM OE IBM. Wrote the paper: TD EJS. Revised the paper for important intellectual content: TD EJS IAM OE IBM. Approved the final version: TD EJS IAM OE IBM.

References

1. Tschop M, Morrison KM (2001) Weight loss at high altitude. Adv Exp Med Biol 502: 237–247.
2. Kayser B, Verges S (2013) Hypoxia, energy balance and obesity: from pathophysiological mechanisms to new treatment strategies. Obes Rev 14: 579–592.
3. Westerterp-Plantenga MS, Westerterp KR, Rubbens M, Verwegen CR, Richelet JP, et al. (1999) Appetite at "high altitude" [Operation Everest III (Comex-'97)]: a simulated ascent of Mount Everest. J Appl Physiol 87: 391–399.
4. Rose MS, Houston CS, Fulco CS, Coates G, Sutton JR, et al. (1988) Operation Everest. II: Nutrition and body composition. J Appl Physiol (1985) 65: 2545–2551.
5. Hackett PH, Roach RC (2001) High-altitude illness. N Engl J Med 345: 107–114.
6. Riepl RL, Fischer R, Hautmann H, Hartmann G, Muller TD, et al. (2012) Influence of acute exposure to high altitude on basal and postprandial plasma levels of gastroenteropancreatic peptides. PLoS One 7: e44445.
7. Shukla V, Singh SN, Vats P, Singh VK, Singh SB, et al. (2005) Ghrelin and leptin levels of sojourners and acclimatized lowlanders at high altitude. Nutr Neurosci 8: 161–165.
8. Wasse LK, Sunderland C, King JA, Batterham RL, Stensel DJ (2012) Influence of rest and exercise at a simulated altitude of 4,000 m on appetite, energy intake, and plasma concentrations of acylated ghrelin and peptide YY. J Appl Physiol 112: 552–559.
9. Benso A, Broglio F, Aimaretti G, Lucatello B, Lanfranco F, et al. (2007) Endocrine and metabolic responses to extreme altitude and physical exercise in climbers. Eur J Endocrinol 157: 733–740.
10. Snyder EM, Carr RD, Deacon CF, Johnson BD (2008) Overnight hypoxic exposure and glucagon-like peptide-1 and leptin levels in humans. Appl Physiol Nutr Metab 33: 929–935.
11. Tschop M, Strasburger CJ, Hartmann G, Biollaz J, Bartsch P (1998) Raised leptin concentrations at high altitude associated with loss of appetite. Lancet 352: 1119–1120.
12. Sierra-Johnson J, Romero-Corral A, Somers VK, Johnson BD (2008) Effect of altitude on leptin levels, does it go up or down? J Appl Physiol (1985) 105: 1684–1685.
13. Broglio F, Gottero C, Prodam F, Gauna C, Muccioli G, et al. (2004) Non-acylated ghrelin counteracts the metabolic but not the neuroendocrine response to acylated ghrelin in humans. J Clin Endocrinol Metab 89: 3062–3065.
14. Schubert MM, Sabapathy S, Leveritt M, Desbrow B (2013) Acute Exercise and Hormones Related to Appetite Regulation: A Meta-Analysis. Sports Med.
15. Stensel D (2010) Exercise, appetite and appetite-regulating hormones: implications for food intake and weight control. Ann Nutr Metab 57 Suppl 2: 36–42.
16. Russel RR, Willis KS, Ravussin E, Larson-Meyer ED (2009) Effects of endurance running and dietary fat on circulating ghrelin and peptide YY. J Sports Sci Med 8: 574–583.
17. Martins C, Kulseng B, King NA, Holst JJ, Blundell JE (2010) The effects of exercise-induced weight loss on appetite-related peptides and motivation to eat. J Clin Endocrinol Metab 95: 1609–1616.
18. Guelfi KJ, Donges CE, Duffield R (2013) Beneficial effects of 12 weeks of aerobic compared with resistance exercise training on perceived appetite in previously sedentary overweight and obese men. Metabolism 62: 235–243.
19. Debevec T, Amon M, Keramidas ME, Kounalakis SN, Pisot R, et al. (2010) Normoxic and hypoxic performance following 4 weeks of normobaric hypoxic training. Aviat Space Environ Med 81: 387–393.
20. Wiesner S, Haufe S, Engeli S, Mutschler H, Haas U, et al. (2010) Influences of normobaric hypoxia training on physical fitness and metabolic risk markers in overweight to obese subjects. Obesity (Silver Spring) 18: 116–120.
21. Netzer NC, Chytra R, Kupper T (2008) Low intense physical exercise in normobaric hypoxia leads to more weight loss in obese people than low intense physical exercise in normobaric sham hypoxia. Sleep Breath 12: 129–134.
22. Wenger RH (2002) Cellular adaptation to hypoxia: O2-sensing protein hydroxylases, hypoxia-inducible transcription factors, and O2-regulated gene expression. FASEB J 16: 1151–1162.
23. Semenza GL (2001) Hypoxia-inducible factor 1: control of oxygen homeostasis in health and disease. Pediatr Res 49: 614–617.
24. Katayama K, Goto K, Ishida K, Ogita F (2010) Substrate utilization during exercise and recovery at moderate altitude. Metabolism 59: 959–966.
25. Haufe S, Wiesner S, Engeli S, Luft FC, Jordan J (2008) Influences of normobaric hypoxia training on metabolic risk markers in human subjects. Med Sci Sports Exerc 40: 1939–1944.

26. Morishima T, Kurihara T, Hamaoka T, Goto K (2014) Whole body, regional fat accumulation, and appetite-related hormonal response after hypoxic training. Clin Physiol Funct Imaging 34: 90–97.
27. Mackenzie R, Maxwell N, Castle P, Elliott B, Brickley G, et al. (2012) Intermittent exercise with and without hypoxia improves insulin sensitivity in individuals with type 2 diabetes. J Clin Endocrinol Metab 97: E546–555.
28. Roach RC, Bartsch P, Hackett PH, Oelz O (1993) The Lake Louise AMS Scoring Consensus Committee. The Lake Louise acute mountain sickness scoring system. In: Sutton JR, Houston CS, Coates G, Burlington VT, editors. Hypoxia and Molecular Medicine: Queen City Printers. pp. 272–274.
29. Mifflin MD, St Jeor ST, Hill LA, Scott BJ, Daugherty SA, et al. (1990) A new predictive equation for resting energy expenditure in healthy individuals. Am J Clin Nutr 51: 241–247.
30. Jequier E, Constant F (2010) Water as an essential nutrient: the physiological basis of hydration. Eur J Clin Nutr 64: 115–123.
31. Debevec T, Pialoux V, Mekjavic IB, Eiken O, Mury P, et al. (2014) Moderate exercise blunts oxidative stress induced by normobaric hypoxic confinement. Med Sci Sports Exerc 46: 33–41.
32. Debevec T, McDonnell AC, Macdonald IA, Eiken O, Mekjavic IB (2014) Whole body and regional body composition changes following 10-day hypoxic confinement and unloading-inactivity. Appl Physiol Nutr Metab 39: 386–395.
33. Hind K, Oldroyd B, Truscott JG (2011) In vivo precision of the GE Lunar iDXA densitometer for the measurement of total body composition and fat distribution in adults. Eur J Clin Nutr 65: 140–142.
34. Forster CD, Macdonald IA (1999) The assay of the catecholamine content of small volumes of human plasma. Biomedical Chromatography 13: 209–215.
35. Stubbs RJ, Hughes DA, Johnstone AM, Rowley E, Reid C, et al. (2000) The use of visual analogue scales to assess motivation to eat in human subjects: a review of their reliability and validity with an evaluation of new hand-held computerized systems for temporal tracking of appetite ratings. British Journal of Nutrition 84: 405–415.
36. Gibbons C, Caudwell P, Finlayson G, King N, Blundell J (2011) Validation of a new hand-held electronic data capture method for continuous monitoring of subjective appetite sensations. International Journal of Behavioral Nutrition and Physical Activity 8: 57.
37. Matthews DR, Hosker JP, Rudenski AS, Naylor BA, Treacher DF, et al. (1985) Homeostasis model assessment: insulin resistance and beta-cell function from fasting plasma glucose and insulin concentrations in man. Diabetologia 28: 412–419.
38. Anini Y, Brubaker PL (2003) Role of leptin in the regulation of glucagon-like peptide-1 secretion. Diabetes 52: 252–259.
39. Martins C, Morgan LM, Bloom SR, Robertson MD (2007) Effects of exercise on gut peptides, energy intake and appetite. J Endocrinol 193: 251–258.
40. Bailey DM, Davies B, Castell LM, Newsholme EA, Calam J (2001) Physical exercise and normobaric hypoxia: independent modulators of peripheral cholecystokinin metabolism in man. J Appl Physiol (1985) 90: 105–113.
41. Chen SM, Lin HY, Kuo CH (2013) Altitude Training Improves Glycemic Control. Chin J Physiol 56.
42. Zoll J, Ponsot E, Dufour S, Doutreleau S, Ventura-Clapier R, et al. (2006) Exercise training in normobaric hypoxia in endurance runners. III. Muscular adjustments of selected gene transcripts. J Appl Physiol (1985) 100: 1258–1266.
43. Brooks GA, Butterfield GE, Wolfe RR, Groves BM, Mazzeo RS, et al. (1991) Increased dependence on blood glucose after acclimatization to 4,300 m. J Appl Physiol (1985) 70: 919–927.
44. Seals DR, Johnson DG, Fregosi RF (1991) Hypoxia potentiates exercise-induced sympathetic neural activation in humans. J Appl Physiol (1985) 71: 1032–1040.
45. Bailey DM, Davies B, Baker J (2000) Training in hypoxia: modulation of metabolic and cardiovascular risk factors in men. Med Sci Sports Exerc 32: 1058–1066.
46. Dinmore AJ, Edwards JS, Menzies IS, Travis SP (1994) Intestinal carbohydrate absorption and permeability at high altitude (5,730 m). J Appl Physiol 76: 1903–1907.
47. Kalson NS, Hext F, Davies AJ, Chan CW, Wright AD, et al. (2010) Do changes in gastro-intestinal blood flow explain high-altitude anorexia? Eur J Clin Invest 40: 735–741.
48. King JA, Wasse LK, Ewens J, Crystallis K, Emmanuel J, et al. (2011) Differential acylated ghrelin, peptide YY3-36, appetite, and food intake responses to equivalent energy deficits created by exercise and food restriction. J Clin Endocrinol Metab 96: 1114–1121.
49. Hamad N, Travis SP (2006) Weight loss at high altitude: pathophysiology and practical implications. Eur J Gastroenterol Hepatol 18: 5–10.
50. Faiss R, Pialoux V, Sartori C, Faes C, Deriaz O, et al. (2013) Ventilation, Oxidative Stress and Nitric Oxide in Hypobaric vs. Normobaric Hypoxia. Med Sci Sports Exerc 45: 253–260.

10

Near Infrared Spectroscopy (NIRS) as a New Non-Invasive Tool to Detect Oxidative Skeletal Muscle Impairment in Children Survived to Acute Lymphoblastic Leukaemia

Francesca Lanfranconi[1]*, Luca Pollastri[1], Alessandra Ferri[1], Donatella Fraschini[2], Giuseppe Masera[2], Giuseppe Miserocchi[1]

1 Department of Health Sciences, Laboratory of Clinical Physiology and Sport Medicine, University of Milano-Bicocca, Monza, Italy, **2** Department of Pediatrics, University of Milano-Bicocca, San Gerardo Hospital, Monza, Italy

Abstract

Background: Separating out the effects of cancer and treatment between central and peripheral components of the O_2 delivery chain should be of interest to clinicians for longitudinal evaluation of potential functional impairment in order to set appropriate individually tailored training/rehabilitation programmes. We propose a non-invasive method (NIRS, near infrared spectroscopy) to be used in routine clinical practice to evaluate a potential impairment of skeletal muscle oxidative capacity during exercise in children previously diagnosed with acute lymphoblastic leukaemia (ALL). The purpose of this study was to evaluate the capacity of skeletal muscle to extract O_2 in 10 children diagnosed with ALL, 1 year after the end of malignancy treatment, compared to a control group matched for gender and age (mean$\pm$SD = 7.8$\pm$1.5 and 7.3$\pm$1.4 years, respectively).

Methods and Findings: Participants underwent an incremental exercise test on a treadmill until exhaustion. Oxygen uptake ($\dot{V}O_2$), heart rate (HR), and tissue oxygenation status (Δ[HHb]) of the *vastus lateralis* muscle evaluated by NIRS, were measured. The results showed that, in children with ALL, a significant linear regression was found by plotting $\dot{V}O_2$ *vs* Δ[HHb] both measured at peak of exercise. In children with ALL, the slope of the HR *vs* $\dot{V}O_2$ linear response (during sub-maximal and peak work rates) was negatively correlated with the peak value of Δ[HHb].

Conclusions: The present study proves that the NIRS technique allows us to identify large inter-individual differences in levels of impairment in muscle O_2 extraction in children with ALL. The outcome of these findings is variable and may reflect either muscle atrophy due to lack of use or, in the most severe cases, an undiagnosed myopathy.

Editor: Guillermo López Lluch, Universidad Pablo de Olavide, Centro Andaluz de Biología del Desarrollo-CSIC, Spain

Funding: All the sources of funding are related to the Department of health sciences of University of Milano-Bicocca. The senjor researcher, prof. G. Miserocchi, who provided this fund, was involved in study design and preparation of the manuscript.

Competing Interests: The authors have declared that no competing interests exist.

* Email: francesca.lanfranconi@unimib.it

Introduction

Approximately 1500 children under 15 years of age are diagnosed with cancer each year in Italy, of which acute lymphoblastic leukaemia (ALL) is the most common malignancy accounting for 38% of all childhood cancers [1]. In the last few decades progress in treatment has considerably increased the survival rates of children with ALL and a 70% cure rate for children with standard-risk disease is provided by the Italian Association of Paediatric Haematology and Oncology (*AIEOP, Associazione Italiana Emato Oncologia Pediatrica*) [2], [3]. It has been estimated that 1 out of 900 persons (aged 18–34 years), has been treated for cancer during their childhood [3], [4]. Among the potential consequences of childhood cancer therapy are death, neuro-psychiatric adverse events and myopathy, pain, fatigue, obesity, osteoporosis, cardiomyopathy and neuromuscular complications [5–8]. Therefore, in order to better understand the consequences of ALL or malignancy treatments, a long-term follow up in a large number of young people will assist to evaluate the resiliency and health-related quality of life [3], [4].

The main system of energy supply within cells is *via* oxidative metabolism. Any impairment along the "O_2 transport and utilization chain" significantly affects skeletal muscle function and exercise capacity. Peak O_2 uptake ($\dot{V}O_{2peak}$), considered as an individual index of aerobic fitness, was found to be reduced in children with ALL because malignancy treatments can lead to chronic pulmonary disease [9] and/or to cardiovascular impairment [10], [11]. The reduced $\dot{V}O_{2peak}$ in children with ALL has been attributed principally to the inability of the cardiovascular system to deliver O_2 to skeletal muscles (the "central" component of the O_2 transport chain) [5]. However, restricting the focus solely to O_2 delivery may not be appropriate and could cloud understanding of the physiological basis of aerobic fitness as originally proposed by the Fick equation [12]. Indeed, muscle O_2 extraction in children with ALL might be damaged both by a decrease in O_2 delivery as well as by an impairment in O_2 tissue utilization (a "peripheral" component of the O_2 transport chain). Some authors have suggested that the reduced exercise capacity in children with ALL might also reflect drug-induced side effects such as myopathy, osteonecrosis (often asymptomatic), impairment of the peripheral nervous system, and/or a decrease in skeletal muscle oxidative metabolism [5], [8], [13–17]. Furthermore, a sedentary life style could also affect the aerobic fitness of this population [5]: a lower level of functioning of the skeletal muscle pump and of the vasodilatatory capacity, as seen in unfit persons, could affect the ability of tissue O_2 extraction due to malignancy treatment [12].

Although several studies have reported muscle atrophy in long-term survivors of ALL, there is a paucity of data regarding the time-course of functional impairment in children with ALL. Following up on metabolic impairments along the O_2 transport utilization chain, after ALL treatment, or on the effect of specific rehabilitation programmes, a non-invasive evaluation approach is desirable. This could be obtained by near infrared spectroscopy (NIRS), a non-invasive methodology which provides an estimate of O_2 utilization of the peripheral muscles [18], [19]. Oxygenation NIRS indices are the result of the balance between O_2 delivery and muscle $\dot{V}O_2$ in the portion of tissue under consideration, being therefore conceptually similar to muscle O_2 extraction [20]. The changes in NIRS light absorption in working muscles reflect adjustments in oxygenation at the level of the microcirculation and intracellular sites of O_2 transport and uptake. More specifically, for a given $\dot{V}O_2$, a decrease in O_2 extraction (deoxygenation) relative to O_2 delivery decreases the NIRS signal, while the opposite is true for an increase in O_2 extraction: therefore this technique has been previously utilized to evaluate the efficiency of the peripheral component of aerobic fitness [18–20].

The purpose of this study was to evaluate non-invasively the potential limitations of the O_2 transport and utilization chain in children with ALL. We contend that an evaluation of the efficiency of the central and peripheral components of $\dot{V}O_2$ in children with ALL (above and beyond the information provided by $\dot{V}O_{2peak}$), extending from the onset of malignancy treatment through to long term follow up, would be of particular interest considering that: 1) a decreased exercise capacity could be related to muscle atrophy due to lack of use or, in the most severe cases, has to raise suspicions about an underlying metabolic myopathy; 2) rehabilitation and training programmes are specifically focused on skeletal muscle reconditioning. Our study hypothesized that NIRS would allow us to identify and quantify any impairment of muscle O_2 extraction during an incremental exercise test, especially at submaximal workloads. Indirect evidence in favour of this hypothesis would derive from the observation of significant correlations between the NIRS-derived index of O_2 extraction, $\dot{V}O_2$ and the extent of cardiovascular response to submaximal exercise.

Materials and Methods

Participants

Children with ALL (n = 10) were compared to an equal number of healthy children (CTRL), the latter group recruited as peers from different schools in the same geographical area, matched for age (mean ± standard deviation (SD) = 7.8±1.5 and 7.3±1.4 years, respectively), gender and sexual maturity. Sexual maturity was assessed by medical doctors using the indices of pubic hair and male genital or female breast development as described by Tanner (stage 1, 80% and stage 2 20% of participants in each group). Experienced medical doctors specialized in sports medicine collected details concerning the physical activities reported by children (daily life, leisure activities and recreational actvities). All the children were at limit for being considered physically active as defined by the 2008 physical activities guidelines for Americans: they performed recreational activities (aerobic, muscle-strengthening and bone-strengthening exercise) less than 3 days a week, these activities were appropriate and enjoyable for their age and did not require experience of exhaustive exercise. The clinical characteristics and weekly recreational activities performed by children with ALL as well as CTRL, are shown in Table 1. Inclusion criteria were absence of anaemia, neuropathy, orthopaedic, pulmonary and/or cardiovascular disorders. There were no exclusions on medical ground for infective diseases. Every attempt to avoid any unnecessary discomfort and disturbance to all participants and parents was made according to the ERICE statement about the cure and care of long-term survivors of childhood cancer [21]. All children and their parent(s) provided informed assent and written consent to participate in the project, which was approved by the University of Milano Bicocca (Milano – Italy) ethics committee. Personal data was treated according to standard principles of confidentiality.

Risk group definitions and final stratification

Children with ALL, all consecutive clinical attendees, came to the laboratory after attending their routine follow up, for a complete physical examination by the paediatricians at the Department of Paediatrics, S. Gerardo Hospital (Monza –Italy). To stratify ALL patients in prospective studies, a standardized quantitative assessment of minimal residual disease (MRD), based on immunoglobulin and T-cell receptor gene rearrangements as polymerase chain reaction targets at 2 time points, was introduced by AIEOP and the Berlin Frankfurt Munster (BFM) ALL study in 2000 [3]. The oncologists of the Department of Paediatrics classified patients with precursor B ALL in MRD as standard risk (MRD-SR) if MRD was already negative at day 33 (analyzed by 2 markers, with a sensitivity of at least 10^{-4}), as MRD high risk (MRD-HR) if MRD was 10^{-3} or more at day 78 and as MRD intermediate risk (MRD-IR) for all the others.

Our MRD-SR patients were 41%, MRD-IR were 50% and 1 patient was defined MRD-HR. The time period elapsed from the end of treatment in children with ALL, against MRD–SR, MRD–IR and MRD-HR following the AIEOP BFM ALL 2000 study protocol, until the exercise test session was approximately 1 year (11.3±4.3 months, range 6–20 months). One patient received cranial irradiation for MRD-HR.

AIEOP-BFM ALL 2000 Treatment protocol: induction and consolidation phase

The backbone of contemporary multiagent chemotherapeutic regimens is formed by 4 elements: induction, central nervous system (CNS)-directed treatment and consolidation, reinduction and maintenance. All patients underwent 7 days of prephase with steroid therapy (prednisone) and 1 intrathecal dose of methotrexate (intrathecal MTX), followed by induction phase IA and induction consolidation phase IB; from day 8, patients were randomized to continue steroid treatment with either prednisone (60 mg $(m^2)^{-1}$ per day) or dexamethasone (10 mg $(m^2)^{-1}$ per day) until day 28 with subsequent tapering of dose within a week; ***Protocol M and reinduction phases***. MRD-SR and IR patients received 4 cycles of high-dose MTX (5 g $(m^2)^{-1}$); at the beginning of the reinduction phase, patients were randomized to receive either protocol II or reduced-intensity protocol III in MRD-SR group, or protocol II versus reduced-intensity protocol

Table 1. Clinical characteristics and recreational activities of children with acute lymphoblastic leukemia (ALL) and controls (CTRL).

ALL	Gender	Age	Risk factor	Time elapsed since diagnosis of ALL	Clinical events during maintenance therapy	Recreational activities
		yrs		*months*		*minutes, weekly, last 6 months*
A1	M	10	S	31	none	swimming 50′×2
A2	M	6	I	32	none	soccer 50′×2
A3	F	10	I	37	none	swimming 50′
A4	M	8	H	34	none	/
A5	F	8	S	43	none	swimming 50′
A6	M	7	I	30	none	soccer 70′
A7	M	6	S	35	none	judo 50′
A8	M	6	I	41	none	swimming 50′×2
A9	F	8	S	35	Leishman.	kick boxing 70′
A10	M	9	I	35	none	soccer 70′×2
CTRL						
C1	M	7				climbing 70′, swimming 50′
C2	F	9				volleyball 50′, swimming 50′
C3	F	6				artistic gymnastic 50′×2
C4	M	9				athletics 70′
C5	F	7				swimming 50′×2
C6	M	7				savate 50′
C7	F	6				swimming 50′
C8	M	6				savate 50
C9	M	6				savate 50′
C10	M	10				karate 50′×2

S = standard risk; I = intermediate risk; H = high risk (see text for further explanation).

III given twice in the MRD-IR group. MRD-HR patient were randomized to receive 3 blocks of non–cross-resistant drugs followed by protocol III given 3 times versus 3 blocks followed by protocol II given twice in the AIEOP group; ***Maintenance therapy***. Maintenance therapy consisted of daily 6-mercaptopurine together with weekly MTX until 24 months after diagnosis; ***CNS-directed therapy***. CNS-directed therapy consisted of repeated intrathecal MTX administration during each treatment phase. Cranial radiotherapy was given (dosage by age) to patients at MRD-HR or with CNS involvement at diagnosis.

Exercise protocol

Before starting the test session individual body mass index (BMI) was calculated for children and was plotted on the American Academy of Pediatrics BMI for-age growth charts to obtain a percentile ranking. All exercise tests were conducted under close medical supervision and with 12-lead electrocardiography monitoring (Quark C12x: Cosmed, Roma, Italy). Children were allowed time to gain familiarity with the researchers and the experimental protocol by means of short preliminary practice runs on a treadmill. Parents were allowed to be present during the test session. A careful assessment that the participants were in a resting condition was carried out before the tests by measuring heart rate (HR), pulmonary ventilation ($\dot{V}E$, in BTPS) and observation of the child. An incremental exercise test was performed on a treadmill (Pulsar: h/p/Cosmos, Dusseldorf, Germany). After 2 minutes of walking at 1.5 km h^{-1} at 0% gradient, a constant-load exercise was conducted at 2.5 km h^{-1} at 5% slope for 4 minutes, thereafter the speed and gradient were increased by 0.1 km h^{-1} and 0.5% every 30 seconds until voluntary exhaustion was reached. Peak efforts were considered to have been given if, in addition to subjective indications, such as sweating, hyperpnea, and facial flushing, there was a consistent reduction in walking cadence, despite strong verbal encouragement. The exercise was stopped by the supervisor on the basis of subjective exhaustion feeling showed by the participant. The peak work rate was defined as the work rate attained at the point of test termination [11]. Uphill running offers the chance to estimate the external mechanical work done by participants to increase the potential energy of the body calculated by $W = weight*\Delta H$, where ΔH is the vertical distance given by $\Delta H = D*\sin\alpha$, where D is the distance run on the incline and α is the angle between zero level and the treadmill inclination. The average duration of the treadmill test for children with ALL and CTRL was 10.0±0.8 and 10.1±2.5 minutes respectively. $\dot{V}E$, $\dot{V}O_2$, and CO_2 output ($\dot{V}CO_2$) were determined breath-by-breath by a computerized metabolic cart (Vmax SPECTRA 229: SensorMedics Corporation Yorba Linda, California, USA). Expiratory flow was determined by a mass flow sensor (hot wire anemometer). $\dot{V}O_2$ and $\dot{V}CO_2$ were determined through continuous monitoring of PO_2 and PCO_2 at the mouth throughout the respiratory cycle and from established mass balance equations. Ventilatory efficiency was estimated by the slope of $\dot{V}E$ *vs* $\dot{V}CO_2$ below the ventilatory compensation point for exercise metabolic acidosis [22]. HR was determined from a 12-lead electrocardiographic signal interfaced to SensorMedics metabolic cart. Arterial blood O_2 saturation (SaO_2) was monitored continuously through pulse oximetry at the finger (RAD 9 Signal

Extraction Pulse Oximeter: Masimo Corporation, Irvine - California, USA). The environmental temperature during exercise was standardised to 20°C using an air-conditioning system and the current barometric pressure was recorded. The rated perceived exertion (RPE) was collected through the Borg scale aid.

NIRS technique

NIRS is a non-invasive method that allows the monitoring of muscle oxygenation on the principle that the near-infrared (NIR) light absorption characteristics of haemoglobin (Hb) and myoglobin (Mb) depend on their O_2 saturation. The absorption characteristics of light at 780 and 850 nm depend on the relative oxygenation of Hb and Mb. Mb has similar absorption spectra to Hb. In human skeletal muscle, however, the ratio [Hb]/[Mb] is higher than 5.19 so the signal is usually considered as deriving mainly from Hb. In view of these facts, it is appropriate to refer to NIRS measurements as indices of overall tissue oxygenation, with the understanding that ~70% of underlying vascular beds are composed of venous blood. In the present study data were expressed as a variation of absolute units, $\Delta[O_2Hb]$ and Δ[HHb], from the baseline value recorded after a 2 minutes light warm up and as a function of time. Therefore, decreases in $\Delta[O_2Hb]$ and corresponding increases in Δ[HHb] were interpreted as evidence of relative muscle deoxygenation and, conversely, as evidence of improved oxygenation [19;20]. Since Δ[HHb] is closely associated with changes in venous O_2 content, it is believed to be a sensitive measure of relative tissue deoxygenation due to O_2 extraction.

The NIRS probe (Nimo: Nirox, Brescia, Italy), composed of an emitter and detector pair, was firmly placed on the skin over the lower third of the right *vastus lateralis* muscle (~10 cm above the proximal border of patella and 3 cm lateral to the midline of the thigh), and secured with a small belt of Velcro straps. Elastic bandages were put around the muscle probe to prevent contamination from localised light. Pen-marks were made over the skin to indicate the margins of the plastic spacer in order to check for any downward sliding of the probe during running. Once secured in place, no sliding of the probe was detected. According to the Monte Carlo method of simulation, based on skin and muscle scattering and absorption characteristics for NIR light, in in-vivo measurements, a source-detector spacing of 20 mm is enough for the NIR light passing through the muscle layer, even when the adipose tissue thickness is 15 mm. Skinfold thickness at the site of application of the NIRS probe was determined before the exercise protocol by a calliper (C10 Plicometer Tanner – Whitehouse; Holtain, Ltd., Crymych, UK): the measured average values of skin and subcutaneous thigh tissue thickness in children with ALL and CTRL were 11.0±1.0 *vs* 9.9±0.9 mm, respectively and not statistically different. Statistically significant correlation between skinfold thickness and muscle O_2 extraction did not hold for both children with ALL and CTRL (slope −6.10, r^2 0.10 and p = 0.65 and slope −6.33, r^2 0.02 and p = 0.68, respectively). The probe was connected to a personal computer for data acquisition, A/D conversion, and subsequent analysis. Data were recorded at 2 Hz. Muscle Δ[HHb] data were expressed as a percentage of the maximal deoxygenation reference point obtained by a post exercise leg-cuff ischemia technique (Δ[HHb]/Δ[HHb]isch). Ischemia was obtained by inflating a cuff at 150–250 mmHg (depending on the child's BMI) for 2–3 minutes while children were sitting on the medical bed. The final reading was taken when detection of simultaneous increase of Δ[HHb] and corresponding decrease in $\Delta[O_2Hb]$ reached a plateau.

Statistical analysis

We applied the Shapiro-Wilk test for normality. For normal distributions we provided mean ± standard deviation (SD) and used Student t test to estimate statistical significant difference between groups. The level of significance was set at $p<0.05$. Regression and correlation analyses were performed using the least squared residuals method. All statistical analyses were performed by utilizing a commercially available software package (Prism 4.0: GraphPad, San Diego, California).

Results

Based on Shapiro-Wilk test, we found that for both groups the data were drawn from normally distributed populations at the 0.05 level of significance. We therefore evaluated the significance of the differences between groups by Student t test. The mean BMI was 18.4±3.35 kg $(m^2)^{-1}$ in children with ALL and was not significantly different from CTRL (16.3±1.60). Nevertheless 40% of children with ALL had a percentile BMI>85th while only 1 children in the CTRL group fell in this range (10%) (Figure 1).

Table 2 presents the mean (± SD) basal and peak values of the main variables obtained at rest and at the end of the exercise. The only apparent difference between CTRL and ALL groups concerned the $\Delta[HHb]_{peak}$ values: on average, at peak speed, O_2 extraction in children with ALL was 50% lower than in CTRL, the difference being highly significant (p = 0.018). The coefficient of variation was 55% higher in children with ALL than in CTRL.

The average $\dot{V}O_{2peak}$, relative to predicted value [23], was about 10% lower - although this was not significant - in children with ALL compared to the CTRL. For CTRL children this ratio was higher than 1 (1.12±0.20) and was statistically greater compared to the ALL group (0.95±0.09). Additionally, the coefficient of variation for children with ALL was remarkably lower than in CTRL (10.2 *vs* 18.2%, respectively), as showed also in Figure 2. Table 2 also shows that no difference in $\dot{V}E$, $PetO_2$, $PetCO_2$, and SaO_2 was noticed between the children with ALL and CTRL.

The RPE, evaluated by Borg's scale at peak exercise, was not significantly different for children with ALL (16.1±2.4) compared to CTRL (14.5±4.1), the coefficient of variation being 48% lower for children with ALL. The r^2 values of the correlations between HR and BORG values throughout the execution of the test, were

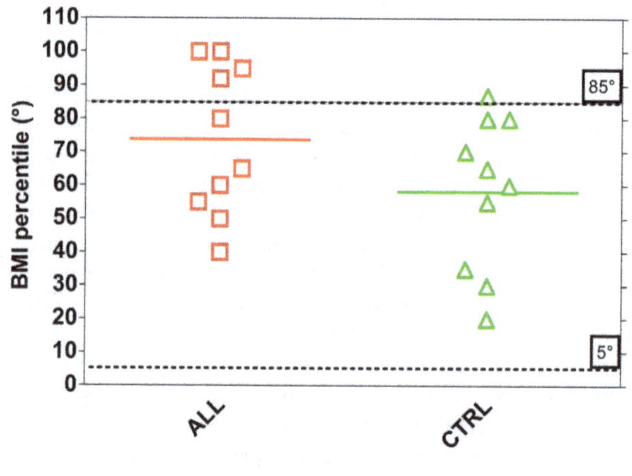

Figure 1. Individual and mean values of body mass index percentile (BMI) in ALL (n = 10) and CTRL (n = 10) children. Statistical significance level was defined as p<0.05.

Table 2. Mean±SD of basal and peak values (with coefficient of variation) of the investigated variables in the two groups of children.

	$\dot{V}O_2$	$\dot{V}O_2$	$\dot{V}E$ (BTPS)	Pet O_2	Pet CO_2	SaO_2	Δ[HHb]
	(L*min^{-1})	(mL*kg^{-1}*min^{-1})	(L*min^{-1})	mmHg	mmHg		% of ischemia
CTRL							
baseline values							
mean	0.15	5.91	7.24	105.99	35.34	97.21	\
SD	*0.03*	*0.84*	*1.27*	*3.34*	*2.63*	*1.71*	\
peak values							
mean	1.06	40.54	38.90	109.78	35.73	95.70	30.40
SD	*0.34*	*8.40*	*12.85*	*4.56*	*3.96*	*2.32*	*11.90*
coef.var.(%)	*31.89*	*20.71*	*33.03*	*4.15*	*11.08*	*2.43*	*39.14*
Children with ALL							
baseline values							
mean	0.20	6.48	8.72	106.73	32.69	97.46	\
SD	*0.08*	*1.05*	*3.20*	*6.12*	*3.75*	*1.53*	\
peak values							
mean	1.13	37.02	37.00	109.07	36.58	96.03	15.32*
SD	*0.37*	*4.71*	*9.15*	*2.18*	*1.77*	*3.01*	*13.30*
coef.var.(%)	*32.63*	*12.73*	*24.74*	*2.00*	*4.84*	*3.13*	*86.70*

$\dot{V}O_2$: O2 uptake; $\dot{V}E$: pulmonary ventilation; PetO2: pulmonary end tidal of O2; Pet CO2: pulmonary end tidal of CO2; Sa O2: arterial blood saturation; Δ[HHb]: skeletal muscle O2 extraction.

* $p<0.05$ significantly different from CTRL peak values.

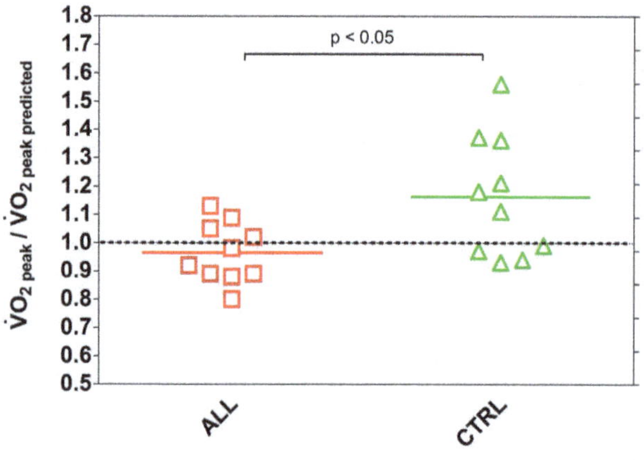

Figure 2. Individual and mean values of $\dot{V}O_{2peak}$ relative to predicted $\dot{V}O_{2peak}$ in ALL (n = 10) and CTRL (n = 10) children. Statistical significance level was defined as $p<0.05$.

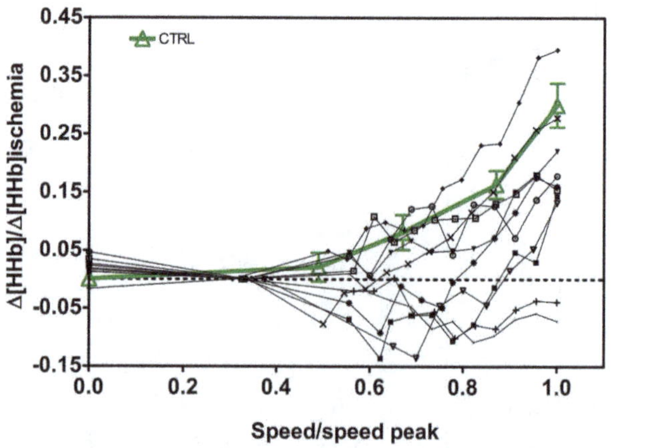

Figure 3. Individual skeletal muscle O_2 extraction, Δ[HHb], expressed as the ratio of the values obtained during limb ischemia, are presented for children with ALL as a function of speed. CTRL values (thick line) are shown as mean±SE. Speed is expressed relative to peak value. Statistical significance level was defined as $p<0.05$.

respectively 0.46 ($p<0.0001$) for ALL and 0.13 ($p<0.008$) for CTRL.

The average peak workload was the same for children with ALL and CTRL. The treadmill inclination was 15.0±0.9 *vs* 15.2±1.8% and velocity 4.4±0.2 *vs* 4.4±0.5 km h^{-1}, respectively and not statistically different. The peak external mechanical work was 56.30±6.35 *vs* 53.48±6.14 watt respectively and was not significantly different in children with ALL *vs* CTRL. The slopes of the $\dot{V}O_2$ *vs* workload linear response, taken as an index of the energy cost of locomotion, were not significantly different between the 2 groups (12.2±1.1 ml O_2 min^{-1} $watt^{-1}$ in children with ALL, *vs* 15.6±0.7 ml O_2 min^{-1} $watt^{-1}$ in CTRL, comparison of slopes by covariance analysis $p>0.05$).

Individual data for O_2 extraction at the skeletal muscle level, as measured by NIRS and expressed as the fraction of the values obtained during limb ischemia, are presented in Figure 3 for children with ALL as a function of speed, along with the mean (± SE) values obtained in CTRL. The speed values are expressed relative to peak speed, to allow a comparison of the muscle extraction values of O_2 obtained at the same relative velocity among individuals with varying exercise capacity. Children with ALL present a high variability in terms of O_2 extraction, ranging from normal to severe deficiency in O_2 extraction (2 cases).

In Figure 4, a statistically significant linear regression was found in children with ALL between $\dot{V}O_{2peak}$ and $\Delta[HHb]_{peak}$, note that the value of r^2 reveals that essentially only about 50% of the variance of $\dot{V}O_{2peak}$ is explained by $\Delta[HHb]_{peak}$ as independent variable. No such correlation did hold for CTRL (slope −23.2, r^2 0.09 and $p = 0.41$) so only the average value of $\dot{V}O_{2peak}$ and corresponding $\Delta[HHb]_{peak}$ is reported in the Figure. Figure 5 (A) shows, as an example, that the HR *vs* $\dot{V}O_2$ response during exercise was displaced upward and displayed a greater slope on comparing an ALL to a CTRL. Figure 5 (B) shows that for children with ALL there was indeed a statistically significant linear regression with a negative slope between the individual slopes of the HR *vs* O_2 correlation and muscle O_2 extraction. Therefore this regression reveals that a greater cardiac response occurs the lower is the peripheral O_2 extraction capacity. Such correlation was not found for CTRL (slope 1.21; r^2 0.08 and $p = 0.42$) and therefore we only present an average value of slopes of the HR *vs* O_2 correlation and muscle O_2 extraction.

The mean $\dot{V}E$ *vs* $\dot{V}CO_2$ slope in children with ALL was 27.1±2.92 and was not significantly different from CTRL (28.4±2.78).

Discussion

It has been suggested but not demonstrated that there is O_2 extraction impairment in children with ALL [5]. This is the first study, to our knowledge, to perform measurements of skeletal muscle O_2 extraction by NIRS in children with ALL during exercise. This technique was previously adopted by different authors as a non-invasive approach in clinical practice, even in the case of severe diseases, to demonstrate a potential impairment in the O_2 extraction capabilities of skeletal muscle during exercise [20], [24], [25]. A further novelty of this study is that we provide data on the peripheral O_2 extraction 1 year on average after the end of malignancy treatment.

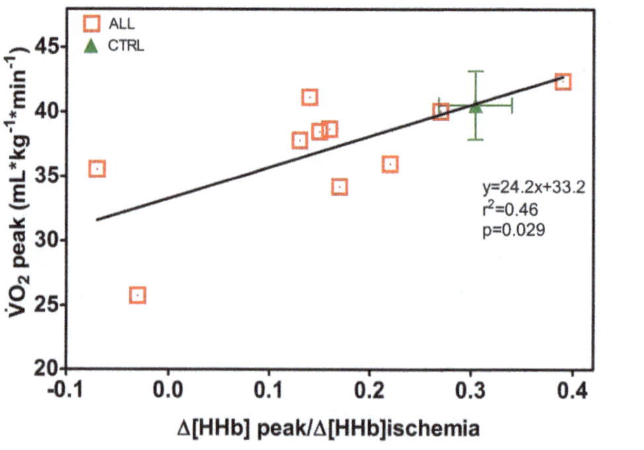

Figure 4. Regression between $\dot{V}O_{2peak}$ and skeletal muscle O_2 extraction at peak of exercise, $\Delta[HHb]_{peak}$, expressed as the ratio of the values obtained during limb ischemia for children with ALL (n = 10). CTRL values are shown as mean±SE. Statistical significance level was defined as $p<0.05$.

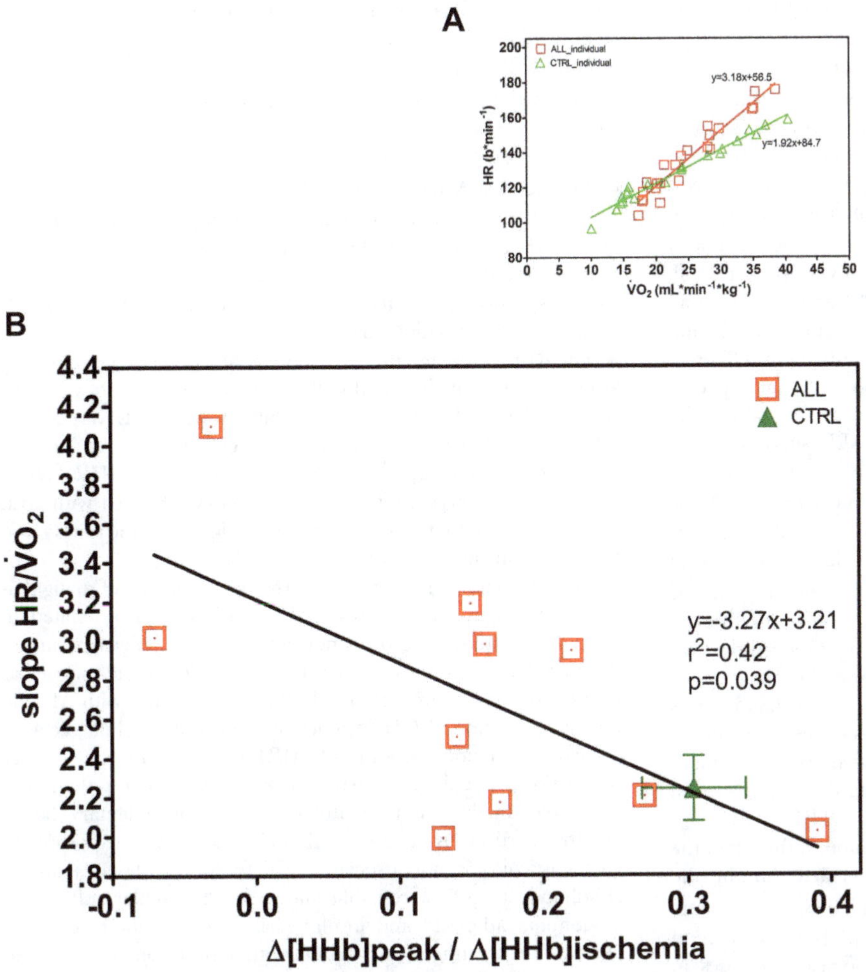

Figure 5. Individual regression for heart rate (HR) *vs* the corresponding $\dot{V}O_2$ for one ALL and one CTRL child (A graph). Regression between the individual slopes of the HR *vs* $\dot{V}O_2$ relationship, obtained in children with ALL (n = 10) and skeletal muscle O_2 extraction at peak of exercise $\Delta[HHb]_{peak}$, expressed as the ratio of the values obtained during limb ischemia with the corresponding regression line (B graph). CTRL values are given as mean±SE. Statistical significance level was defined as $p<0.05$.

The present findings indicate that muscle O_2 extraction ability during exercise was about 50% lower in ALL, as compared to CTRL, revealing an impairment of various degree in microvascular perfusion and/or the O_2 shuttle system. Figure 2 shows that an impairment in oxidative muscle extraction could be detected in children with ALL even at submaximal running speeds compared to the CTRL. The same is true at peak workout. In particular, in 2 children with ALL (1 MRD-SR and 1 MRD-IR) O_2 muscle extraction was so low, at submaximal and maximal exercise rates, as to raise suspicions about an underlying metabolic myopathy. A similar observation was reported in severe disease conditions, such as after heart transplant and in metabolic myopathy, supporting the relevance of the peripheral component in limiting the increase in O_2 consumption [24–26]. Marchese et al. [24] reported a decreased skeletal muscle function in children with ALL early in their course of treatment, with the weakest muscle strength occurring on the 28th day of the delayed intensification phase. Murat et al. [17] found reliable data indicating that muscle weakness is a relevant clinical manifestation in patient with ALL also in the maintenance phase of ALL therapy. Our present data are consistent with the idea that impaired muscle function could be a relevant manifestation in children with ALL and further extend this notion to children after 1 year from the end of malignancy treatment. A limitation of the capacity of muscle fibres to consume O_2 in leukaemia survivors may be explained at least in part by muscle atrophy due to the catabolic effects of malignancy treatment such as vincristine or corticosteroids. Glucocorticoids inhibit overall protein synthesis in skeletal muscle causing muscle atrophy and loss of muscle function, the effect of corticosteroids being to blunt the stimulatory effect of insulin and amino acids on protein synthesis [14], [15]. Also, the muscle connective tissue undergoes a gene suppression leading to a collagen degradation, especially in fast muscles [14]. There may also be an altered metabolic function of muscle fibres, as in metabolic myopathy, due to immunosuppressive therapy (particularly in female patients). The muscle weakness due to oxidative inefficiency may be subnormal for many years after therapy for childhood leukemia [27], [28]. An additional explanation is that muscle atrophy and altered muscle function may be further worsened by bed rest and sedentary habits [5]. Although aerobic activities could prevent muscle atrophy, exercise may not to be able to compensate for the changes observed during corticosteroid treatment [15]. As a result, when physical exercise is kept low, muscle atrophy and early fatigue become self-perpetuating conditions [6]. To compensate for these deficiencies, the possible benefits of prophylactic and individually planned exercise should be studied [28].

A mild average difference in relative $\dot{V}O_{2peak}$ – which is however not statistically significant – was seen when comparing children with ALL with CTRL, indicating a reduced exercise capacity only in some children with ALL. This finding is at variance with data from van Brussels et al. [5] meta analysis, based on a systematic review of the literature, indicating a reduced $\dot{V}O_{2peak}$ in children with ALL. However, some heterogeneity among the studies considered was admitted by van Brussels et al. [5] in their meta analysis: Vizinova et al. [29] and Hauser et al. [30] did not find significant differences between ALL survivors and CTRL participants, the possible explanation residing in differences in the level of physical activity. Also in our study an expected grade of variability in level of aerobic fitness was shown by children with ALL, due to the fact that ALL survivors were vigorously encouraged to be physically active by the oncologists (as were demonstrated by the ratios of $\dot{V}O_{2peak}$ to predicted $\dot{V}O_{2peak}$ near 100% in more than half of the cases). Additionally, the most important difference in previous studies regarding a decrease in $\dot{V}O_2$ in children with ALL, as compared with findings in our study, relates to the lapse of time between the end of the therapy and the date of the functional evaluation. Our study was performed within 1 year on average from the end of malignancy treatment, while in other studies the functional evaluation was done over a period extending up to 5 years after the end of therapy. It appears difficult to predict how sedentary habits might affect exercise capacity after such a long time, during the crucial teenage years both in children with ALL and CTRL.

In healthy people, the maximum cardiac output rather than the maximal rate of tissue O_2 extraction, is the main factor limiting the $\dot{V}O_{2peak}$ for exercise involving large muscle mass,. The same phenomenon is confirmed by McNarry et al. [31] in a population of healthy girls, suggesting the same physiological responses in children. We confirm this same pattern in our CRTL. However, in children with ALL there was a tendency to show a greater increase in HR with increasing $\dot{V}O_2$ when the muscle O_2 extraction was reduced. The limitation in $\dot{V}O_{2peak}$ children with ALL may reflect both a decrease in muscle O_2 extraction (Figure 4) and/or a decrease in O_2 delivery [Figure 5). Considering HR as a proxy of muscle blood flow (and presumably O_2 delivery) in some children with ALL there was a compensatory behaviour of the central component, in order to increase convective O_2 delivery to the muscle. Our data showed a decrease in muscle oxygen extraction as well as a greater slope of the HR vs $\dot{V}O_2$ relationship. Interestingly, the strongest cardiac response occurs in children with the lowest extraction capacity at skeletal muscle level. Whereas higher HR values for the same $\dot{V}O_2$ are generally considered a sign of poor exercise capacity, the leftward shift with a higher slope of regression in the children with ALL reveals an enhanced cardiovascular response for a given metabolic response (Figure 5 A). Note, that compared to a normal O_2 extraction seen in CTRL at peak of exercise, 70% of children with ALL showed an extraction rate at least 30% lower than CTRL. The negative correlation between muscle O_2 extraction and the slopes of the HR *vs* $\dot{V}O_2$ relationships has been previously reported for patients with metabolic myopathies [20]. Thus, contrary to what happens with healthy participants, in some children with ALL, the decreased muscle O_2 extraction capacity that seriously limits $\dot{V}O_{2peak}$ may reflect a state of myopathy possibly due to corticosteroids treatment, and/or to sedentary life habits [5], [16]. A potential correlation between the severity of disease, as based on the MRD risk, and our functional variables, namely the slope of the HR vs VO_2 relationship and muscle O_2 extraction (Figure 5 B) appears critical. Indeed in 2 children with ALL categorized as MRD-S and MRD-I risk, the $\dot{V}O_{2peak}$ was equally strongly decreased, and the highest cardiac response reflected an extreme reduction of oxygen muscle capacity. Conversely in 1 child graded as MRD-H, the $\dot{V}O_{2peak}$ was essentially normal, the extraction was partially maintained and higher than in MRD-S and MRD-I children, while the cardiac response was essentially normal. We therefore conclude that in our study the severity of MRD is poorly correlated to the potential limitation of the O_2 transport and utilisation chain.

The RPE, estimated using the Borg Scale, is not commonly used among healthy children and in fact a great coefficient of variation was found in CTRL. Interestingly, children with ALL were able to rate perceived exertion in a real convincing way as the index of fatigue correlated persuasively with the increase in HR values. Our personal consideration is that, probably, children with ALL are more used to the experience of fatigue or uneasiness and therefore can rate it better as a subjective feeling.

Excessive fatness is another reported consequence of malignancy treatment in children with ALL. This has been related to cranial irradiation or growth hormone (GH) insufficiency and to the cumulative doses of anthracyclines or corticosteroids, as well as to the type of corticosteroid used [32]. Our children with ALL do not have a reported GH insufficiency and only 1 child received cranial irradiation because of MRD-HR, so that a greater proportion of ALL participants with a BMI greater than 85th percentile, might again be attributed to their sedentary habits and/or corticosteroid use. Although short-term exposure to glucocorticoids is not associated with coronary diseases during childhood, it is of interest that known cardiovascular risk factors (abdominal adiposity and insulin resistance) are increased even after a short treatment, and the magnitude of the changes induced is proportional to the dosage of the drug [33]. Long-term corticosteroids effects, and the small amount of leisure-time dedicated to physical activity could be a hard inheritance for leukemia survivors reaching adult age. In fact, as confirmed by a recent study, survivors of leukemia were more likely than the general population to report no leisure-time physical activity, combined with unhealthy diet habits, contributing to altered body composition parameters in adulthood [6].

Children with ALL were all subjected to the same treatment, receiving standard doses of cardiotoxic drugs, such as anthracyclines (<300 mg $(m^2)^{-1}$, and none was subjected to thoracic irradiation. A study performed by our Department of Paediatrics shows that in the absence of any signs or symptoms of heart failure, female ALL survivors treated with low cumulative anthracycline doses showed a reduced left ventricular mass and wall thickness [34]. It should also be pointed out that we consider HR merely as a substitute for O_2 delivery, but we are anyway inclined to believe that impaired cardiac function is responsible, at least partly, for the reduced exercise capacity of some of our children with ALL. According to van Brussel et al. [5], even more interestingly, a greater coefficient of variation in $\dot{V}O_{2peak}$ and of the ratio of $\dot{V}O_{2peak}$ to predicted $\dot{V}O_{2peak}$ in CTRL children may be interpreted as resulting from a variable state of fitness (where children followed either a sedentary lifestyle or were engaged in recreational activities). Conversely, a lower coefficient of variation in children with ALL may reflect a more homogeneous lifestyle reflecting sedentary habits only as compared to their healthy peers.

SaO_2 during exercise, an index of efficiency of the central component in the O_2 transport and utilization chain from the lung to tissues, remained normal in our children with ALL. Also $PetCO_2$ values and the slope of $\dot{V}E$ *vs* $\dot{V}CO_2$, which are not different in children with ALL compared with CTRL, indicate normal lung diffusion function and appropriate ventilatory efficiency during exercise [22], [25]. This finding is to some extent in conflict with the reported impairments in lung function [9] due to the late effects of MTX and cyclophosphamide in children aged 14.6 years (which is older than our children, who are mostly pre-pubertal). However in Jenney et al. study [9], the evaluation was performed more than 4 years after the end of therapy (which is later than our children, who were evaluated 1 year after the end of malignancy treatment). In fact, prolonged immunosuppression during maintenance chemotherapy may lead to an increased frequency of lower respiratory tract infections. It is indeed known that children who suffer from acute respiratory diseases in early life (even without immunosuppression) may develop more chronic problems as they get older [9].

Conclusions

The present study shows that the NIRS technique allows us to identify large inter-individual differences in levels of impairment in muscle O_2 extraction in children with ALL. The outcome of these findings is variable and may reflect either muscle atrophy due to lack of use or, in the most severe cases, an undiagnosed myopathy. Our data support the argument that the impaired O_2 extraction in children with ALL may be partly compensated by a central component (i.e. a greater increase in HR when increasing $\dot{V}O_2$). Compensation reflects the balance between the extent of the impairment on peripheral O_2 extraction and the functional condition of the heart. This multifaceted interaction may justify controversies about the $\dot{V}O_{2peak}$ reported by different research groups [5]. Separating out the effects of cancer and treatment between central and peripheral components of the O_2 delivery chain should be of interest to clinicians for longitudinal evaluation of potential functional impairment in order to set appropriate individually tailored training/rehabilitation programmes [35–38]. The long-term objective of the cure and care of children with cancer is that they become resilient, efficient and autonomous adults with a high health-related quality of life.

Acknowledgments

We are grateful to the "brave children" who underwent the tests as well as to their parents. We also thank: Drs. Valentina Scotti and Nino Lania for technical assistance; Dr. Hayley Vergani, Dr. Damian Randle and Dr. David Bishop as native speaker consultants; Dr. Alessandra Lanfranconi as English full proficiency consultant.

Author Contributions

Conceived and designed the experiments: FL AF G. Masera G. Miserocchi. Performed the experiments: FL LP AF. Analyzed the data: FL LP. Contributed reagents/materials/analysis tools: FL DF. Wrote the paper: FL LP AF DF G. Miserocchi. Revised the article: G. Miserocchi. Provided useful discussion of the results: G. Masera.

References

1. Dama E, Rondelli R, De Rosa M, Aricò M, Carli M, et al. (2008) Patterns of domestic migration and access to childhood cancer care centres in Italy: a report from the hospital based registry of the Italian Association of Pediatric Haematology and Oncology (AIEOP). Eur J Canc 44: 2101–105.
2. Aricò M, Valsecchi MG, Rizzari C (2008) Long-term results of the AIEOP-ALL-95 Trial for Childhood Acute Lymphoblastic Leukemia: insight on the prognostic value of DNA index in the framework of Berlin-Frankfurt-Muenster based chemotherapy. J Clin Oncol 26(2): 283–9.
3. Conter V, Bartram CR, Valsecchi MG, Schrauder A, Panzer-Grumayer R, et al. (2010) Molecular response to treatment redefines all prognostic factors in children and adolescents with B-cell precursor acute lymphoblastic leukemia: results in 3184 patients of the AIEOP-BFM ALL 2000 study. Blood 115(16): 3206–14.
4. Benedetti G, Camnasio M, Fioredda F, Fraschini D, Haupt R, et al. (2003) A system for the informatics charge of the follow up of recovered cancer child. CILEA bulletin 86: 15–16.
5. van Brussel M, Takken T, Lucia A, van der Net J, Helders PJM (2005) Is physical fitness decreased in survivors of childhood leukemia? A systematic review. Leukemia 19: 13–17.
6. Cox CL, Montgomery M, Oeffinger KC, Leisering W, Zelter L, et al. (2009) Promoting physical activity in childhood cancer survivors. Cancer 115:642–54.
7. Hartman A, Winkel ML, van Beek RD, de Muinck Keizer-Schrama SM, et al. (2009) A randomized trial investigation an exercise program to prevent reduction of bone mineral density and impairment of motor performance during treatment for childhood acute lymphoblastic leukemia. Pediatr Blood Cancer 53: 64–71.
8. Teuffel O, Kuster SP, Hunger SP, Conter V, Hitzler J, et al. (2011) Dexamethasone versus prednisone for induction therapy in childhood acute lymphoblastic leukemia: a systematic review and meta-analysis. Leukemia 25: 1232–1238.
9. Jenney ME, Faragher EB, Jones PH, Woodcock A (1995) Lung function and exercise capacity in survivors of childhood leukaemia. Med Pediatr Oncol 24(4): 222–230.
10. Hogarty A (2000) Longitudinal evaluation of cardiopulmonary performance during exercise after bone marrow transplantation in children. J Ped 136(3): 311–317.
11. San Juan AF, Chamorro-Viña C, Maté-Muñoz JL, Fernández del Valle M, Cardona C, et al. (2008) Functional capacity of children with leukemia. Int J Sports Med 29(2): 163–7.
12. Rowland TW (2005) Circulatory responses to exercise: are we misreading Fick? Chest 127: 1023–1030.
13. Harila-Saari AH, Vainionpaa LK, Kovala TT, Tolonen E, Lanning BM (2000) Nerve lesions after therapy for childhood acute lymphoblastic leukemia. Cancer 82: 200–207.
14. Long W, Liping W, Barrett EJ (2001) Dexamethasone inhibits the stimulation of muscle protein synthesis and PHAS-I and p/ = S6-kinase phosporylation. Am J Physiol Endocrnol Metab 280: E570–E575.
15. Ahticosky AM, Riso E-M, Koskinen SOA, Risteli J, Takala TES (2004) Regulation of type IV collagen gene expression and degradation in fast and slow muscle during dexamethasone treatment and exercise. Pflugers Arch – Eur J Physiol 448: 123–130.
16. Marchese VG, Connolly BH, Able C, Boten AR, Bowen P, et al. (2008) Relationships among severity of osteonecrosis, pain, range of motion, and functional mobility in children, adolescent, and young adults with acute lymphoblastic leukemia. Phys Therapy 88(3): 341–350.
17. Murat MD, Perondi MB, D'Andrea Greve JM, Roschel H, Lucia de Sa Pinto A, et al. (2011) Strength capacity in young patients who are receiving maintenance therapy for acute lymphoblastic leukemia: a case control study. Clinics 66(7): 1277–1281
18. McCully KK, Hamaoka H (2000) Near-infrared spectroscopy: what can it tell us about oxygen saturation in skeletal muscle? Exer Sport Sci Rev 28: 123–127.
19. Ferrari M, Mottola L, Quaresima V (2004) Principles, technique and limitations of near infrared spectroscopy. Can. J. Appl. Physiol 29:463–487.
20. Grassi B, Marzorati M, Lanfranconi F, Ferri A, Longaretti M, et al. (2007) Impaired oxygen extraction in metabolic myopathies: detection and quantification by near-infrared spectroscopy. Muscle Nerve 35:510–520.
21. Haupt R, Spinetta JJ, Ban I (2007) Long term survivors of childhood cancer: cure and care. The ERICE Statement. Eur J Canc 43:1778–780.
22. Gitt AK, Wasserman K, Kilkowski C, Kleemann T, Kilkowski A, et al. (2002) Exercise anaerobic threshold and ventilatory efficiency identify heart failure patients for high risk of early death. Circulation 106:3079–3084.
23. Cooper DM, Weiler-Ravell D, Whipp BJ (1984) Aerobic parameters of exercise as function of body size during growth in children. J Appl Physiol 56: 628–634
24. Mancini DM (1997) Application of near infrared spectroscopy to the evaluation of exercise performance and limitations in patients with heart failure. J Biomed Optics 2: 22–30.
25. Lanfranconi F, Borrelli E, Ferri A, Porcelli S, Maccherini M, et al. (2006) Non-invasive evaluation of skeletal muscle oxidative metabolism after heart transplant. Med Sci Sports Exerc 38(8): 1374–83.
26. Porcelli S, Marzorati M, Lanfranconi F, Vago P, Pisot R, et al. (2010) Role of skeletal muscles impairment and brain oxygenation in limiting oxidative metabolism during exercise after bed rest. J Appl Physiol 109(1): 101–11.
27. Marchese VG, Chiarello LA, Lange BJ (2004) Effects of physical therapy intervention for children with acute lymphoblastic leukemia. Pediatr Blood Cancer 42: 127–133.
28. Hovi L, Era P, Rautonene J, Siimes MA (1993) Impaired muscle strenght in female adolescents and young adults surviving leukemia in childhood. Cancer 72(1): 276–81.

29. Vizinova H, Malincikova J, Klaskova E, Wiederman I (2002) Exercise cardiorespiratory indexes in children motivated to physical activity after treatment for acute lymphoblastic leukemia. Cas Lek Cesk 141: 491–493.
30. Hauser M, Gibson BS, Wilson N (2001) Diagnosis of anthracycline induced late cardiomyopathy by exercise spiroergometry and stress echocardiography. Eur J Pediatr 160: 607–610.
31. McNarry MA, Welsman JR, Jones AM (2011) Influence of training maturity status on the cardiopulmonary responses to ramp incremental cycle and upper body exercise in girls. J Appl Physiol 110: 375–381
32. Wallace AM, Tuckert P, Williams DM, Hughest IA, Ahmed SF (2003) Short term effects of prednisolone and dexamethasone on circulating concentrations of leptin and sex hormone_binding globulin in children being treated for acute lymphoblastic leukaemia. Clin Endocrin 58: 770–776.
33. Nysom K, Holm K, Michaelsen KF, Hertz H, Müller J, et al. (1999) Degree of fatness after treatment for acute lymphoblastic leukemia in childhood. J Clin Endocrinol Metab 84(12): 4591–6.
34. Amigoni M, Giannattasio C, Fraschini D (2010) Low Anthracyclines Doses-Induced Cardiotoxicity in Acute Lymphoblastic Leukemia Long-Term Female Survivors. Pediatr Blood Cancer 55: 1343–1347.
35. Wright MJ, Hanna SE, Halton JM (2003) Maintenance of ankle range of motion in children treated for acute lymphoblastic leukemia. Pediatr Phys Ther 15: 146–152.
36. San Juan AF, Chamorro-Viña C, Moral S, Fernández Del Valle M, et al. (2008) Benefits of intrahospital exercise training after pediatric bone marrow transplantation. Int J Sports Med 29(5): 439–46.
37. Takken T, van der Torre P, Zwerink M, Bierings M, Helders PJ, et al. (2009) Development and feasibility and efficacy of a community-based exercise training program in pediatric cancer survivors. Psycho Oncology 18: 440–448.
38. Speyer E, Herbinet A, Vuillemin A, Briancon S, Chastagner P (2010) Effect of adapted physical activity session in the hospital on health-related quality of life for children with cancer: a cross-over randomized trial. Pediatr Blood Cancer 55: 1160–1166.

11

Reproducibility of Fat_{max} and Fat Oxidation Rates during Exercise in Recreationally Trained Males

Ilaria Croci[1,2*], Fabio Borrani[3,4], Nuala Byrne[5,6], Rachel Wood[5], Ingrid Hickman[1,7,8], Xavier Chenevière[3,9], Davide Malatesta[3,4]

1 The University of Queensland Diamantina Institute, The University of Queensland, Translational Research Institute, Brisbane, Australia, **2** School of Human Movement Studies, University of Queensland, Brisbane, Australia, **3** Institute of Sport Sciences University of Lausanne, University of Lausanne, Lausanne, Switzerland, **4** Department of Physiology, University of Lausanne, Lausanne, Switzerland, **5** Institute of Health and Biomedical Innovation, Queensland University of Technology, Brisbane, Australia, **6** Bond Institute of Health and Sport, Bond University, Robina, Australia, **7** Department of Nutrition and Dietetics, Princess Alexandra Hospital, Brisbane, Australia, **8** Mater Medical Research Institute, Mater Mother's Hospital, Brisbane, Australia, **9** Department of Medicine, University of Fribourg, Fribourg, Switzerland

Abstract

Aerobic exercise training performed at the intensity eliciting maximal fat oxidation (Fat_{max}) has been shown to improve the metabolic profile of obese patients. However, limited information is available on the reproducibility of Fat_{max} and related physiological measures. The aim of this study was to assess the intra-individual variability of: a) Fat_{max} measurements determined using three different data analysis approaches and b) fat and carbohydrate oxidation rates at rest and at each stage of an individualized graded test. Fifteen healthy males [body mass index 23.1±0.6 kg/m^2, maximal oxygen consumption ($\dot{V}O_{2\,max}$) 52.0±2.0 ml/kg/min] completed a maximal test and two identical submaximal incremental tests on ergocycle (30-min rest followed by 5-min stages with increments of 7.5% of the maximal power output). Fat and carbohydrate oxidation rates were determined using indirect calorimetry. Fat_{max} was determined with three approaches: the sine model (SIN), measured values (MV) and 3rd polynomial curve (P3). Intra-individual coefficients of variation (CVs) and limits of agreement were calculated. CV for Fat_{max} determined with SIN was 16.4% and tended to be lower than with P3 and MV (18.6% and 20.8%, respectively). Limits of agreement for Fat_{max} were −2±27% of $\dot{V}O_{2\,max}$ with SIN, −4±32 with P3 and −4±28 with MV. CVs of oxygen uptake, carbon dioxide production and respiratory exchange rate were <10% at rest and < 5% during exercise. Conversely, CVs of fat oxidation rates (20% at rest and 24–49% during exercise) and carbohydrate oxidation rates (33.5% at rest, 8.5–12.9% during exercise) were higher. The intra-individual variability of Fat_{max} and fat oxidation rates was high (CV>15%), regardless of the data analysis approach employed. Further research on the determinants of the variability of Fat_{max} and fat oxidation rates is required.

Editor: Reury F.P. Bacurau, University of Sao Paulo, Brazil

Funding: These authors have no support or funding to report.

Competing Interests: The authors have declared that no competing interests exist.

* E-mail: ilaria.croci@uqconnect.edu.au

Introduction

Carbohydrate and fat are the two main sources of energy that sustain oxidative metabolism. Their relative utilization during aerobic exercise depends largely on exercise intensity [1,2]. The whole-body carbohydrate oxidation rate (CHO_{ox}) increases with the workload, whereas the whole-body fat oxidation rate (F_{ox}) increases from low to moderate exercise intensities, and then markedly declines at high intensities. The exercise intensity at which the maximal fat oxidation (MFO) rate occurs has been defined as Fat_{max} [3]. Aerobic exercise training performed at Fat_{max} has the potential to increase F_{ox} and insulin sensitivity in obese patients [4] and in individuals with metabolic syndrome [5]. In patients with type 2 diabetes, aerobic training targeted at Fat_{max} was shown to have a greater effect on body composition and glucose control than high intensity interval training [6].

To determine Fat_{max}, a submaximal graded exercise test using indirect calorimetry is performed, and data is analyzed with two main steps. First, F_{ox} and CHO_{ox} at each stage of the test are calculated from indirect calorimetry measures [oxygen consumption ($\dot{V}O_2$) and carbon dioxide production ($\dot{V}CO_2$)] by means of the stoichiometric equations [7]. Subsequently, F_{ox} values are plotted as a function of exercise intensity and Fat_{max} is identified with one of the following four commonly used methods: a) the determination of the maximal value of measured F_{ox} reached during each stage of the graded exercise test and identification of the corresponding intensity (measured values approach, MV) [3,8–10], b) the construction of a 3rd polynomial fitting curve (P3) [11], c) the Sine model (SIN) [12] and d) the non-protein "respiratory quotient technique" [13].

Knowledge of the reproducibility of Fat_{max} is necessary for establishing its usefulness as a parameter for training prescription and for adequately interpreting outcomes from research studies. To date, there has been limited research into the reproducibility of testing Fat_{max}, and findings to date are conflicting and have methodological limitations [8,13,14]. Achten *et al.* [8] found a coefficient of variation (CV) for Fat_{max} of 9.6% in 10 endurance athletes tested on three occasions and concluded that Fat_{max} measurements are reliable. Perez-Martin *et al.* [13] tested 10

Table 1. Subject characteristics.

	n = 15
Age (years)	27.4±4.0
Height (cm)	180±5
Weight (kg)	74.5±7.6
BMI (kg·m^2)	23.1±2.3
Body fat (%)	14.4±2.9
Fat-free mass (kg)	63.7±5.9
$\dot{V}O_{2max}$ (mL·kg^{-1}·min^{-1})	52.0±7.7
HR_{max} (beats·min^{-1})	185±11
$\dot{W}_{max}$ (Watts)	322±51

Values are means ± SD. *n*, number of subjects; BMI, body mass index; $\dot{V}O_{2max}$, maximal oxygen uptake; HR_{max}, maximal heart rate; $\dot{W}_{max}$, maximal aerobic power output.

healthy males on two occasions, reported a CV for Fat_{max} of 11.4% and suggested this to be a "satisfactory result". Conversely, Meyer *et al.* [14] studied 21 recreationally trained men and women who completed the test twice. The limits of agreement (LoA) for oxygen consumption at Fat_{max} corresponded to a heart rate (HR) difference of 35 bpm between the two tests, which lead them to conclude that the intra-individual variability in Fat_{max} measurements is too large to recommend using this parameter for prescribing exercise training. In addition to coming to different conclusions, these studies had methodological limitations in terms of testing protocol and data analysis approach. Data analysis to determine Fat_{max} was performed using the MV [8,14] or the "respiratory quotient technique" [13] approaches. However, Chenevière *et al.* [12] recently showed that the employment of a mathematical model (SIN) provides a more complete description of the Fat_{ox} kinetics as a function of exercise intensity and more accurate Fat_{max} measures than the "respiratory quotient technique" approach. Secondly, in two of these studies [8,14], the starting workload of the graded test occurred on average at ~45% of the maximal oxygen uptake ($\dot{V}O_{2max}$), therefore not providing information on substrate metabolism at low intensities, while in the other [13], the protocol included a limited number of exercise stages, therefore limiting information for determining Fat_{max}. Furthermore, the statistical approach to assess reliability used by Achten *et al.* and Perez-Martin *et al.* was not comprehensive given that only CVs were reported [15]. Other measures of variability such as the LoA were not calculated.

Crucially, even though Fat_{max} is calculated from F_{ox} values at each stage of a submaximal graded test, the reproducibility of F_{ox} over a wide range of exercise intensities has not been assessed. Some studies have evaluated the intra-individual variability of the physiological parameters used to determine substrate oxidation ($\dot{V}O_2, \dot{V}CO_2$and respiratory exchange ratio or RER). The authors reported that $\dot{V}O_2$ and $\dot{V}CO_2$ were reliable in resting conditions [16,17] and that CVs for $\dot{V}O_2, \dot{V}CO_2$ and RER were lower than 5% in response to each stage of an incremental exercise test [8,18,19]. However, while CVs of $\dot{V}O_2, \dot{V}CO_2$ and RER are often reported to inform on the variability in substrate oxidation rates, this might be misleading. The relationship existing between those CVs and the variability of F_{ox} and CHO_{ox} has not been established.

Limited information is available on the reproducibility of Fat_{max} and on the reproducibility of CHO_{ox} and F_{ox} at each stage of a graded test. It was therefore the aim of this study to assess the intra-individual variability of: a) Fat_{max} measurements determined using three different data analysis approaches (SIN, P3 and MV), and b) CHO_{ox} and F_{ox} at rest and in response to each stage of an individualized graded test. A further aim was to investigate how the CVs of $\dot{V}O_2, \dot{V}CO_2$ and RER are related to the CV of F_{ox}.

Methods

Ethics Statement

The study was conducted in accordance with ethical principles of the 1964 World medical Declaration of Helsinki and was approved by the human research ethics committee of the University of Lausanne (Switzerland). All test procedures, risks and benefits associated with the experiment were fully explained, and written informed consent was obtained from all participants.

Subjects

Fifteen healthy, moderately trained male volunteers (see Table 1 for anthropometric and physical characteristics) were recruited to participate in this study. All participants were of normal weight according to the World Health Organization (Body Mass Index< 25 kg·m^{-2}), non-smokers and disease-free. They were not taking regular medications and were screened for the absence of electrocardiographic abnormalities at rest and during exercise.

General Design

Each participant completed three test sessions. In the first session anthropometric measurements (*i.e.*, stature, body mass and body composition) were taken and a maximal incremental test on a cycle ergometer was performed. In the remaining two sessions the subjects performed an identical submaximal incremental test (Test 1 and Test 2). The two tests were performed in the morning (start of exercise between 7 and 8 am) after a10-hour overnight fast. They were separated by 3 to 7 days and performed at the same time of day to avoid circadian variance. The volunteers were asked to fill in a 1-day food diary on the day before Test 1 and to repeat this diet before Test 2. Furthermore, participants were asked to refrain from vigorous exercise and alcohol and caffeine consumption in the 24 hours prior to testing. Participants were familiarized with the equipment prior to testing.

Anthropometric Measurements

Body composition (fat mass and percentage of body fat) was estimated from skin-fold thickness measurements at four sites according to the methods of Durnin and Womersley [20].

Maximal Exercise Test

A maximal incremental test on a cycle ergometer (Ebike Basic BPlus, General Electric, Niskayuna, NY, USA) to determine maximal oxygen uptake ($\dot{V}O_{2max}$) and maximal aerobic power output ($\dot{W}_{max}$) was performed. After a 5-min rest period and a 5-min warm-up at 60 W, output was increased by 30 W every minute until volitional exhaustion. $\dot{V}O_2$was considered as maximal when at least three of the following four criteria were met [21]: 1) a plateauing of $\dot{V}O_2$ (defined as an increase of no more than 2 mL·kg^{-1}·min^{-1} with an increase in workload) during the latter stages of the exercise test, 2) an HR>90% of the age-predicted maximum (220-age), 3) an RER>1.1 and 4) an inability to maintain the minimal required pedaling frequency (*i.e.* 60 rpm) despite maximum effort and verbal encouragement. $\dot{V}O_{2max}$was calculated as the average $\dot{V}O_2$ over the last 20 seconds of the last stage of the test.

Submaximal Graded Exercise Tests (Test 1 and Test 2)

Test 1 and Test 2 were characterized by two phases: a pre-exercise resting phase (rest) and a submaximal incremental exercise test. They were carried out under identical circumstances with an identical protocol. Data from these two tests were subsequently employed for reliability calculations.

In the pre-exercise resting phase (rest), participants were seated for 30-min on the cycle ergometer and respiratory measures were collected during the last 15-min of this sitting period. Subsequently, a submaximal incremental exercise test to determine whole-body F_{ox} kinetics was performed. After a 10-min warm-up at 20% $\dot{W}_{max}$, the power output was increased by 7.5% $\dot{W}_{max}$ every 5-min until RER was >1.0 during the last minute of the stage.

Indirect Calorimetry and Calculations

Oxygen uptake ($\dot{V}O_2$), carbon dioxide output ($\dot{V}CO_2$) and ventilation ($\dot{V}_E$) were measured continuously using a breath-by-breath system (Oxycon Pro, Jaeger, Würzburg, Germany). Before each test the gas analyzers were calibrated with gases of known concentration (16.00% O_2 and 5.02% CO_2), and the volume was automatically calibrated at two different flow rates (0.2 $L \cdot s^{-1}$ and 2 $L \cdot s^{-1}$). The HR was recorded continuously using an HR monitor (S810i, Polar Electro OY, Kempele, Finland).

During Test 1 and Test 2, HR and gas exchange data ($\dot{V}O_2$,$\dot{V}CO_2$) collected during the final 5-min of the pre-exercise resting phase and during the last 2-min of each stage of the submaximal incremental exercise test were averaged and used for calculations. RER was calculated as the ratio between $\dot{V}CO_2$ and $\dot{V}O_2$, while F_{ox} and CHO_{ox} were calculated using stoichiometric equations [7], with the assumption that the urinary nitrogen excretion rate was negligible:

$$F_{ox}(g \cdot min^{-1}) = 1.67\dot{V}O_2(L \cdot min^{-1}) - 1.67\dot{V}CO_2(L \cdot min^{-1}) \quad (1)$$

$$CHO_{ox}(g \cdot min^{-1}) = 4.55\dot{V}CO_2(L \cdot min^{-1}) - 3.21\dot{V}O_2(L \cdot min^{-1}) \quad (2)$$

(1-RER) was also calculated given that the equation to calculate F_{ox} can be simplified to:

$$F_{ox}(g \cdot min^{-1}) = 1.67(1\text{-}RER)\dot{V}O_2. \quad (3)$$

F_{ox} as a function of exercise intensity is reflected by two different linear relationships: a progressive decrease of (1–RER) and a linear increase of $\dot{V}O_2$ as power output is increased. The percentages of total energy expenditure derived from fat (% ENE_{fat}) and CHO (% ENE_{CHO}) were calculated [22]:

$$\%ENE_{fat} = [(1 - RER/0.29)] \cdot 100 \quad (4)$$

$$\%ENE_{CHO} = [(RER - 0.71)/0.29)] \cdot 100 \quad (5)$$

Data Analysis Approaches to Determine Fat_{max}

F_{ox} values obtained at each stage of the submaximal graded exercise test (which was terminated when RER was >1) were graphically depicted as a function of exercise intensity. Then, Fat_{max} and MFO (and subsequently RER, $\%HR_{max}$ at Fat_{max}, % $\dot{W}_{max}$ at Fat_{max}) were determined using three different data analysis approaches (SIN, MV and P3). The "respiratory quotient technique" was not used in this study since it has been shown to be less accurate than the other methods [12].

SIN model. The SIN model [12] was used to model and characterize whole-body F_{ox} kinetics:

$$\%MFO = Sin\left(\left[\frac{\pi^{\frac{1}{s}}}{\pi + 2d}(K \cdot \%\dot{V}o_{2\,max} + d + t)\right]^{s}\right) \quad (6)$$

Dilatation (*d*), *symmetry* (*s*) and *translation* (*t*) are the three independent variables representing the main modulations of the curve. *K* is the constant of intensity and corresponds to (π/100). To fit the experimental data (*i.e.* F_{ox} rates) and to model the F_{ox} kinetics, the three variables were independently changed using an iterative procedure by minimizing the sum of the mean squares of the differences between the estimated energy derived from fat based on the SIN model and the energy derived from fat calculated from the raw F_{ox} data, as described in a previous study [12]. For each subject, Fat_{max} was calculated by differentiation of the SIN model equation. The Fat_{max} zone was determined as the range of exercise intensities with F_{ox} rates within 10% of MFO [3].

P3. Graphical depiction of F_{ox} values as a function of exercise intensity was performed by constructing a third polynomial curve with intersection at (0;0) [11]. Fat_{max} was calculated by differentiation of the P3 equation, and corresponded to the intensity at which the value of the differentiated equation was equal to zero.

Measured values. From the graphical representation of F_{ox} values as a function of exercise intensity, the stage at which the value of measured F_{ox} rates was maximal was determined, and the corresponding intensity was identified [3,8–10,23].

Theoretical Example to Study how the CVs of $\dot{V}O_2$ and $\dot{V}CO_2$ are Related to the CVs of RER and the CV of F_{ox}

In order to investigate how the CV of $\dot{V}O_2$ and $\dot{V}CO_2$ are linked to the CVs of parameters informing of substrate utilization (RER, F_{ox}, CHO_{fat}, 1-RER, ENE_{fat}) three theoretical scenarios were created. $\dot{V}O_2$ and $\dot{V}CO_2$values for Test 1 and Test 2 were generated so that CVs of $\dot{V}O_2$ and $\dot{V}CO_2$ between Test 1 and Test 2 were ≤3%. A CV of ≤3% for $\dot{V}O_2$ and $\dot{V}CO_2$ was chosen in line with results from previous studies [8,18].

Statistical Analysis

Data are expressed as the means ± standard deviation (SD) for all variables. Intra-individual CVs and LoA were calculated to test the variability between Test 1 and Test 2 for the following measures: a) Fat_{max} and physiological measures at Fat_{max} (MFO, RER, % HR_{max} and % $\dot{W}_{max}$) determined with three different data analysis approaches (SIN, MV and P3) and b) gas exchange data, HR and substrate oxidation rates at rest and during the first six stages of the submaximal incremental tests (from 20% to 57.5% of $\dot{W}_{max}$). Intra-individual CVs were calculated for the physiological variables studied in the three theoretical scenarios.

Two-factorial analysis of variance for repeated measures (RMANOVA) was carried out to test for systematic changes in:

Table 2. Average values, limits of agreement and CVs for Fat_{max} and physiological measures at Fat_{max} determined with three approaches: SIN, P3 and MV.

		SIN	*P3*	*MV*
Fat_{max}	Test 1	46.9±9.0	44.2±10.2	45.7±9.0
(% $\dot{V}O_{2max}$)	Test 2	48.9±12.2	48.6±13.1	49.6±12.6
	LoA	−29.7, 25.7	−36.7, 28.0	−32.0, 24.0
	CV (%)	16.4	20.8	18.6
MFO	Test 1	0.28±0.08	0.28±0.08	0.29±0.08
($g \cdot min^{-1}$)	Test 2	0.29±0.13	0.29±0.13	0.30±0.12
	LoA	−0.27, 0.24	−0.25, 0.23	−0.26, 0.26
	CV (%)	25.3	22.8	26
RER Fat_{max}	Test 1	0.91±0.02	0.91±0.02	0.91±0.02
	Test 2	0.91±0.02	0.91±0.02	0.91±0.02
	LoA	−0.05, 0.04	−0.06, 0.04	−0.06, 0.05
	CV (%)	1.6	1.7	1.6
% HR_{max} Fat_{max}	Test 1	60.9±8.3	58.7±9.3	58.8±8.9
	Test 2	63.0±10.0	62.7±10.5	63.3±11.0
	LoA	−23.9, 19.7	−30.0, 22.2	−29.4, 20.4
	CV (%)	10	12.8*	12.8*
% $\dot{W}_{max}$ Fat_{max}	Test 1	34.9±8.9	32.4±10.4	39.0±10.6
	Test 2	36.7±11.8	36.3±12.8	32.0±11.7
	LoA	−26.4, 22.6	−33.4, 25.6	−18.1, 32.1
	CV (%)	19.8	26.4*	24.9*

Values are means ± SD. LoA, limits of agreement; CV, coefficient of variation; SIN, sine model; MV, measured values; P3, 3rd polynomial curve; Fat_{max}, exercise intensity at which maximal fat oxidation rate occurs; MFO, maximal fat oxidation rate; RER Fat_{max}, respiratory exchange ratio at Fat_{max}; % HR_{max} Fat_{max}, % maximal heart rate at Fat_{max}; % $\dot{W}_{max}$ Fat_{max}, % maximal aerobic power output at Fat_{max}.
*$P<0.05$ between SIN and the other approaches (P3 and MV).

a) Fat_{max}, and physiological measures at Fat_{max} (factor 1: tests, factor 2: data analysis approaches), and b) gas exchange data, HR and substrate oxidation rates (factor 1: tests; factor 2: exercise intensity). For the same outcome measures, one-way RMANOVA was carried out to test for systematic changes in the intra-individual CV at Fat_{max}.

Bland-Altman scatterplots are presented for Fat_{max} and MFO determined with SIN, P3 and MV. They show the difference between two corresponding measurements plotted against the mean of the measurements. Reference lines for the mean difference±1.96 SD are given. For all statistical analyses, the level of significance was set at $P \leq 0.05$. Statistical analysis was performed with the software SPSS 17.0 for Windows (SPSS, Chicago, IL) and Graph Pad Prism version 5.0 for Mac (GraphPad Software, San Diego, CA).

Results

Fat_{max} and Physiological Measures at Fat_{max} Determined with SIN, P3 and MV

Fat_{max} and physiological measures at Fat_{max} determined with three data analysis approaches (SIN, P3 and MV) are presented in Table 2. For all parameters, average values (n = 15) obtained from Test 1 and Test 2 were not significantly different (i.e. for Fat_{max}: $P=0.37$ for factor test and $P=0.20$ for factor interaction between test and approach), indicating that no habituation or training effects occurred between testing sessions. Average values for Fat_{max} and related measures obtained with the three different approaches were also not significantly different (*i.e.* for Fat_{max}: $P=0.13$ for factor approach).

On the other hand, the within-individual CVs for Fat_{max} determined with SIN was 16.4% and tended to be lower ($P=0.10$) than with P3 and MV (20.8% and 18.6% respectively). Similarly, the intra-individual CVs of % HR at Fat_{max} and % $\dot{W}_{max}$ at Fat_{max} determined with SIN were significantly lower than with the other approaches ($P=0.043$ and $P=0.05$, respectively).

The Bland–Altman scatterplots for Fat_{max} and MFO (Figure 1) reveal considerable intra-individual variability. The LoA for Fat_{max} were −2±27% of $\dot{V}O_{2max}$ with SIN, −4±32% with P3, and −4±28% with MV. For MFO they were −0.01±0.25 g/min with SIN, 0.01±0.24 g/min with P3, and 0±0.26 g/min with MV (Table 2). A large between-individual difference in the variability between Test 1 and Test 2 was also seen. Accordingly, the CV at Fat_{max} ranged from 0 to 48%. For seven subjects it was under 10%, for two subjects it was between 10 and 15%, while for six subjects it was over 20%. However, the size of the difference between Test 1 and Test 2 appeared to be independent of the average value between the two measurements.

The difference in the HR at Fat_{max} between test 1 and 2 was < 10 bpm in six participants, between 10 and 25 bpm in eight participants and was >25 bpm in one. In both tests, the range of HR frequencies corresponding to the Fat_{max} zone was broad (it was 38±8 bpm, and ranged from 95±16 to 133±20 bpm).

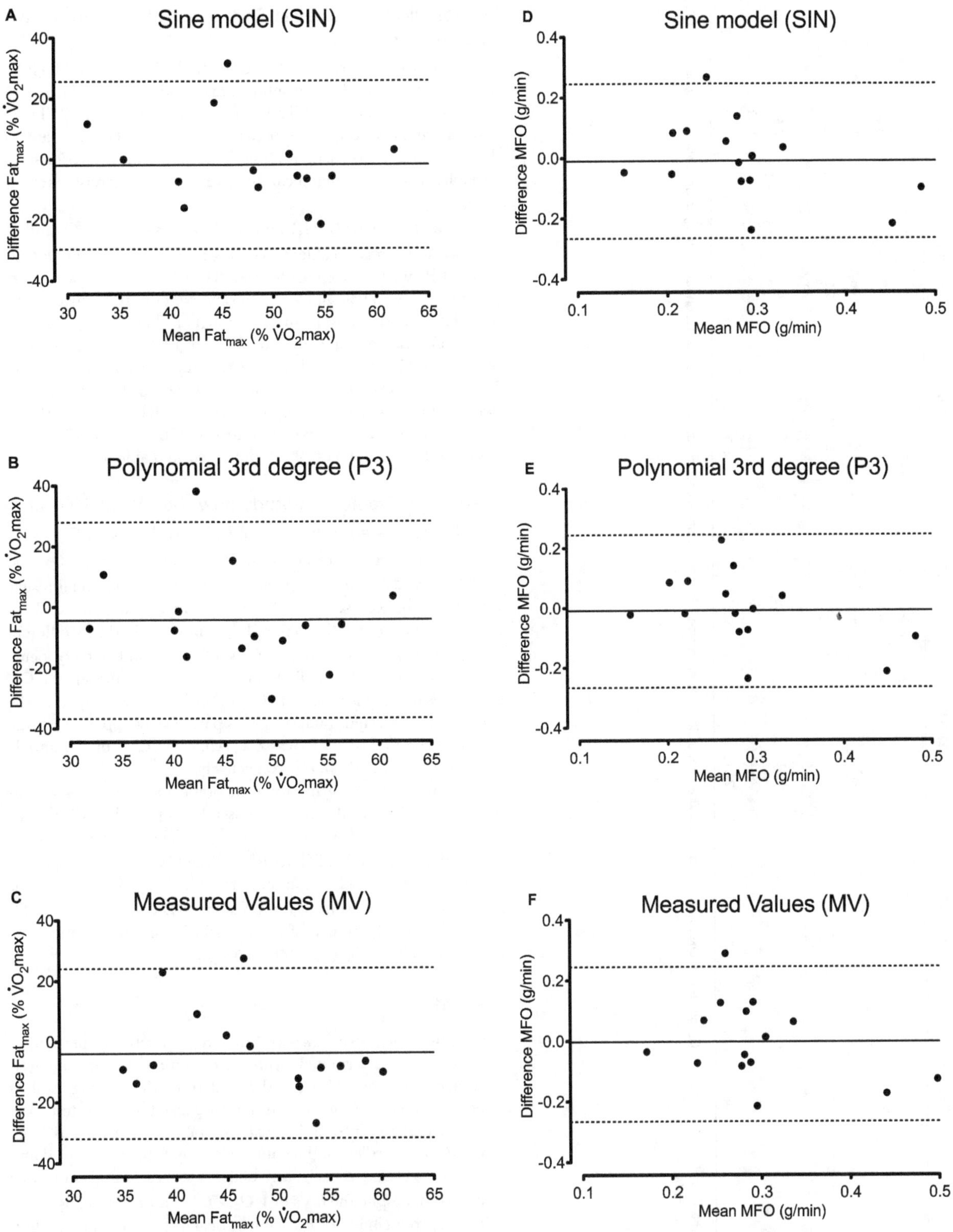

Figure 1. Bland-Altman plots of Fat$_{max}$ and MFO determined with SIN, P3 or MV. SIN, sine model. P3, polynomial 3rd degree; MV, measured values; Fat$_{max}$, exercise intensity at which maximal fat oxidation rate occurs; $\dot{V}O_{2max}$, maximal oxygen uptake; MFO, maximal fat oxidation rate; Biases (*solid lines*) and 95% limits agreement (*dashed lines*).

Table 3. Coefficients of variation (%) for respiratory values and substrate oxidation rates in reponse to a submaximal graded exercise test.

	Rest	$\dot{W}_{max}$20%	$\dot{W}_{max}$27.5%	$\dot{W}_{max}$35%	$\dot{W}_{max}$42.5%	$\dot{W}_{max}$50%	$\dot{W}_{max}$57.5%
$\dot{V}O_2$ (ml·min^{-1})	7.5	4.0	3.0	2.9	3.3	3.1	2.6
$\dot{V}CO_2$ (ml·min^{-1})	9.1	3.4	3.1	3.0	2.5	3.0	3.0
HR (bpm)	5.7	3.7	4.2	4.4	3.6	2.6	2.5
RER	3.8	2.8	2.9	2.6	2.6	2.5	2.1
Fat_{ox} (g·min^{-1})	20.6	24.1	29.5	32	38.1	49.2	45.1
CHO_{ox} (g·min^{-1})	33.5	12.9	12.1	10.9	9.3	9.1	8.5
(1-RER)	20.6	20.9	24.1	28.0	30.8	36.6	47.9
ENE_{fat} (%)	20.6	20.9	24.1	28.0	30.8	36.6	47.9

Values are means. $\dot{W}_{max}$, maximal aerobic power output; $\dot{V}O_2$, oxygen uptake; $\dot{V}CO_2$, carbon dioxide production; HR, heart rate; RER, respiratory exchange ratio; Fat_{ox}, fat oxidation rate; CHO_{ox}, carbohydrate oxidation rate; ENE_{fat}, % energy expenditure derived from fat.

Physiological Measures at Each Stage of a Submaximal Graded Test

The course of average $\dot{V}O_2, \dot{V}CO_2$, RER, HR, F_{ox} and CHO_{ox} in response to two identical submaximal graded test performed on separate days (Test 1 and Test 2) is presented in Figure 2. There was no significant difference between Test 1 and Test 2 in any of the parameters assessed. Average values of most physiological variables (except F_{ox}) significantly increased with exercise intensity ($P<0.001$).

CVs of $\dot{V}O_2, \dot{V}CO_2$, HR and RER were <10% at rest and < 5% during exercise (Table 3). For instance, CVs for $\dot{V}O_2, \dot{V}CO_2$ and RER were 7.5%, 9.1% and 3.8% at rest and were, on average, 3.1%, 3.0% and 2.5% during exercise. In contrast, CVs for CHO_{ox} and F_{ox} were markedly higher. The CV for F_{ox} was 20.6% at rest and ranged from 24.1 to 49.2% during exercise, while for CHO_{ox}, it was 33.5% at rest and ranged from 8.5% to 12.9% during exercise. Interestingly, although the CV of RER was <4% under each condition, the CV of 1-RER was markedly higher (>20%), and was equal to the CV of the % of ENE_{fat}. LoA between Test 1 and Test 2 are presented in Table 4.

Theoretical Example to Study how the CVs of $\dot{V}O_2$ and $\dot{V}CO_2$ are Related to the CVs of RER and the CV of F_{ox}

Three theoretical scenarios in which the CVs of $\dot{V}O_2$ and $\dot{V}CO_2$ were ≤3% are presented in Table 5 and additional results with mathematical explanations are presented in appendix S1. In case scenario 1 and 2, the CVs of F_{ox} from were markedly different (3.1% *vs.* 38.2%) despite the CVs of $\dot{V}O_2$ and $\dot{V}CO_2$ being identical (3%) (see Appendix S1, eq. 7, 8 and 9). Further, the CV of 1-RER was higher than the CV of RER, and was equal to the CV of %ENE_{fat}. This difference was particularly apparent in case 2, where the CV of RER was 6%, while the CVs of F_{ox} and 1-RER were 38.2 and 35.3%, respectively.

From the analysis of the three theoretical scenarios (as well as from the analysis of the whole dataset of 15 participants) we also observed that the CV of F_{ox} can be calculated from sum or subtraction of the CV of (1-RER) and the CV of $\dot{V}O_2$ (Appendix S1, eq. 10 and 11). For example, in case 2, the CV of F_{ox} was 38.2% and was the sum of the CVs of 1-RER (35.3%) and $\dot{V}O_2$ (3.0%). In case 3, the CV of F_{ox} was 15.3%, and equaled the CV of 1-RER (15.3%) ± CV $\dot{V}O_2$ (0.0%).

Discussion

In this study we assessed the reproducibility of Fat_{max} measurements determined with three different data analysis approaches and of CHO_{ox} and F_{ox} at rest (while sitting) and in response to each stage of an individualized graded test. We observed that the intra-individual variability of Fat_{max} was large (CV>16%) regardless of the data analysis approach employed and that F_{ox} at rest and at each stage of a graded test was also variable (CV>20%), despite the CVs of $\dot{V}O_2, \dot{V}CO_2$and RER being <5%.

The reproducibility of F_{ox} values at each stage of a graded test, despite being a key aspect in the determination of Fat_{max}, was previously unexplored. In the current study, the CVs found for the parameters from which Fat_{ox} is calculated ($\dot{V}O_2, \dot{V}CO_2$ and RER) were in line with previous observations. At rest, the CV for RER was 3.8%, which closely mirrors the CV of 3.5% found by Roffey *et al.* [17]. In the present study the resting assessment was performed with the individuals in a seated position and this needs to be taken into consideration when making comparisons with studies in which resting metabolism was assessed with participants

Table 4. Limits of agreement between Test 1 and Test 2 for respiratory values and substrate oxidation rates in response to a submaximal graded exercise test.

	Rest	$\dot{W}_{max}$20%	$\dot{W}_{max}$27.5%	$\dot{W}_{max}$35%	$\dot{W}_{max}$42.5%	$\dot{W}_{max}$50%	$\dot{W}_{max}$57.5%
$\dot{V}O_2$ (ml·min^{-1})	−142,102	−139, 191	−117, 185	−146, 178	−206, 263	−241, 298	−225, 283
$\dot{V}CO_2$ (ml·min^{-1})	−118, 89	−132, 155	−118, 151	−134, 178	−150, 186	188, 274	−236, 301
HR (bpm)	−16, 11	−11, 10	−15, 12	−19, 17	−18, 10	−16, 11	−20, 14
RER	−0.11, 0.12	−0.10, 0.07	−0.10, 0.07	−0.09, 0.10	−0.09, 0.08	−0.09, 0.10	−0.09, 0.09
Fat_{ox} (g·min^{-1})	−0.09, 0.07	−0.16, 0.21	−0.19, 0.25	−0.28, 0.26	−0.29, 0.33	−0.37, 0.32	−0.31, 0.30
CHO_{ox} (g·min^{-1})	−0.18, 0.18	−0.47, 0.40	−0.55, 0.48	−0.60, 0.69	−0.67, 0.65	−0.75, 0.95	−0.88, 0.99

Lower and higher limit of agreement are separated by a comma. $\dot{W}_{max}$, maximal aerobic power output; $\dot{V}O_2$, oxygen uptake; $\dot{V}CO_2$, carbon dioxide production; HR, heart rate; RER, respiratory exchange ratio; Fat_{ox}, fat oxidation rate; CHO_{ox}, carbohydrate oxidation rate.

lying supine. During exercise, the average CVs for $\dot{V}O_2$,$\dot{V}CO_2$ and RER were 3.1%, 3.0% and 2.5%, respectively, and were similar or lower than those reported in previous investigations [8,13,18,19]. Despite this, the CVs found for F_{ox} were >20%. This shows that even though CHO_{ox} and F_{ox} are calculated from $\dot{V}O_2$ and $\dot{V}CO_2$ by means of the stoichiometric equations [7], a low variability in those parameters is not necessarily indicative of low variability in CHO_{ox} and F_{ox}.

To further study how the CVs of $\dot{V}O_2$ and $\dot{V}CO_2$ are related to the CVs of RER and the CV of F_{ox}, three theoretical scenarios were created. At present, scientific reports as well as companies validating calorimeters tend to draw information on the variability of substrate oxidation from the CVs of $\dot{V}O_2$, $\dot{V}CO_2$ and RER. The results of the theoretical scenarios (Table 5) and the mathematical explanations presented in the appendix S1 illustrate that those CVs do not provide sufficient information on the variability of substrate oxidation rates.

As can be seen in case 2, when the $\dot{V}O_2$ and $\dot{V}CO_2$ vary in different directions between two tests (increase in $\dot{V}O_2$ and decrease in $\dot{V}CO_2$ or *viceversa*), the variability of F_{ox} is high. This is because in such conditions, the standard deviation of F_{ox} results from the sum of the standard deviations of $\dot{V}O_2$ and $\dot{V}CO_2$, multiplied by a factor 1.67. Therefore, in addition to the size of the change in $\dot{V}O_2$ and $\dot{V}CO_2$ between tests, it is crucial to know whether they change in the same or opposite sense between measurements.

The RER is the ratio between $\dot{V}CO_2$ and $\dot{V}O_2$ and, therefore, provides information on the relationship between those measurements. However, in the theoretical scenarios the CV of RER remains low (<6%) also when the variability in F_{ox} is high (> 30%), showing that the CV of RER is not a parameter adequately informing on the variability in the proportion of nutrients utilized. This is because the RER is value bounded in an interval separate from zero (0.7–1.0) and therefore the CV is not an adequate measure to assess the variability of RER. On the other hand, the CV of 1-RER appears to be an informative marker on the variability in F_{ox} rates: it provides the same results as the CV of ENE_{fat}, it accounts for a large proportion of the CV of F_{ox}, and it is simple to calculate.

In this study, as well as in other studies investigating the reproducibility of indirect calorimetry measures [8,13,14,16–19], the total variation observed between Test 1 and Test 2 is the sum of both biological and equipment variation. It was beyond the scope of this study to assess the relative contribution of each. However, the average variation of the equipment (gas analysis system) used in this study is known. It was assessed using a portable metabolic simulator (which excludes any biological variability) and the average CV for $\dot{V}O_2$ and $\dot{V}CO_2$ was 1.9±0.6% and 1.3±0.5% respectively [18].

In addition to investigating the variability in F_{ox} and related parameters at each stage of a graded test, a novel feature of this study was the assessment of the intra-individual variability in Fat_{max} determined with the SIN model and its comparison with the variability of Fat_{max} measures obtained using different data analysis approaches. All the approaches to determine Fat_{max} presented in the literature were compared in this analysis, except the "respiratory quotient technique", since it has previously been shown to be less accurate [12]. The comparison revealed that the intra-individual CV at Fat_{max} was higher than 16% with any of the data analysis approaches employed and that there was a relatively small difference between approaches. However, the CVs of Fat_{max}, % $\dot{W}_{max}$ at Fat_{max} and of % HR_{max} determined with SIN were

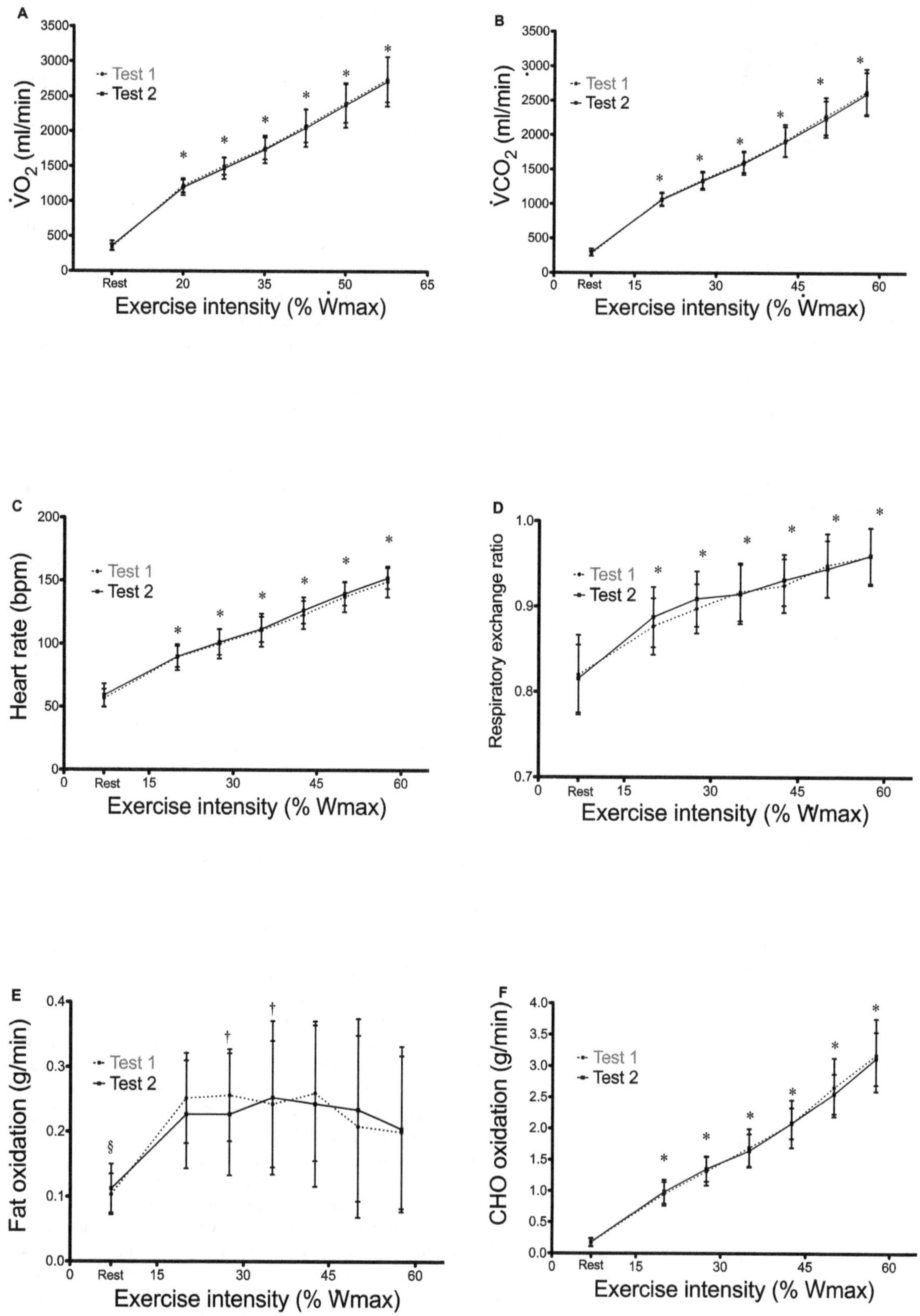

Figure 2. Course of average $\dot{V}O_2$, $\dot{V}CO_2$, HR, RER, F_{ox} and CHO_{ox} during two identical submaximal incremental tests (mean and SD).
$1\dot{W}_{vmax}$, maximal aerobic power output; $\dot{V}O_2$, oxygen uptake; $\dot{V}CO_2$, carbon dioxide production; RER, respiratory exchange ratio; HR, heart rate; F_{ox}, fat oxidation rate; CHO_{ox}, carbohydrate oxidation rate. *significantly increases with exercise intensity, §rest significantly different than exercise (20–57.5% $1\dot{W}_{vmax}$\), † significantly different than 57.5% $\dot{W}_{max}$.

Table 5. Three case scenario in which CV for $\dot{V}O_2$ and $\dot{V}CO_2$ are≤3%.

	Case 1			Case 2			Case 3		
	Test 1	**Test 2**	**CV (%)**	**Test 1**	**Test 2**	**CV (%)**	**Test 1**	**Test 2**	**CV (%)**
<b>$\dot{V}O_2$ </b>(ml·min^{-1})	**1699**	**1628**	**3.0**	**1699**	**1628**	**3.0**	**1699**	**1699**	**0.0**
$\dot{V}CO_2$(ml·min^{-1})	**1450**	**1390**	**3.0**	**1390**	**1450**	**3.0**	**1390**	**1450**	**3.0**
RER	0.85	0.85	0.0	0.82	0.89	6.0	0.82	0.85	3.0
Fat$_{ox}$ (g·min^{-1})	0.42	0.40	3.1	0.52	0.30	38.2	0.52	0.42	15.3
CHO$_{ox}$ (g·min^{-1})	1.15	1.10	3.0	0.87	1.37	31.7	0.87	1.15	19.2
1-RER	0.15	0.15	0.1	0.18	0.11	35.3	0.18	0.15	15.3
% ENE$_{fat}$	50.4	50.4	0.0	62.7	37.6	35.3	62.7	50.4	15.3

$\dot{V}O_2$ and $\dot{V}CO_2$, the values generated for the purpose of this study, are presented in bold. RER, Fatox, CHOox, 1-RER and % ENEfat were calculated. Case 1: CVs of $\dot{V}O_2$ and $\dot{V}CO_2$ are 3% and the correlation coefficient between $\dot{V}O_2$ and $\dot{V}CO_2$ is positive; case 2: CVs of $\dot{V}O_2$ and $\dot{V}CO_2$ are 3% and the correlation coefficient between $\dot{V}O_2$ and $\dot{V}CO_2$ is negative; case 3: CV $\dot{V}O_2$ is 0% and CV $\dot{V}CO_2$ is 3%. When assuming CV $\dot{V}CO_2$ 0% and CV $\dot{V}O_2$ 3%, similar results as for case 3 are obtained (data not shown). $\dot{V}O_2$, oxygen uptake; $\dot{V}CO_2$, carbon dioxide production; RER, respiratory exchange ratio; Fatox, fat oxidation rate; CHOox, carbohydrate oxidation rate; % ENEfat, % energy derived from fat.

lower than with P3 and MV, possibly because the SIN model provides an accurate and more complete description of the F$_{ox}$ kinetics as a function of exercise intensity than the other data analysis approaches. These results support the use of SIN over other approaches in future studies given that it is more reliable and provides more detailed information.

The intra-individual variability of Fat$_{max}$ and related parameters found in this study was in line with those of Meyer *et al.* [14]. In the present study the LoA for Fat$_{max}$ determined with SIN were -2.0 ± 27.7 of $\dot{V}O_{2max}$, while in the study from Meyer *et al.* LoA for Fat$_{max}$ of -3.9 ± 27.7 of $\dot{V}O_{2max}$ were observed. Further, also consistent with the results published by Meyer *et al.* [14], the within-individual variability was markedly different between individuals. On the other hand, the CV for Fat$_{max}$ observed in this study, on average, was slightly higher than those reported in other studies [8,13,24]. The lower CV found by Achten *et al.* [8] (9.6%) could be due to the fact that measurements were repeated three times [and the CV generally decreases when the number of measurements increases [25]] and were performed in trained athletes, who may have a less variable response to exercise than individuals with a lower training level. Overall, the differences in the results obtained between studies are difficult to interpret, particularly because most studies only report average results, and do not present "individual responses" and/or ranges. This highlights the need for a better understanding of the determinants of intra-individual variability in Fat$_{max}$.

Previous studies in the field considered an intra-individual variability of ±10 bpm in the HR at Fat$_{max}$ acceptable, since this value reflects a realistic margin in individuals who use HR for the monitoring of training intensity [8,14]. In the present study this target was met by the majority, but not all, participants. However, the range of intensities at which F$_{ox}$ is within 10% of MFO (Fat$_{max}$ zone) was broad and this was consistent with previous observations [3,26]. Therefore, despite its variability, training prescription at Fat$_{max}$ ensures that high rates of F$_{ox}$ are elicited on different days.

The determination of F$_{ox}$ and Fat$_{max}$ (and therefore the determination of their variability) is influenced by a number of methodological factors including the exercise test design, the data analysis approach and the pre-test conditions. In this study, a robust methodological approach was employed. The submaximal graded exercise was individualized based upon the results of a maximal test. It started at 20% of $\dot{W}_{max}$ and the workload was subsequently increased by 7.5% $\dot{W}_{max}$ every 5-min. This ensured the reaching of a steady state [27] and allowed to study F$_{ox}$ at several intensities (participants performed at least six exercise stages with an RER<1). Further, the statistical analysis was carried out in accordance with the recommendations for reliability assessment in sport medicine [15].

Pre-test conditions included a 10-hour overnight fast and 24 hours of standardization in diet and physical activity prior to each submaximal graded exercise test. This level of standardization was adopted because it appears to be the most commonly employed approach in our research field [3,8,28–32] and because more rigorous standardization is difficult to achieve both in out-clinic and research settings. Despite the standardization adopted, in some individuals a high intra-individual variability in Fat$_{max}$ and related variables was found, suggesting that a longer period of standardization (≥2 days prior to testing) might be needed to improve the reproducibility of those measures. However, while more strict pre-test standardization leads to greater internal validity, it also leads to poorer external validity (i.e harder translation of the results into practice). More generally, while the validity of using a graded exercise tests to determine Fat$_{max}$ has been reported in a number of studies [3,13,33,34], a recent study questions the usefulness using this approach to prescribe training in populations such as highly trained athletes [35]".

A number of questions on the reproducibility of substrate metabolism during exercise are still to be answered. Further research is required to: a) describe how standardization in physical activity and diet prior to testing impact on reliability of measurements, b) study the determinants of the variability in CHO_{ox} and F_{ox} and c) explore the reproducibility in F_{ox} in other cohorts including overweight and untrained individuals.

In summary, we have shown here that the intra-individual variability in Fat_{max} is high (CV>16%) and is highly variable between individuals, regardless of the data analysis approach employed. The intra-individual variability at rest and in response to an individualized graded test is high for F_{ox} measures (CV> 20% for F_{ox}) although it is low for $\dot{V}O_2$, $\dot{V}CO_2$ and RER (CV< 5%). The CV of (1-RER) appears to be a more representative measure of the variability in substrate oxidation than CV of RER. Training prescription at Fat_{max} can be useful clinically given that, despite its variability, it results in Fat_{ox} rates within 90% of MFO on different days. In a research setting, differences in Fat_{max} and F_{ox} within and between groups can be detected as long as a sufficiently large number of participants is recruited. Further research in this area is required.

Acknowledgments

The authors would like to thank Aleš Neubert for mathematical inputs, and Graeme Macdonald and John Prins for helpful suggestions and criticisms.

Author Contributions

Conceived and designed the experiments: IC FB NB RW IH XC DM. Performed the experiments: IC FB XC DM. Analyzed the data: IC FB XC DM. Contributed reagents/materials/analysis tools: IC FB NB RW IH XC DM. Wrote the paper: IC. Revised the manuscript for important intellectual content and approved the final version: IC FB NB RW IH XC DM.

References

1. van Loon LJ, Greenhaff PL, Constantin-Teodosiu D, Saris WH, Wagenmakers AJ (2001) The effects of increasing exercise intensity on muscle fuel utilisation in humans. J Physiol 536: 295–304.
2. Romijn JA, Coyle EF, Sidossis LS, Gastaldelli A, Horowitz JF, et al. (1993) Regulation of endogenous fat and carbohydrate metabolism in relation to exercise intensity and duration. Am J Physiol 265: E380–391.
3. Achten J, Gleeson M, Jeukendrup AE (2002) Determination of the exercise intensity that elicits maximal fat oxidation. Med Sci Sports Exerc 34: 92–97.
4. Venables MC, Jeukendrup AE (2008) Endurance training and obesity: effect on substrate metabolism and insulin sensitivity. Med Sci Sports Exerc 40: 495–502.
5. Dumortier M, Brandou F, Perez-Martin A, Fedou C, Mercier J, et al. (2003) Low intensity endurance exercise targeted for lipid oxidation improves body composition and insulin sensitivity in patients with the metabolic syndrome. Diabetes Metab 29: 509–518.
6. Maurie J, Brun J-F, Jean E, Romain A-J, Mercier J (2011) Comparison of Square-Wave Endurance Exercise Test (SWEET) training and endurance training targeted at the level of maximal lipid oxidation in type 2 diabetics. Science & Sports 26: 92–96.
7. Frayn KN (1983) Calculation of substrate oxidation rates in vivo from gaseous exchange. J Appl Physiol 55: 628–634.
8. Achten J, Jeukendrup AE (2003) Maximal fat oxidation during exercise in trained men. Int J Sports Med 24: 603–608.
9. Achten J, Venables MC, Jeukendrup AE (2003) Fat oxidation rates are higher during running compared with cycling over a wide range of intensities. Metabolism 52: 747–752.
10. Venables MC, Achten J, Jeukendrup AE (2005) Determinants of fat oxidation during exercise in healthy men and women: a cross-sectional study. J Appl Physiol 98: 160–167.
11. Stisen AB, Stougaard O, Langfort J, Helge JW, Sahlin K, et al. (2006) Maximal fat oxidation rates in endurance trained and untrained women. Eur J Appl Physiol 98: 497–506.
12. Cheneviere X, Malatesta D, Peters EM, Borrani F (2009) A mathematical model to describe fat oxidation kinetics during graded exercise. Med Sci Sports Exerc 41: 1615–1625.
13. Perez-Martin A, Dumortier M, Raynaud E, Brun JF, Fedou C, et al. (2001) Balance of substrate oxidation during submaximal exercise in lean and obese people. Diabetes Metab 27: 466–474.
14. Meyer T, Folz C, Rosenberger F, Kindermann W (2009) The reliability of fat. Scand J Med Sci Sports 19: 213–221.
15. Atkinson G, Nevill AM (1998) Statistical methods for assessing measurement error (reliability) in variables relevant to sports medicine. Sports Med 26: 217–238.
16. Gasic S, Schneider B, Waldhausl W (1997) Indirect calorimetry: variability of consecutive baseline determinations of carbohydrate and fat utilization from gas exchange measurements. Horm Metab Res 29: 12–15.
17. Roffey DM, Byrne NM, Hills AP (2006) Day-to-day variance in measurement of resting metabolic rate using ventilated-hood and mouthpiece & nose-clip indirect calorimetry systems. JPEN J Parenter Enteral Nutr 30: 426–432.
18. Carter J, Jeukendrup AE (2002) Validity and reliability of three commercially available breath-by-breath respiratory systems. Eur J Appl Physiol 86: 435–441.
19. Michallet AS, Tonini J, Regnier J, Guinot M, Favre-Juvin A, et al. (2008) Methodological aspects of crossover and maximum fat-oxidation rate point determination. Diabetes Metab 34: 514–523.
20. Durnin JV, Womersley J (1973) Total body fat, calculated from body density, and its relationship to skinfold thickness in 571 people aged 12–72 years. Proc Nutr Soc 32: 45A.
21. Wood RE, Hills AP, Hunter GR, King NA, Byrne NM (2010) Vo2max in overweight and obese adults: do they meet the threshold criteria? Med Sci Sports Exerc 42: 470–477.
22. Brandou F, Savy-Pacaux AM, Marie J, Bauloz M, Maret-Fleuret I, et al. (2005) Impact of high- and low-intensity targeted exercise training on the type of substrate utilization in obese boys submitted to a hypocaloric diet. Diabetes Metab 31: 327–335.
23. Croci I, Byrne NM, Choquette S, Hills AP, Chachay VS, et al. (2013) Whole-body substrate metabolism is associated with disease severity in patients with non-alcoholic fatty liver disease. Gut 62: 1625–1633.
24. Gmada N, Marzouki H, Haboubi M, Tabka Z, Shephard RJ, et al. (2011) Crossover and maximal fat-oxidation points in sedentary healthy subjects: methodological issues. Diabetes Metab 38: 40–45.
25. Hopkins WG (2000) Measures of reliability in sports medicine and science. Sports Med 30: 1–15.
26. Cheneviere X, Malatesta D, Gojanovic B, Borrani F (2010) Differences in whole-body fat oxidation kinetics between cycling and running. Eur J Appl Physiol 109: 1037–1045.
27. MacRae HS, Noakes TD, Dennis SC (1995) Role of decreased carbohydrate oxidation on slower rises in ventilation with increasing exercise intensity after training. Eur J Appl Physiol Occup Physiol 71: 523–529.
28. Achten J, Jeukendrup AE (2004) Relation between plasma lactate concentration and fat oxidation rates over a wide range of exercise intensities. Int J Sports Med 25: 32–37.
29. Brandou F, Dumortier M, Garandeau P, Mercier J, Brun JF (2003) Effects of a two-month rehabilitation program on substrate utilization during exercise in obese adolescents. Diabetes Metab 29: 20–27.
30. Tolfrey K, Jeukendrup AE, Batterham AM (2010) Group- and individual-level coincidence of the 'Fatmax' and lactate accumulation in adolescents. Eur J Appl Physiol 109: 1145–1153.
31. Aucouturier J, Rance M, Meyer M, Isacco L, Thivel D, et al. (2009) Determination of the maximal fat oxidation point in obese children and adolescents: validity of methods to assess maximal aerobic power. Eur J Appl Physiol 105: 325–331.
32. Kang J, Rashti SL, Tranchina CP, Ratamess NA, Faigenbaum AD, et al. (2009) Effect of preceding resistance exercise on metabolism during subsequent aerobic session. Eur J Appl Physiol 107: 43–50.
33. Takagi S, Sakamoto S, Midorikawa T, Konishi M, Katsumura T (2014) Determination of the exercise intensity that elicits maximal fat oxidation in short-time testing. J Sports Sci 32: 175–182.
34. Crisp NA, Guelfi KJ, Licari MK, Braham R, Fournier PA (2012) Does exercise duration affect Fatmax in overweight boys? Eur J Appl Physiol 112: 2557–2564.
35. Schwindling S, Scharhag-Rosenberger F, Kindermann W, Meyer T (2013) Limited Benefit of Fatmax-Test to Derive Training Prescriptions. Int J Sports Med.

12

Sling Exercise for Chronic Low Back Pain

Yu-Shan Yue[1], Xu-Dong Wang[2], Bin Xie[3], Zhong-Han Li[4], Bing-Lin Chen[5], Xue-Qiang Wang[5]*, Yi Zhu[1]*

1 Second School of Clinical Medical, Nanjing University of Chinese Medicine, Nanjing, Jiangsu, China, **2** Institute of Literature in Chinese Medicine, Nanjing University of Chinese Medicine, Nanjing, Jiangsu, China, **3** First School of Clinical Medical, Nanjing University of Chinese Medicine, Nanjing, Jiangsu, China, **4** Applied Health Science Department, University of Waterloo, Waterloo, Ontario, Canada, **5** Department of Sport Rehabilitation, Shanghai University of Sport, Shanghai, China

Abstract

Background: Trials on sling exercise (SE), commonly performed to manage chronic low back pain (LBP), yield conflicting results. This study aimed to review the effects of SE on chronic LBP.

Methods: The randomized controlled trials comparing SE with other treatments or no treatment, published up to August 2013, were identified by electronic searches. Primary outcomes were pain, function, and return to work. The weighted mean difference (WMD) and 95% confidence interval (CI) were calculated, using a random-effects model.

Results: Risk of bias was rated as high in 9 included trials, where some important quality components such as blinding were absent and sample sizes were generally small. We found no clinically relevant differences in pain or function between SE and other forms of exercise, traditional Chinese medical therapy, or in addition to acupuncture. Based on two trials, SE was more effective than thermomagnetic therapy at reducing pain (short-term: WMD −13.90, 95% CI −22.19 to −5.62; long-term: WMD −26.20, 95% CI −31.32 to −21.08) and improving function (short-term: WMD −10.54, 95% CI −14.32 to −6.75; long-term: WMD −25.75, 95% CI −30.79 to −20.71). In one trial we found statistically significant differences between SE and physical agents combined with drug therapy (meloxicam combined with eperisone hydrochloride) but of borderline clinical relevance for pain (short-term: WMD −15.00, 95% CI −19.64 to −10.36) and function (short-term: WMD −10.00; 95% CI −13.70 to −6.30). There was substantial heterogeneity among the two trials comparing SE and thermomagnetic therapy; both these trials and the trial comparing SE with physical agents combined with drug therapy had serious methodological limitations.

Interpretation: Based on limited evidence from 2 trials, SE was more effective for LBP than thermomagnetic therapy. Clinically relevant differences in effects between SE and other forms of exercise, physical agents combined with drug therapy, traditional Chinese medical therapy, or in addition to acupuncture could not be found. More high-quality randomized trials on the topic are warranted.

Editor: Matthias Briel, University Hospital Basel, Switzerland

Funding: This work was supported by Key Laboratory of Exercise and Health Sciences of Ministry of Education, Shanghai University of Sport; Ministry of Education, the First-class Disciplines of Shanghai Colleges and Universities (Psychology), Supporting Program of the Ministry of Science and Technology of China (2009BAK62B02-002), Performance (SUS) (11DZ2261100). The funders had no role in study design, data collection and analysis, decision to publish, or preparation of the manuscript.

Competing Interests: The authors have declared that no competing interests exist.

* E-mail: qiang897@163.com (X-QW); zhuyi1010@163.com (YZ)

Introduction

Low back pain (LBP) is a very common disorder [1], with approximately 84% of adults experiencing an episode of LBP at some point during their lifetimes [2] and variable recurrence rates (5% to 60%) [3]. LBP, identified as the leading disability contributor [4], may result in a reduced level of physical capacity [5–9], negative psychological effects [10–17], and reduction in the quality of life; as such, LBP is one of the most common reasons that patients opt to undergo health care [18,19]. In the United States, back pain-related lost productive work time in workers aged between 40 and 65 years costs employers an estimated $7.40 billion per year [20]; and an estimated $50 billion is spent annually on LBP treatments [21]. In Australia, direct medical costs associated with LBP treatments are estimated at more than $1 billion per year, with additional $8 billion covering indirect expenses [22]. Although the outcomes for many individuals with first-episode LBP are positive, 20% of these cases may develop into chronic LBP, which is defined as a chronic condition of LBP lasting for at least three months or longer [3,23–26]. And chronic LBP accounts for three-quarters of the total direct and indirect costs of medical care and lost productivity associated with LBP [27]. Hence, it is essential to improve the efficiency of treatment of chronic LBP.

In clinical guidelines, exercise therapy is considered as an effective treatment to reduce self-reported pain and improve the back pain specific functional status of participants with chronic LBP [28]. Sling exercise (SE) is a specific form of exercise established by Meier [29] to rehabilitate professional German sportsmen and later developed by Kirkesola to treat motor problems [30]. SE supports or suspends the pelvis and lower extremities in a sling, and allows an individual to use his or her body weight to provide resistance [31,32]. This exercise minimizes the use of global muscles without pain as local muscles are activated. This procedure can be performed easily by using a sling and an elastic cord to offset body weight; however, this procedure is difficult when an unstable surface is used [31]. SE has been claimed to reduce pain, normalize muscle response patterns, retrain muscle motor units, re-operate inhibited actions, and improve damaged postural adjustment abilities [33].

Published randomized controlled trials (RCTs) have assessed the effects of SE on the treatment of chronic LBP [34–42]. However, RCTs that assess the effects of SE compared with other forms of exercise on self-reported pain in patients with chronic LBP have presented conflicting findings [34,35,38,41]. In some of these studies, no differences between SE and other forms of exercise have been found [34,41]. In other studies, SE exhibits more advantages than other forms of exercise [35,38]. Studies examining back pain specific functional status between SE and other forms of exercise have also yielded inconsistent results [34,36,38]. Some studies have found no differences between patients receiving SE and other forms of exercise [34,38]. The remaining trial has demonstrated an increased improvement in patients receiving SE [36]. In two randomized trials, in which SE is compared with traditional Chinese medical therapies [37,42], one trial has shown that pain is reduced when SE is used [37]; the other trial has demonstrated that SE produced less pain reduction compared with a specific traditional Chinese medical therapy [42]. To the best of our knowledge, no published systematic review or guideline on the efficacy of SE for subjects with chronic LBP has been conducted. Therefore, the effectiveness of SE compared with other treatments remains unclear. Clinicians may also be undecided whether or not SE should be prescribed in patients with chronic LBP. It is necessary to conduct a systematic evaluation of RCTs focusing on SE for patients with chronic LBP in this case.

We performed a systematic review to assess the efficacy of SE in participants with chronic LBP. The results of this study provided information to help clinicians come up with evidence-based decisions on the use of SE for patients with chronic LBP.

Methods

Literature Search

The following databases were searched from the earliest available date to August 2013: Cochrane Library; Cumulative Index to Nursing and Allied Health Literature; Pubmed; the Web of Science; Embase; the Physiotherapy Evidence Database; Chinese Biomedical Literature Database; Wanfang Database; and China National Knowledge Infrastructure. We used "LBP", "SE", and "RCTs" as search terms (full details of the search in File S1). To increase the chance of finding all relevant publications describing the effects of SE on LBP, we did not set limitations on language, year, or status during the initial search.

To identify gray literature, we contacted experts and inquired regarding materials not listed in these databases. The International Controlled Trials Registry Platform was also searched, in which "SE" and "LBP" were used as key words, to obtain relevant registered trials, which may contain additional data, but did not have any published papers. The reference lists of identified articles were screened manually for additional studies.

Inclusion Criteria

Types of studies. Only RCTs investigating the use of SE as treatment for chronic LBP were included. No language or publication date restrictions were applied.

Types of participants. The study samples included patients with chronic LBP affected for longer than three months. Unless an adequate washout period was described, patients who were exposed to similar treatments prior to the study were not included.

Types of interventions. We included articles in which SE was compared with no or placebo treatment, as well as any other treatment for chronic LBP. In the SE training program, the neuromuscular activation was induced to regain normal functional movement patterns in patients with musculoskeletal disorders [33]. SE was performed using specially designed devices, such as Record Trainer or TerapiMaster [34,43]. Trials in which a treatment was applied with concomitant therapy were accepted as long as similar treatments were applied in the control conditions.

Types of outcome measures. The findings were analyzed in three primary outcome categories: (1) self-reported pain; (2) back pain specific functional status; and (3) return to work (expressed as the number of days of sick leave or the proportion of patients returned to work). Secondary outcomes of this review include global improvement, health-related quality of life, satisfaction with treatment, and adverse events. We categorized outcomes as long term (≥12 months), intermediate (closer to 6 months), or short term (post-treatment assessment no longer than 12 weeks).

Selection of Studies

Two reviewers (Yue YS, Zhu Y) independently screened for potentially relevant titles and abstracts based on the pre-specified criteria; full-text articles were retrieved whenever necessary. Any disagreements were resolved by discussion or consultation with a third independent reviewer (Wang XQ) if necessary.

Data Extraction

Two independent reviewers (Yue YS, Zhu Y) abstracted and cross-checked the data obtained from the included trials. These data were then compiled in a pre-designed data extraction form. The data extraction form included study design (treatment allocation, concealed allocation, blinding, intention-to-treat analysis, etc.), participant characteristics (mean age, group distribution, etc.), description of control and treatment interventions (SE style and practices, type of control intervention, frequency, total duration, etc.), outcome measures used, and follow-up period. Any disagreements were resolved by discussion to obtain a consensus. The authors were also contacted to provide further information when deemed necessary.

Quality Assessment

The two independent reviewers (Yue YS, Zhu Y) used the Cochrane Collaboration's risk of bias tool to evaluate the methodological quality of all included studies. The following domains were evaluated: random sequence generation, allocation concealment, blinding of participants and personnel, blinding of outcome assessments, incomplete outcome data, selective reporting, and other bias [44]. For each domain, each study's description of methods was examined and the judgment regarding potential bias was made, according to three categories: low risk, high risk and unclear risk [45]. The overall risk of bias of individual study was rated as low (low risk of bias for all domains), high (high risk of bias for one or more domains) or unclear (unclear risk of bias for one or more domains) [46]. A third independent reviewer (Wang XQ) was consulted to resolve disagreements.

Statistical Analysis

Data were analyzed with the Review Manager statistical software (RevMan version 5.2) by using a random-effects model. Random effects meta-analysis was performed to combine the results because we predicted that study characteristics and other factors were different, suggesting that the effects may differ across studies. Chi-square test was performed to detect statistically significant heterogeneity [47]. We then estimated the amount of heterogeneity among studies by using the I^2 statistic: <25%, low; <50%, moderate heterogeneity; and >50%, substantial heterogeneity [48]. Heterogeneity was further investigated by checking data extracted from outlier studies and exploring the effects of study exclusion in sensitivity analyses. No funnel plots or assessments for publication bias were performed because of the small number of trials (maximum five trials) that were pooled in the comparisons included in this literature.

The control conditions were divided into five groups: other forms of exercise; traditional Chinese medical therapy; thermomagnetic therapy; physical agents in combination with drug therapy; and no treatment. We then performed separate meta-analyses for short-term, intermediate, and long-term follow-up time points. One study included two different control groups, which were individually considered during analysis [49].

Analyses were only possible for self-reported pain and back pain specific functional status because of absence of data for return to work, global improvement, health-related quality of life, satisfaction with treatment, and adverse events. In the included studies, several outcome measures were used to assess the constructs of self-reported pain, including a 10 mm or 100 mm visual analogue scale (VAS) [43] or 0-point to 10-point numerical pain rating scale (NPRS) [34], and the back pain specific functional status, such as 100-point Oswestry disability index (ODI) [40] or modified Oswestry disability index (M-ODI) [34]. Moderate to high correlations between the different measures of the two constructs were obtained [50]. In this literature, the individual trial outcomes for self-reported pain and back pain specific functional status were linearly rescaled to a 0 to 100 scoring system, in which lower scores indicated better outcomes, to facilitate the comparison and interpretability of the syntheses [49,51,52]. For example, we rescaled a NPRS pain score of 2.3±1.1 points (mean ± SD) out of 10 points to 23±11 points out of 100 points, where positive mean effect sizes indicated an improvement that is decreased pain. All of the variables included in the analysis were continuous; as such, the inverse variance method was used to calculate the weighted mean differences (WMDs) and the corresponding 95% confidence intervals (95% CIs) for each study based on the post-intervention means of each group and the pooled standard deviation. Two-sided statistical tests were performed. $P<0.05$ or 95% confidence interval that excluded a null result was considered statistically significant [53]. On the basis of current research on minimal clinically significant differences, a 20-point (of 100 points) improvement in pain [54] and a 10-point (of 100 points) improvement in functional outcomes [55] were considered as clinically meaningful.

Results

Study Selection

Our initial search yielded 7,128 records. Among these data, 5,197 were retained after duplicates were removed. A total of 4,646 articles were excluded because these studies did not use randomized controlled trial designs, the recruited sample populations comprised patients without chronic LBP, or no adequate intervention group was used. The 551 remaining articles were assessed in detail for eligibility. Among these remaining articles, 542 were excluded. A total of 450 articles were non-RCTs or studies of unrelated intervention conditions. A total of 86 studies used participants without chronic LBP or reported on results not included in the predefined outcomes. Six articles [56–61] were not available for full text [56,59–61] or had incomplete outcome data [57,58], and the authors of these studies [56–61] did not respond to our repeated contacts. Thus, nine RCTs [34–42] with a total of 706 participants were included in this study. Figure 1 shows the flow chart from initial results of publication searches to final inclusion or exclusion.

Description of Included Studies

We included 9 single center randomized controlled trials [34–42] aiming to examine the efficacy of SE on chronic LBP. Of these, one trial [34] was conducted in a primary care setting in Norway, seven trials [36–42] were done in Chinese hospitals, and one trial [35] was from Republic of Korea. Trials [34–42] were published between 2008 and 2012, and all [34–42] but two [34,35] were published in Chinese language. The summarized characteristics of the studies [34–42] included in our systematic review are presented in Table 1.

Participants. Data from a total of 706 participants (ranging from 29 to 246, only 3 studies [34,38,40] enrolled ≥100 individuals) were extracted of whom 98 received SE alone and 203 received SE combined with other therapies (151 combined with back school, 12 combined with magnetic field warmer vibration synthetic therapy, 20 combined with intermediate frequency electrotherapy, 10 combined with acupuncture therapy). 46% of the participants included in 8 trials [34,36–42] were men, and sex was not reported for one trial [35]. The mean age of study patients ranged from 20.30 to 49.94 years. Six studies [36–41] were done with hospital patients, one [34] with primary care and hospital patients, one [42] with community and hospital patients, and one [35] with university students. Subjects were included according to various inclusion criteria (non-specific LBP, specific LBP or both).

SE. The intervention was primarily SE based, and five [38–42] of the 9 trials [34–42] involved the application of concomitant therapy (eg. back school, 3 [38,40,41]/5 [38–42]; intermediate frequency electrotherapy, 1 [39]/5 [38–42]; acupuncture therapy, 1 [42]/5 [38–42]) alongside the intervention and control. Intervention duration ranged from 1 week to 8 weeks with an average length of 5.89 weeks, and intervention frequency was various, ranging from once a week to seven times a week. Eight trials [34,36–42] were done in hospital, and in one [35], the setting was unclear. In 1 study [39], participants spent 20 minutes per session doing SE. In 2 studies [38,41], participants spent 30 minutes per session doing SE. In 2 studies [34,36], participants spent 40 minutes per session doing SE. In 1 study [42], participants spent 30 to 60 minutes per session doing SE. And the time spent on the SE per session was unclear in 3 studies [35,37,40].

Control conditions. Regarding control conditions, one study [37] used a traditional Chinese medical therapy, four studies [34–36,41] used other forms of exercise, two studies [39,40] used thermomagnetic therapies, and two trials [38,42] used two separate control interventions, of which one trial [38] used another form of exercise and physical factor therapy combined with drug therapy (meloxicam combined with eperisone hydrochloride tablet) and the remaining one trial [42] used no treatment and a traditional Chinese medical therapy.

Outcomes. Outcome measures were self-reported pain (9 trials [34–42]), back pain specific functional status (6 trials

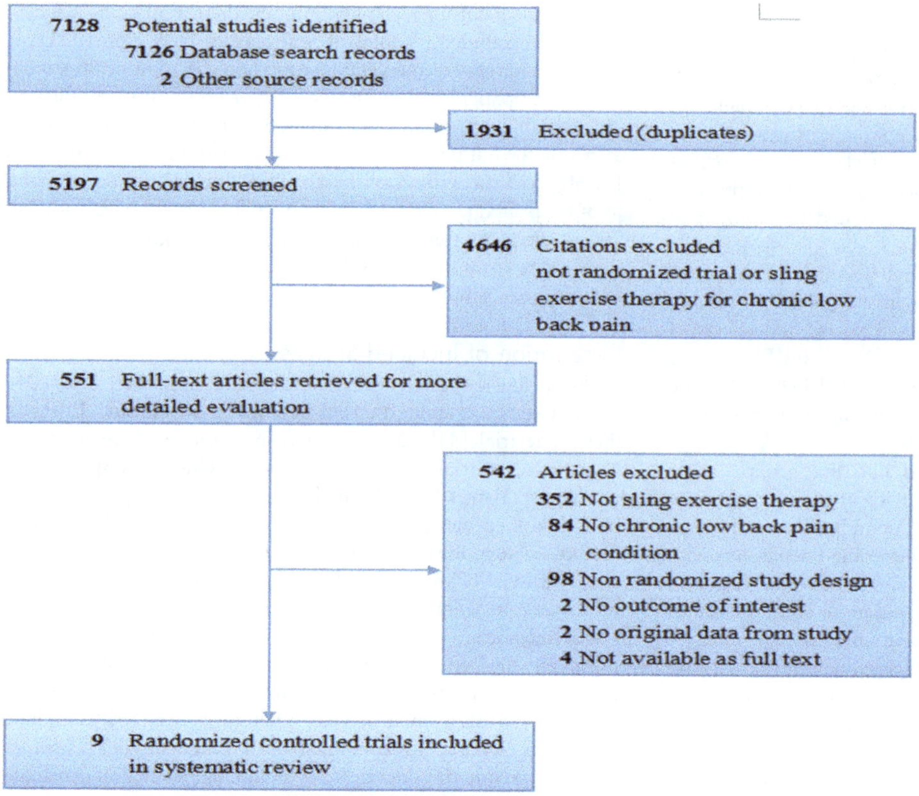

Figure 1. Review flow diagram.

[34,36,38–41]), disability (1 trial [42]), skeletal muscle metabolism (1 trial [37]), fear of physical activity and work (1 trial [34]), trunk flexion (1 trial [34]), health care utilization (1 trial [34]), clinical effect (1 trial [39]), anxiety state (1 trial [39]), ability of daily life (1 trial [39]), joint function (1 trial [39]), and trunk extensor strength (1 trial [35]). Of these, the methods used to assess self-reported pain and back pain specific function status among all trials [34–42] were different. The pain was measured by VAS (6 [35,37,39–42]/ 9 [34–42] trials) or NPRS (3 [34,36,38]/9 [34–42] trials), and back pain specific function status was measured by ODI (4 [36,39–41]/ 6 [34,36,38–41] trials) or M-ODI (2 [34,38]/6 [34,36,38–41] trials). However, none of the included trials [34–42] reported data for return to work, global improvement, health-related quality of life, satisfaction with treatment or adverse events. Data from 9 included studies [34–42] were collected at short-term period (9 [34–42]/9 [34–42] trials), intermediate period (2 [36,41]/9 [34–42] trials) or long-term period (2 [34,40]/9 [34–42] trials). All included trials [34–42] reported mean rather than median data for continuous outcomes and reported number of events and total for dichotomous outcomes.

Conflict of interest. One study [34] was financed by the Norwegian Fund for Post-Graduate Training in Physiotherapy, and sponsorship of other studies [35–42] was not mentioned.

Methodological Quality of Included Trials

Only 4 trials [34,38–40] adequately reported allocation sequence generation. The remaining 5 trials [35–37,41,42] were randomized, but no details were provided. One trial [34] had adequate allocation concealment, but we could not determine the allocation concealment in the remaining 8 trials [35–42]. None of the 9 included trials [34–42] met the blinding of participants, personnel and outcome assessors criterion. Given the direct participant-personnel involvement due to the nature of therapeutic trials, and self-reported outcome measures such as VAS and NPRS, it was not feasible to blind participants, personnel and outcome assessors. While the blinding in 9 included trials [34–42] was not feasible, it was still an inherent source of bias that must be highlighted for every trial. The risk of incomplete outcome data was low for only 6 included trials [34–37,39,42]. Selective outcome reporting was at a low risk of bias in all 9 included trials [34–42]. Sources of other bias were unclear in 9 included trials [34–42]. Overall, nine included trials [34–42] were adjudicated to be of high risk of bias. Table 2 shows the detailed results of the quality assessment of individual characteristics.

Effectiveness

SE compared with other forms of exercise. Five trials (457 patients) [34–36,38,41] randomly assigned patients to undergo SE (164 patients) or other forms of exercise (199 patients), and reported data regarding self-reported pain. Among these trials [34–36,38,41], three [34,36,38] evaluated self-reported pain by using NPRS and two trials [35,41] used VAS. In four studies (427 patients) [34,36,38,41], data regarding back pain specific functional status were reported, in which SE for 149 patients and other forms of exercise for 184 patients were assessed. Among these four studies, two [36,41] used ODI to measure back pain specific functional status, whereas two [34,38] utilized M-ODI. Figures 2 and 3 show the overall meta-analysis results of the comparison of SE with other forms of exercise.

The trials [34–36,38,41] comparing SE with other forms of exercise failed to reveal significant differences in self-reported pain at short-term [−7.30 point (CI = −14.86 to 0.25)], interme-

Table 1. Characteristics of trials included in systematic review.

Article, Year	Patients Characteristic, Sample Size	Intervention	Duration of trial period	Outcomes	Time point
Gao Baolong (2008)	Source: hospital 29 patients (G1 = 15, G2 = 14); Mean age (SD): G1 = 37.0y (4.28), G2 = 35.0y (3.99).	G1: SE; G2: Massage.	five times a week for 8 weeks.	Self-reported pain (VAS 0–10); Skeletal muscle metabolism (Serum CK, Serum LDH).	8 weeks.
Unsgaard-Tondel (2010)	Source: primary care and hospital 109 patients (G1 = 36, G2 = 36, G3 = 37); Mean age (SD): G1 = 43.4y (10.2), G2 = 40.9y (11.5), G3 = 36.0y (10.3).	G1: SE; G2: Motor control exercise; G3: General exercise.	once a week for 8 weeks.	Self-reported pain (NPRS 0–10); Back pain specific functional status (M-ODI); Fear of physical activity and work (FABQ); Trunk flexion (FTF); Health care utilization (Low back pain therapy, Low back pain medication).	8 weeks; 14 months.
Guo Xianfeng (2010)	Source: hospital 246 patients (G1 = 82, G2 = 82, G3 = 82); Mean age (SD): G1 = 34.1y (6.5), G2 = 33.3y (6.5), G3 = 33.5y (5.0).	G1: Intensive therapy: Back school+SE+Health ball exercise; G2: Home exercise: Back school+Aerobic training+Freestanding exercise; G3: Conventional therapy: Back school+Physical agents+Drug therapy.	SE: three times a week for the first 8 weeks; Health ball exercise: four times a week for the last 4 weeks; Aerobic training: three times a week for 12 weeks; Freestanding exercise: four times a week for 12 weeks; Physical agents: five times a week for the first 4 weeks; Drug therapy: Meloxicam - once a day for the first 4 weeks, Eperisone hydrochloride tablet - three times a day for the first 4 weeks.	Self-reported pain (NPRS 0–10); Back pain specific functional status (M-ODI).	4 weeks; 12 weeks; 24 weeks.
Qin Jiang (2010)	Source: hospital 34 patients (G1 = 12, G2 = 12, G3 = 10); Mean age (SD): 49.94y (11.90).	G1: SE; G2: SE+Magnetic field warmer vibration synthetic therapy; G3: Immobilized with waistline+Williams gymnastics training.	SE: once every two days for 6 weeks; Magnetic field warmer vibration synthetic therapy: once every two days for 6 weeks; Williams gymnastics training: three times a day for 6 weeks.	Self-reported pain (NPRS 0–10); Back pain specific functional status (ODI).	6 weeks; 18 weeks.
Jin Miao (2011)	Source: hospital 60 patients (G1 = 20, G2 = 20, G3 = 20); Mean age (SD): G1 = 45.97y (2.68), G2 = 44.74y (2.54), G3 = 44.79y (2.80).	G1: Intermediate frequency electrotherapy+SE; G2: Intermediate frequency electrotherapy+Thermomagnetic therapy; G3: Drug therapy.	Intermediate frequency electrotherapy: once a day for a week; SE: once a day for a week; Thermomagnetic therapy: once a day for a week; Drug therapy: Gentongping capsule - two times a day for a week, Mecobalamin - three times a day for a week.	Clinical effect (Criteria of diagnostic efficacy on syndrome of traditional Chinese medicine); Self-reported pain (VAS 0–10); Anxiety state (HAMD); Ability of daily life (ADLRS); Back pain specific functional status (ODI); Joint function (ROM).	1 week; 5 weeks.
Hu Yuan (2011)	Source: hospital 100 patients (G1 = 50, G2 = 50); Mean age (SD): G1 = 40.39y (10.68), G2 = 39.13y (9.38)[based on completed cases].	G1: Back school+SE; G2: Back school+Thermomagnetic therapy.	three times a week for 6 weeks.	Self-reported pain (VAS 0–10); Back pain specific functional status (ODI).	6 weeks; 13.5 months.
Yoo (2012)	Source: university 30 patients (G1 = 15, G2 = 15); Mean age (SD): G1 = 20.1y (0.7), G2 = 20.5y (0.5).	G1: SE; G2: Mat exercise.	three times a week for 4 weeks.	Self-reported pain (VAS 0–10); Trunk extensor strength (The Tergumed Device).	4 weeks.
Wang Cong (2012)	Source: hospital 38 patients (G1 = 19, G2 = 19); Mean age (SD): G1 = 36.95y (11.78), G2 = 36.05y (10.80).	G1: Back school+SE; G2: Back school+Freestanding exercise+Health ball training.	three times a week for 8 weeks.	Self-reported pain (VAS 0–10); Back pain specific functional status (ODI [exclude sexual life item]).	8 weeks; 12 weeks; 20 weeks.

Table 1. Cont.

Article, Year	Patients Characteristic, Sample Size	Intervention	Duration of trial period	Outcomes	Time point
Liu Pan (2012)	Source: community and hospital 60 patients (G1 = 20, G2 = 20, G3 = 20); Mean age (SD): G1 = 46.73y (11.58), G2 = 44.60y (10.57), G3 = 43.28y (10.34).	G1: SE; G2: Acupuncture therapy; G3: Acupuncture therapy+SE.	seven times a week for 4 weeks.	Self-reported pain (VAS 0–10); Disability (JOA).	the first day; 2 weeks; 4 weeks.

Abbreviations G: Group; SD: Standard deviation; SE: Sling exercise; VAS: Visual analog scale; CK: Creatine kinase; LDH: Lactate dehydrogenase; NPRS: Numeric pain rating scale; M-ODI: Modified oswestry disability index; FABQ: Fear-avoidance beliefs questionnaire; FTF: the Fingertip-to-Floor test (in centimeters); ODI: Oswestry disability index; HAMD: Hamilton rating scale for depression; ADLRS: Activity of daily living rating scale; ROM: Range of motion; JOA: Japanese Orthopedic Association scores for assessment of low back pain.

diate [−3.81 point (CI = −16.98 to 9.36)], and long-term [3.70 point (CI = −3.16 to 10.55)] follow-up periods.

However, significant heterogeneities for short-term and intermediate self-reported pain were derived when SE was compared with other forms of exercise. The heterogeneity for short-term self-reported pain was substantially high ($I^2 = 88\%$). A visual inspection of the forest plot indicated that two studies [36,38], in which the control treatment was mainly conducted by patients at home, were the most likely source of heterogeneity. A meta-analysis excluding these two studies [36,38] indicated a substantially reduced heterogeneity ($I^2 = 39\%$) and revealed a statistically non-significant effect size [−3.01 point (CI = −7.22 to 1.21)]. For intermediate self-reported pain, high I^2 value ($I^2 = 62\%$) derived in the random effects analysis also suggested a substantial heterogeneity between the included studies [36,41]. This result may be due to the fact that the included trials [36,41] differed in patient populations and treatment durations. The baseline scores of pain obtained by Qin et al. [36] were >1.5 points higher than those in Wang et al. [41]; by comparison, the treatment duration presented by Qin et al. [36] was two weeks shorter than that reported by Wang et al. [41]. However, neither of the studies [36,41] yielded statistically significant effects of SE on the decrease in intermediate self-reported pain compared with other forms of exercise. This result is consistent with that of the pooled analysis.

No significant differences were observed in short-term back pain specific functional status between SE and other forms of exercise [−6.57 point (CI = −14.09 to 0.96)]. We also observed a statistically, but probably not clinically meaningful difference in the intermediate back pain specific functional status [−8.81 point (CI = −13.82 to −3.80)] in favor of SE compared with other forms of exercise.

The statistical heterogeneity for short-term back pain specific functional status was substantially high ($I^2 = 91\%$). This result may be attributed to the inclusion of one trial [34], in which SE was performed less frequently than in remaining trials [36,38,41]. Eliminating this study [34] from the analysis, we no longer observed heterogeneity ($I^2 = 0\%$). Nevertheless, the result was statistically significant, which differed from the conclusion of no statistically significant differences in short-term back pain specific functional status. A subgroup analysis based on the frequency of SE was then performed, and the result showed that smaller effect sizes were achieved in trials, in which SE was performed less frequently.

SE compared with traditional chinese medical therapies. Among the included trials [34–42], two (89 patients) [37,42] demonstrated SE and traditional Chinese medical therapies with randomly assigning patients (35 and 34 patients, respectively); the results regarding self-reported pain were determined using VAS. The results of our meta-analysis are shown in Figure 4.

The meta-analysis of two trials [37,42] showed that SE and traditional Chinese medical therapies were different in terms of the short-term self-reported pain [−5.29 point (CI = −20.27 to 9.70)], but this result was not significant.

The pooled studies [37,42] demonstrated substantially high levels of heterogeneity ($I^2 = 56\%$), probably because of the differences between the two included trials [37,42] in terms of participant populations and treatment durations. The baseline scores of pain observed by Liu et al. [42] were higher than those of Gao et al. [37] by more than two points. By comparison, the treatment duration obtained by Liu et al. [42] was four weeks shorter than that observed by Gao et al. [37]. Neither of the studies [37,42] indicated the positive effects of SE on the decrease in short-term self-reported pain compared with traditional Chinese medical therapies. This result is similar to that obtained in pooled analysis.

SE compared with thermomagnetic therapy. Two studies (160 patients) [39,40] assessed SE performed by 70 patients and thermomagnetic therapy conducted by 70 patients; data on self-reported pain and back pain specific functional status were presented. For the two studies [39,40], self-reported pain was determined using VAS [39,40], and both studies [39,40] assessed back pain specific functional status by using ODI. The weighted mean difference (95% CI) results of the included trials [39,40] are shown in Figures 5 and 6.

We observed significant differences between SE and thermomagnetic therapy for self-reported pain at either short-term [−13.90 point (CI = −22.19 to −5.62)] or long-term [−26.20 point (CI = −31.32 to −21.08)] follow-up periods.

The heterogeneity of short-term self-reported pain was substantially high ($I^2 = 62\%$). This result may be due to differences in the frequency of SE between the two included trials [39,40]. SE was performed less frequently as revealed by Jin et al. [39] than by Hu et al. [40]. The two studies [39,40] comparing SE with thermomagnetic therapy both reported the positive effects of SE on the reduction of short-term self-reported pain. This result is consistent with that of the pooled analysis.

We recorded both statistically and clinically significant differences between SE and thermomagnetic therapy for back pain specific functional status at either short-term [−10.54 point (CI = −14.32 to −6.75)] or long-term [−25.75 point (CI = −30.79 to −20.71)] follow-up periods.

Table 2. Methodological quality of trials included in systematic review.

Article, Year	Random sequence generation	Allocation concealment	Blinding of Participants and personnel	Blinding of outcome assessments	Incomplete outcome data	Selective reporting	Other bias	Risk of bias
Gao Baolong (2008)	Unclear	Unclear	High	High	Low	Low	Unclear	High
Unsgaard-Tondel (2010)	Low	Low	High	High	Low	Low	Unclear	High
Guo Xianfeng (2010)	Low	Unclear	High	High	Unclear	Low	Unclear	High
Qin Jiang (2010)	Unclear	Unclear	High	High	Low	Low	Unclear	High
Jin Miao (2011)	Low	Unclear	High	High	Low	Low	Unclear	High
Hu Yuan (2011)	Low	Unclear	High	High	High	Low	Unclear	High
Yoo (2012)	Unclear	Unclear	High	High	Low	Low	Unclear	High
Wang Cong (2012)	Unclear	Unclear	High	High	Unclear	Low	Unclear	High
Liu Pan (2012)	Unclear	Unclear	High	High	Low	Low	Unclear	High

SE compared with the combination of physical agents and drug therapy. Self-reported pain and back pain specific functional status were evaluated in a randomized controlled trial [38], in which 82 patients receiving SE and another 82 patients receiving physical agents combined with drug therapy were included. In this trial [38], self-reported pain was determined using NPRS, and back pain specific functional status was determined using M-ODI.

This trial [38] showed significant differences between SE and physical agents combined with drug therapy for either self-reported pain [−15.00 point (CI = −19.64 to −10.36)] or back pain specific functional status [−10.00 point (CI = −13.70 to −6.30)] at short-term follow-up period.

SE combined with acupuncture therapy versus acupuncture therapy alone. One randomized controlled trial [42] with 20 participants receiving acupuncture therapy and another 20 participants receiving acupuncture therapy combined with SE reported data for self-reported pain, which was measured by VAS.

This trial [42] indicated no difference between SE in addition to acupuncture therapy and the acupuncture therapy alone for self-reported pain at short-term follow-up period [−6.30 point (CI = −16.85 to 4.25)].

Discussion

Systematic reviews [62,63] have been conducted to evaluate the effects of exercise therapy in participants with chronic LBP. To the best of our knowledge, this study is the first systematic review and meta-analysis that evaluated the effects of SE on chronic LBP management. We derived the following points to provide useful information for caregivers as a guide for patient management, to assist guideline developers in creating guidelines for the use of SE in the chronic LBP treatment, and to allow policy makers in tailoring intervention options towards the desired outcome, available resources, and local healthcare context.

1. The meta-analysis showed no statistically significant or clinically relevant differences in self-reported pain at short-term, intermediate, and long-term follow-up periods between SE and other forms of exercise. SE is no more efficacious than other forms of exercise in improving back pain specific functional status at short-term follow-up period among patients with chronic LBP. However, there is a small, clinically irrelevant benefit of SE over other forms of exercise on intermediate back pain specific functional status, based on an evaluation of less than 60 patients in 2 trials, which both did not perform allocation concealment or blinded outcome assessment, and intention-to-treat analysis was only performed in one of which.
2. SE is as effective as traditional Chinese medical therapies in decreasing short-term self-reported pain, which is consistent with the findings of some published systematic reviews [62,63] which suggest that exercise therapy and massage are equally effective for chronic LBP.
3. The results indicated that SE was more effective than thermomagnetic therapy for self-reported pain and back pain specific functional status in short- or long-term follow-up periods, but the substantial heterogeneity for short-term self-reported pain comparing SE with thermomagnetic therapy was recorded.
4. In one trial, significant differences between SE and physical agents combined with drug therapy were derived for self-reported pain and back pain specific functional status in the

Study or Subgroup	SET Mean	SET SD	SET Total	Non SET Mean	Non SET SD	Non SET Total	Weight	Mean Difference IV, Random, 95% CI
1.1.1 Short term								
Guo Xianfeng 2010	28	14	80	47	12	74	19.3%	-19.00 [-23.11, -14.89]
Qin Jiang 2010	40.8	18.8	12	58	13.2	10	12.4%	-17.20 [-30.62, -3.78]
Unsgaard-Tondel 2010 (1)	23.4	22.6	36	17.6	15.4	36	15.9%	5.80 [-3.13, 14.73]
Unsgaard-Tondel 2010 (2)	23.4	22.6	36	27.3	23.2	37	14.7%	-3.90 [-14.41, 6.61]
Wang Cong 2012	28.9	9.9	18	33.7	8.1	19	18.2%	-4.80 [-10.65, 1.05]
Yoo 2012	13	5	15	18	6	15	19.4%	-5.00 [-8.95, -1.05]
Subtotal (95% CI)			**197**			**191**	**100.0%**	**-7.30 [-14.86, 0.25]**
Heterogeneity: Tau² = 72.58; Chi² = 41.53, df = 5 (P < 0.00001); I² = 88%								
Test for overall effect: Z = 1.89 (P = 0.06)								
1.1.2 Intermediate								
Qin Jiang 2010	40	22.2	12	53	16.4	10	34.8%	-13.00 [-29.16, 3.16]
Wang Cong 2012	40.6	9.1	18	39.5	7.6	19	65.2%	1.10 [-4.32, 6.52]
Subtotal (95% CI)			**30**			**29**	**100.0%**	**-3.81 [-16.98, 9.36]**
Heterogeneity: Tau² = 61.60; Chi² = 2.63, df = 1 (P = 0.10); I² = 62%								
Test for overall effect: Z = 0.57 (P = 0.57)								
1.1.3 Long term								
Unsgaard-Tondel 2010 (1)	27	22.2	36	20.1	19.4	36	50.7%	6.90 [-2.73, 16.53]
Unsgaard-Tondel 2010 (2)	27	22.2	36	26.6	20.3	37	49.3%	0.40 [-9.37, 10.17]
Subtotal (95% CI)			**72**			**73**	**100.0%**	**3.70 [-3.16, 10.55]**
Heterogeneity: Tau² = 0.00; Chi² = 0.86, df = 1 (P = 0.35); I² = 0%								
Test for overall effect: Z = 1.06 (P = 0.29)								

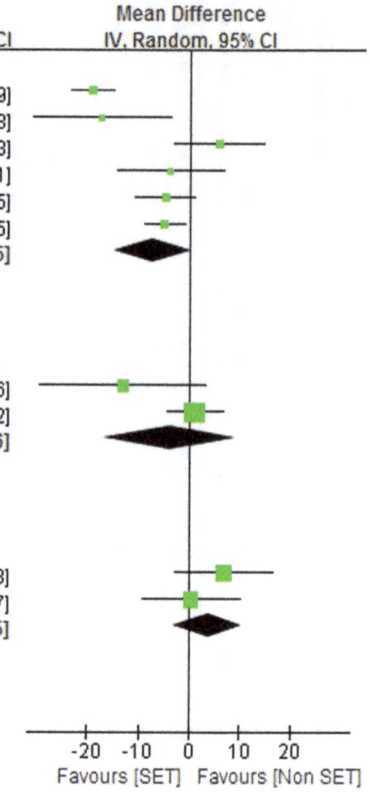

Figure 2. Self-reported pain for sling exercise versus other forms of exercise. Unsgaard-Tondel 2010(1), sling exercise versus motor control exercise; Unsgaard-Tondel 2010(2), sling exercise versus general exercise.

short-tern, which was consistent with the findings of some published trials [64,65,66,67] where exercise therapy is more effective than physical agents or drug therapy in pain relief and functional improvement, and systematic reviews [62,63] where exercise therapy is more effective than usual care by a general practitioner for chronic LBP.

5. Concerning short-term self-reported pain, no significant differences between SE combined with acupuncture therapy and acupuncture therapy alone were found in one trial.

Study or Subgroup	SET Mean	SET SD	SET Total	Non SET Mean	Non SET SD	Non SET Total	Weight	Mean Difference IV, Random, 95% CI
1.2.1 Short term								
Guo Xianfeng 2010	23	10	80	37	11	74	21.5%	-14.00 [-17.33, -10.67]
Qin Jiang 2010	12.42	7.34	12	21.9	8.12	10	19.2%	-9.48 [-16.00, -2.96]
Unsgaard-Tondel 2010 (1)	16.18	10.88	36	12.78	7.62	36	20.9%	3.40 [-0.94, 7.74]
Unsgaard-Tondel 2010 (2)	16.18	10.88	36	17.75	9.63	37	20.6%	-1.57 [-6.29, 3.15]
Wang Cong 2012	31.58	12.8	18	43.47	12	19	17.9%	-11.89 [-19.90, -3.88]
Subtotal (95% CI)			**182**			**176**	**100.0%**	**-6.57 [-14.09, 0.96]**
Heterogeneity: Tau² = 65.74; Chi² = 46.11, df = 4 (P < 0.00001); I² = 91%								
Test for overall effect: Z = 1.71 (P = 0.09)								
1.2.2 Intermediate								
Qin Jiang 2010	12.58	7.79	12	21.7	6.7	10	68.3%	-9.12 [-15.18, -3.06]
Wang Cong 2012	40.28	14.29	18	48.42	13.27	19	31.7%	-8.14 [-17.04, 0.76]
Subtotal (95% CI)			**30**			**29**	**100.0%**	**-8.81 [-13.82, -3.80]**
Heterogeneity: Tau² = 0.00; Chi² = 0.03, df = 1 (P = 0.86); I² = 0%								
Test for overall effect: Z = 3.45 (P = 0.0006)								

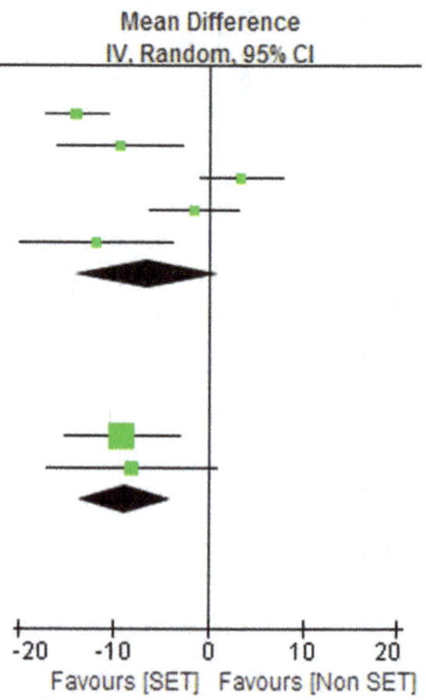

Figure 3. Back pain specific functional status for sling exercise versus other forms of exercise. Unsgaard-Tondel 2010(1), sling exercise versus motor control exercise; Unsgaard-Tondel 2010(2), sling exercise versus general exercise.

Study or Subgroup	SET Mean	SET SD	SET Total	Non SET Mean	Non SET SD	Non SET Total	Weight	Mean Difference IV, Random, 95% CI	Year
2.1.1 Short term									
Gao Baolong 2008	17.6	15.8	15	30.8	23.5	14	48.3%	-13.20 [-27.88, 1.48]	2008
Liu Pan 2012	28.8	24.1	20	26.7	19.5	20	51.7%	2.10 [-11.49, 15.69]	2012
Subtotal (95% CI)			35			34	100.0%	-5.29 [-20.27, 9.70]	
Heterogeneity: Tau² = 64.97; Chi² = 2.25, df = 1 (P = 0.13); I² = 56%									
Test for overall effect: Z = 0.69 (P = 0.49)									

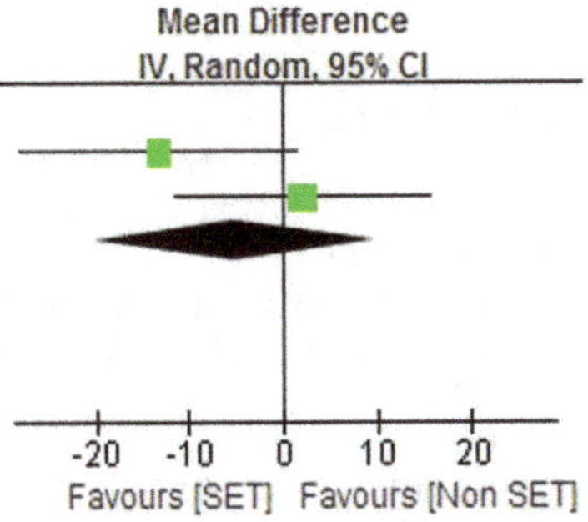

Figure 4. Self-reported pain for sling exercise versus traditional Chinese medical therapies.

Strengths

Our study presented several strengths. We collected data by using a broad search strategy with the following procedures: searching multiple citation databases; soliciting experts for published or unpublished studies; searching trial registries; and screening the references of identified trials. Also, no language restriction was applied. This strategy suggested that our synthesis represented the current state of related studies. We also performed our review according to previously published protocol and methodological guidelines. The consistency of self-reported pain and back pain specific functional status, which were primary outcomes of our review, was satisfactory. All of the studies [34–42] in this literature included a measure of self-reported pain and two-thirds [34,36,38–41] of the studies [34–42] included a measure of back pain specific functional status.

Limitations

First, our systematic review is limited because all of the studies [34–42] included in our literature contain methodological drawbacks, which may lead to an overestimated effect. Risk of bias was rated as high in all included trials [34–42]. The most frequent methodological shortcoming in included trials [34–42] was lack of blinding of patients, caregivers and assessors, due to the nature of the therapeutic interventions indicating that the blinding of patients and caregivers was almost impossible and patient-reported outcomes such as self-reported pain.

Second, the implementation of outcome measures is notably limited. Although the data for self-reported pain and back pain specific functional status were available for the majority of studies [34–42], the evaluations of self-reported pain and back pain specific functional status were not standardized, indicating that different trials would use different pain surveys or back pain functional status measures as outcome measures, which could lead to the heterogeneity derived among the trials [34–42]. Few researchers reported return to work, global improvement, health-related quality of life, satisfaction with treatment or adverse events; hence, no interpretations on the differences in these outcomes based on the treatment type used were presented. Data for any outcome at intermediate or long-term follow-up period were sparse, suggesting that the efficacy of SE at intermediate and long-term follow-up periods is not well known. Only two of the included studies [36,41] assessed the intermediate efficacy, and long-term data were only available for one study [34] included in our review.

Third, all included studies [35–42], except one study [34] which was sponsored by the Norwegian Fund for Post-Graduate Training in Physiotherapy, did not report sponsoring agent. This serves to limit the study as it could lead to an overestimation of the efficacy of SE in participants with chronic LBP. For example, the inclusion of only trials [35,36,38,41], the sponsorship of which was not mentioned, substantially changed the conclusion of no difference in self-reported pain and back pain specific functional status at short-term follow-up between SE and other forms of exercise.

Study or Subgroup	SET Mean	SET SD	SET Total	Non SET Mean	Non SET SD	Non SET Total	Weight	Mean Difference IV, Random, 95% CI	Year
3.1.1 Short term									
Jin Miao 2011	14.2	13.2	20	33.2	15.5	20	40.7%	-19.00 [-27.92, -10.08]	2011
Hu Yuan 2011	19.6	12.5	46	30	12.8	45	59.3%	-10.40 [-15.60, -5.20]	2011
Subtotal (95% CI)			66			65	100.0%	-13.90 [-22.19, -5.62]	
Heterogeneity: Tau² = 23.10; Chi² = 2.66, df = 1 (P = 0.10); I² = 62%									
Test for overall effect: Z = 3.29 (P = 0.001)									
3.1.2 Long term									
Hu Yuan 2011	18.9	12	46	45.1	12.9	45	100.0%	-26.20 [-31.32, -21.08]	2011
Subtotal (95% CI)			46			45	100.0%	-26.20 [-31.32, -21.08]	
Heterogeneity: Not applicable									
Test for overall effect: Z = 10.03 (P < 0.00001)									

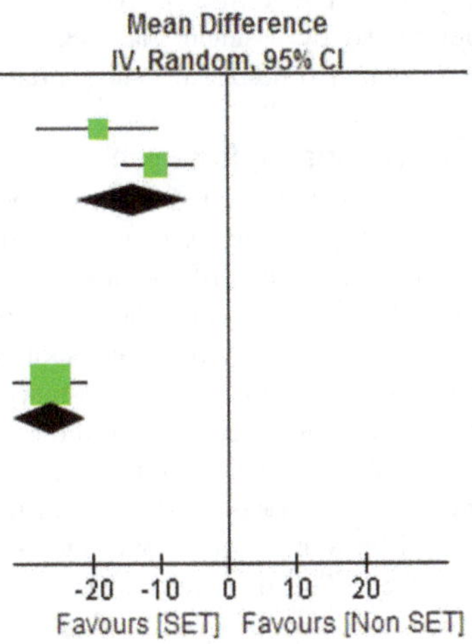

Figure 5. Self-reported pain for sling exercise versus thermomagnetic therapies.

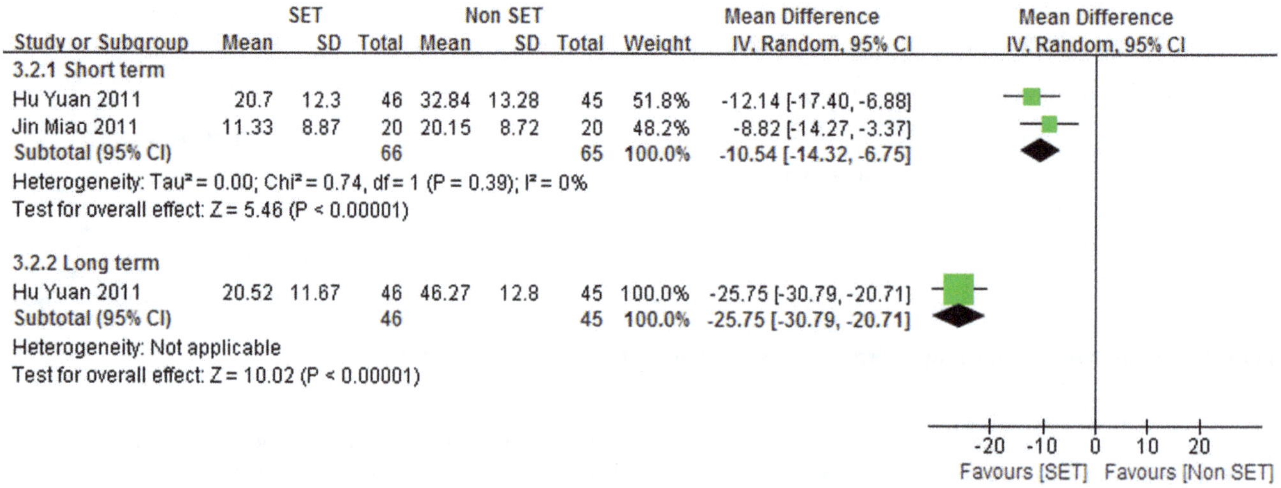

Figure 6. Back pain specific functional status for sling exercise versus thermomagnetic therapies.

Fourth, we were unable to retrieve four full-text studies [56,59–61] that may be suitable for the analysis; these studies were then considered to limit the review because whether or not the results of these trials [56,59–61] alter the conclusions derived in this review remains unknown.

Fifth, the sample sizes of trials [34–42] included in our systematic review were relatively small, such that only one third [34,38,40] of the studies [34–42] in our review enrolled 100 or more patients. Several trials [35–37,39,41,42] with small sample sizes (<100 participants) are likely to be underpowered to detect relatively small disparities between the effects of SE and that of the control conditions; these studies may overestimate the efficacy of SE in participants with chronic LBP. However, the inclusion of only small trials (<100 participants) [34–36,41] influenced neither the direction nor the significance of the result of our study that no statistically or clinically significant differences in self-reported pain and back pain specific functional status at short-term follow-up between SE and other forms of exercise were derived.

Lastly, the limited number of RCTs [34–42] published in this study area might raise the possibility of publication bias. Nine trials [34–42] conducted is significantly low in therapeutic research, such that the outcome comparisons included only a few trials [34–42], and the results of certain comparisons can easily be dominated by a single trial [38,40,42]. No unpublished studies were obtained despite the substantial search.

Implications for Research

Well-designed and sufficiently powered studies with larger sample sizes should be conducted to clarify whether or not SE improves chronic LBP because of limitations in included trials [34–42]. And we identified several implications for further research. First, future trials should adequately use random sequence generation and random concealment, and completely report outcome data. Second, future studies should be conducted in populations that best represent patients with chronic LBP; hence, patient selection should be carefully considered. Third, SE should be well designed, and interventions should be thoroughly described. The treatment affected short-term back pain specific functional status between SE and other forms of exercise at a less extent in trials in which SE was performed less frequently [34]. Hence, studies should evaluate the frequency at which SE is more effective than others for the treatment of chronic LBP. Fourth, the outcome measures for future studies should include pain intensity, functional status, and general health. This recommendation is based on the standard use of outcome measures in back pain research in 1998, including a minimum of pain intensity, functional status, and general health measures [68]. We believe that the intermediate or long-term efficacy associated with SE should be accurately assessed, particularly with standardized methods to report outcomes based on published recommendations. Fifth, further studies should also be conducted regarding the relative cost effectiveness of SE and the potential active mechanisms of SE for chronic LBP. Sixth, researchers should register RCTs and adhere to the CONSORT guidelines to improve the quality of studies. Journals on the field of back pain should adopt reporting guidelines and apply these guidelines in their review process to improve the quality of future reports in this field [51,69].

Conclusions

SE is no more efficacious in reducing self-reported pain or improving back pain specific functional status compared with other forms of exercise or traditional Chinese medical therapies with the exception of a statistically significant, but clinically probably irrelevant improvement in intermediate back pain specific functional status between SE and other forms of exercise. In comparison to thermomagnetic therapy or the combination of physical agents and drug therapy, SE more effectively decreased self-reported pain or improved back pain specific functional status. SE in addition to acupuncture therapy is as effective as acupuncture therapy alone for reduction of self-reported pain and improvement of back pain specific functional status. However, the interpretation of our findings is required to be made with caution due to limitations in included trials such as methodological drawbacks and small sample sizes.

Author Contributions

Conceived and designed the experiments: YSY XQW YZ. Performed the experiments: YSY XQW. Analyzed the data: BX ZHL. Contributed reagents/materials/analysis tools: XDW ZHL BLC. Wrote the paper: YSY XQW YZ.

References

1. Woolf AD, Pfleger B (2003) Burden of major musculoskeletal conditions. Bull World Health Organ 81: 646–656.
2. Goubert L, Crombez G, De Bourdeaudhuij I (2004) Low back pain, disability and back pain myths in a community sample: prevalence and interrelationships. Eur J Pain 8: 385–394.
3. Weiner SS, Nordin M (2010) Prevention and management of chronic back pain. Best Pract Res Clin Rheumatol 24: 267–279.
4. Lim SS, Vos T, Flaxman AD, Danaei G, Shibuya K, et al. (2013) A comparative risk assessment of burden of disease and injury attributable to 67 risk factors and risk factor clusters in 21 regions, 1990–2010: a systematic analysis for the Global Burden of Disease Study 2010. Lancet 380: 2224–2260.
5. van Dieën JH, Selen LP, Cholewicki J (2003) Trunk muscle activation in low-back pain patients, an analysis of the literature. J Electromyogr Kinesiol 13: 333–351.
6. Hodges P, van den Hoorn W, Dawson A, Cholewicki J (2009) Changes in the mechanical properties of the trunk in low back pain may be associated with recurrence. J Biomech 42: 61–66.
7. Leeuw M, Goossens ME, Linton SJ, Crombez G, Boersma K, et al. (2007) The fear-avoidance model of musculoskeletal pain: current state of scientific evidence. J Behav Med 30: 77–94.
8. Wang XQ, Pi YL, Chen PJ, Chen BL, Liang LC, et al. (2014) Whole body vibration exercise for chronic low back pain: study protocol for a single-blind randomized controlled trial. Trials 15: 104.
9. O'Sullivan P (2005) Diagnosis and classification of chronic low back pain disorders: maladaptive movement and motor control impairments as underlying mechanism. Man Ther 10: 242–255.
10. Gatchel RJ, Peng YB, Peters ML, Fuchs PN, Turk DC (2007) The biopsychosocial approach to chronic pain: scientific advances and future directions. Psychol Bull 133: 581–624.
11. Nicholas MK, Linton SJ, Watson PJ, Main CJ (2011) Early identification and management of psychological risk factors ("yellow flags") in patients with low back pain: a reappraisal. Phys Ther 91: 737–753.
12. Tan G, Jensen MP, Robinson-Whelen S, Thornby JI, Monga TN (2001) Coping with chronic pain: a comparison of two measures. Pain 90: 127–133.
13. Turk DC, Okifuji A (2002) Psychological factors in chronic pain: evolution and revolution. J Consult Clin Psychol 70: 678–690.
14. Manchikanti L, Pampati V, Beyer C, Damron K, Barnhill RC (2002) Evaluation of psychological status in chronic low back pain: comparison with general population. Pain Physician 5: 149–155.
15. Pincus T, Burton AK, Vogel S, Field AP (2002) A systematic review of psychological factors as predictors of chronicity/disability in prospective cohorts of low back pain. Spine (Phila Pa 1976) 27: E109–E120.
16. Burns JW, Bruehl S, Quartana PJ (2006) Anger management style and hostility among patients with chronic pain: effects on symptom-specific physiological reactivity during anger- and sadness- recall interviews. Psychosom Med 68: 786–793.
17. Carson JW, Keefe FJ, Lowry KP, Porter LS, Goli V, et al. (2007) Conflict about expressing emotions and chronic low back pain: associations with pain and anger. J Pain 8: 405–411.
18. Deyo RA, Mirza SK, Martin BI (2006) Back pain prevalence and visit rates: estimates from U.S. national surveys, 2002. Spine (Phila Pa 1976) 31: 2724–2727.
19. Haldeman S, Dagenais S (2008) A supermarket approach to the evidence-informed management of chronic low back pain. Spine J 8: 1–7.
20. Ricci JA, Stewart WF, Chee E, Leotta C, Foley K, et al. (2006) Back pain exacerbations and lost productive time costs in United States workers. Spine (Phila Pa 1976) 31: 3052–3060.
21. Deyo RA, Weinstein JN (2001) Low back pain. N Engl J Med 344: 363–370.
22. Ostelo RW, Deyo RA, Stratford P, Waddell G, Croft P, et al. (2008) Interpreting change scores for pain and functional status in low back pain: towards international consensus regarding minimal important change. Spine (Phila Pa 1976) 33: 90–94.
23. Pengel LH, Herbert RD, Maher CG, Refshauge KM (2003) Acute low back pain: systematic review of its prognosis. BMJ 327: 323.
24. Wang XQ, Zheng JJ, Yu ZW, Bi X, Lou SJ, et al. (2012) A meta-analysis of core stability exercise versus general exercise for chronic low back pain. PLoS One 7: e52082.
25. Wang XQ, Zheng JJ, Bi X, Liu J (2012) Effect of core stability training on patients with chronic low back pain. Healthmed 6: 754–759.
26. Wang XQ, Zheng JJ, Chen PJ. (2013) Clinical pilates versus general exercise for chronic low back pain. Med Sci Sports Exerc 45: 603.
27. Fourney DR, Andersson G, Arnold PM, Dettori J, Cahana A, et al. (2011) Chronic low back pain: a heterogeneous condition with challenges for an evidence-based approach. Spine (Phila Pa 1976) 36: S1–S9.
28. Hayden JA, van Tulder MW, Malmivaara A, Koes BW (2005) Exercise therapy for treatment of non-specific low back pain. Cochrane Database Syst Rev: CD000335.
29. Meier HP (2006) Neue aspekte der gelenkstabilisation-das sling-training. Leistungssport 2: 19–23.
30. Kirkesola G (2001) Sling exercise therapy (SET)-ein konzept zur behandlung von beschwerden am bewegungssystem. Krankengymnastik 53: 428–439.
31. Saliba SA, Croy T, Guthrie R, Grooms D, Weltman A, et al. (2010) Differences in transverse abdominis activation with stable and unstable bridging exercises in individuals with low back pain. N Am J Sports Phys Ther 5: 63–73.
32. Huang JS, Pietrosimone BG, Ingersoll CD, Weltman AL, Saliba SA (2011) Sling exercise and traditional warm-up have similar effects on the velocity and accuracy of throwing. J Strength Cond Res 25: 1673–1679.
33. Kirkesola G (2009) Neurac-a new treatment method for long-term musculoskeletal pain. J Fysioterapeuten 76: 16–25.
34. Unsgaard-Tondel M, Fladmark AM, Salvesen O, Vasseljen O (2010) Motor control exercises, sling exercises, and general exercises for patients with chronic low back pain: a randomized controlled trial with 1-year follow-up. Phys Ther 90: 1426–1440.
35. Yoo YD, Lee YS (2012) The effect of core stabilization exercises using a sling on pain and muscle strength of patients with chronic low back pain. J Phys Ther Sci 24: 671–674.
36. Qin J, Hu Y, Tang JS, Hou SX (2010) Sling exercise therapy combined with hot magner instrument for chronic nonspecific low back pain. Chinese Journal of Bone and Joint 9: 437–440.
37. Gao BL, Rong XJ, Liang DD, Li L (2008) The effect of sling exercise therapy on low back pain caused by exercises training. Chinese Journal of Rehabilitation Medicine 23: 1095–1097.
38. Guo XF, Zhang DC, Tao L (2010) Efficacy of rehabilitation on 216 patients with nonspecific low back pain. Chinses Journal of Rehabilitation Theory and Practice 16: 556–559.
39. Jin M (2011) The clinical efficacy of sling exercise therapy on CLBP [Master]: Kunming Medical University.
40. Hu Y, Qin J, Tang JS (2011) Evaluation of stabilizing exercise of the lumbar spine in the treatment of chronic non-specific low back pain. Chinese Journal of Pain Medicine 17: 146–149.
41. Wang C, Guo XF (2012) Effect of sling exercise for chronic non-specific low back pain. Chinese Journal of Rehabilitation Medicine 27: 760–762.
42. Liu P (2012) Clinical observation of acupuncture combined with scale of exercise therapy in the treatment of nonspecific chronic low back pain [Master]: Shandong University of Traditional Chinese Medicine.
43. Ljunggren AE, Weber H, Kogstad O, Thom E, Kirkesola G (1997) Effect of exercise on sick leave due to low back pain. A randomized, comparative, long-term study. Spine (Phila Pa 1976) 22: 1610–1616; discussion 1617.
44. Higgins JP, Altman DG, Gotzsche PC, Juni P, Moher D, et al. (2011) The Cochrane Collaboration's tool for assessing risk of bias in randomised trials. BMJ 343: d5928.
45. Orrow G, Kinmonth AL, Sanderson S, Sutton S (2012) Effectiveness of physical activity promotion based in primary care: systematic review and meta-analysis of randomised controlled trials. BMJ 344: e1389.
46. Bafeta A, Dechartres A, Trinquart L, Yavchitz A, Boutron I, et al. (2012) Impact of single centre status on estimates of intervention effects in trials with continuous outcomes: meta-epidemiological study. BMJ 344: e813.
47. Bowering KJ, O'Connell NE, Tabor A, Catley MJ, Leake HB, et al. (2013) The effects of graded motor imagery and its components on chronic pain: a systematic review and meta-analysis. J Pain 14: 3–13.
48. Jamal SA, Vandermeer B, Raggi P, Mendelssohn DC, Chatterley T, et al. (2013) Effect of calcium-based versus non-calcium-based phosphate binders on mortality in patients with chronic kidney disease: an updated systematic review and meta-analysis. Lancet 382: 1268–1277.
49. Bystrom MG, Rasmussen-Barr E, Grooten WJ (2013) Motor control exercises reduces pain and disability in chronic and recurrent low back pain: a meta-analysis. Spine (Phila Pa 1976) 38: E350–E358.
50. Larroy C (2002) Comparing visual-analog and numeric scales for assessing menstrual pain. Behav Med 27: 179–181.
51. Hayden JA, van Tulder MW, Malmivaara AV, Koes BW (2005) Meta-analysis: exercise therapy for nonspecific low back pain. Ann Intern Med 142: 765–775.
52. Bussing A, Ostermann T, Ludtke R, Michalsen A (2012) Effects of yoga interventions on pain and pain-associated disability: a meta-analysis. J Pain 13: 1–9.
53. Parkes MJ, Maricar N, Lunt M, LaValley MP, Jones RK, et al. (2013) Lateral wedge insoles as a conservative treatment for pain in patients with medial knee osteoarthritis: a meta-analysis. JAMA 310: 722–730.
54. Salaffi F, Stancati A, Silvestri CA, Ciapetti A, Grassi W (2004) Minimal clinically important changes in chronic musculoskeletal pain intensity measured on a numerical rating scale. Eur J Pain 8: 283–291.

55. Bombardier C, Hayden J, Beaton DE (2001) Minimal clinically important difference. Low back pain: outcome measures. J Rheumatol 28: 431–438.
56. Gürsoy C, Filiz C (2012) Effects of dynamic and static stabilization exercises on pain and functionality in chronic low back pain. Fizyoterapi Rehabilitasyon 23: 65–72.
57. Vasseljen O, Fladmark AM (2010) Abdominal muscle contraction thickness and function after specific and general exercises: a randomized controlled trial in chronic low back pain patients. Man Ther 15: 482–489.
58. Vasseljen O, Unsgaard-Tondel M, Westad C, Mork PJ (2012) Effect of core stability exercises on feed-forward activation of deep abdominal muscles in chronic low back pain: a randomized controlled trial. Spine (Phila Pa 1976) 37: 1101–1108.
59. Carvalho ACA, da Rocha ASM, Gonçalves KOF, Hespanhol Jr LC, Girotto N, et al. (2010) The utilization of the exercises for central stabilization in chronic low back pain-a clinical trail. Revista Terapia Manual 8: 497–500.
60. Nam H, Park K, Choi M (2007) The influence of sling and mat exercise to have on lumbar stability in patients with chronic low back pain. J KSSPT 3: 47–61.
61. Martin PR, Rose MJ, Nichols PJ, Russell PL, Hughes IG (1986) Physiotherapy exercises for low back pain: process and clinical outcome. Int Rehabil Med 8: 34–38.
62. van Tulder MW, Malmivaara A, Esmail R, Koes BW (2000) Exercise therapy for low back pain: a systematic review within the framework of the cochrane collaboration back review group. Spine (Phila Pa 1976) 25: 2784–2796.
63. van Tulder MW, Malmivaara A, Esmail R, Koes BW (2000) Exercise therapy for low back pain. Cochrane Database Syst Rev: CD000335.
64. Qiu YC (2007) Biomechanical changes in the muscle and lumbar vertebrae tissue in patients with low back pain caused by sport training. Journal of Clinical Rehabilitative Tissue Engineering Research 11: 9906–9909.
65. Gao MX, Liu XY, Zhen P, Wang P, Wang XM, et al. (2006) Evaluation of the efficacy of exercise program in the remission of low back pain in manage tank soldiers. Chinese Journal of Clinical Rehabilitation 10: 32–34.
66. Zhu DM (2003) Study of curative effects of sports therapy emphasized on trunk muscles in female patients with chronic low back pain [Master]: Soochow University.
67. Deyo RA, Walsh NE, Martin DC, Schoenfeld LS, Ramamurthy S (1990) A controlled trial of transcutaneous electrical nerve stimulation (TENS) and exercise for chronic low back pain. N Engl J Med 322: 1627–1634.
68. Deyo RA, Battie M, Beurskens AJ, Bombardier C, Croft P, et al. (1998) Outcome measures for low back pain research. A proposal for standardized use. Spine (Phila Pa 1976) 23: 2003–2013.
69. Begg C, Cho M, Eastwood S, Horton R, Moher D, et al. (1996) Improving the quality of reporting of randomized controlled trials. The CONSORT statement. JAMA 276: 637–639.

13

Patterns of Leisure-Time Physical Activity Participation in a British Birth Cohort at Early Old Age

Kathryn R. Martin[1,2,3]*, Rachel Cooper[2], Tamara B. Harris[3], Soren Brage[4], Rebecca Hardy[2], Diana Kuh[2], and on behalf of the NSHD scientific and data collection team¶

1 Epidemiology Group, School of Medicine and Dentistry, University of Aberdeen, Aberdeen, United Kingdom, **2** Medical Research Council Unit for Lifelong Health and Ageing at University College London, London, United Kingdom, **3** Laboratory of Epidemiology and Population Sciences, National Institute of Aging, National Institutes of Health, Bethesda, Maryland United States of America, **4** Medical Research Council Epidemiology Unit, School of Clinical Medicine, Institute of Metabolic Science, University of Cambridge, Cambridge, United Kingdom

Abstract

Using data from a nationally representative British birth cohort we characterized the type and diversity of leisure-time physical activity that 2,188 participants (age 60–64 years) engaged in throughout the year by gender and obesity. Participants most commonly reported walking (71%), swimming (33%), floor exercises (24%) and cycling (15%). Sixty-two percent of participants reported ≥2 activities in the past year and 40% reported diversity on a regular basis. Regular engagement in different types of activity (cardio-respiratory, balance/flexibility and strength) was reported by 67%, 19% and 11% of participants, respectively. We found gender differences, as well as differences by obesity status, in the activities reported, the levels of activity diversity and activity type. Non-obese participants had greater activity diversity, and more often reported activities beneficial for cardio-respiratory health and balance/flexibility than obese participants. These findings may be used to inform the development of trials of physical activity interventions targeting older adults, and those older adults with high body mass index.

Editor: Hemachandra Reddy, Oregon Health & Science University, United States of America

Funding: This research was supported in part by the Intramural Research Program of the National Institute on Aging, NIH, and was carried out while KRM was an IRTA postdoctoral research fellow in the Laboratory of Epidemiology and Population Sciences at the National Institute of Aging, National Institutes of Health. This work was supported by the UK Medical Research Council (programme codes MC_UU_12019/1 and MC_UU_12015/3). The funders had no role in study design, data collection and analysis, decision to publish, or preparation of the manuscript.

Competing Interests: The authors have declared that no competing interests exist.

* E-mail: kathryn.martin@abdn.ac.uk

¶ Membership of the NSHD scientific and data collection teams is provided in the Acknowledgments.

Introduction

Leisure-time physical activity (LTPA) can be defined as volitional activity obtained through participation in sports, exercise and recreation at a moderate and/or vigorous intensity level, independent of other key physical activity (PA) domains, i.e., active transport (purposeful walking or cycling), domestic and occupational activity [1,2]. In most high-income nations, modern technology and amenities have reduced the necessity for regular higher-level intensity activity via housework, physically demanding occupations, and active transport [3]. This is reflected in time-trend data showing declines in the average amount of time spent in domestic and work activity domains over recent decades [4,5]; trends in active transport have been mixed, indicating both a decline [4] and an increase in this domain [6,7]. Unlike other domains, time spent in LTPA has either remained stable [7,8] or increased in several countries [2,6], including the United Kingdom (UK) [9,10]. Despite this population-level increase in LTPA, the proportion of UK adults meeting the minimum recommended PA guidelines (≥30 minutes of moderate or vigorous intensity PA on ≥5 days a week) was low in the Health Survey for England 2008 [10,11]. Among older (≥65 years) UK adults, only 16% of men and 12% of women met the guidelines [10,11], with exercise and fitness activities constituting only a small proportion of time spent in moderate-to-vigorous PA [11]. Data from Sport England's 2012/13 Active People Survey suggest that, of English adults aged 55–64 and ≥65 years, 61.6% and 73.9%, respectively, do not play any sports [12]. However, to achieve recommended levels of PA, LTPA is thought to be the domain most amenable to intervention especially in later life because other domains (e.g. occupational activity) are unlikely to be viable targets due to factors including retirement. Medical and public health professionals, as well as policymakers, have therefore focused intently on increasing the levels of activity obtained through LTPA at all ages, including older adults, in efforts to improve population health [13,14].

Physical inactivity is associated with increased risk of numerous chronic conditions, cognitive decline and physical disability, as well as premature mortality [15–19]. Given the health benefits of PA, previous research has explored and identified numerous real and/or perceived personal and environmental barriers to initiating and maintaining PA [20,21]. In older adults, barriers to PA can include current health status, availability of social support, and access to safe and affordable resources [21–24]. Additionally, a narrower range of different types of LTPAs may be acceptable and/or feasible in older adults because of increasing chronic disease burden and perceived and real injury risk. To help health promotion programs to be successful in improving levels of LTPA, it may also be useful to examine what sports and exercises adults in early old age organically engage in during their leisure-time, identifying the types and diversity of activity that are most acceptable and therefore potentially amenable to intervention.

Only a few nationally representative studies have examined the type and diversity of LTPA self-reported by community-dwelling older adults. Walking for exercise was the most commonly reported LTPA among older Americans (≥60 years) [25], Australians (≥65 years) [26], European Union citizens (≥55 years) [3], and English adults (≥65 years) [11]. After walking, activities such as cycling, golf, aerobics, swimming/water sports, and stretching were most often reported [3,25]. Less than a third of older Australians reported two or more LTPA activities and only 2.6% reported engaging in a combination of aerobic, balance and flexibility exercises, as well as strength activities [26].

Health promotion programs also need to take account of how gender and obesity may influence type and diversity of LTPA. Studies of younger adults have highlighted notable gender differences in LTPA type, with men engaging in sports, jogging/running, cycling, and golf more often than women [27–29], however gender differences may change with increasing age. Previous research suggests that non-obese individuals are more likely to engage in LTPA than obese individuals [3,29] but it is less clear whether type and diversity of activity are also influenced by obesity status in older age.

The aim of this study was to use data from the Medical Research Council (MRC) National Survey of Health and Development (NSHD) (1946 British Birth Cohort) to describe the types and diversity of leisure-time sports and exercise activities that adults aged 60–64 years report undertaking by gender and obesity status.

Particpants And Methods

Sample

The MRC NSHD is an ongoing birth cohort study of a socially-stratified sample of 5,362 males and females who have been followed up regularly since their birth in England, Scotland and Wales in 1946 [30,31]. The most recent data collection took place between 2006 and 2010 when participants were aged 60–64 years. In 2006, the target sample consisted of 3,163 participants; 718 had previously died, 567 were living abroad, 594 had withdrawn from the study and 320 had been untraceable for more than 10years [31,32]. Study members received postal questionnaires and were invited to attend a clinic visit or receive a nurse home visit. Information was obtained from the postal questionnaire and/or visits from 2,662 (84%) of the target sample. Of these, 2,224 participants (1,062 men and 1,162 women) completed a postal pre-assessment questionnaire prior to the clinic or home visit that included questions on physical activity. Data from 2,188 (1,046 men and 1,142 women) with no missing data on LTPA or body mass index (BMI) were used in the current analyses.

Ethical approval for the data collection at 60–64 years was obtained from the Central Manchester Local Research Ethics Committee and the Scotland A Research Ethics Committee. Written informed consent was obtained from study members at each stage of data collection. Bona fide researchers can apply to access the NSHD data via a standard application procedure (further details available at: http://www.nshd.mrc.ac.uk/data.aspx).

Assessment of Type and Diversity of Leisure-Time Physical Activity

Physical activity was assessed using the EPIC-Norfolk Physical Activity Questionnaire (EPAQ2), which is a previously validated self-completed questionnaire that assesses activity in different domains of life – work, home and leisure [33]. In the current study, we used a modified version of this questionnaire which included the addition of two 'free text boxes' for participants to record other physical activities not in the pre-defined lists. LTPA was assessed by self-report of the frequency and duration of time spent in each of 30 pre-defined sports and exercise activities. Participants indicated the frequency of activity (choice of eight frequency categories ranging from 'not done in last year' to 'six times a week/every day') and gave the average time per episode in hours and minutes. We followed established methodology for data handling [27,33,34]. A duration variable (minutes/week) was derived for each leisure-time activity. For each of the activities, two variables were created: 'report of any participation in the last year' and 'report of regular weekly participation of at least 30 minutes per episode.' Ten activities were grouped to create five summary activities: swimming (leisure swimming and competitive swimming), running/jogging (jogging and competitive running), cycling (leisure cycling and racing cycling), aerobics (high-impact and other) and racquet sports (tennis and squash). In addition, we quantified the number of participants reporting zero, one, two, three, or four or more activities to assess level of activity diversity. Finally, we examined regular participation by 'activity type' categorized as: (1) cardio-respiratory, which included: walking for pleasure; back-packing/hill-walking; running/jogging; golf; swimming; cycling; aerobics; rowing; racquet sports; netball/volleyball/basketball; football; cricket; horse-riding; ice-skating; winter-sports (e.g. skiing); (2) activities beneficial for balance and flexibility, which included: martial arts; dancing; floor exercises; (3) activities beneficial for strength, which included: exercises with weights; conditioning exercises; and (4) all combinations, defined as a combination of cardio-respiratory, balance and flexibility and strength activity types [26].

Covariates

Gender and body mass index (BMI) were explored as potential explanatory factors. Height and weight were measured by nurses using a standardized protocol; BMI was calculated (weight (kg)/height(m)^2) and categorized as non-obese (<30 kg/m^2) and obese (≥30 kg/m^2).

Statistical analysis

We examined the percent of participants reporting each sport and exercise activity in the past year and calculated the corresponding mean (SD) number of minutes per week among those who reported each activity. We formally tested whether differences in participation existed by gender for each activity reported in the last year and also on a regular basis (i.e. ≥30 min/week). We also tested whether participation in each of the activities differed by BMI status within gender. We then examined the difference between gender, as well as BMI status within gender, with regard to the number of different activities (i.e. diversity) and activity type (cardio-respiratory, balance and flexibility, and strength). Tests of difference were conducted using chi-squared and Fisher's exact tests; Ns, percent participation (%), mean minutes per week (SD), and 95% confidence intervals are reported and we list top 10 activities by gender and BMI status (stratified by gender). All statistical analyses were conducted using STATA v13.0 (STATA Corp. – College Station, Texas).

Results

The percentage of participants reporting participation in each sport and exercise activity in the past year, as well as the mean number of minutes per week participants reported undertaking an activity are given in Table 1. Overall, 71% of participants reported walking for pleasure in the past year for an average of 192.7 minutes per week. Other activities were less frequently reported; the top 10 most commonly reported activities in the last year were swimming (33%), floor exercises (24%), conditioning exercises (16%), cycling (15%), backpacking/hill-walking (14%), dancing (14%), golfing (12%), exercises with weights (11%), and aerobics (8%). Walking for pleasure was also the most common activity reported on a regular basis (≥30 minutes per week), as it was reported by 59% of women and 52% of men (test of gender difference, $p = 0.002$). While similarities existed between men and women with regard to the top 10 activities reported on a regular basis, gender differences were observed in the percentage of individuals reporting each given activity. Briefly, women more often participated in walking for pleasure, swimming, aerobics, floor exercises, and dancing on a regular basis (Figure 1), whereas men more often engaged in backpacking/hill-walking, jogging and running, cycling and golfing.

Among men (Figure 2A), the top 10 regular reported activities were similar by obesity status, however differences were observed in the percentage of individuals reporting each given activity. A greater percentage of non-obese men regularly engaged in walking for pleasure (55% vs. 46%, $p = 0.02$) and floor exercises (12% vs. 5%, $p = 0.002$) than obese men. A trend for non-obese men to more often report cycling (8% vs. 5%, $p = 0.08$) than obese men was also observed. Similar to men, among women the top 10 regular activities were comparable by obesity status but again differences were observed in the reported percentages. Among women (Figure 2B), those who were non-obese more often reported regularly walking for pleasure (64% vs.47%, $p < 0.001$), engaging in floor exercises (23% vs. 17%, $p = 0.02$), as well as backpacking/hill-walking (7% vs. 3%, $p = 0.01$), and golfing (5% vs 2%, $p = 0.01$) when compared to obese women. However, obese women more frequently reported taking part in conditioning exercises (12% vs. 8%, $p = 0.04$) than non-obese women.

Overall, 16% of participants reported no engagement in any of the activities at least once within the past year, while approximately 21% engaged in one, 19% in two, 15% in three and 28% in four or more activities; the distribution across groups was comparable by gender ($p = 0.2$) (Table 2). When restricting analyses to activities participants engaged in on a regular basis, there was less activity diversity; nearly 27% of participants reported no regular engagement in any of the activities, 34% reported one activity, 20% reported two, 11% reported three, and just 9% of participants reported regular engagement in four or more different activities. Diversity of regular activity was comparable by gender ($p = 0.9$). The majority of activity was classified as cardio-respiratory and the percentage engaging in cardio-respiratory activity was comparable by gender, both at least once throughout the year ($p = 0.2$) and on a regular basis ($p = 0.3$). However, when compared to men, women were more likely to engage in activities beneficial for balance and flexibility at least once throughout the year and on a regular basis (both $p < 0.001$). A

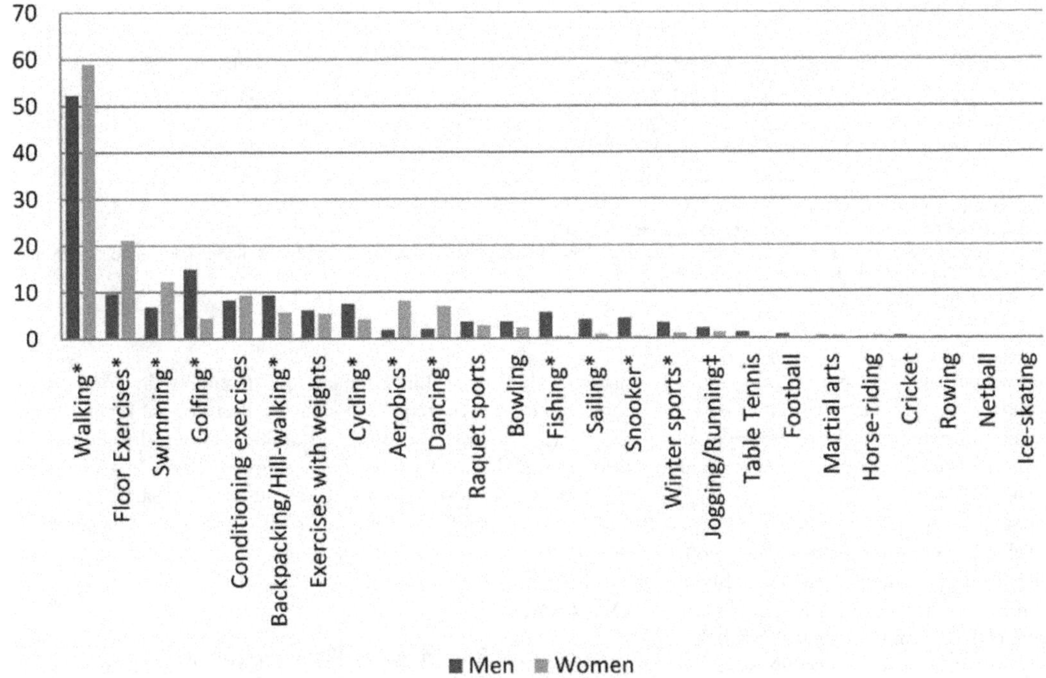

Figure 1. The percentage (%) of participants, (n§ = 2188) reporting sport and exercise activities on a regular basis‡, by gender.
§ Percentages reported are based on available n for each specific activity; ‡'report of weekly participation in 'x' activity of minimum duration, 30 minutes per episode'. *p<0.05; ‡p<0.10: test of gender difference. *Note*: No difference by gender existed for exercises with weights and conditioning exercises either in the last year or report of regular participation; N's were not robust to examine football, horse-riding, cricket, ice-skating, martial arts, and netball by gender due to low number of participants reporting these activities. Activity order was determined by the most frequent activity in both genders combined. Top ten most frequently reported activities by gender (where '1' indicates most frequently reported activity): *Men*: 1) walking for pleasure, 2) golfing, 3) floor exercises, 4) backpacking/hill-walking, 5) conditioning exercises, 6) cycling, 7) swimming, 8) exercises with weights, 9) fishing and 10) snooker. *Women*: 1) walking for pleasure, 2) floor exercises, 3) swimming, 4) conditioning exercises, 5) aerobics, 6) dancing, 7) backpacking/hill-walking, 8) exercises with weights, 9) golfing and 10) cycling.

Table 1. The percentage (%) of participants reporting each sport and exercise activity in the past year and mean (SD) time (minutes per week) spent in each activity.

	N*	% reporting participation in past year (N)	Mean minutes per week (SD)‡
Walking for pleasure	2187	71 (1555)	192.7 (300.5)
Swimming[a]	2187	33 (725)	33.3 (61.1)
Floor exercises	2176	24 (524)	66.3 (84.7)
Conditioning exercises	2176	16 (342)	53.7 (57.1)
Cycling[b]	2187	15 (328)	70.4 (158.2)
Backpacking/Hill-walking	2187	14 (310)	85.0 (167.6)
Dancing	2170	14 (296)	56.6 (112.3)
Golfing	2175	12 (266)	309.1 (298.5)
Exercises with weights	2176	11 (236)	53.4 (77.8)
Aerobics[c]	2176	8 (163)	66.1 (76.7)
Bowling	2175	7 (161)	100.6 (166.6)
Snooker	2175	6 (130)	70.5 (115.8)
Racquet sports[d]	2175	5 (113)	100.1 (123.8)
Fishing	2170	4 (92)	171.2 (65.2)
Sailing	2170	4 (85)	160.3 (409.1)
Jogging/running[e]	2187	3 (71)	58.1 (69.8)
Table Tennis	2175	3 (59)	36.1 (75.2)
Winter sports (e.g., skiing)◇	2170	3 (57)	444.9 (790.1)
Rowing	2170	1 (26)	27.1 (43.4)
Football◇	2175	<1 (20)	43.1 (42.7)
Horse-riding	2170	<1 (17)	169.6 (205.5)
Ice-skating	2170	<1 (14)	20.4 (37.5)
Cricket◇	2175	<1 (13)	104.8 (137.7)
Martial arts	2170	<1 (9)	113.3 (66.7)
Netball, volleyball, basketball	2170	<1 (4)	22.7 (17.7)

*N varies due to missing data for specific activities.
‡Represents mean time spent in activity among those reporting activity participation in past year.
[a]: Combined swimming leisurely and competitive swimming; [b]: Combined cycling recreational and competitive cycling; [c]: Combined high-impact aerobics and other aerobics; [d]Combined tennis and squash; [e]Combined jogging and competitive running.
◇Values represent time spent in activity during the season.

lower percentage of men and women engaged in all combinations of activity on a regular basis than at any point throughout the year. When compared to men, women were more likely to engage in all combinations of activity at least once throughout the year ($p = 0.02$) and on a regular basis ($p = 0.04$).

BMI was associated with both activity diversity and activity type for both men and women (Table 2). A greater percentage of non-obese men reported engaging in four or more activities, while a greater percentage of obese men reported no participation in any of the activities at any point throughout the year ($p = 0.03$). Diversity was not significantly associated with obesity status among men when examining activity on a regular basis ($p = 0.3$), though trends remained. In women, however, diversity of activity was associated with obesity status both throughout the year and on a regular basis (both $p<0.001$). When examining the activity type reported, a greater percentage of non-obese men and women reported cardio-respiratory activity at some point throughout the year ($p = 0.01$ and $p<0.001$, respectively) and on a regular basis ($p = 0.02$ and $p<0.001$, respectively), than did obese participants. In addition, a greater percentage of non-obese men also reported activities beneficial for balance and flexibility at some point throughout the year ($p = 0.04$), as well as on a regular basis ($p = 0.01$). This was also observed among women throughout the year ($p = 0.03$), as well as on a regular basis ($p = 0.01$). No difference was observed by BMI status for participation in activities beneficial for strength or all combinations of activities among men and women (all $p>0.05$).

Discussion

Using data from a nationally representative study, we have characterized the types and diversity of LTPA that British adults in early old age reported undertaking in the past year. We found gender differences, as well as differences by obesity status, in the activities reported, the levels of activity diversity and activity types. Walking for pleasure was the most commonly reported LTPA among both men and women, and these findings are consistent with the literature [3,11,25,26]. In addition to walking, we found that 62% of participants reported diversity (i.e. ≥2 unique activities) of leisure-time activities at least once throughout the year, but only 40% reported doing so on a regular basis. Levels of

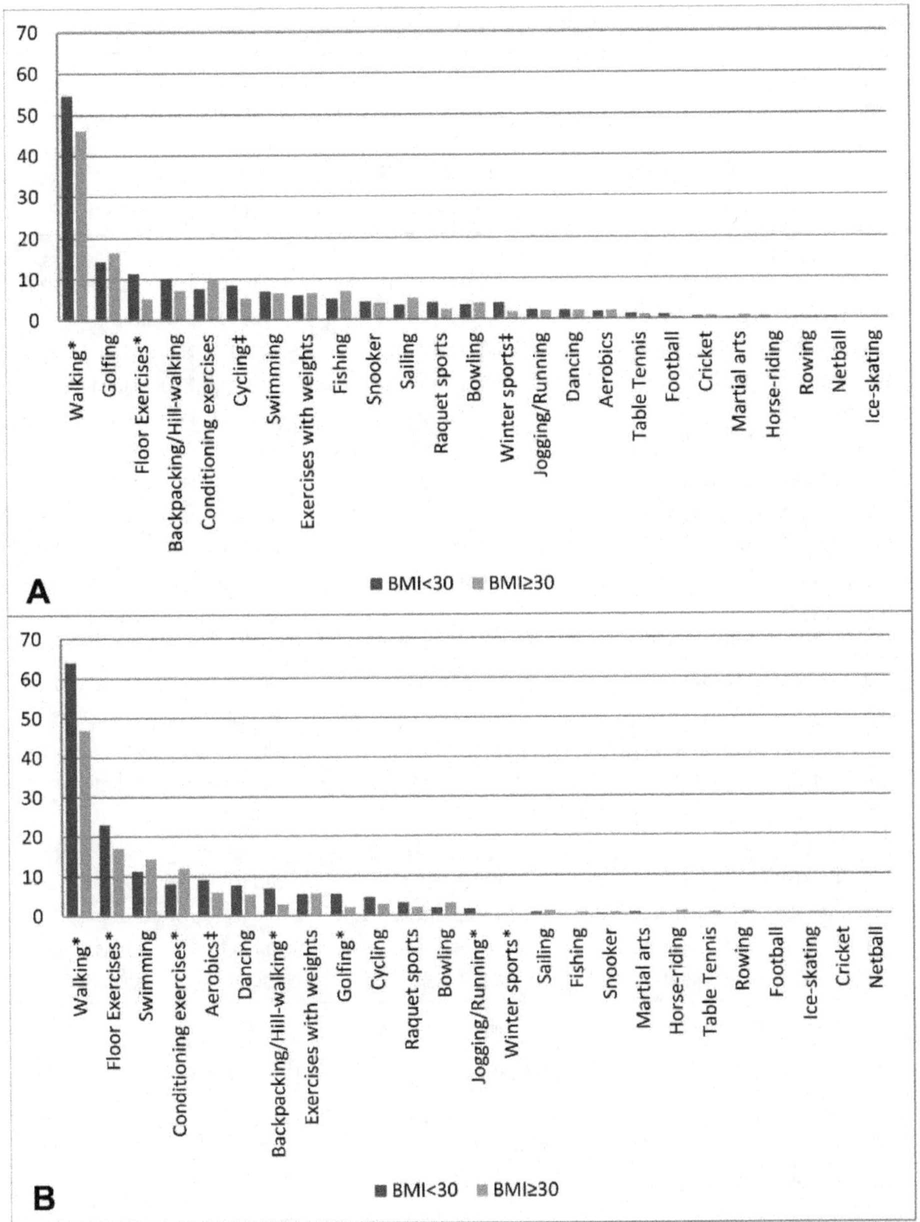

Figure 2. The percentage (%) of men (n[§] = 1046) and women (n[§] = 1142) reporting sport and exercise activities on a regular basis[‡], by obesity status. [§] Percentages reported are based on available n for each specific activity; [‡]'report of weekly participation in 'x' activity of minimum duration, 30 minutes per episode'. [*]p<0.05; [‡]p<0.10: test of difference by obesity status. (A) Activity order was determined by the most frequent activity among men. Top ten most frequently reported activities among men (where '1' indicates most frequently reported activity): *BMI< 30 kg/m²*: 1) walking for pleasure, 2) golfing, 3) floor exercises, 4) backpacking/hill-walking, 5) conditioning exercises, 6) cycling, 7) swimming, 8) fishing, 9) exercises with weights and 10) snooker. *BMI≥30 kg/m²*: 1) walking for pleasure, 2) golfing, 3) conditioning exercises, 4) backpacking/hill-walking, 5) fishing, 6) exercises with weights, 7) swimming, 8) floor exercises, 9) sailing and 10) cycling. (B) Activity order was determined by the most frequent activity among women. Top ten most frequently reported activities among women (where '1' indicates most frequently reported activity): *BMI<30 kg/m²*: 1) walking for pleasure, 2) floor exercises, 3) swimming, 4) aerobics, 5) conditioning exercise, 6) dancing,7) backpacking/hill-walking, 8) exercises with weights, 9) golfing and 10) cycling. *BMI≥30 kg/m²*: 1) walking for pleasure, 2) floor exercises, 3) swimming, 4) conditioning exercise, 5) aerobics, 6) exercises with weights, 7) dancing, 8) bowling, 9) backpacking/hill-walking and 10) cycling.

participation diversity were higher in this study than previously reported in a sample of older Australians (≥65years) [26].

There were gender differences found in the activities reported. Among the list of the top 10 activities undertaken on a regular basis, a greater percentage of men reported golfing, cycling, and backpacking/hill-walking, whereas more women reported walking for pleasure, floor exercises, aerobics, dancing and swimming. The activities men more often reported engaging in are of greater intensity and have higher associated metabolic equivalent (MET) values [35,36] yet high-impact team activities (e.g. football) that are often popular in earlier adulthood, especially among men [28], are noticeably absent from the top 10 list in this study. Indeed, football was one of the most frequently reported activities among men in the NSHD at age 36 years [37]. Swimming (in both sexes)

Table 2. Diversity in leisure-time physical activity and participation in different activity-types, % (CI), by gender and obesity status.

	Men			Women		
	Total (n = 1,046)	BMI <30 (n = 754)	BMI ≥30 (n = 292)	Total (n = 1,142)	BMI <30 (n = 801)	BMI ≥30 (n = 341)
	% (CI)	% (CI)	% (CI)	% (CI)	% (CI)	% (CI)
Diversity within year□						
0 activities	16.1 (13.9, 18.4)	13.9 (11.5, 16.6)*	21.6 (17.0, 26.7)	15.9 (13.8, 18.1)	12.9 (10.6, 15.4)*	22.9 (18.5, 27.7)
1 activity	21.6 (19.1, 24.2)	22.7 (19.7, 25.8)	18.8 (14.5, 23.8)	21.1 (19.0, 23.8)	20.9 (18.2, 24.0)	22.3 (17.9, 27.1)
2 activities	18.8 (16.5, 21.3)	18.6 (15.9, 21.5)	19.5 (15.1, 24.5)	20.4 (17.8, 22.5)	20.1 (17.4, 23.0)	19.9 (15.8, 24.6)
3 activities	14.0 (12.0, 16.3)	14.7 (12.3, 17.5)	12.3 (8.8, 16.7)	16.0 (14.8, 19.2)	18.0 (15.4, 20.8)	14.3 (10.8, 18.5)
4+ activities	29.5 (26.7, 32.3)	30.1 (26.8, 33.5)	27.7 (22.7, 33.3)	26.6 (23.3, 28.5)	28.1 (25.0, 31.3)	20.5 (16.4, 25.2)
Diversity on a regular basis¥						
0 activities	26.7 (24.0, 29.5)	24.8 (21.8, 28.0)	31.5 (26.2, 37.2)	26.4 (23.8, 29.0)	22.2 (19.4, 25.3)*	36.1 (31.0, 41.4)
1 activity	33.3 (30.4, 36.2)	33.8 (30.4, 37.3)	31.8 (26.5, 37.5)	34.5 (31.7, 37.3)	35.4 (32.0, 38.8)	32.6 (27.6, 37.8)
2 activities	19.6 (17.2, 22.1)	20.2 (17.4, 23.2)	18.2 (13.9, 23.1)	19.5 (17.3, 21.9)	21.8 (19.0, 24.9)	14.1 (10.6, 18.2)
3 activities	10.7 (8.9, 12.7)	10.9 (8.7, 13.3)	10.3 (7.0, 14.3)	11.1 (9.4, 13.1)	11.5 (9.4, 13.9)	10.3 (7.3, 14.0)
4+ activities	9.8 (8.0, 11.7)	10.3 (8.3, 12.7)	8.2 (5.3, 12.0)	8.5 (6.9, 10.3)	9.1 (7.2, 11.3)	7.0 (4.6, 10.3)
Activity-type within year□						
Cardio-respiratory[a]	77.8 (75.2, 80.3)	79.8 (76.8, 82.6)*	72.6 (67.1, 77.6)	80.3 (77.9, 82.6)	83.6 (80.9, 86.1)*	72.4 (67.4, 77.1)
Balance and flexibility[b]	23.9 (21.3, 26.6)*	25.6 (22.5, 28.9)*	19.5 (15.1, 24.5)	39.6 (36.7, 42.5)	41.7 (38.3, 45.2)*	34.6 (29.6, 39.9)
Strength[c]	17.5 (15.2, 19.9)	17.1 (14.5, 20.0)	18.5 (14.2, 23.4)	19.4 (17.2, 21.9)	19.1 (16.4, 22.0)	20.2 (16.1, 24.9)
All combinations[d]	10.5 (8.7, 12.5)*	10.6 (8.5, 13.0)	10.3 (7.0, 14.3)	13.9 (12.0, 16.1)	14.1 (11.8, 16.7)	13.5 (10.0, 17.6)
Activity-type on a regular basis¥						
Cardio-respiratory[a]	65.8 (62.8, 68.6)	67.9 (64.4, 71.2)*	60.3 (54.4, 65.9)	67.9 (65.1, 70.6)	72.5 (69.3, 75.6)*	56.9 (51.4, 62.2)
Balance and flexibility[b]	11.3 (9.4, 13.4)*	12.9 (10.6, 15.5)*	7.2 (4.5, 10.8)	25.7 (23.2, 28.4)	27.8 (24.8, 31.1)*	20.8 (16.6, 25.5)
Strength[c]	10.8 (9.0, 12.8)	10.3 (8.3, 12.7)	12.0 (8.5, 16.3)	11.8 (10.0, 13.8)	10.7 (8.7, 13.1)	12.9 (9.5, 16.9)
All combinations[d]	3.8 (2.7, 5.2)*	4.1 (2.8, 5.8)	3.1 (1.4, 5.8)	5.7 (4.4, 7.2)	5.5 (4.0, 7.3)	6.2 (3.9, 9.3)

Note: Values for football, cricket and winter sports (e.g., skiing) represented time spent in activity during the season.
□Any report of activity (activities) in last year.
¥Report of average participation in activity (activities) for 30+ min per week; note that values used for skiing, winter sport football and cricket represented time spent in season.
[a]cardio-respiratory, which included: walking for pleasure; backpacking/hill-walking; running/jogging; golfing; swimming; cycling; aerobics; rowing; racquet sports; netball/volleyball/basketball; football; cricket; horse-riding; ice-skating; winter-sports (e.g., skiing); [b]Martial arts, dancing, floor exercises; [c]Exercises with weights, conditioning exercises; [d]Combination of Cardio-respiratory, Balance and flexibility and Strength.
*Indicates $p<0.05$ for chi-squared test of association by BMI status within gender.

and golf (in men) were among the most frequently reported activities at both ages [37], suggesting that such lower intensity activities may be more likely to be maintained with increasing age than more vigorous activities such as football and running. That more of the activities frequently reported among women at age 36 years (e.g. swimming and dancing) were also in the top 10 most frequently reported activities at age 60–64 years [37], suggests that greater changes in activity type may occur among men than women with increasing age.

Study results also suggest that activity diversity and activity type varied by obesity status among men and women. Non-obese women reported greater activity diversity on a regular basis than obese women, though this relationship was not observed among men. These results are in line with findings from a Canadian study that found the prevalence of physical inactivity increased with increasing BMI among women, but not in men and that the largest difference between BMI status occurred among the oldest age group (50–64 years) [38]. In the current study, lower BMI was associated with more regular participation in cardio-respiratory activity, as well as balance and flexibility activity for both men and women. To our knowledge, this study is the first to examine the relationship between leisure-time sport and exercise activity, gender and BMI in this way. Despite different PA measurement and operationalization (e.g., leisure METS), our findings are also supported by prior research suggesting an association between higher levels of recreational activity and lower BMI, as well as no association for vigorous active recreation (time spent in any activity of ≥5METS) among men by BMI status [29].

Although walking is often recommended to adults, especially those overweight and/or older, as a way to increase PA levels through low-impact activity, our study found that regular weekly walking for pleasure varied by BMI status among both men and women. This difference was not observed among another low-impact activity, swimming, which is commonly recommended to older and/or overweight populations as a low weight-bearing, joint-friendly activity [39,40]. While the difference in reports observed by BMI status may reflect lower BMI as a result of regular walking for pleasure during one's lifetime or adulthood, our findings may also indicate that obese individuals face additional barriers to walking for pleasure (e.g. pain, physical disability, embarrassment) that go beyond, but are also related to body size and weight [41]. Indeed, findings from the EPIC-Norfolk cohort suggest that weight status and weight gain are associated with both contemporaneous levels and subsequent changes in physical inactivity [42]. Combined with findings from the current study, this may suggest that the benefits of walking should be promoted within a context that acknowledges personal, social, and/or environmental barriers among older adults with higher BMI, so as to increase engagement in walking for pleasure as a LTPA and reduce the observed difference by BMI status.

Previous research has found that, in contrast to domestic activities, leisure pursuits, outdoor pursuits, sports (team and non-team), and exercise and fitness contributed very little towards the proportion of total time per week spent in moderate-to-vigorous physical activity among English adults aged 65 years and older [11]. We extend these observations through our examination of diversity and activity type in the current study. While fewer than 10 percent of older adults reported high activity diversity, i.e. four or more different leisure sport and exercise activities on a regular basis, nearly a third were found to have high diversity throughout the year. Seasonality of activity participation may play a role in the finding of higher diversity when considering activity undertaken at any point throughout the year, as some activities can only be undertaken in specific seasons and better conditions exist for many activities (e.g., reduced access/transportation barriers, increased daylight, fairer weather conditions), especially those conducted outdoors, in spring and summer. However, these findings do suggest that older adults have varied activity interests and that there may be great potential for increasing the time older adults spend in sport and exercise activities by encouraging regular participation in a variety of diverse activities. That nearly 60 percent of participants reported either none or participation in just one of the activities on a regular basis represents an opportunity for public health practitioners and clinicians to discuss and encourage older adults to increase their PA through a varied and diverse routine of sport and exercise activities. Engagement in a greater number of different activities may be a strategy that results in greater time spent in overall activity, especially for older adults who are either overweight or obese.

Our study has several strengths. It is a nationally representative sample of adults in early old age, with good characterization of LTPA as measured by a validated questionnaire, the EPAQ2. However, some limitations should be noted. In general, self-report PA, as measured by questionnaire, is noted to suffer from recall bias, especially among older adults [43–45]. For example, participants may have difficulty remembering whether or not they engaged in a particular activity in the past, as well as the average length of time per episode. Self-report PA is also prone to social desirability bias, as participants might feel compelled to over-report activity levels knowing the benefits of PA on health. However, self-reported questionnaires are currently the best method for ascertaining information on participation in different types of activity, as these parameters of PA are not yet easily captured by objective monitoring. Further, we purposefully chose to focus on sport and exercise activities that are of higher intensity (moderate-to-vigorous) partly because they are reported with greater reliability and validity than lower intensity (light) activities [46,47]. Additionally, higher intensity activities are often thought to enable older adults to meet the currently recommended PA levels. We were unable to explore reasons for choice of activity and explanations of non-participation, as we did not ask participants whether or not non-participation or low participation frequency was due to lack of interest, lack of opportunity/resources, or physical inability to engage in a specific activity. Nor did we ask participants if they independently engaged in an activity, if they were active with a group or someone in their social network, or even their preference for solo or group activity. Therefore, we suggest that these factors are explored in future research, as well as in advance of development/implementation of interventions to increase PA among older men and women.

Conclusion

In conclusion, there is considerable variation in types and diversity of leisure sports and exercise activities in this population of British adults in early old age, and different patterns of activity were observed by gender and obesity status. While 40 percent engaged in two or more types of activity on a regular basis, the majority reported no diversity or regular participation in any of the activities queried. In general, walking for pleasure is the activity most often reported among older adults, perhaps due in part to its ease, convenience, lack of associated risk and inexpensive nature, as well as perhaps increased likelihood of exposure to an outdoor environment. Clinicians, public health professionals and researchers might capitalize on this knowledge when developing trials of PA interventions tailored and targeted to older men and women, and those with high BMI.

Acknowledgments

The authors are grateful to NSHD study members who took part in this latest data collection for their continuing support. We thank Professor Michael Wadsworth, Suzie Clennell, and members of the NSHD scientific and data collection team at the following centres: MRC Unit for LHA, MRC Human Nutrition Research, Cambridge; MRC Epidemiology Unit, Cambridge; MRC Lifecourse Epidemiology Unit, Southampton; Wellcome Trust (WT) Clinical Research Facility (CRF) Manchester, the Manchester Heart Centre, and the Department of Clinical Radiology at the Central Manchester University Hospitals NHS Foundation Trust; WTCRF, Medical Physics and the Department of Cardiology at the Western General Hospital in Edinburgh; WTCRF, Department of Nuclear Medicine and the Department of Cardiology at University Hospital Birmingham; WTCRF and the Department of Nuclear Medicine at University College London Hospital; CRF, the Department of Medical Physics and the Department of Cardiology at the University Hospital of Wales; CRF and Twin Research Unit at St Thomas' Hospital London; Vascular Physiology Unit, Institute of Child Health, London; National Heart and Lung Institute, Imperial College London; Institute of Cardiovascular & Medical Sciences, University of Glasgow, Glasgow; Cardiovascular Institute, Sahlgrenska Academy, Gothenburg University; National Centre of Social Research (NatCen).

Members of the NSHD scientific and data collection teams (lead Diana Kuh; email: d.kuh@ucl.ac.uk) are:

Rachel Cooper (MRC Unit for Lifelong Health and Ageing at UCL, London, UK), Rebecca Hardy (MRC Unit for Lifelong Health and Ageing at UCL, London, UK), Diana Kuh (MRC Unit for Lifelong Health and Ageing at UCL, London, UK), Mary Pierce (MRC Unit for Lifelong Health and Ageing at UCL, London, UK), Marcus Richards (MRC Unit for Lifelong Health and Ageing at UCL, London, UK), Jane Abington (MRC Unit for Lifelong Health and Ageing at UCL, London, UK), Andrew Wong (MRC Unit for Lifelong Health and Ageing at UCL, London, UK), Judith E. Adams (Clinical Radiology, Manchester Royal Infirmary, Manchester, UK), Mike Machin (Clinical Radiology, Manchester Royal Infirmary, Manchester, UK), Alison M. Stephens (MRC Human Nutrition Research, Cambridge, UK), Kerina Bonar (MRC Human Nutrition Research, Cambridge, UK), Susan Bryant (MRC Human Nutrition Research, Cambridge, UK), Darren Cole (MRC Human Nutrition Research, Cambridge, UK), Wing Nip (MRC Human Nutrition Research, Cambridge, UK), Gina Ambrosini (MRC Human Nutrition Research, Cambridge, UK), Denis Pellerin (Department of Echocardiography, The Heart Hospital, London, UK), Nishi Chaturvedi (International Centre for Circulatory Health (ICCH), National Heart and

Lung Institute, Imperial College London, London, UK), Alun Hughes (International Centre for Circulatory Health (ICCH), National Heart and Lung Institute, Imperial College London, London, UK), Arjun Ghosh (International Centre for Circulatory Health (ICCH), National Heart and Lung Institute, Imperial College London, London, UK), Katherine March (International Centre for Circulatory Health (ICCH), National Heart and Lung Institute, Imperial College London, London, UK), Peter Macfarlane (Institute of Cardiovascular & Medical Sciences, University of Glasgow, Glasgow, UK), Louise Inglis (Institute of Cardiovascular & Medical Sciences, University of Glasgow, Glasgow, UK), Peter Friberg (Cardiovascular Institute, Sahlgrenska University Hospital, Göteborg, Sweden), Walter Osika (Cardiovascular Institute, Sahlgrenska University Hospital, Göteborg, Sweden), Soren Brage (MRC Epidemiology Unit, Cambridge, UK), Ulf Ekelund (MRC Epidemiology Unit, Cambridge, UK), Stefanie Mayle (MRC Epidemiology Unit, Cambridge, UK), Kate Westgate (MRC Epidemiology Unit, Cambridge, UK), John Deanfield (Vascular Physiology Unit, Institute of Child Health, University College London, London, UK), Ann Donald (Vascular Physiology Unit, Institute of Child Health, University College London, London, UK), Sarah Kok (Vascular Physiology Unit, Institute of Child Health, University College London, London, UK), Stefano Masi (Vascular Physiology Unit, Institute of Child Health, University College London, London, UK), Ravneet Phalora (Vascular Physiology Unit, Institute of Child Health, University College London, London, UK), John Woodside (Vascular Physiology Unit, Institute of Child Health, University College London, London, UK), Ian Bruce (Wellcome Trust Clinical Research Facility, Manchester, UK), Nikki Harwood (Wellcome Trust Clinical Research Facility, Manchester, UK), Emma Oughton (Wellcome Trust Clinical Research Facility, Manchester, UK), Alison Chapman (Department of Clinical Radiology, Central Manchester University Hospitals NHS Foundation Trust, Manchester, UK), Rajdeep S Khattar (The Manchester Heart Centre, Central Manchester University Hospitals NHS Foundation Trust, Manchester, UK), Satheesh Balakrishnan Nair (The Manchester Heart Centre, Central Manchester University Hospitals NHS Foundation Trust, Manchester, UK), Jayne Franklyn (Wellcome Trust Clinical Research Facility, Birmingham, UK), Sue Palmer (Wellcome Trust Clinical Research Facility, Birmingham, UK), Karen Boardman (Wellcome Trust Clinical Research Facility, Birmingham, UK), Nicola Crabtree (Department of Nuclear Medicine, University Hospital Birmingham, Birmingham, UK), Ross Clements (Department of Cardiology, University Hospital Birmingham, Birmingham, UK), Michael Suvari (Department of Cardiology, University Hospital Birmingham, Birmingham, UK), Rick Steeds (Department of Cardiology, University Hospital Birmingham, Birmingham, UK), Kathrine Craig (Wellcome Trust Clinical Research Facility, Cardiff, UK), Emma Howard (Wellcome Trust Clinical Research Facility, Cardiff, UK), Terese Morley (Wellcome Trust Clinical Research Facility, Cardiff, UK), Maurice Scanlon (Wellcome Trust Clinical Research Facility, Cardiff, UK), Rebecca Petit (Department of Medical Physics, University Hospital of Wales, Cardiff, UK), Wil Evans (Department of Medical Physics, University Hospital of Wales, Cardiff, UK), Alan Fraser (Department of Cardiology, University Hospital of Wales, Cardiff, UK), Julie Edwards (Department of Cardiology, University Hospital of Wales, Cardiff, UK), Emma Reece (Department of Cardiology, University Hospital of Wales, Cardiff, UK), David Newby (Wellcome Trust Clinical Research Facility, Edinburgh, UK), Fiona Marshall (Wellcome Trust Clinical Research Facility, Edinburgh, UK), Jim Hannan (Department of Medical Physics, Western General Hospital, Edinburgh, UK), Carol Miller (Department of Medical Physics, Western General Hospital, Edinburgh, UK), Audrey White (Department of Cardiology, Western General Hospital, Edinburgh, UK), Raymond MacAllister (Wellcome Trust Clinical Research Facility, University College London, London, UK), Joanne Harris (Wellcome Trust Clinical Research Facility, University College London, London, UK), Roldan Singzon (Wellcome Trust Clinical Research Facility, University College London, London, UK), Peter Ell (Department of Nuclear Medicine, University College London Hospital, London, UK), Caroline Townsend (Department of Nuclear Medicine, University College London Hospital, London, UK), Camelia Demetrescu (Department of Echocardiography, The Heart Hospital, London, UK), Philip Chowienczyk (Wellcome Trust Clinical Research Facility, St. Thomas' Hospital, London, UK), Paula Darroch (Wellcome Trust Clinical Research Facility, St. Thomas' Hospital, London, UK), Karen McNeill (Wellcome Trust Clinical Research Facility, St. Thomas' Hospital, London, UK), Tim Spector (Twin Research Unit, St Thomas' Hospital, London, UK), Gail Clements (Twin Research Unit, St Thomas' Hospital, London, UK), Benyu Jiang (Twin Research Unit, St Thomas' Hospital, London, UK), Carli Lessof(NatCen, London, UK), Hayley Cheshire(NatCen, London, UK).

Author Contributions

Conceived and designed the experiments: KRM RC DK RH. Analyzed the data: KRM. Contributed to the writing of the manuscript: KRM RC. Acquisition of data: DK KRM RH RC SB. Interpretation of data: KRM RC TBH SB RH DK. Revising the article critically for important intellectual content: KRM RC TBH SB RH DK.

References

1. Moore SC, Patel AV, Matthews CE, Berrington de GA, Park Y, et al. (2012) Leisure time physical activity of moderate to vigorous intensity and mortality: a large pooled cohort analysis. PLoS Med 9: e1001335.
2. Palacios-Cena D, Alonso-Blanco C, Jimenez-Garcia R, Hernandez-Barrera V, Carrasco-Garrido P, et al. (2011) Time trends in leisure time physical activity and physical fitness in elderly people: 20 year follow-up of the Spanish population national health survey (1987–2006). BMC Public Health 11:799. doi: 10.1186/1471-2458-11-799.
3. Vaz de Almeida MD, Graca P, Afonso C, D'Amicis A, Lappalainen R, et al. (1999) Physical activity levels and body weight in a nationally representative sample in the European Union. Public Health Nutr 2: 105–113.
4. Brownson RC, Boehmer TK, Luke DA (2005) Declining rates of physical activity in the United States: what are the contributors? Annu Rev Public Health 26:421–443.
5. Church TS, Thomas DM, Tudor-Locke C, Katzmarzyk PT, Earnest CP, et al. (2011) Trends over 5 decades in U.S. occupation-related physical activity and their associations with obesity. PLoS One 6: e19657.
6. Juneau CE, Potvin L (2010) Trends in leisure-, transport-, and work-related physical activity in Canada 1994–2005. Prev Med 51: 384–386.
7. Hallal PC, Knuth AG, Reis RS, Rombaldi AJ, Malta DC, et al. (2011) Time trends of physical activity in Brazil (2006-2009). Rev Bras Epidemiol 14 Suppl 1:53–60.
8. Moore LV, Harris CD, Carlson SA, Kruger J, Fulton JE (2012) Trends in no leisure-time physical activity—United States, 1988-2010. Res Q Exerc Sport 83: 587–591.
9. Stamatakis E, Chaudhury M (2008) Temporal trends in adults' sports participation patterns in England between 1997 and 2006: the Health Survey for England. Br J Sports Med 42: 901–908.
10. Craig R, Mindell J, Hirani V (2009) Health Survey for England 2008. Volume 1: Physical Activity and Fitness. Health Survey for England 8–395.
11. Belanger M, Townsend N, Foster C (2011) Age-related differences in physical activity profiles of English adults. Prev Med 52: 247–249.
12. Sport England (2014) Active People Survey 2012/2013. Available: http://activepeople.sportengland.org/Querty. Accessed 2014 Mar 05.
13. Department of Health PAHIaP (2011) Start Active, Stay Active: a report on physical activity for health from the four home countries' Chief Medical Officers. Available: http://www.dh.gov.uk/en/Publicationsandstatistics/Publications/PublicationsPolicyAndGuidance/DH_128209.
14. NICE (2013) Physical activity: brief advice for adults in primary care. Public Health Guidance 44.
15. Warburton DE, Nicol CW, Bredin SS (2006) Health benefit of physical activity: the evidence. CMAJ 174: 801–809.
16. Paterson DH, Warburton DE (2010) Physical activity and functional limitations in older adults: a systematic review related to Canada's Physical Activity Guidelines. Int J Behav Nutr Phys Act 7:38. doi: 10.1186/1479-5868-7-38.
17. Boyle PA, Buchman AS, Wilson RS, Bienias JL, Bennett DA (2007) Physical activity is associated with incident disability in community-based older persons. J Am Geriatr Soc 55: 195–201.
18. Xue QL, Bandeen-Roche K, Mielenz TJ, Seplaki CL, Szanton SL, et al. (2012) Patterns of 12-year change in physical activity levels in community-dwelling older women: can modest levels of physical activity help older women live longer? Am J Epidemiol 176: 534–543.
19. Andersen LB, Schnohr P, Schroll M, Hein HO (2000) All-cause mortality associated with physical activity during leisure time, work, sports, and cycling to work. Arch Intern Med 160: 1621–1628.
20. Wendel-Vos W, Droomers M, Kremers S, Brug J, van LF (2007) Potential environmental determinants of physical activity in adults: a systematic review. Obes Rev 8: 425–440.
21. Chipperfield JG, Newall NE, Chuchmach LP, Swift AU, Haynes TL (2008) Differential determinants of men's and women's everyday physical activity in later life. J Gerontol B Psychol Sci Soc Sci 63: S211–S218.
22. Moschny A, Platen P, Klaassen-Mielke R, Trampisch U, Hinrichs T (2011) Barriers to physical activity in older adults in Germany: a cross-sectional study. Int J Behav Nutr Phys Act 8:121. doi: 10.1186/1479-5868-8-121.

23. Salmon J, Owen N, Crawford D, Bauman A, Sallis JF (2003) Physical activity and sedentary behavior: a population-based study of barriers, enjoyment, and preference. Health Psychol 22: 178–188.
24. Finch C, Owen N, Price R (2001) Current injury or disability as a barrier to being more physically active. Med Sci Sports Exerc 33: 778–782.
25. Hughes JP, McDowell MA, Brody DJ (2008) Leisure-time physical activity among US adults 60 or more years of age: results from NHANES 1999-2004. J Phys Act Health 5: 347–358.
26. Merom D, Carmen C, Kamalesh V, Adrian B (2012) How diverse was the leisure time physical activity of older Australians over the past decade? J Sci Med Sport 15: 213–219.
27. Parsons TJ, Thomas C, Power C (2009) Estimated activity patterns in British 45 year olds: cross-sectional findings from the 1958 British birth cohort. Eur J Clin Nutr 63: 978–985.
28. Deaner RO, Geary DC, Puts DA, Ham SA, Kruger J, et al. (2012) A sex difference in the predisposition for physical competition: males play sports much more than females even in the contemporary U.S. PLoS One 7: e49168.
29. Livingstone MB, Robson PJ, McCarthy S, Kiely M, Harrington K, et al. (2001) Physical activity patterns in a nationally representative sample of adults in Ireland. Public Health Nutr 4: 1107–1116.
30. Wadsworth M, Kuh D, Richards M, Hardy R (2006) Cohort Profile: The 1946 National Birth Cohort (MRC National Survey of Health and Development). Int J Epidemiol 35: 49–54.
31. Kuh D, Pierce M, Adams J, Deanfield J, Ekelund U, et al. (2011) Cohort profile: updating the cohort profile for the MRC National Survey of Health and Development: a new clinic-based data collection for ageing research. Int J Epidemiol 40: e1–e9.
32. Stafford M, Black S, Shah I, Hardy R, Pierce M, et al. (2013) Using a birth cohort to study ageing: representativeness and response rates in the National Survey of Health and Development. Eur J Ageing 10: 145–157.
33. Wareham NJ, Jakes RW, Rennie KL, Mitchell J, Hennings S, et al. (2002) Validity and repeatability of the EPIC-Norfolk Physical Activity Questionnaire. Int J Epidemiol 31: 168–174.
34. Espana-Romero V, Golubic R, Martin KR, Hardy R, Ekelund U, et al. (2014) Comparison of the EPIC Physical Activity Questionnaire with Combined Heart Rate and Movement Sensing in a Nationally Representative Sample of Older British Adults. PLoS One 9: e87085.
35. Ainsworth BE, Haskell WL, Leon AS, Jacobs DR Jr., Montoye HJ, et al. (1993) Compendium of physical activities: classification of energy costs of human physical activities. Med Sci Sports Exerc 25: 71–80.
36. Ainsworth BE, Haskell WL, Whitt MC, Irwin ML, Swartz AM, et al. (2000) Compendium of physical activities: an update of activity codes and MET intensities. Med Sci Sports Exerc 32: S498–S504.
37. Kuh DJ, Cooper C (1992) Physical activity at 36 years: patterns and childhood predictors in a longitudinal study. J Epidemiol Community Health 46: 114–119.
38. Chen Y, Mao Y (2006) Obesity and leisure time physical activity among Canadians. Prev Med 42: 261–265.
39. Waumsley J, Mutrie N (2011) Physical Activity and Exercise Psychology: Our role in healthy weight management for adults. Obesity in the UK: A psychological perspective 5–15.
40. Young A, Dinan S (1994) ABC of sports medicine. Fitness for older people. BMJ 309: 331–334.
41. Ball K, Crawford D, Owen N (2000) Too fat to exercise? Obesity as a barrier to physical activity. Aust N Z J Public Health 24: 331–333.
42. Golubic R, Ekelund U, Wijndaele K, Luben R, Khaw KT, et al. (2013) Rate of weight gain predicts change in physical activity levels: a longitudinal analysis of the EPIC-Norfolk cohort. Int J Obes (Lond) 37: 404–409.
43. Prince SA, Adamo KB, Hamel ME, Hardt J, Connor GS, et al. (2008) A comparison of direct versus self-report measures for assessing physical activity in adults: a systematic review. Int J Behav Nutr Phys Act 5:56. doi: 10.1186/1479-5868-5-56.
44. Loney T, Standage M, Thompson D, Sebire SJ, Cumming S (2011) Self-report vs. objectively assessed physical activity: which is right for public health? J Phys Act Health 8: 62–70.
45. Colbert LH, Matthews CE, Havighurst TC, Kim K, Schoeller DA (2011) Comparative validity of physical activity measures in older adults. Med Sci Sports Exerc 43: 867–876.
46. Bonnefoy M, Normand S, Pachiaudi C, Lacour JR, Laville M, et al. (2001) Simultaneous validation of ten physical activity questionnaires in older men: a doubly labeled water study. J Am Geriatr Soc 49: 28–35.
47. Lee IM, Shiroma EJ (2014) Using accelerometers to measure physical activity in large-scale epidemiological studies: issues and challenges. Br J Sports Med 48: 197–201.

14

Usefulness of Decrease in Oxygen Uptake Efficiency to Identify Gas Exchange Abnormality in Patients with Idiopathic Pulmonary Arterial Hypertension

Xiaoyue Tan[1,4]✉, Wenlan Yang[1], Jian Guo[1], Yan Zhang[1,2], Changwei Wu[1]✉, Rikesh Sapkota[3], Shailendra Prasad Kushwaha[3], Sugang Gong[3], Xingguo Sun[4]*, Jinming Liu[1,3]*

1 Department of Pulmonary Function Test, Shanghai Pulmonary Hospital Affiliated to Tongji University, Shanghai, China, 2 Respiratory Division, Hangzhou, Zhejiang Provincial Hospital of traditional Chinese Medicine, The First Affiliated Hospital of Zhejiang Chinese Medicine University, Hangzhou, China, 3 Department of Pulmonary Circulation, Shanghai Pulmonary Hospital Affiliated to Tongji University, Shanghai, China, 4 State Key Laboratory of Cardiovascular Disease, Heart-Lung Function Testing Center, Fuwai Hospital, National Center for Cardiovascular Diseases, Chinese Academy of Medical Sciences and Peking Union Medical College, Beijing, China

Abstract

Background: Decline in oxygen uptake efficiency (OUE), especially during exercise, is found in patients with chronic heart failure. In this study we aimed to test the validity and usefulness of OUE in evaluating gas exchange abnormality of patients with idiopathic pulmonary arterial hypertension (IPAH).

Methods: We retrospectively investigated the cardiopulmonary exercise test (CPET) with gas exchange measurements in 32 patients with confirmed IPAH. All patients also had resting hemodynamic measurements and pulmonary function test (PFT). Sixteen healthy subjects, matched by age, sex, and body size were used as controls, also had CPET and PFT measurements.

Results: In IPAH patients, the magnitude of absolute and percentage of predicted (%pred) oxygen uptake efficiency slope (OUES) and oxygen uptake efficiency plateau (OUEP), as well as several other CPET parameters, were strikingly worse than healthy subjects ($P<0.0001$). Pattern of changes in OUE in patients is similar to that in controls, In IPAH patients, OUE values at rest, warming up, anaerobic threshold and peak exercise were all significantly lower than in normal ($P<0.0001$). OUEP%pred, better than OUES%pred, correlated significantly with New York Heart Association (NYHA) functional Class ($r=-0.724$, $P<0.005$), Total Pulmonary Vascular Resistance (TPVR) ($r=-0.694$, $P<0.005$), diffusing capacity for carbon monoxide (DL_{CO}) ($r=0.577$, $P<0.05$), and the lowest ventilation versus CO_2 output ratio during exercise (Lowest$\dot{V}E/\dot{V}CO_2$) ($r=-0.902$, $P<0.0001$). In addition, the coefficient of variation (COV) of OUEP was lower (20.9%) markedly than OUES (34.3%) ($P<0.0001$).

Conclusions: In patients with IPAH, OUES and OUEP are both significantly lower than the healthy subjects. OUEP is a better physiological parameter than OUES in evaluating the gas exchange abnormality of patients with IPAH.

Editor: James West, Vanderbilt University Medical Center, United States of America

Funding: This retrospective CPET data reanalysis is partially supported by Chinese Academy of Medical Sciences (No. 2012-YJR02), Key Project Starting Grant from National Center for Cardiovascular Diseases. CPET data collected at Shanghai Pulmonary Hospital were partially supported from Chinese Medicine Association (No. 08020420120) and science and technology commission of shanghai municipality (NO. 11411951302 and 114119a3000). The funders had no role in study design, data collection and analysis, decision to publish, or preparation of the manuscript.

Competing Interests: The authors have declared that no competing interests exist.

* E-mail: xgsun@labiomed.org (XGS); jinmingliu2013@163.com (JML)

✉ These authors contributed equally to this work.

Introduction

Idiopathic pulmonary arterial hypertension (IPAH) is a progressive and fatal disease caused by pulmonary vasculopathy [1–2]. Low perfusion to the lungs due to inability of the right ventricle to adequately increase pulmonary blood flow (cardiac output [CO]) for O_2 exercise demand, gives rise to mismatching of ventilation/perfusion (V/Q) and inefficient lung gas exchange. Cardiopulmonary exercise test (CPET) with gas exchange measurements has proved to be a powerful tool to detect abnormalities in patients with IPAH during exercise [3]. Patients with IPAH can safely undergo noninvasive cycle ergometer testing to their maximal tolerance [4]. The key CPET characteristics in these patients include a diminished aerobic capacity, an impaired ventilatory efficiency and a decreased minute O_2 uptake versus heart rate at peak exercise (peak $\dot{V}O_2$/HR) etc [4–8]. These CPET parameters have been widely utilized to grade the severity of exercise limitation, to detect exercise-induced right-to-left shunting, to assess responses to therapy, and to predict prognosis in IPAH patients [5–8]. Because of the increasing recognition of potential value of CPET in patients with IPAH, more CPET indexes are required in clinical practice.

Oxygen uptake efficiency (OUE) is a recently emerging parameter which is not obvious in the traditional Wasserman

CPET 9-panel plots [9]. OUE measures the change in minute oxygen uptake ($\dot{V}O_2$) relative to minute ventilation ($\dot{V}E$). The most widely studied index of OUE is the oxygen uptake efficiency slope (OUES), which ordinarily mathematically describes a near-linear relationship for $\dot{V}O_2$ versus $\dot{V}E$ after transforming $\dot{V}E$ from a linear to log scale. Thus OUES defines the slope of $\dot{V}O_2$-vs-log$\dot{V}E$ during an entire exercise period [10]. It was used initially in young patients (mean age 12 yrs) with cardiac disease and then later in adults with heart disease to assess exercise capacity, severity and prognosis [11–13]. Recently, the other index of OUE, oxygen uptake efficiency plateau (OUEP) was added. It is well known that the relationship between $\dot{V}O_2$ and $\dot{V}E$ during an incremental exercise test is curvilinear due to hyperventilation stimulated by the excess [H^+] of the acidosis of heavy exercise [14]. We found that $\dot{V}O_2/\dot{V}E$ when plotted against time normally reached its highest and briefly stable values (plateau) near the anaerobic threshold (AT), before declining due to hyperventilation stimulated by the metabolic acidosis [14]. We defined the highest 90 sec average of $\dot{V}O_2/\dot{V}E$ as OUEP. In our CHF patients and normal subjects, we found that the OUEP had less variability and higher predictability and test-retest reproducibility than the OUES. It follows that OUEP may have the potential to better assess severity of dysfunction and to better prognosticate mortality and morbidity in patients with either chronic left or right heart failure [15].However, previously we did not investigate this issue in our patients with pulmonary hypertension .

OUE representing the change in $\dot{V}_2$ as related to $\dot{V}E$, could be affected by cardiac output (CO), difference between systemic and pulmonary arterial blood O_2 contents, lung gas exchange, and changes in pH. OUES is the most widely studied index of OUE, but OUEP, which has not been previously studied in IPAH patients, may have advantages. We had already shown $\dot{V}O_2/\dot{V}E$ is lower and can decline in the transition from rest to exercise in patients with left heart failure [15–16]. We hypothesized that OUEP in IPAH patients could be lower than the normals and decline in the transition from rest to exercise due to inability to adequately increase cardiac output during exercise.

Methods

Patients and control subjects

We retrospectively investigated the exercise pathophysiology in 32 patients with IPAH referred for evaluation and treatment in Shanghai Pulmonary Hospital between 2009 and 2012. For comparison purposes, the CPET and pulmonary function test (PFT) data of 16 healthy subjects of similar age, sex, and body size were also analyzed (6 men and 10 women; mean age 37.88±16.76 yrs). All CPET study participants signed written informed consent. This study was approved by the Institution of Human Subjects Committee at Shanghai Pulmonary Hospital. The diagnosis of IPAH was based on clinical and laboratory data, including right heart catheterization (RHC), according to currently accepted diagnostic criteria (Dana Point, 2008) [17]. Patients with disorders other than IPAH were excluded according to the recommended diagnostic guidelines for IPAH [17]. The patients were non-smokers at the time of study and most had never smoked. The data included only the first PFT and CPET measurements made after referral to our hospital, nearly always prior to the initiation of pulmonary vasodilator therapy.

PFT Measurements

Each patient and normal subject underwent resting measurements of forced vital capacity (FVC), forced expiratory volume in 1 sec (FEV_1), maximum voluntary ventilation (MVV), diffusing capacity for carbon monoxide (DL_{CO}) and total lung capacity (TLC) using standard methodology[18–19] and equipments (Masterscreen-PFT, Jaeger, Hoechberg, Germany; Masterscreen-plethysmography, Jaeger, Hoechberg, Germany). All PFT values were reported in absolute terms and normalized to percentage of predicted (%pred). Predicted spirometry values, TLC and DL_{CO} were calculated using accepted equations for Chinese adults [20].

CPET Procedure and Data Collection

Each patient performed PFT and CPET, after familiarization with the exercise apparatus, on the same day. Before each test, the equipment was calibrated according to manufacturer's specifications using reference and calibration gases. Standard 12 lead electrocardiograms (ECGs) and pulse oximetry were continuously monitored. Blood pressure at the brachial artery was measured every two minutes with an automatic cuff. The exercise protocol consisted of 3 min of rest, 3 min of unloaded cycling at 60 rpm, followed by uniform increase in resistance of 5 to 15 W/min for the patients and 20 to 25 W/min for the normal subjects to maximal tolerance on an electromagnetically braked cycle ergometer (Ergoselect 100, ergoline GmbH, Bitz, Germany) [9]. The rate of increasing work depended on the estimated exercise capacity of the subjects. Subjects were encouraged to exercise to the limits of their functional capacities or until the physician stopped the test because of severe adverse events, such as chest pain, light-headedness, potentially life-threatening arrhythmias, ST-segment changes, or marked systolic hypotension. Most CPET values were reported in absolute terms and normalized to percentage of predicted (%pred). Predicted values were calculated using accepted equations [9].

CPET data Calculations

Carbon dioxide output ($\dot{V}CO_2$, ml/min, STPD), $\dot{V}O_2$ (ml/min, STPD), $\dot{V}E$ (l/min, BTPS), tidal volume (l, BTPS), were measured continuously on a breath-by-breath basis using a CPX Metabolic Measurement Cart (Masterscreen-CPX, Jaeger, Hoechberg, Germany) that was equipped with rapidly-responding O_2 and CO_2 analyzers. Data were averaged every 10 sec. Peak $\dot{V}O_2$ was defined as the highest 30 sec average of $\dot{V}O_2$, and other peak parameters were calculated at the same time. Each AT was determined by the V-slope method [21]. $\dot{V}E$-$\dot{V}CO_2$ slope was determined by linear regression analysis of the relation between $\dot{V}E$ and $\dot{V}CO_2$ during exercise, excluding data above the ventilatory compensation point [22]. Lowest $\dot{V}E/\dot{V}CO_2$ was determined by averaging the lowest consecutive 90 sec data points [22].

In addition, to show patterns of gas exchange change in patients as related to time and exercise intensity during CPET, $\dot{V}O_2/\dot{V}E$, $\dot{V}E/\dot{V}CO_2$ and $P_{ET}CO_2$ values at 4 periods were respectively averaged: the last minute of rest, last minute of unloaded cycling, 1 min before the AT was reached (only for $\dot{V}O_2/\dot{V}E$), 1 min after the AT was reached (only for $\dot{V}E/\dot{V}CO_2$ and $P_{ET}CO_2$) and for 30 sec at peak exercise.

OUE definitions and measurements

The OUES was defined as the regression slope "a" in $\dot{V}O_2 = a \times \log_{10}\dot{V}E + b$. A steeper slope or higher OUES represents a more efficient oxygen uptake per volume of ventilation (Figure 1). The OUEP was defined as the 90 sec average of the highest consecutive measurements of $\dot{V}O_2/\dot{V}E$ near the AT (Figure 2) [14].

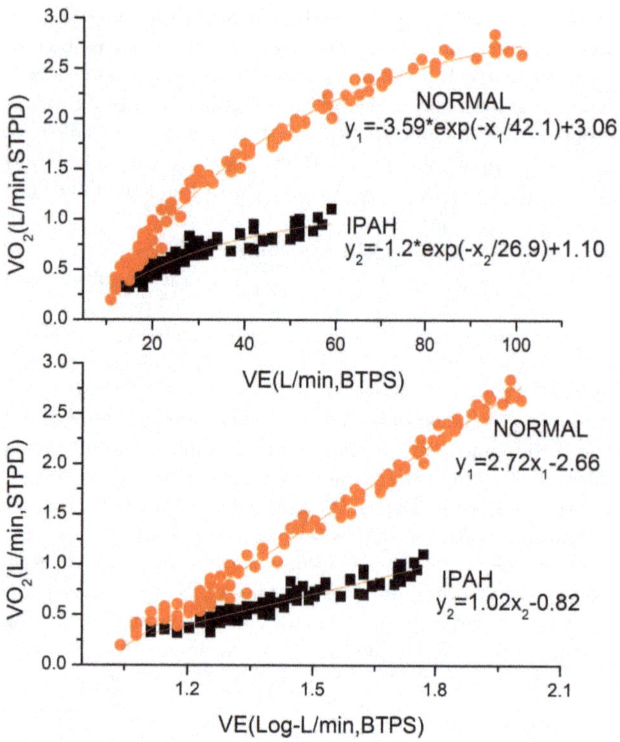

Figure 1. Difference of OUES between a typical IPAH patient and a control subject. Linear (upper panel) and single-segment logarithmic (lower panel) relation between $\dot{V}O_2$ (ml/min) and $\dot{V}E$ (ml/min) for 2 different subjects. Steeper slopes represents more efficient oxygen uptake. The control subject (steeper slopes, aged 24 years; height, 158 cm; weight, 45 kg), has an oxygen uptake efficiency slope (OUES) of 2.72 whereas the IPAH patient (shallower slopes, aged 21 years; height, 161 cm; weight, 47 kg) has an OUES of 1.02.

Statistical analysis

Microsoft Office-2000, SPSS-10.0 and Origin-7.0 computer software were used. Data are expressed as mean ±SD, except where specifically noted. Most PFT and CPET values are expressed in absolute terms and %pred. $P<0.05$ was considered significant. Unpaired Student *t*-test was used for comparison between IPAH patients and normal subjects, whereas X^2 test was performed for gender analysis. The differences in OUE, $\dot{V}E/\dot{V}CO_2$ and $P_{ET}CO_2$ at each time period were respectively assessed by repeated-measures analysis of variance (ANOVA). Correlations between OUE and other variables were determined by Pearson's correlation test, except for NYHA functional classification by Spearman rank correlation test.

Results

Baseline clinical and demographic characteristics

Characteristics of patients and healthy subjects are detailed in Table 1. The female-to-male ratio of the IPAH patients and healthy subjects in this study were about 2:1. The PFT and CPET parameters of the healthy group were within normal limits. The DL_{CO} values were significantly lower in the IPAH patients compared with the normals. The FEV_1/FVC in the IPAH group was significantly lower than the control group, but still within normal limit. Other PFT values were normal. 69% of IPAH patients were NYHA functional class 2 while 75% had cardiac index below 2.5.

All individuals completed their CPET studies without accident or untoward effects. Nearly all patients stopped exercise because of fatigue and/or acute shortness of breath; uncommonly, patients noted palpitations or light-headedness and recovered after resting for several minutes. All subjects declared they had done their best. In IPAH group, except for peak heart rate and peak ventilation, the magnitude of the absolute and percentage of all CPET parameters of oxygen uptake and ventilatory efficiency were strikingly abnormal.

Decrease of OUES in IPAH

As shown in Figure 1, the typical case of IPAH had a lower OUES than the matched normal subject. The OUES of IPAH group was 1.08±0.37 which was significantly lower than 1.98±0.44 of control (p<0.0001).

Changes and contributions in OUE and $\dot{V}E/\dot{V}CO2$ during CPET

As shown in Figure 2, the OUE response of IPAH patient to exercise was clearly different from that of the matched normal subject. At all times, the OUE values of IPAH patient were lower than those of control.

The left top portion of Figure 3 shows OUE values for patients and normal subjects at four time periods. OUE values at all time periods were markedly lower in IPAH patients than in normal subjects ($P<0.001$). In control group, the differences in OUE values at four time periods were significant ($P<0.001$), and changes between adjacent periods were evident ($P<0.001$). However in IPAH group, the differences in OUE values at four time periods were also significant ($P=0.023$), but the magnitude of OUE changes was much smaller than the control group.

Figure 3 left center, shows $\dot{V}E/\dot{V}CO_2$ values at similar times. IPAH patients had significantly greater $\dot{V}E/\dot{V}CO_2$ than normal subjects at all activity levels ($P<0.001$). From rest to the AT, $\dot{V}E/\dot{V}CO_2$ values in control group reduced greatly, however in IPAH group decreased hardly. Compared with $\dot{V}E/\dot{V}CO_2$ values at AT, there was no obvious reduction at peak either for controls or patients.

Figure 3 left bottom, shows the significantly reduced $P_{ET}CO_2$ values at all levels of activity in the IPAH group compared with the control group ($P<0.001$). In the control group, $P_{ET}CO_2$ values distinctively increased with increasing level of activity until AT, thereafter decreased mildly at peak. On the contrary, $P_{ET}CO_2$ values in IPAH patients did not increase at all from resting values.

Figure 3 right side, shows the similarities of both IPAH and Control groups for $\dot{V}O_2$ and $\dot{V}CO_2$ at rest and warm-up ($P>0.05$). There were significant differences at AT ($P<0.05$) and peak exercise ($P<0.001$). However, for $\dot{V}E$, IPAH patients had higher values than those of Control subjects at rest ($P<0.05$) and warm-up ($P<0.001$), but no difference at AT and peak exercise ($P>0.05$). This indicates that at any required metabolic rate (as $\dot{V}O_2$ and $\dot{V}CO_2$), the ventilation is over driven by lung compensation for a limited heart function, i.e. mismatched Q/VA. The low and unchanged $P_{ET}CO_2$ is the evidence of hyperventilation in patients with IPAH.

OUE as related to key abnormal parameters for IPAH patients

The correlations between OUE and other key parameters for IPAH patients are shown in Table 2. OUEP %pred correlated significantly with NYHA functional Class ($r=-0.724$, $P<0.005$), Total Pulmonary Vascular Resistance (TPVR) ($r=-0.694$, $P<0.005$), DLco %pred ($r=0.577$, $P<0.05$), peak $P_{ET}CO_2$ ($r=0.68$,

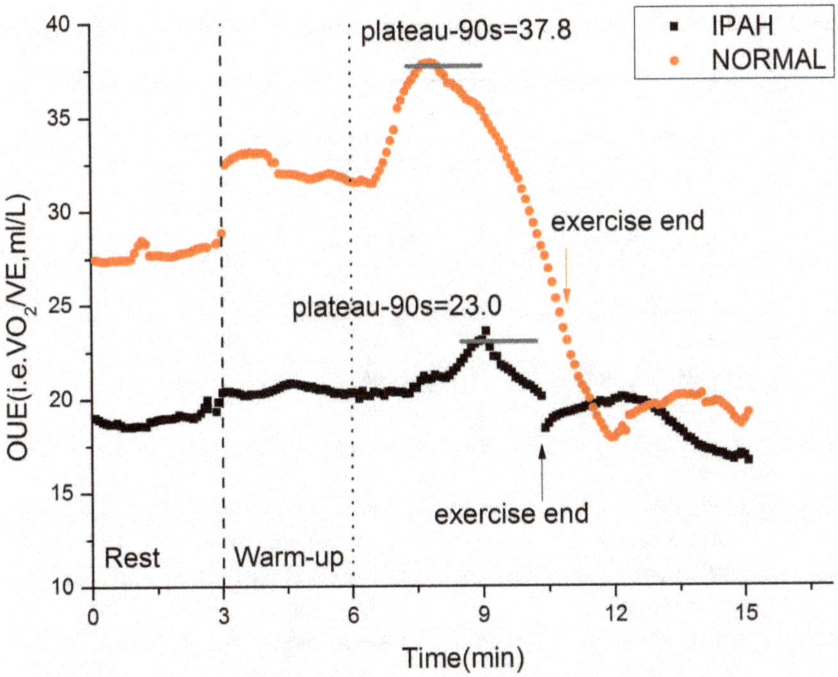

Figure 2. Difference of OUEP and OUE between a typical IPAH patient and a control subject. The kinetics of changes in oxygen uptake efficiency (OUE) for the same tests and subjects as depicted in Figure 1. OUE typically increase during exercise from rest to plateau in normal subjects and then decrease gradually until exercise end. It then decreases further in the immediate recovery period and begin stabilizing after about 2 minutes. In IPAH patients, OUE changes in a similar way as the controls, but is always lower than the controls in the transition from rest to exercise end.

$P<0.005$), and lowest $\dot{V}E/\dot{V}CO_2$ ($r=-0.902$, $P<0.0001$). In contrast, the OUES %pred did not correlate significantly with above parameters ($r=0.125$, -0.015, 0.493, 0.179, -0.136, all $P>0.05$).

Comparison between OUEP and OUES for IPAH patients

Table 3 compares the mean and variability of the OUEP and OUES values in the 32 IPAH patients. The coefficient of variation(COV) of the OUEP (20.9%) was significantly lower than that of the OUES (34.3%) ($P<0.0001$).

Discussion

Although previous studies have demonstrated the clinical utility of CPET in patients with IPAH [3], our study is the first to evaluate the value of OUE measurements driven from CPET in these patients. In addition, our study is the first to show that the decreased OUE can also be a marker representing impaired gas exchange in patients with IPAH. Moreover, we have shown that, beyond the traditional measurements of exercise capacity and ventilatory efficiency, OUEP is better than OUES, because it is less variable and is more significantly correlated with resting pulmonary hemodynamics in these patients.

In the present study, the usual parameters of exercise capacity and gas exchange ($\dot{V}$peak O_2, peak work rate, anaerobic threshold, peak heart rate, peak O_2 pulse, peak $P_{ET}CO_2$, $\dot{V}E$-$\dot{V}CO_2$ slope and lowest $\dot{V}E/\dot{V}CO_2$) were all abnormal in the IPAH patients (Table 1). Peak $\dot{V}O_2$, anaerobic threshold, $\dot{V}E$-$\dot{V}CO_2$ slope, lowest $\dot{V}E/\dot{V}CO_2$, and $P_{ET}CO_2$ are the most commonly used clinical parameters for diagnostic and prognostic information [8,15]. Peak $\dot{V}O_2$ is reduced in patients with higher total pulmonary vascular resistance and lower cardiac index and is highly correlated with the amount of functional pulmonary vascular bed [23]. However, it is strongly influenced by the patients' motivation and supervisors' subjective choice of ending test. In searching for more objective, reliable sub-maximal variables, anaerobic threshold (AT) has been tested. Although AT is significantly correlated with peak $\dot{V}O_2$ [24], it is often not easy to identify, as was the case with 5 of our patients. The AT is also subject to substantial inter-observer and intra-observer variability [25]. Recently, the values of $\dot{V}E/\dot{V}CO_2$ during moderate exercise have been demonstrated as diagnostic and prognostic values in heart failure patients [26].The mechanism responsible for elevated $\dot{V}E/\dot{V}CO_2$ in IPAH patients is considered to be multifactorial. In normal subjects, the ventilatory response ($\dot{V}E$) is approximately linear with the CO_2 output ($\dot{V}CO_2$) during exercise before ventilatory compensation point [22]. In IPAH patients, elevated $\dot{V}E/\dot{V}CO_2$ levels manifest that the ventilation of underperfused alveoli causes an increase in dead space ventilation [4]. Increased $\dot{V}E/\dot{V}CO_2$ levels have also been significantly correlated with decreased cardiac output, elevated pulmonary arterial pressures, decreased alveolar-capillary membrane conductance, and diminished heart rate variability [27–29]. In patients with severe IPAH, the $\dot{V}E/\dot{V}CO_2$ ratio correlates significantly with pulmonary vascular resistance but not with mean pulmonary arterial pressure or cardiac index [30]. Additionally, both resting and peak exercise $P_{ET}CO_2$ values have prognostic value in patients with heart failure [31–32]. However $P_{ET}CO_2$ values are susceptible to multiple factors such as acute hyperventilation, increased dead space (due to emphysema or other lung diseases), or rapid shallow breathing patterns, all of which will reduce the $P_{ET}CO_2$ independently of cardiac function [3]. Compared with all of the above CPET variables, the analysis of OUE has been limited, especially in patients with IPAH.

Table 1. Demographics, hemodynamics, Pulmonary Function Testing and Cardiopulmonary Exercise Testing parameters in IPAH patients and Control subjects.

	IPAH patients (n = 32)	Control subjects (n = 16)
Age, yrs	40.3±14.8	37.9±16.8
Gender, F/M	20/12	10/6
Height, cm	162±7.8	160±9.0
Weight, kg	60.3±13.7	53.2±9.9
Body mass index, kg/m^2	22.8±3.9	20.7±2.2
NYHA functional class	2.3±0.48	NA
mPAP, mm Hg	59.0±14.2	NA
mRAP, mm Hg	11.2±4.8	NA
mPWP, mmHg	8.6±4.4	NA
TPVR, mm Hg/L/min	13.1±5.7	NA
Cardiac index, L/min/m^2	2.48±0.85	NA
FVC, L (%pred)	3.30±0.85 (95±20)	3.45±0.84 (100±14)
FEV_1, L (%pred)	2.56±0.61(87±17)	2.93±0.62(101±15)
FEV_1/FVC (%pred)	78.1±6.7(96±5) *	85.6±5.9(101±6)
MVV, L/min (%pred)	86±25 (98±19)	98±30 (116±18)
DL_{CO}, ml/mm Hg/min (%pred)	17.1±6.5 (79±23) ‡	23.9±5.2(117±15)
TLC, L (%pred)	5.14±0.92 (99±11)	5.13±1.17 (100±12)
Peak $\dot{V}O_2$, ml/min (%pred)	920±298(49±14) ‡	1617±547 (95±15)
Peak work rate, W (%pred)	72±26(54±16) ‡	137±52(102±26)
AT, ml/min (%pred)	615±165(76±14) ‡	937±255(111±10)
Peak heart rate, beats/min (%pred)	146±17(80±7) †	166±12(90±7)
Peak O_2 pulse, ml/beat (%pred)	6.2±1.7(63±17) ‡	9.6±2.8(97±7)
Peak $\dot{V}E$, L/min (%MVV)	49±13(59±16)	61±23(62±7)
Peak $P_{ET}CO_2$, mm Hg	23.2±8.0‡	40.9±2.9
$\dot{V}E$-$\dot{V}CO_2$ slope	51.7±28.1*	27.9±5.9
Lowest $\dot{V}E/\dot{V}CO_2$, (%pred)	49.4±14.9(183±49) ‡	27.7±2.2(106±9)
OUES, L/min/log(L/min) (%pred)	1.08±0.37(58±19) ‡	1.98±0.44(98±13)
OUEP, ml/L (%pred)	23.4±4.9(60±12) ‡	37.8±4.8(98±12)

Values are expressed as mean ± SD and percentage of measured to predicted values (%pred).
*$p<0.05$, †$p<0.005$, ‡$p<0.0001$, vs. controls using unpaired *t* test. NA = not applicable.
NYHA = New York Heart Association functional classification; mPAP = mean pulmonary artery pressure; mRAP = mean right atrial pressure; mPWP = mean pulmonary artery wedge pressure; TPVR = total pulmonary vascular resistance; FVC = forced vital capacity; FEV_1 = forced expiratory volume in 1 second; MVV = maximum voluntary ventilation; DL_{CO} = gas transfer index or diffusing capacity for carbon monoxide; TLC = total lung capacity; AT = anaerobic threshold; %MVV = percentage of maximum voluntary ventilation; $P_{ET}CO_2$ = partial pressure of end-tidal carbon dioxide; OUES = oxygen uptake efficiency slope; OUEP = oxygen uptake efficiency plateau; IPAH = idiopathic pulmonary arterial hypertension; %pred = percent of predicted; $\dot{V}O_2$ = peak oxygen uptake, STPD = standard temperature pressure dry; $\dot{V}E$ = minute ventilation, BTPS = body temperature pressure saturated; $\dot{V}CO_2$ = carbon dioxide output, STPD.

Neither OUES nor OUEP is included in the traditional 9-panel plots [9]. However, they can be measured noninvasively without additional patient effort [4–6]. The OUE may have important prognostic value in exercise physiology in patients with chronic heart failure [15,33]. Davies et al[33] assessed OUES in 243 patients with chronic heart failure and found that only OUES was identified as the sole significant independent prognostic variable in a multivariable model, compared with standard exercise variables. We calculated reference values for OUEP and found that OUEP was the best predictor of mortality ($P<0.0001$) in a study of patients with left heart failure, better than OUES or any other CPET variables. When combined with oscillatory breathing, the odds ratio for death in 6 months increased to 56.3[14–15].

The OUE during exercise in normal subjects is mainly impacted by several factors including cardiac output; alveolar and dead space ventilation; and the matching of the changes in cardiac output and pulmonary blood flow with the increase in alveolar ventilation [14]. We postulate that decreased OUE during CPET in IPAH patients in our present study might be due to an abnormally high pulmonary vascular resistance, leading to the greater right ventricular afterload and reducing cardiac output as well as pulmonary blood flow. The highest OUE usually occurs near AT in normal subjects, because at that time ventilation is often most efficient and matching of perfusion to ventilation is optimal. However, in IPAH patients the volume of pulmonary capillary bed is reduced and the distal pulmonary arteries lose their ability to dilate during exercise. The lower ratio of $\dot{V}O_2$ to $\dot{V}E$ during CPET may be predominantly attributed to the inability to improve ventilation/perfusion match and distribution of blood flow to the metabolizing muscles for IPAH patients. Furthermore, we found that OUEP was sub-maximal exercise parameter, better than the OUES, and did not require maximal exertion, so the

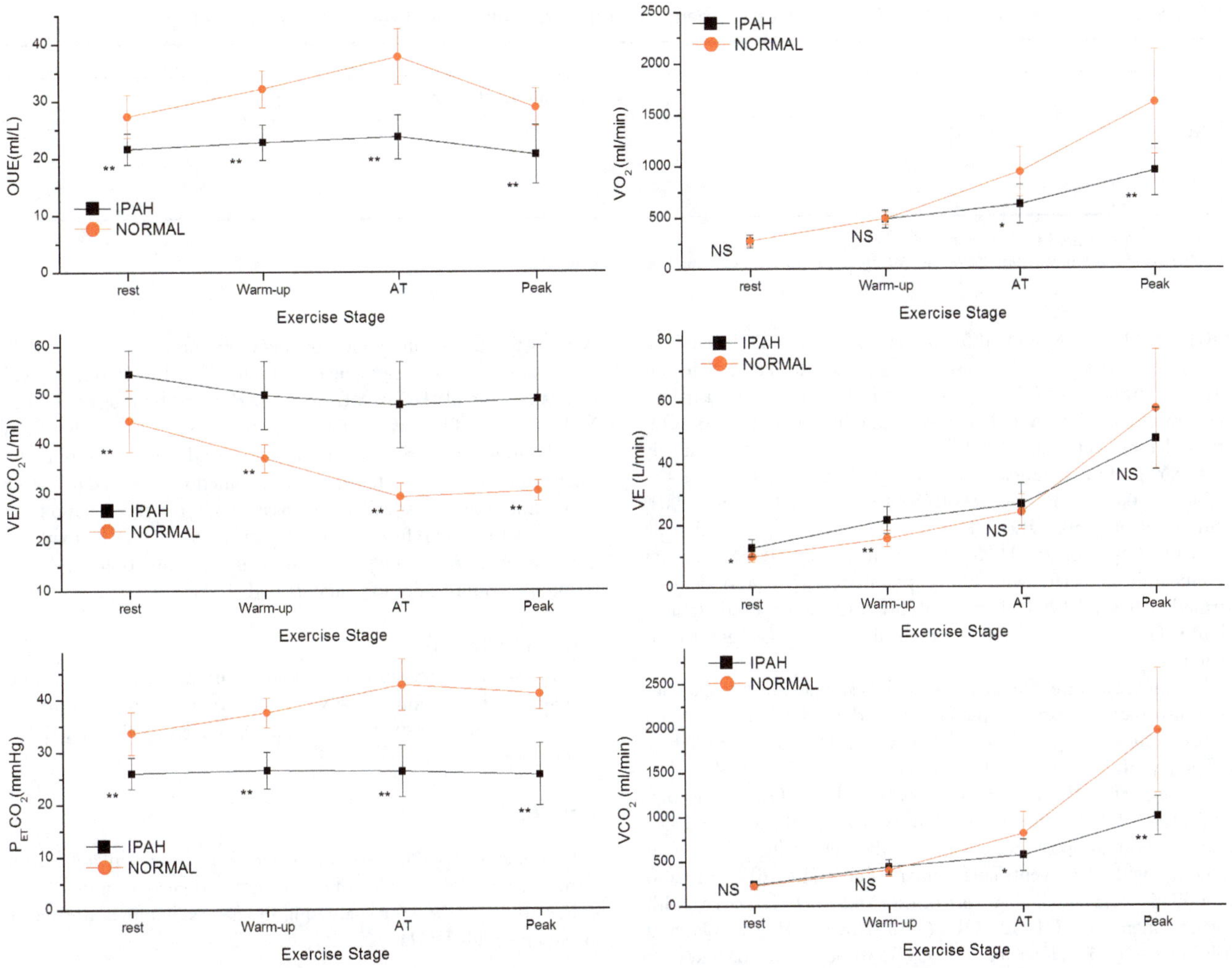

Figure 3. Difference of CPET parameters between IPAH and control groups at different stages of exercise. The group mean±SD Values of IPAH) and control (NORMAL) groups are shown at stages of rest, unloaded cycling, AT, and peak exercise during incremental cycle ergometry tests. Values are. On the left side from top to bottom, they are OUE, $\dot{V}E/\dot{V}CO_2$ and $P_{ET}CO_2$.; on the right side from top to bottom they are $\dot{V}O_2$, $\dot{V}CO_2$ and $\dot{V}E$. Statistically significant differences between groups at the same stage are shown as NS for no significance, * for P<0.05, ** for *P*<0.005, below value symbol.

Table 2. Correlations between OUE and key abnormal parameters for IPAH patients (N = 32).

	OUEP %pred	OUES %pred
NYHA	−0.724**	0.125
mPAP, mm Hg	−0.338	−0.351
TPVR, mm Hg/L/min	−0.694**	−0.015
CI, L/min/m^2	0.295	0.047
DLco, ml/mm Hg/min	0.577*	0.493
Peak$\dot{V}O_2$, (%pred)	0.460	0.009
Peak $P_{ET}CO_2$, mm Hg	0.680**	0.179
Lowest $\dot{V}E/\dot{V}CO_2$ (%pred)	−0.902**	−0.136

*P<0.05, **P<0.005.
The abbreviation definitions are same as Table 1.

Table 3. Mean, SD, range and COV of OUE measurements during Cardiopulmonary Exercise Testing in IPAH patients (N = 32).

	OUEP (ml/L)	OUES [L/min/log(L/min)]
Mean±SD	23.4±4.9	1.1±0.4
Range	11.0-31.0	0.51-1.76
COV	20.9%***	34.3%

***P<0.0001 by paired t test, versus OUES.
COV = coefficient of variation (SD/mean); all other abbreviation definitions are same as Table 1.

OUEP might be more fitted for IPAH patients unable to perform maximal exercise test. As shown in figure 2 and Table 3 in our present study, the OUEP was relatively easier to visualize, recognize, calculate and had less variability than OUES. Our study demonstrated that OUEP %pred was correlated negatively with NYHA functional class ($r = -0.724$, $P<0.005$), TPVR ($r = -0.694$, $P<0.005$), and lowest $\dot{V}E/\dot{V}CO_2$ ($r = -0.902$, $P<0.0001$) and positively with DLco %pred ($r = 0.577$, $P<0.05$) and peak $P_{ET}CO_2$ ($r = 0.68$, $P<0.005$). In contrast, the OUES did not significantly correlate with above parameters. We also demonstrated that OUEP had less variability and higher predictability than OUES for normal subjects regardless of the age, gender, or height[14].

Recently,we were the first one to investigate the full exercise response pattern, exercise physiology and predictions of oxygen uptake efficiency (OUE, i.e. $\dot{V}O_2/\dot{V}E$, ml/L) and ventilatory efficiency of carbon dioxide elimination ($\dot{V}E/\dot{V}CO_2$), their key measurements OUEP and the lowest $\dot{V}E/\dot{V}CO_2$, in normal subjects[14,22] and described their pathophysiological evidence and prognostic importance of early death, specifically as %pred, in patients with left ventricular heart failure[14–16]. We also identified that oscillatory breathing did not interfere with measurements of OUEP, OUE@AT, lowest $\dot{V}E/\dot{V}CO_2$ and $\dot{V}E/\dot{V}CO_2$@AT. However, the OUE response during exercise and the OUEP and OUE@AT were not investigated for IPAH patients. As shown in Figure 3 in our present study, both OUE and $\dot{V}E/\dot{V}CO_2$ abnormalities indicate lower ventilatory efficiency of oxygen uptake and carbon dioxide elimination in IPAH patients. They result from the compensative over driven hyperventilation in order to maintain the required metabolic rate of $\dot{V}O_2$ and $\dot{V}CO_2$ mainly due to the limitation of blood flow perfusion, i.e. Q/VA mismatch. This is a similar mechanism as we previously described in patients with left ventricular heart failure and IPAH[4,6,14–16]. This gas exchange pathophysiology is more clear and easy understanding after we created the new theoretical system of "Holistic Integrative Physiology and Medicine", which demonstrates the intra-coupling pulmonary and cardiovascular systems for the maintenance of metabolic homeostasis in whole body, and gas exchange measurement of CPET is one typical clinical example[34–35]. $\dot{V}E$ can be performed by lungs only, but $\dot{V}O_2$ and $\dot{V}CO_2$ gas exchange needs lung-heart to work in coordination. In primary cardiovascular diseases without the malfunction of other systems, the heart function is limited (as lower $\dot{V}O_2$) and the lungs will compensate with hyperventilation (as higher $\dot{V}E$). Therefore in this regard, the OUEP may be advantageous in evaluating cardiovascular function and gas exchange abnormality for patients with IPAH.

Study Limitations

It is a single center study with smaller sample size; a higher ratio of female distribution (F20/M12). So we plan to do a future investigation to retrospectively and prospectively analyze all IPAH patients from our center.

Conclusion

In conclusion, the OUEP, which can be calculated from retrospective data could offers a new, objective and effort-independent method for evaluating the gas exchange abnormality in patients with IPAH.

Acknowledgments

The authors thank Hai-Jian Liu and Shu-Juan Chen for invaluable support and collaboration in this study. The authors thank Dr. James E. Hansen at Los Angeles Biomedical Research Institute at Harbor-UCLA Medical Center, Torrance, CA, USA for his generous and professional editing.

Author Contributions

Conceived and designed the experiments: JML XGS WLY XYT. Performed the experiments: XYT WLY JG YZ CWW RS SP SGG. Analyzed the data: JML XGS XYT. Contributed reagents/materials/analysis tools: JML XGS. Wrote the paper: JML XYT JG XGS.

References

1. Rich S, Dantzker DR, Ayres SM, Bergofsky EH, Brundage BH, et al (1987) Primary pulmonary hypertension: a national prospective study. Ann Intern Med 107: 216–223.
2. Rubin LJ (1997) Current concepts: primary pulmonary hypertension. N Engl J Med 336: 111–117.
3. American Thoracic Society, American College of Chest Physicians (2003) ATS/ACCP statement on cardiopulmonary exercise testing. Am J Respir Crit Care Med 167: 211–277.
4. Sun XG, Hansen JE, Oudiz RJ, Wasserman K (2001) Exercise pathophysiology in patients with primary pulmonary hypertension. Circulation 104: 429–435.
5. Yasunobu Y, Oudiz RJ, Sun XG, Hansen JE, Wasseeman K (2005) End-tidal Pco_2 abnormality and exercise limitation in patients with primary pulmonary hypertension. Chest 127: 1637–1646.
6. Sun XG, Hansen JE, Oudiz RJ, Wasseeman K (2002) Gas exchange detection of exercise-induced right-to-left shunt in patients with primary pulmonary hypertension. Circulation 105: 54–60.
7. Oudiz RJ, Roveran G, Hansen JE, Sun XG, Wasserman K (2007) Effect of sildenafil on ventilatory efficiency and exercise tolerance in pulmonary hypertension. Eur J Heart Fail 9: 917–921.
8. Oudiz RJ, Middle R, Hovanesyan A, Sun XG, Roveran G, et al (2010) Usefulness of right-to-left shunting and poor exercise gas exchange for predicting prognosis in patients with pulmonary arterial hypertension. Am J Cardiol 105(8): 1186–1191.
9. Wasserman K, Hansen JE, Sue DY, Stringer WW, Whipp BJ (2011) Principles of Exercise Testing and Interpretation, 5th ed. Philadelphia: Lippincott, Williams & Wilkins 568.
10. Baba R, Nagashima M, Goto M, Nagano Y, Yokota M, et al (1996) Oxygen uptake efficiency slope: a new index of cardiorespiratory functional reserve derived from the relation between oxygen uptake and minute ventilation during incremental exercise. J Am Coll Cardiol 28:1567–1572.

11. Hollenberg M, Tager IB (2000) Oxygen uptake efficiency slope: an index of exercise performance and cardiopulmonary reserve requiring only submaximal exercise. J Am Coll Cardiol. 36: 194–201.
12. Baba R, Tsuyuki K, Kimura Y, Ninomiya K, Aihara M, et al. (1999) Oxygen uptake efficiency slope as a useful measure of cardiorespiratory functional reserve in adult cardiac patients. Eur J Appl Physiol Occup Physiol 80: 397–401.
13. Van Laethem C, Van De Veire N, De SJ, Bartunek J, De Backer G, et al. (2006) Prospective evaluation of the oxygen uptake efficiency slope as a submaximal predictor of peak oxygen uptake in aged patients with ischemic heart disease. Am Heart J 152: 297–315.
14. Sun XG, Hansen JE, Sringer WW (2012) Oxygen uptake efficiency plateau: physiology and reference values. Eur J Appl Physiol 112: 919–928.
15. Sun XG, Hansen JE, Sringer WW (2012) Oxygen uptake efficiency plateau best predicts early death in heart failure. Chest 141: 1284–1294.
16. Sun XG, Hansen JE, Sringer WW (2012) A simple new visualization of exercise data discloses pathophysiology and severity of heart failure. J Am Heart Assoc 1:e001883.
17. Simonneau G, Robbins IM, Beghetti M, Channick RN, Delcroix M, et al. (2009) Updated clinical classification of pulmonary hypertension. J Am Coll Cardiol 54: S43–S54.
18. Cotes JE, Chinn DJ, Quanjer PH, Roca J, Yernault JC (1993) Standardization of the measurement of transfer factor (diffusing capacity). Report Working Party Standardization of Lung Function Tests, European Community for Steel and Coal. Official Statement of the European Respiratory Society. Eur Respir J 6: Suppl. 16, S41–S52.
19. Stocks J, Quanjer PH (1995) Reference values for residual volume, functional residual capacity and total lung capacity. ATS workshop on lung volume measurements. Official Statement of the European Respiratory Society. Eur Respir J 8: 492–506.
20. Mu K, Liu S (1990) Summary of Chinese pulmonary function normal values. Beijing Medical University and Peking Union Medical College Press 2: 83–86.
21. Beaver WL, Wasserman K, Whipp BJ (1986) A new method for detecting anaerobic threshold by gas exchange. J Appl Physiol 60: 2020–2027.
22. Sun XG, Hansen JE, Garatachea N, Storer TW, Wasserman K (2002) Ventilatory efficiency during exercise in healthy subjects. Am J Respir Crit Care Med 166: 1443–1448.
23. Guazzi M, Myers J, Arena R (2005) Cardiopulmonary exercise testing in the clinical and prognostic assessment of diastolic heart failure. J Am Coll Cardiol 46: 1883–1890.
24. Itoch H, Taniguchi K, Koike A, Doi M (1990) Evaluation of severity of heart failure using ventilatory gas analysis. Circulation 81 suppl:31–7.
25. Shimizu M, Myers J, Buchanan N (1991) The ventilatory threshold: method, protocol, and evaluator agreement. Am Heart J 122: 509–516.
26. Arena R, Myers J, Guazzi M (2008) The clinical and research applications of aerobic capacity and ventilatory efficiency in heart failure: an evidence-based review. Heart Fail Rev 13: 245–269.
27. Reindl I, Werneck KD, Opitz C (1998) Impaired ventilatory efficiency in chronic heart failure: possible role of pulmonary vasoconstriction. Am Heart J 136: 778–85.
28. Mortara A, La Rovere MT, Pinna GD (1997) Arterial baroreflex modulation of heart rate in chronic heart failure: clinical and hemodynamic correlates and prognostic implications. Circulation 96: 3450–8.
29. Ponikowski P, Anker SD, Chua TP (1997) Depressed heart rate variability as an independent predictor of death in chronic congestive heart failure secondary to ischemic or idiopathic dilated cardiomyopathy. Am J Cardiol 79: 1645–50
30. Ting H, Sun XG, Chuang ML, Lewis DA, Hansen JE, et al. (2011) A noninvasive assessment of pulmonary perfusion abnormality in patients with primary pulmonary hypertension. Chest 119: 824–832.
31. Arena R, Myers J, Abella J, Pinkstaff S, Brubaker P, et al. (2008) The partial pressure of resting end-tidal carbon dioxide predicts major cardiac events in patients with systolic heart failure. Am Heart J 156: 982–988.
32. Arena R, Guazzi M, Myers J (2007) Prognostic value of end-tidal carbon dioxide during exercise testing in heart failure. Int J Cardiol 117: 103–108
33. Davies LC, Wensel R, Georgiadou P, Cicoira M, Coats AJ (2006) Enhanced prognostic value from cardiopulmonary exercise testing in chronic heart failure by non-linear analysis: oxygen uptake efficiency slope. Eur Heart J 27: 684–690.
34. Sun XG (2013) New theoretical system of holistic integrative physiology and medicine: integrative control and regulation of human functions in whole body. Chinese Circulation Journal 28: 88–92
35. Sun XG (2013) New theoretical system of holistic control and regulation for life and cardiopulmonary exercise testing. Medicine and Philosophy 34: 22–27

15

Acute Aerobic Exercise Increases Cortical Activity during Working Memory: A Functional MRI Study in Female College Students

Lin Li[1,2], Wei-Wei Men[3], Yu-Kai Chang[4], Ming-Xia Fan[3], Liu Ji[1,2]*, Gao-Xia Wei[5,6]*

1 Key Laboratory of Adolescent Health Assessment and Exercise Intervention, Ministry of Education, Shanghai, China, **2** Physical Education and Health School, East China Normal University, Shanghai, China, **3** Shanghai Key Laboratory of Magnetic Resonance, East China Normal University, Shanghai, China, **4** Graduate Institute of Athletics and Coaching Science, National Taiwan Sport University, Taiwan, **5** Key Laboratory of Mental Health, Institute of Psychology, Chinese Academy of Sciences, Beijing, China, **6** Key Laboratory of Behavioral Science, Institute of Psychology, Chinese Academy of Sciences, Beijing, China

Abstract

There is increasing evidence that acute aerobic exercise is associated with improved cognitive function. However, neural correlates of its cognitive plasticity remain largely unknown. The present study examined the effect of a session of acute aerobic exercise on working memory task-evoked brain activity as well as task performance. A within-subjects design with a counterbalanced order was employed. Fifteen young female participants (M = 19.56, SD = 0.81) were scanned using functional magnetic resonance imaging while performing a working memory task, the N-back task, both following an acute exercise session with 20 minutes of moderate intensity and a control rest session. Although an acute session of exercise did not improve behavioral performance, we observed that it had a significant impact on brain activity during the 2-back condition of the N-back task. Specifically, acute exercise induced increased brain activation in the right middle prefrontal gyrus, the right lingual gyrus, and the left fusiform gyrus as well as deactivations in the anterior cingulate cortexes, the left inferior frontal gyrus, and the right paracentral lobule. Despite the lack of an effect on behavioral measures, significant changes after acute exercise with activation of the prefrontal and occipital cortexes and deactivation of the anterior cingulate cortexes and left frontal hemisphere reflect the improvement of executive control processes, indicating that acute exercise could benefit working memory at a macro-neural level. In addition to its effects on reversing recent obesity and disease trends, our results provide substantial evidence highlighting the importance of promoting physical activity across the lifespan to prevent or reverse cognitive and neural decline.

Editor: Yijun Liu, University of Florida, United States of America

Funding: This work was supported by grants from Open Research Fund of the Key Laboratory of Adolescent Health Assessment and Exercise Intervention (7823005E), the Research Fund for the Doctoral Program of Higher Education (20110076120029), large instruments Open Foundation of East China Normal University (2013-46), the National Natural Science Foundation of China (31200794, 91132728 to GXW), the Open Research Fund of the Key Laboratory of Mental Health of the Chinese Academy of Sciences (to GXW). The funders had no role in study design, data collection and analysis, decision to publish, or preparation of the manuscript.

Competing Interests: The authors have declared that no competing interests exist.

* E-mail: lji@tyxx.ecnu.edu.cn (LJ); weigx@psych.ac.cn (GXW)

Introduction

The effect of a single session of exercise, also known as acute exercise, on cognition has received growing interest since the pioneering review conducted by Tomporowski [1]. Although there have been some inconsistent findings, subsequent research has generally acknowledged an improvement of cognitive performance following exercise [2]. These facilitative effects of acute exercise on cognitive function have been further established by recent meta-analytical reviews [3,4]. Despite being significantly positive, the magnitude of the detected impact (i.e., the effect sizes) of acute exercise on cognition has varied widely, suggesting that there are factors that moderate the relationship between acute exercise and cognitive function.

The type of cognitive function has been recognized as a primary moderator of exercise and cognition, most likely because exercise training leads, in particular, to more benefits on executive function relative to other cognitive categories (i.e., speed, spatial, and controlled) [5]. Executive function refers to a higher order of cognitive processes that supervise control over several lower levels of cognitive processes and guide the optimal behavior for achieving goal-directed behaviors [6]. These characteristics are responsible for the essential role that executive function plays in daily life. Remarkably, a disproportionate beneficial effect of exercise training has recently also been found for acute exercise. Specifically, although acute exercise improves multiple aspects of cognitive function, executive function receives the greatest positive effect, reflecting that acute exercise results in both general and specific improvements [7]. Notably, rather than acting as a unitary construct, executive function is composed of distinct sub-components, including working memory, inhibition, and shifting [8], and Etnier and Chang [9] postulated that acute exercise would have different influences on specific aspects of executive function. Nevertheless, the majority of studies addressing acute exercise have emphasized the inhibitory aspects of executive function [10,11], leading to an insufficient overall understanding. Therefore, the present study attempted to examine other primary aspects of executive function, particularly working memory, to advance our understanding.

Working memory reflects an executive system involving limited resources that temporarily and simultaneously stores, maintains, and updates complex action-related information [12]. The maximum amount of information that an individual can retain, also known as the working memory capacity, is believed to serve a vital role underlying many cognitive processes and even other aspects of executive function [8]. Previous studies have indicated that working memory reacts sensitively to environmental changes, and improved performance has been observed after intensive cognitive training [13,14]. However, only a few studies have investigated the impact of acute exercise on working memory, with inconsistent results. Specifically, these studies either found that acute exercise resulted in improvements in long-term memory, rather than working memory [15], or showed that exercise improved working memory, depending on the exercise modality (e.g., aerobic exercise) [16] and individual differences (e.g., individuals with a lower working memory) [17]. These few, but diverse studies make it difficult to formulate concrete hypotheses, and further investigation is needed.

In addition to behavioral measures, researchers utilize neuroimaging techniques to investigate the neural correlates underlying the improvement of cognition following acute exercise. Studies examining event-related potential (ERP) found that acute exercise is associated with an increased P300 amplitude and shortened P300 latency, indicating that acute exercise enhances attentional resource allocation as well as speeds the efficiency of classification for stimulus evaluation, thus providing the mechanism at the neural level [18,19]. Such ERP studies have undoubtedly established a better understanding of the effects of acute exercise on cognition. However, ERP tends to be temporally oriented and provides limited information regarding the spatial locations of brain activity during certain cognitive tasks. Recently, functional magnetic resonance imaging (functional MRI) has been applied as a promising technique for observing changes in global cortical activity elicited by cognitive tasks [20,21]. This technique measures the blood oxygenation that accompanies neuronal activity and establishes a bridge between cognitive function and brain activity, elucidating the neural systems related to exercise and cognition. Indeed, individuals with higher fitness show greater activation or more extensive neural networks in specific brain regions (e.g., the frontal and parietal cortices), which might, in turn, play a mediating role in the improvement of cognitive function. This technique can advance exercise-cognition research [20–22]. However, to our knowledge, studies investigating the effect of acute exercise on cognitive performance have yet to use functional MRI, and it remains largely unknown whether neural activity related to working memory is altered by acute exercise. Therefore, the use of functional MRI to explore the functional alterations of brain activity induced by acute exercise should receive more attention [23].

The present study aimed to investigate the effect of acute aerobic exercise on the working memory aspect of executive function while simultaneously investigating the underlying neural mechanism, as assessed through functional MRI. This technique was aimed at obtaining new insight linking exercise, executive function, and the brain. We hypothesized that acute aerobic exercise would improve working memory and change the functional pattern of brain activity associated with working memory.

Materials and Methods

Ethics Statement

The experimental procedure was approved by the Institutional Review Board of the East China Normal University and met the standards of the Declaration of Helsinki. Each participant was informed of the discomfort associated with acute exercise and provided written informed consent.

Participants

Fifteen healthy female college students, aged 19 to 22 years, were voluntarily recruited through advertisements and fliers at East China Normal University. The sample size satisfied the criteria of a power analysis from a 2×4 mixed design with a power of 0.8, an alpha of 0.05, and an effect size of $g = 1.41$, where these parameters were based upon a recent meta-analysis that specifically focused on acute exercise and working memory [24]. The gender of the participants and their education level were restricted to avoid potential confounders of neural activation [25,26]. The participants' demographic characteristics were as follows: height (cm), $M = 161.56$, $SD = 3.12$; weight (kg), $M = 50.75$, $SD = 3.44$; body mass index, $M = 19.45$, $SD = 1.38$; and education (years), $M = 14$, $SD = 0.00$. All participants were first screened by the University's Mental Counselling Center to ensure that they had no mental problems or disorders. Their medical and neurological histories were also screened, and individuals with a history of hearing or vision problems, physical injury, seizures, metal implants, head trauma with loss of consciousness, or substance abuse were excluded. The additional inclusion criteria were being right handed (Edinburgh Handedness Questionnaire), not currently menstruating (self-report question), and not pregnant. Importantly, participants were required to report their involvement in physical activities. As a result, none of the participants included in this study engaged in regular physical exercise. Furthermore, we requested that the participants get adequate sleep and not drink stimulating caffeine-containing beverages within 24 hours before the examination. In addition, we confirmed the usual MRI contraindications prior to functional MRI scanning (e.g., metallic objects or tattoos on the body).

Working Memory Measures

A modified N-back task was programmed using E-Prime to assess working memory [27]. The N-back task consists of a sequence of stimuli, in which participants are asked to identify whether the current stimulus matches the stimulus from N steps earlier in the sequence, and the cognitive load is elevated with the operating number of N. The N-back task applied in the present study, designed using E-Prime software, consisted of 0-back, 1-back, and 2-back conditions, in which a letter stimulus (e.g., A to Z) was presented in a red, green, or yellow color, respectively. Each block condition included 18 trials (6 target trials and 12 non-target trials) in random order. Each letter stimulus was displayed on the screen for 2,000 ms. The participant was instructed to respond to the target trial by pressing a button on the keyboard with her right finger.

In the 0-back condition, the target trial consisted of a stimulus presented as the letter "X". In the 1-back condition, the target trial was a letter stimulus that was identical to the letter that immediately preceded it (i.e., the letter presented one trial back), whereas in the 2-back condition, the target trial was a letter stimulus that was identical to the letter presented two positions before it (i.e., the letter presented two trials back). The participants were asked to complete six alternating blocks, in the order 0-back, 1-back, and 2-back, twice, with 50-second resting intervals

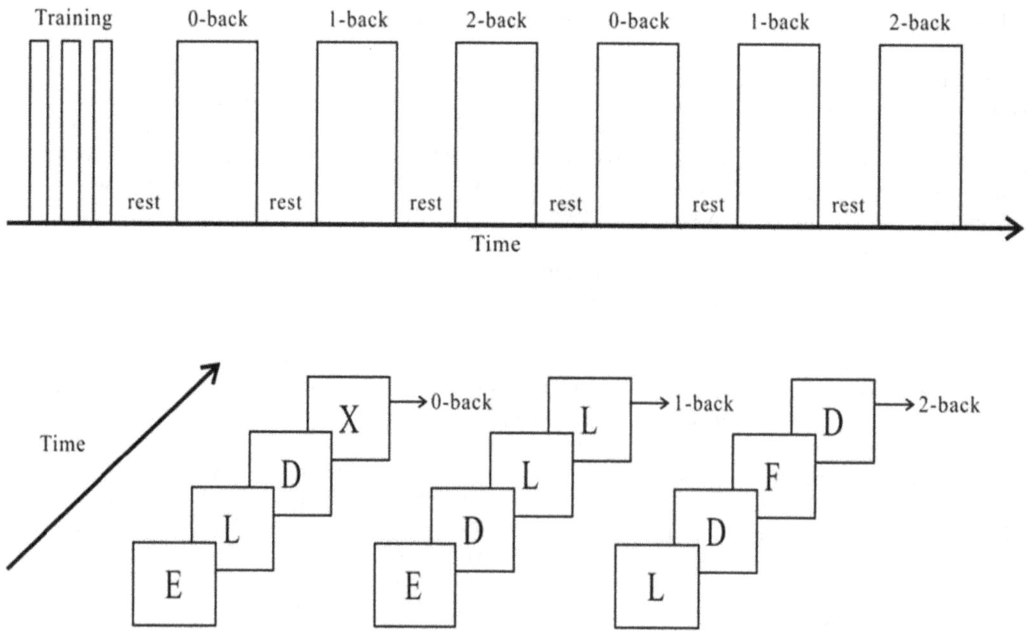

Figure 1. Schematic illustration of the experimental procedure and an example of the resultant stimulation under the three conditions of the N-back task.

between each block (Figure 1). The total experiment duration was 422 seconds. Reaction time and accuracy were further identified as behavioral measures for each trial.

Experimental Procedure

The present study employed a within-subjects design with a counterbalanced order to minimize the learning effect. The participants were tested individually in the laboratory and conducted the working memory task during functional MRI scans in two separate sessions, with a seven-day interval. The participants were also instructed to not undertake any physical activity or physical education course, and the sessions occurred at the same time of day at both visits.

During the first session, the participants were screened using the inclusion criteria, provided their demographic data, completed an ethical procedure, and went through a practice trial of the N-back task. The participants then underwent an acute session of aerobic exercise, including a 5-minute warm-up, cycling ergometer exercise for 20 minutes, and a 5-minute cool-down. The intensity of exercise was set at a heart rate of 120 beats/min on a cycling ergometer, with a graded work load of a 60–70 rpm/min pedaling rate. The work rate of the acute exercise, corresponding to 60% to 70% of the estimated maximal heart rate (calculated based on 220-age), has been shown to improve multiple aspects of cognitive function [18,28]. Following the acute exercise session, the participants were instructed to conduct the N-back task while undergoing a functional MRI scan within 15 minutes after the cessation of exercise.

The second session was a control session that consisted of 20 minutes of quiet, seated resting. The participants were then scanned while performing the N-back task again, in an manner identical to the first session. Their heart rates were assessed with a heart rate monitor (Suunto t6, Serial No. 60502677, Finland) with recordings set to occur at 10-second intervals throughout the experimental process. At the end of the experimental protocol, the participants were briefly informed of the purpose of the research.

Functional MRI Data Acquisition and Scanning Protocol

All brain images were acquired using a 3T Trio Tim scanner (Siemens, Erlangen, Germany) with a 32-channel head matrix coil. The N-back task was presented with ESys by Invivo Company. Functional images were obtained using an echo-planar imaging (EPI) sequence, with the following scan parameters: TR = 2,000 ms, TE = 30 ms, flip angle (FA) = 90°, slice thickness = 3.75 mm, field of view (FOV) = 192×192 mm^2, and voxel size = $3.0 \times 3.0 \times 3.75$ mm^3. The resulting data included 243 brain volumes with 32 axial slices. During the functional MRI scans, all of the subjects were instructed to keep their eyes closed, relax, and move as little as possible. High-resolution structural images were acquired using a magnetization-prepared rapid gradient echo (MPRAGE) three-dimensional T1-weighted sequence (TR = 2530 ms, TE = 2.34 ms, T1 = 1100 ms, FA = 7°, thickness = 1 mm, field of view (FOV) = 256×256 mm^2, voxel size = $1.0 \times 1.0 \times 1.0$ mm^3).

Statistical Analysis of Functional MRI Data

Functional image preprocessing and statistical analyses were carried out using SPM8 (http://www.fil.ion.ucl.ac.uk/spm/software/spm8/). The first five images of each time series were excluded to account for T1-stabilization effects. For each participant, EPI images were slice-time corrected and realigned to the first image, followed by normalization to the standard Montreal Neurological Institute EPI template and spatial smoothing using a Gaussian kernel (8 mm^3 full width at half maximum). Contrast images were generated for each participant for the contrasts of interest (0-back > rest, 1-back > rest, 2-back > rest, respectively, in the control and exercise sessions), representing the pair-wise comparison of parameter estimates for the conditions, and then, separate single-group t tests were used to identify within-group contrasts of interest. Differences between any of the two groups were examined using two-sample t tests, masked by the single-sample t test results. All statistical maps were set at a level of an uncorrected cluster significance threshold of $p = 0.001$ ($Z > 2.3$) and a cluster size >5 voxels [29–31]. Activation maps were overlaid on the group mean high-resolution images for display purposes.

Results

Behavioral Performance

Table 1 presents the detailed behavioral measures obtained based on the treatment session and the N-back condition. A 2 (session: control versus exercise) ×3 (N-back task condition: 0-back, 1-back, versus 2-back) repeated-measures ANOVA of reaction time revealed a significant main effect of the N-back task condition (F (2, 28) =8.18, p<.01, partial eta square =.37). A follow-up post-hoc analysis revealed that the reaction time under the 2-back condition was significantly longer than that under the 1-back and 0-back conditions. However, no significant differences were found for the main effect of session or the interaction of the session and condition (p>.05).

Similar to the results for the reaction time, a 2×3 ANOVA of accuracy revealed that there was a significant main effect of the N-back task condition (F (2, 28) =16.40, p<.01, partial eta square =.54). Follow-up post-hoc analysis revealed that the accuracy under the 2-back was significantly lower than that under the 1-back and 0-back conditions. No significant differences were found for the main effect of session or the interaction of the session and condition (p>.05).

Moreover, the mean heart rate was 83.23±6.36 beats per minute (bpm) in the resting state and 135.37±16.43 bpm during exercise.

Functional MRI Results

A main effect of the N-back condition was generally observed in both the control and exercise sessions. The functional MRI results revealed that the 2-back condition was associated with the most extensive activation of brain regions (i.e., the frontal lobe, subcortical area, occipital lobe, parietal lobe, and temporal lobe), whereas activation in the 0-back condition was associated with the smallest number of brain regions (e.g., the frontal lobe and occipital lobe) in the exercise session (Figure 2, also see Table S1). Similarly, the regional brain activation in the 2-back condition was the most extensive (i.e., frontal lobe, subcortical area, occipital lobe, parietal lobe, and temporal lobe), whereas the 0-back condition induced activation of the smallest number of brain regions (e.g., the frontal lobe, subcortical area, occipital lobe, and temporal lobe) in the control session (see Figure 2 and Table S1).

Additional analysis of the brain regions activated under the three N-back conditions revealed that the commonly activated regions were the left precentral gyrus and the left inferior occipital lobe in the exercise session versus the left precentral gyrus, the right cerebellum, and the supplementary motor areas in the control session. Among these regions, the cluster sizes generally corresponded to the cognitive load, with the largest cluster size being found under the 2-back condition and the smallest cluster size under the 0-back condition (Table 2).

Regarding contrasts between the exercise and control sessions, a two-sample t-test revealed a significant difference in activation between the exercise and control sessions under the 2-back condition (p<0.001, uncorrected), whereas no significant differences were observed between the two sessions under the 1-back and 0-back conditions (Figure 2). Specifically, the acute exercise session resulted in greater activation of the right middle frontal gyrus (BA 10), the right lingual gyrus (BA 17), and the left fusiform gyrus (BA 19) and less activation of the anterior cingulate cortex (BA 32), the left inferior frontal gyrus (BA 47), and the right paracentral lobule (BA 4) relative to the control session under the 2-back condition (Figure 3, Table 3).

Discussion

A rapidly growing body of literature indicates that acute aerobic exercise improves cognitive function from both the behavioral and neuroelectric perspectives. However, no study had previously investigated the effect of acute exercise on working memory using functional MRI. To our knowledge, the present study is the first designed to examine the behavioral change of working memory assessed in an N-back task following the cessation of acute exercise and to explore the macro-scale level of the neural system underlying the effect of exercise on working memory. The results are partially consistent with our prediction; although moderate acute exercise failed to improve working memory at the behavioral level, acute exercise significantly influenced brain activation under the 2-back condition, with increased activation of the right middle prefrontal gyrus, the right lingual gyrus, and the left fusiform gyrus and decreased activation of the anterior cingulate cortexes, the left inferior frontal gyrus, and the right paracentral lobule. These results may be of great importance for understanding the neural correlates of the effect of acute exercise on working memory.

The lack of significant differences in behavioral performance found between the exercise and control sessions contradicted our hypothesis. The failure to replicate previous findings may be attributed to the small sample size, as previous studies included sample sizes ranging from 20 to 48 [16,17]. However, the absence of an effect of acute exercise on working memory is not unique to this study. In a study involving a similar number of participants [15], acute exercise only positively impacted long-term memory, whereas there was no improvement in the cognitive task applied to measure working memory. Similarly, a recent study indicated that an acute session of yoga (but not aerobic exercise on a treadmill) improved working memory performance, suggesting that an exercise mode other than aerobic exercise may benefit working memory [32]. Clearly, further research will be required to replicate these findings by increasing sample sizes and examining different types of exercise.

Table 1. Behavioral performances under the N-back task conditions in the control and exercise sessions.

	Control session		Exercise session	
Condition	**Accuracy (%)**	**Reaction Time (ms)**	**Accuracy (%)**	**Reaction Time (ms)**
0-back	95.15±4.13	310.51±22.56	94.09±5.32	304.34±25.68
1-back	92.58±6.26	315.54±21.22	92.62±5.62	312.66±19.14
2-back	84.64±6.19	326.69±19.03	87.96±6.53	318.97±22.01

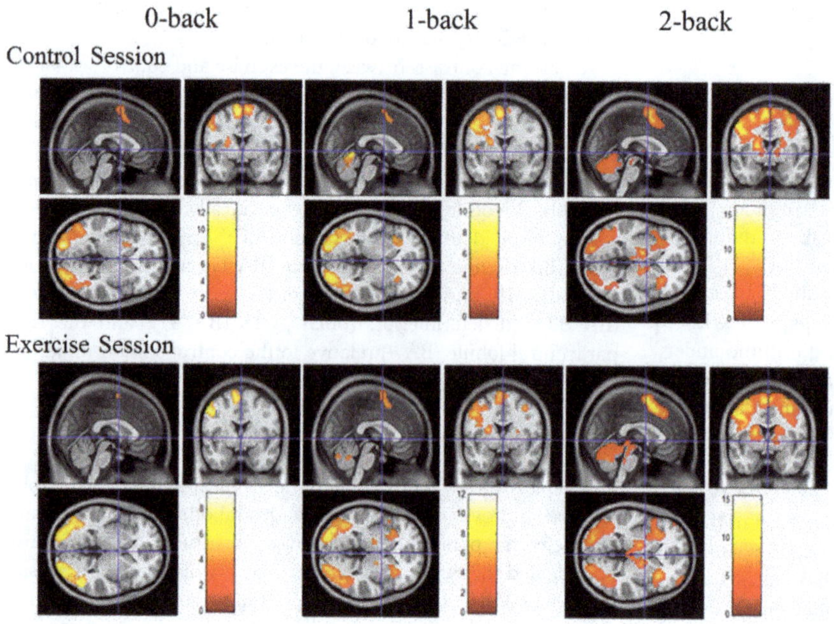

Figure 2. Brain activation maps during the performance of the N-back task in the exercise session and the control session at the level of $p<0.001$ (uncorrected), Z>2.3, and a cluster size >5 voxels for comparisons using cluster detection. Red areas indicate greater activation during the N-back condition relative to the resting condition.

The present study showed that brain activation corresponded to the applied N-back conditions, regardless of the treatment session. Specifically, the 2-back condition resulted in global brain activation, including the frontal lobe, occipital lobe, parietal lobe, temporal lobe, and subcortical area, whereas the 0-back condition activated limited brain regions, such as the frontal and occipital lobes. Additionally, the resultant cluster sizes were generally observed to be larger under the 2-back condition and smallest under the 0-back condition, implying that an increased load of executive control was positively correlated with extensive activated brain regions and with larger cluster sizes. The finding that brain activation reflected the demand for executive control is in agreement with previous studies [33,34] and thus confirms the validity of the applied executive function task and functional MRI modality.

Functional MRI scanning identified differential activation patterns in several brain regions under the 2-back condition in response to exercise relative to the control session. Specifically, acute exercise was positively associated with regional activation in the prefrontal lobe (i.e., the right middle frontal gyrus) and occipital lobe (including the right lingual gyrus and left fusiform gyrus). The prefrontal cortex is considered the brain region that is typically activated during the performance of a working memory task. The right middle frontal gyrus, located in the ventral and frontal pole area, is believed to reflect the coordination and shifting of information among multiple cognitive tasks and functions as an important area for executing and regulating working memory [33,35]. Similarly, the detection of activation in both the lingual and fusiform areas located in the medial occipital cortex distinguished tasks involving different levels of working memory, suggesting that the solving of complex tasks can be attributed to these brain regions [36]. Our finding that acute exercise is associated with these brain regions is consistent not only with our hypothesis but also with recent studies using functional near-infrared spectroscopy (NIRS) [37,38]. Tsujii, Komatsu and Sakatani [38] indicated that moderate acute aerobic exercise increases both working memory and cortical hemodynamic responses in the prefrontal cortex. With an emphasis on other

Table 2. Cluster sizes of commonly activated brain regions under the N-back task conditions in the control and exercise sessions.

		N-back Conditions		
		0-back	**1-back**	**2-back**
Control session				
	Left precentral gyrus	22	68	1031
	Right cerebellum	31	49	584
	Supplementary motor area	163	65	5
Exercise session				
	Left precentral gyrus	33	58	2034
	Left Inferior Occipital lobe	226	391	342

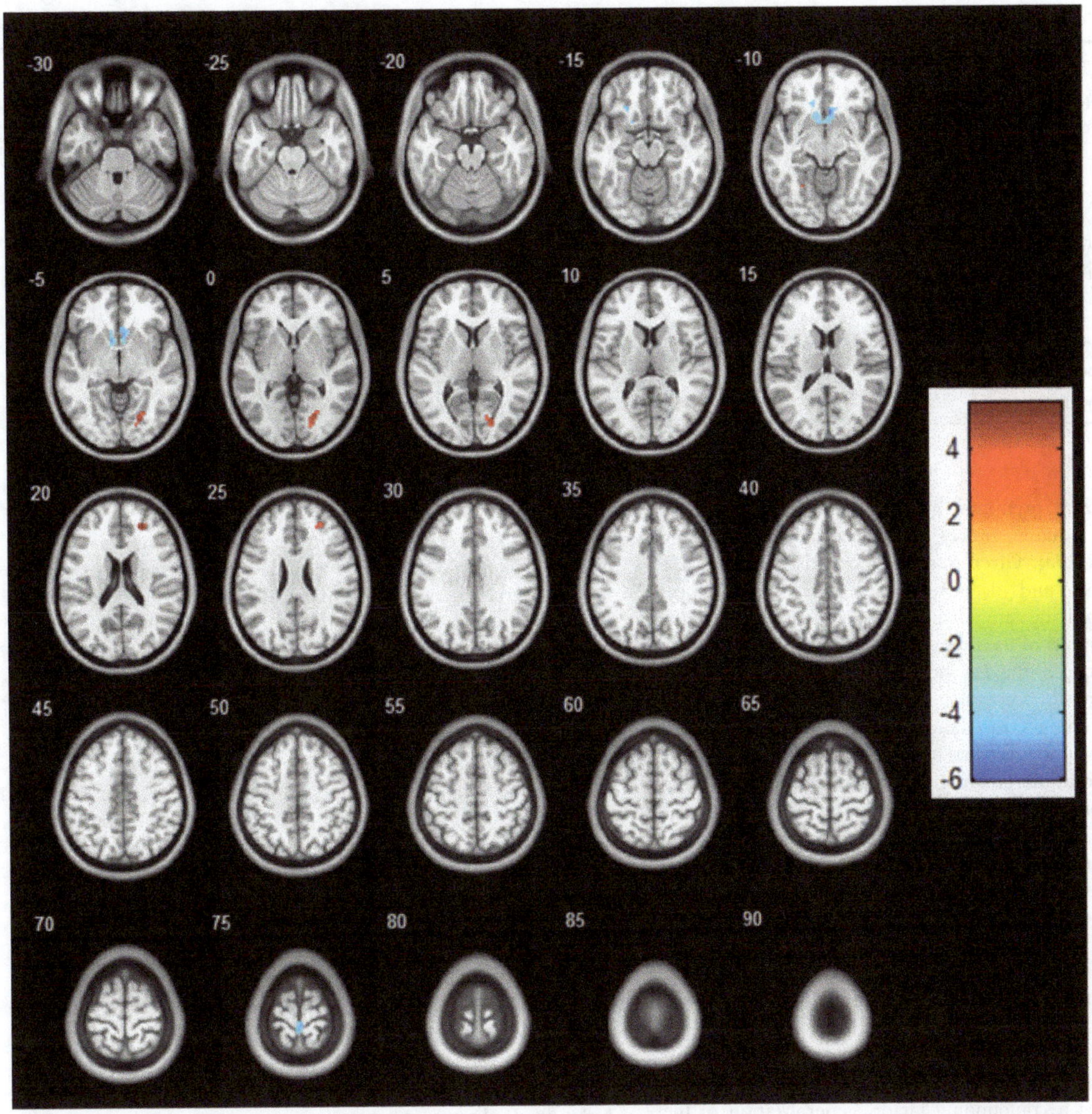

Figure 3. Two-sample t-test analysis: fMRI activation maps under the 2-back condition between the exercise and control sessions (exercise session > control session) at the level of $p<0.001$ (uncorrected), Z>2.3, and a cluster size >5 voxels for comparisons using cluster detection. Red areas indicate greater activation during the 2-back condition in the exercise session relative to the control session. Blue areas indicate greater activation during the 2-back condition in the control session relative to the exercise session.

executive controls (e.g., interference), similar results were also observed, including improved behavioral performance following a short session of aerobic exercise, with the right frontopolar area specifically being activated [37]. These findings suggest that these specific brain cortexes play vital roles in the alteration of executive function induced by acute exercise. The present study also found that these specific regions following acute exercise were markedly activated under the 2-back condition, which involved a higher executive control load, but not under the 1-back or 0-back condition. This result suggests that acute exercise may have greater effect on an executive function task that required a heavier cognitive load. These disproportional effects of acute exercise are in agreement with previous studies using neuroelectric techniques [18,39]. Along with the robust relationship between the prefrontal cortex and executive function, our study extends knowledge regarding the relationship between acute exercise and neuronal activation by providing a spatial perspective at a macro-level using the functional MRI technique.

Interestingly, we also observed deactivation in the anterior cingulate cortexes and the left inferior frontal gyrus following the termination of acute exercise, which may provide an alternative viewpoint to explain the beneficial effect of acute exercise. The anterior cingulate cortex, located in the medial frontal lobe, is believed to reflect the response conflict and adaptation in monitoring the attentional control network [40]. To enhance cognitive processes, reduction of activity in the anterior cingulate cortex occurs during goal-directed cognitive demand [41]. These decreases in brain activation constitute the "default mode of brain function" hypothesis [41,42]. The deactivation in the anterior cingulate cortex observed in the present study agrees with the default mode hypothesis and provides another interpretation of the facilitative effect of acute exercise on cognition at the macro-scale level of the brain. Moreover, the left inferior frontal gyrus, located

Table 3. Brain activation comparisons during the 2-back task in the exercise and control sessions.

Brain region (Brodmann, BA)	Cluster Size	MNI coordinates			Z score	t	p
		X	Y	Z			
Exercise > Control							
Right middle frontal gyrus (BA 10)	19	24	45	21	5.03	3.74	0.000
Right lingual gyrus (BA 17)	50	21	−78	3	5.33	3.88	0.000
Left fusiform gyrus (BA 19)	6	−27	−57	−12	4.12	3.28	0.000
Control > Exercise							
Anterior cingulate cortex (BA 32)	57	6	21	−9	5.92	4.12	0.000
Right paracentral lobule (BA 4)	20	3	−33	75	5.08	3.76	0.000
Left inferior frontal gyrus (BA 47)	17	−15	30	−12	4.82	3.64	0.000

in the ventral lateral prefrontal gyrus, is thought to play an executive role in semantic processing, including encoding and retrieval processing [43]. Given that acute exercise activated the right frontal gyrus and deactivated the left frontal gyrus simultaneously (implying an advantage of the specific frontal hemisphere), the results of the present study possibly indicate that decreased activation in the left hemisphere might represent a reduction of semantic processing or may refer to functional compensation for the increased activation of the contralateral hemisphere. This hypothesis warrants further examination.

Factors limiting our interpretation should be acknowledged, and further investigation is required. The findings of the present work may be restricted by the small sample size, as neuroimaging requires substantial statistical power. Further research with a larger sample size is encouraged; however, the sample examined in the present study could accurately reflect brain activity in accordance with the complexity of the cognitive task and differences in brain activation induced by acute exercise, suggesting that acute exercise does have a positive impact on brain activation. Another limitation could be the gender of participants in the present work. Because our participants were restricted to a specific gender (female) and because this restriction could potentially be a confounding factor, generalization of the current results should be carried out cautiously. However, previous studies investigating acute exercise and cognition have not examined the role of gender or whether gender moderates this relationship. Future research should employ a larger sample size with a proper gender distribution. Finally, future studies should monitor the physiological state or the mental state with objective measurement during scanning to exclude the influence of other potential factors on the results.

In conclusion, the results of the present study indicated that moderate acute aerobic exercise had a limited influence on working memory. Nevertheless, acute exercise activated the prefrontal and occipital cortexes, which are associated with executive control, particularly in the task involving conditions incurring greater cognitive demand. A similar positive influence of acute exercise was also revealed by the deactivation of the anterior cingulate cortex and left frontal hemisphere, implying that acute exercise leads to a default mode status and functional compensation during the performance of complex executive processes. Based on these preliminary positive findings, future research on macro-scale neural network or functional connectivity is warranted to explore the relationships among acute exercise, executive function, and the brain using a functional MRI approach to advance our understanding.

Supporting Information

Table S1 Brain activation of N-back tasks and treatment sessions. It showed the cluster size, coordinates and peak intensity for each activated brain region under 6 conditions (sessions* N-back task).

Acknowledgments

We thank graduate student Mr. Li Xin for his help on performing the experiment and Miss. Li Wei for hard work on data collecting.

Author Contributions

Conceived and designed the experiments: GXW LJ LL. Performed the experiments: LL GXW. Analyzed the data: WWM MXF. Contributed reagents/materials/analysis tools: GXW LJ LL. Wrote the paper: GXW YKC LL.

References

1. Tomporowski PD, Ellis NR (1986) Effects of exercise on cognitive processes: a review. Psychol Bull 99: 338–346.
2. Tomporowski PD (2003) Effects of acute bouts of exercise on cognition. Acta Psychol (Amst) 112: 297–324.
3. Chang YK, Labban JD, Gapin JI, Etnier JL (2012) The effects of acute exercise on cognitive performance: a meta-analysis. Brain Res 1453: 87–101.
4. Lambourne K, Tomporowski PD (2010) The effect of exercise-induced arousal on cognitive task performance: a meta-regression analysis. Brain Res 1341: 12–24.
5. Colcombe SJ, Kramer AF (2003) Fitness effects on the cognitive function of older adults: a meta-analytic study. Psychol Sci 14: 125–130.
6. Jurado MB, Rosselli M (2007) The elusive nature of executive functions: a review of our current understanding. Neuropsychol Rev 17: 213–233.
7. Chang YK, Tsai CL, Huang CC, Wang CC, Chu IH (2014) Effects of acute resistance exercise on cognition in late middle-aged adults: general or specific cognitive improvement? J Sci Med Sports 17: 51–55.
8. Miyake A, Friedman NP, Emerson MJ, Witzki AH, Howerter A, et al. (2000) The unity and diversity of executive functions and their contributions to complex "frontal lobe" tasks: a latent variable analysis. Cogn Psychol 41: 49–100.
9. Etnier JL, Chang YK (2009) The effect of physical activity on executive function: a brief commentary on definitions, measurement issues, and the current state of the literature. J Sport Exerc Psychol 31: 469–483.
10. Kamijo K, Hayashi Y, Sakai T, Yahiro T, Tanaka K, et al. (2009) Acute effects of aerobic exercise on cognitive function in older adults. J Gerontol B Psychol Sci Soc Sci 64: 356–363.

11. Pontifex MB, Hillman CH (2007) Neuroelectric and behavioral indices of interference control during acute cycling. Clin Neurophysiol 118: 570–580.
12. Baddeley AD (2003) Working memory: looking back and looking forward. Nat Rev Neurosci 4: 829–839.
13. Olesen P, Westerberg H, Klingberg T (2004) Increased prefrontal and parietal activity after training of working memory. Nat Neurosci: 75–79.
14. Westerberg H, Klingberg T (2007) Changes in cortical activity after training of working memory-a single-subject analysis. Physiol Behav 92: 186–192.
15. Coles K, Tomporowski PD (2008) Effects of acute exercise on executive processing, short-term and long-term memory. J Sports Sci 26: 333–344.
16. Pontifex MB, Hillman CH, Fernhall B, Thompson KM, Valentini TA (2009) The Effect of acute aerobic and resistance exercise on working memory. Med Sci Sports Exerc 41: 927–934.
17. Sibley BA, Beilock SL (2007) Exercise and working memory: an individual differences investigation. J Sport Exerc Psychol 29: 783–791.
18. Hillman CH, Snook EM, Jerome GJ (2003) Acute cardiovascular exercise and executive control function. Int J Psychophysiol 48: 307–314.
19. Kamijo K, Nishihira Y, Higashiura T, Kuroiwa K (2007) The interactive effect of exercise intensity and task difficulty on human cognitive processing. Int J Psychophysiol 65: 114–121.
20. Voss MW, Erickson KI, Prakash RS, Chaddock L, Malkowski E, et al. (2010) Functional connectivity: a source of variance in the association between cardiorespiratory fitness and cognition? Neuropsychologia 48: 1394–1406.
21. Erickson KI, Colcombe SJ, Wadhwa R, Bherer L, Peterson MS, et al. (2007) Training-induced functional activation changes in dual-task processing: an fMRI study. Cereb Cortex 17: 192–204.
22. Colcombe SJ, Kramer AF, Erickson KI, Scalf P, McAuley E, et al. (2004) Cardiovascular fitness, cortical plasticity, and aging. Proc Natl Acad Sci U S A 101: 3316–3321.
23. Voss MW, Nagamatsu LS, Liu-Ambrose T, Kramer AF (2011) Exercise, brain, and cognition across the lifespan. J Appl physiology 111: 1505–1513.
24. McMorris T, Sproule J, Turner A, Hale BJ (2011) Acute, intermediate intensity exercise, and speed and accuracy in working memory tasks: a meta-analytical comparison of effects. Physiology & behavior 102: 421–428.
25. Lowe PA, Mayfield JW, Reynolds CR (2003) Gender differences in memory test performance among children and adolescents. Archives of Clinical Neuropsychology 18: 865–878.
26. Stratta P, Prosperini P, Daneluzzo E, Bustini M, Rossi A (2001) Educational level and age influence spatial working memory and Wisconsin Card Sorting Test performance differently: a controlled study in schizophrenic patients. Psychiatry research 102: 39–48.
27. Gevins AS, Cutillo BC (1993) Neuroelectric evidence for distributed processing in human working memory. Electroencephalogr Clin Neurophysiol 87: 128–143.
28. Chang YK, Tsai CL, Hung TM, So EC, Chen FT, et al. (2011) Effects of acute exercise on executive function: a study with a Tower of London Task. J Sport Exerc Psychol 33: 847–865.
29. Forman SD, Cohen JD, Fitzgerald M, Eddy WF, Mintun MA, et al. (1995) Improved assessment of significant activation in functional magnetic resonance imaging (fMRI): use of a cluster-size threshold. Magn Reson Med 33: 636–647.
30. Friston KJ, Worsley KJ, Frackowiak RSJ, Mazziotta JC, Evans AC (1993) Assessing the significance of focal activations using their spatial extent. Human brain mapping 1: 210–220.
31. Worsley KJ, Evans AC, Marrett S, Neelin P (1992) A three-dimensional statistical analysis for CBF activation studies in human brain. Journal of cerebral blood flow and metabolism : official journal of the International Society of Cerebral Blood Flow and Metabolism 12: 900–918.
32. Gothe N, Pontifex MB, Hillman C, McAuley E (2012) The acute effects of Yoga on executive function. J Phys Act Health.
33. Owen AM, McMillan KM, Laird AR, Bullmore E (2005) N-back working memory paradigm: a meta-analysis of normative functional neuroimaging studies. Hum Brain Mapp 25: 46–59.
34. Voss B, Thienel R, Reske M, Kellermann T, Sheldrick AJ, et al. (2012) Cholinergic blockade under working memory demands encountered by increased rehearsal strategies: evidence from fMRI in healthy subjects. Eur Arch Psychiatry Clin Neurosci 262: 329–339.
35. Sutton SK, Davidson RJ (1997) Prefrontal brain asymmetry: a biological substrate of the behavioral approach and inhibition systems. Psychol Sci 8: 204–210.
36. Haller S, Bartsch AJ, Radue EW, Klarhöfer M, Seifritz E, et al. (2005) Effect of fMRI acoustic noise on non-auditory working memory task: comparison between continuous and pulsed sound emitting EPI. MAGMA 18: 263–271.
37. Hyodo K, Dan I, Suwabe K, Kyutoku Y, Yamada Y, et al. (2012) Acute moderate exercise enhances compensatory brain activation in older adults. Neurobiol Aging 33: 2621–2632.
38. Tsujii T, Komatsu K, Sakatani K (2013) Acute effects of physical exercise on prefrontal cortex activity in older adults: a functional near-infrared spectroscopy study. In: W. J Welch, F Palm, D. F Bruley and D. K Harrison, editors. Oxygen Transport to Tissue XXXIV. New York: Springer. pp. 293–298.
39. Hillman CH, Pontifex MB, Raine LB, Castelli DM, Hall EE, et al. (2009) The effect of acute treadmill walking on cognitive control and academic achievement in preadolescent children. Neuroscience 159: 1044–1054.
40. Botvinick MM, Braver TS, Barch DM, Carter CS, Cohen JD (2001) Conflict monitoring and cognitive control. Psychol Rev 108: 624–652.
41. Gusnard DA (2005) Being a self: considerations from functional imaging. Conscious Cogn 14: 679–697.
42. Greicius MD, Krasnow B, Reiss AL, Menon V (2003) Functional connectivity in the resting brain: a network analysis of the default mode hypothesis. Proc Natl Acad Sci U S A 100: 253–258.
43. Demb JB, Desmond JE, Wagner AD, Vaidya CJ, Glover GH, et al. (1995) Semantic encoding and retrieval in the left inferior prefrontal cortex: a functional MRI study of task difficulty and process specificity. J Neurosci 15: 5870–5878.

16

Metabolic Implications when Employing Heavy Pre- and Post-Exercise Rapid-Acting Insulin Reductions to Prevent Hypoglycaemia in Type 1 Diabetes Patients: A Randomised Clinical Trial

Matthew D. Campbell[1], Mark Walker[2], Michael I. Trenell[3], Steven Luzio[4], Gareth Dunseath[4], Daniel Tuner[5], Richard M. Bracken[5], Stephen C. Bain[4], Mark Russell[1], Emma J. Stevenson[1], Daniel J. West[1]*

1 Department of Sport, Exercise and Rehabilitation, Faculty of Health and Life Sciences, Northumbria University, Newcastle-upon-Tyne, United Kingdom, **2** Institute of Cellular Medicine, Newcastle University, Newcastle-upon-Tyne, United Kingdom, **3** Institute for Ageing and Health, Faculty of Medicine, Newcastle University, Newcastle-upon-Tyne, United Kingdom, **4** Diabetes Research Group, College of Medicine, Swansea University Swansea, United Kingdom, **5** Applied Sports, Technology, Exercise and Medicine Research Centre, College of Engineering, Swansea University, Swansea, United Kingdom

Abstract

Aim: To examine the metabolic, gluco-regulatory-hormonal and inflammatory cytokine responses to large reductions in rapid-acting insulin dose administered prandially before and after intensive running exercise in male type 1 diabetes patients.

Methods: This was a single centre, randomised, controlled open label study. Following preliminary testing, 8 male patients (24±2 years, HbA1c 7.7±0.4%/61±4 mmol.l^{-1}) treated with insulin's glargine and aspart, or lispro attended the laboratory on two mornings at ~08:00 h and consumed a standardised breakfast carbohydrate bolus (1 g carbohydrate.kg^{-1}BM; 380±10 kcal) and self-administered a 75% reduced rapid-acting insulin dose 60 minutes before 45 minutes of intensive treadmill running at 73.1±0.9% VO_{2peak}. At 60 minutes post-exercise, patients ingested a meal (1 g carbohydrate.kg^{-1}BM; 660±21 kcal) and administered either a **Full** or **50%** reduced rapid-acting insulin dose. Blood glucose and lactate, serum insulin, cortisol, non-esterified-fatty-acids, β-Hydroxybutyrate, and plasma glucagon, adrenaline, noradrenaline, IL-6, and TNF-α concentrations were measured for 180 minutes post-meal.

Results: All participants were analysed. All glycaemic, metabolic, hormonal, and cytokine responses were similar between conditions up to 60 minutes following exercise. Following the post-exercise meal, serum insulin concentrations were lower under **50%** ($p<0.05$) resulting in 75% of patients experiencing hyperglycaemia (blood glucose ≥8.0 mmol.l^{-1}; **50%** n = 6, **Full** n = 3). β-Hydroxybutyrate concentrations decreased similarly, such that at 180 minutes post-meal concentrations were lower than rest under **Full** and **50%**. IL-6 and TNF-α concentrations remained similar to fasting levels under **50%** but declined under **Full**. Under **50%** IL-6 concentrations were inversely related with serum insulin concentrations ($r = -0.484$, $p = 0.017$).

Conclusions: Heavily reducing rapid-acting insulin dose with a carbohydrate bolus before, and a meal after intensive running exercise may cause hyperglycaemia, but does not augment ketonaemia, raise inflammatory cytokines TNF-α and IL-6 above fasting levels, or cause other adverse metabolic or hormonal disturbances.

Trial Registration: ClinicalTrials.gov NCT01531855

Editor: Susanne Breuer Votruba, NIDDK/NIH, United States of America

Funding: This study was funded by Diabetes UK (www.diabetesorg.uk). The funders had no role in study design, data collection and analysis, decision to publish, or preparation of the manuscript.

Competing Interests: The authors have declared that no competing interests exist.

* E-mail: d.j.west@northumbria.ac.uk

Introduction

Cardiorespiratory or endurance-based exercise is promoted as playing an integral role in maintaining a healthy lifestyle for patients with type 1 diabetes because of its utility to enhance cardiovascular fitness, improve anthropometrics and reduce total daily insulin requirements (see Chu et al [1]). Although this form of exercise carries blood glucose lowering effects which may initially offer some therapeutic benefit, reductions in blood glucose following exercise are often excessive, exposing patients to hypoglycaemia [2]. To reduce the incidence of hypoglycaemia during and immediately after exercise, patients are recommended to reduce their pre-exercise rapid-acting insulin dose [2,3]. However, recent evidence also suggests that it is important for patients to reduce the dose of rapid-acting insulin administered with the meal after exercise as well, so that the risk of post-exercise hypoglycaemia is abated [4].

In combining pre and post-exercise rapid-acting insulin dose reductions some patients may be exposed to periods of hyperglycaemia [4]. With this is mind, it is reasonable to speculate that low levels of circulating insulin combined with elevated concentrations of post-exercise counter-regulatory hormones may in fact precipitate a metabolic milieu promoting increased lipolysis [5] and ketogenesis [6]. In addition, inflammatory cytokine responses are related to hyperglycaemia [7–10], lipid oxidation [11], and/or hyperketonaemia [12–14]. Although regular exercise has been demonstrated to reduce systemic inflammation, thus strengthening its therapeutic utility for patients with type 1 diabetes [15], somewhat paradoxically, these long-term adaptations occur despite opposing acute effects in which there is a pronounced increase in inflammatory markers early after exercise [16–21].

Potentially, performing exercise under conditions of concurrent or prior hyperglycaemia and/or hypoinsulinaemia might result in an inappropriately elevated level of inflammation after exercise. Additionally, metabolic disturbances could negate the over-all health benefits of exercise and promote the onset and progression of diabetic complications. Indeed, this may offer some explanation towards conflicting opinion regarding the efficacy of aerobic or endurance-based exercise for improvements in glycaemic control, with some literature demonstrating no improvement or even worsening HbA1c (for review see Tonoli et al [22]).

It is a well-established recommendation that patients reduce their pre-exercise rapid-acting insulin dose to prevent exercise-induced hypoglycaemia, and the metabolic implications of this are well known [23]. However, the deeper metabolic consequences of employing the recently advocated strategy of heavily reducing both pre and post-exercise rapid-acting insulin dose [4] are unknown. Therefore, the aim of this study was to determine whether reducing pre- and also post-exercise rapid-acting insulin dose, as a strategy for preventing post-exercise hypoglycaemia, causes metabolic or hormonal disturbances, influences ketonaemia, or alters inflammatory cytokine concentrations in type 1 diabetes patients, following intensive running exercise.

Methods

Ethics statement

This study was approved by local National Health Service Research Ethics Committee (13/NE/0016); registry details (NCT01531855, ClinicalTrials.gov). All patients who participated provided full written informed consent. All clinical investigations were conducted according to the principles expressed in the Declaration of Helsinki. The study was conducted between 1st March 2013 and 1st September 2013.

Protocol

The protocol for this trial and supporting CONSORT checklist are available as supporting information; see Checklist S1 and Protocol S1. Eight male type 1 diabetes patients (mean ± SEM; age 24±2 years, BMI 22.9±0.7, duration of diabetes 13±2 years, HbA_{1c} 7.7±0.4%/61±4 $mmol.l^{-1}$, $\dot{V}O_{2peak}$ 54±1 $ml.kg.min^{-1}$) volunteered to participate. Female participants were not included due to the potential influence of the menstrual cycle on blood glucose homeostasis [24]. Interested patients who met the eligibility criteria for involvement in the study (aged between 18–35 years with a duration of diabetes greater than 2 years on enrolment, treated with a stable basal-bolus insulin regimen composed of insulin glargine and fast-acting insulin aspart or lispro for a minimum of 6 months, free of diabetes related complications, and receiving no additional medication other than insulin) were screened in-line with the procedures of American College of Sports Medicine's (ACSM) Guidelines for Exercise Testing and Prescription [25]. Screening measures included a comprehensive medical questionnaire and the completion of a cardiopulmonary exercise stress test to assess cardiac function in response to exercise. All patients were regularly and consistently active (self-reporting to participate in aerobic based exercise for at least 30 minutes at a time, 3 times per week), and displayed normal cardio-pulmonary responses to exercise. All patients were familiar with carbohydrate counting. Patients underwent randomisation using a computer programme to determine the sequence of two open label crossover arms.

Upon completion of the screening procedures, patients completed a preliminary incremental treadmill test to quantify peak cardio-respiratory parameters as described previously by our group [2,4]. Following this, patients attended the Newcastle NIHR Clinical Research Facility exercise laboratory on two occasions, once per week at ~08:00 h. Patients replicated their diet (assessed using weighed dietary recording sheets) and maintained a similar insulin regimen (with basal insulin dose standardised i.e. dose, injection site, time of injection) during the 24 hours preceding each trial. Additionally, patients were required to avoid exercise for 24 hours prior to each visit; activity patterns were measured using a pedometer (Omron Healthcare Europe B.V., Netherlands). Patients maintained their usual basal regimen (dose, injection site, time of injection) between trials.

Patients arrived at the laboratory after an overnight fast; if patients experienced a hypoglycaemic episode on the preceding night their trial was rescheduled. Following their arrival, patients assumed a resting position while a 20 gauge cannula (Vasofix, B.Braun Melsungen AG, Germany) was inserted into the antecubital vein of their non-dominant arm. An 11 ml resting venous blood sample was taken, of which 20 µl was analysed immediately for glucose (BG) and lactate (Biosen C-Line, EKF Diagnostic GmbH, Germany), and 10 µl analysed for haemoglobin and haematocrit (Hemo Control, EKF-diagnostic GmbH, Germany) which was used to correct for changes in plasma volume [26]. The remaining sample was dispensed evenly into Lithium-heparin tubes (Vacuette, Greiner Bio-One GmBH, Austria) and serum separation tubes (Vacuette, Greiner Bio-One GmBH, Austria) which were centrifuged for 15 minutes at 3000 $rev.min^{-1}$, and stored at −80°C for later analysis of rapid-acting insulin (Invitron insulin assay, Invitron, UK), glucagon (Glucagon EIA, Sigma-Aldrich, USA), adrenaline and noradrenaline (BI-CAT adrenaline and noradrenaline ELISA, Eagle Biosciences, UK), cortisol (Parameter cortisol ELISA, R & D Systems, Roche Diagnostics, UK), non-esterified-fatty-acids (NEFA; Non-esterified fatty acids colorimetric assay, Randox Laboratories, UK), β-Hydroxybutyrate (D-3-Hydroxybutyrate kinetic enzymatic assay, Randox Laboratories, UK), interleukin-6 (IL-6; Human IL-6 Quantikine ELISA, R & D Systems, Roche Diagnostics, UK) and tumour necrosis factor alpha (TNF-α; Human TNF-alpha Quantikine ELISA, R & D Systems, Roche Diagnostics, UK). The coefficient of variation was <10% for all assays.

Following the resting sample, patients were provided with a standardised cereal-based breakfast-carbohydrate bolus (frosted flakes, semi-skimmed milk, peaches) equating to 1 g $carbohydrate.kg^{-1}BM$ (380±10 kcal; 1.59±0.04 MJ). Immediately before consumption, patients administered a 25% (1.8±0.1 IU) dose (i.e. a 75% reduction) of rapid-acting insulin into the abdomen, as per current recommendations [2,3]. This pre-exercise carbohydrate and insulin strategy was based on previously published methodologies [3,27]. All patients were administering 1.0±0.1 IU of rapid-acting insulin per 10 g of carbohydrate. The injection site was standardised across trials through administration at half the distance between the anterior-superior iliac crest and the naval. Insulin aspart and lispro were administered using Novopen3 (NovoNordisk, UK) and Humapen luxura (Eli Lilly, UK), respectively.

A further blood sample was collected at 60 minutes following the ingestion of the breakfast meal. At 60 minutes, patients performed a 45 minute bout of treadmill running (Woodway, Germany) at a velocity calculated to elicit 70%$\dot{V}O_{2peak}$. During exercise, breath-by-breath respiratory parameters (MetaLyzer 3B; Cortex, Germany) and heart rate (S810; Polar, Finland) were continuously recorded. Immediately upon cessation of exercise, a blood sample was obtained with further blood samples collected at 15, 30, and 60 minutes post-exercise. At 60 minutes post-exercise, patients were provided with a pasta-based lunch (pasta, tomato based sauce, cheddar cheese) equating to 1 g carbohydrate.kg^{-1}BM (660±21 kcal; 2.76±0.09 MJ) to which they administered either a **Full** (7.5±0.3 IU) or **50%** (3.7±0.1 IU) rapid-acting insulin dose immediately before consumption, into the contralateral abdominal site to that which received the pre-exercise rapid-acting insulin dose. Having consumed the meal, patients remained rested for 180 minutes with periodic blood samples every 30 minutes. Hypoglycaemia was defined as a blood glucose concentration of ≤3.9 mmol.1^{-1} and hyperglycaemia as ≥8.0 mmol.1^{-1}. If patients experienced hypoglycaemia during the laboratory period a 20 g carbohydrate bolus was administered (Lucozade, GlaxoSmithKline, UK). Hyperketonaemia was defined as a β-hydroxybutyrate concentration >1.0 mmol.l^{-1} [6].

Data analysis

Sample size was calculated using data from Campbell et al [4] and the methods of Hopkins [28] whereby the number of participants required is based around the precision defined by 95% confidence limits (deriving a power 0.8). The sample size is calculated as $n = 8s^2/d^2$ where n is the samples size, s is the typical error, and d is the smallest worthwhile effect. A sample size of 8 participants was required to achieve 80% power. Statistical analysis was performed using PASW *Statistics* software (IBM PASW version 18; IBM., NY, USA) with significance set at $p \leq 0.05$. Interactions of time and condition were examined using repeated measures ANOVA. Where significant p-values were identified for interaction effects (time*condition), insulin dose was deemed to have influenced the response, and simple main effects analyses were performed. Significant main effects of time were further investigated using BONFERRONI adjusted pairwise comparisons. One-way repeated ANOVA were performed where relevant and relationships were explored using Pearson's product moment correlation coefficient. Data are presented as mean ± SEM.

Results

All patients were analysed for this study. A significant interaction of condition and time were evident when examining serum insulin ($p<0.001$) and blood glucose (condition*time, $p=0.014$). Serum insulin (Figure 1A) and blood glucose (Figure 1B) concentrations were similar between conditions at baseline and immediately before exercise. The performance of exercise was intensive, with patients exercising at a similar % of $\dot{V}O_{2peak}$ (**Full** 74.5±0.01; **50%** 71.6±0.02% $\dot{V}O_{2peak}$, $p=0.329$), and HR_{peak} (**Full** 80±2; **50%** 79±1%HR_{peak}, $p=0.785$). The average respiratory exchange ratio during exercise was similar between conditions (**Full** 0.98±0.01; **50%** 0.96±0.02, $p=0.256$), resulting in similar reductions in blood glucose (**Full** −7.8±0.8; **50%** −7.5±1.11 mmol.l^{-1}, $p=0.453$, Figure 1B) and similar peaks in blood lactate. Serum insulin (Figure 1A) and blood glucose (Figure 1B) concentrations up to 60 minutes post-exercise were similar between conditions, such that blood glucose was comparable immediately prior to the administration of the post-exercise meal (Figure 1B).

Following the post-exercise meal, serum insulin peaked at 60 minutes under both conditions, with mean peak concentrations greater under **Full** (199±47; **50%** 109±28 pmol.l^{-1}, $p=0.021$; Figure 1A). From 60 minutes post-meal, serum insulin under **Full** remained elevated from pre-meal measures, and significantly higher than **50%** ($p<0.05$; Figure 1A). Blood glucose declined under **Full** (Figure 1B), but was preserved under **50%** with concentrations greater than those at pre-meal throughout the three hour observation period (Figure 1B). During this time, 63% of patients (n = 5) experienced hypoglycaemia (BG≤3.9 mmol.l^{-1}) under **Full**, whereas all patients under **50%** were protected. Inversely, fewer patients under **Full** experienced hyperglycaemia (BG≥8 mmol.l^{-1}; **Full** n = 3; **50%** n = 6).

There were no conditional differences in counter-regulatory hormones (Table 1) or metabolites (Table 2) up to 60 minutes post-exercise ($p>0.05$). A significant interaction of condition and time ($p=0.006$) were found when examining plasma glucagon concentrations during the trials (Table 2). Plasma glucagon concentrations following the post-exercise meal were significantly elevated from pre-meal values under both conditions, but were highest under **Full** (Table 1). There were no differences in β-Hydroxybutyrate, adrenaline, noradrenaline, cortisol, blood lactate, or NEFA concentrations between conditions following the post-exercise meal (Table 1 and 2). During this time, there was a transient decline in β-Hydroxybutyrate with concentrations similar to rest under **50%** and lower than rest under **Full** (Table 2).

The IL-6 and TNF-α responses are presented in Figure 2 A–B. Plasma TNF-α concentrations were significantly raised at 15 minutes post-exercise. Following the post-exercise meal, IL-6 concentrations were significantly greater under **50%**. However, TNF-α was similar between conditions. Despite this, both cytokines under **50%** remained similar to pre-meal and resting measures ($p>0.05$; Figure 2A–B). Under **50%** mean IL-6 concentrations over the post-exercise period were positively related to mean TNF-α concentrations ($r=0.676$, $p<0.001$) and serum insulin concentrations were inversely related to IL-6 ($r=-0.484$, $p=0.017$), but not TNF-α ($r=-0.169$, $p=0.430$). No significant relationships existed between mean blood glucose and IL-6 ($r=0.299$, $p=0.155$) or TNF-α ($r=0.005$, $p=0.980$) over the post-meal period under **50%**. No relationships were found between any measures under **Full**.

Discussion

To our knowledge we are the first to demonstrate, that manipulating pre- and also post-exercise rapid-acting insulin dose, as a strategy for preventing post-exercise hypoglycaemia does not cause adverse metabolic or counter-regulatory-hormonal disturbances yet patients remain protected from hypoglycaemia. Specifically, our data indicate that large reductions in rapid-acting insulin dose administered before and also after intensive running exercise may cause post-exercise hyperglycaemia, but this strategy

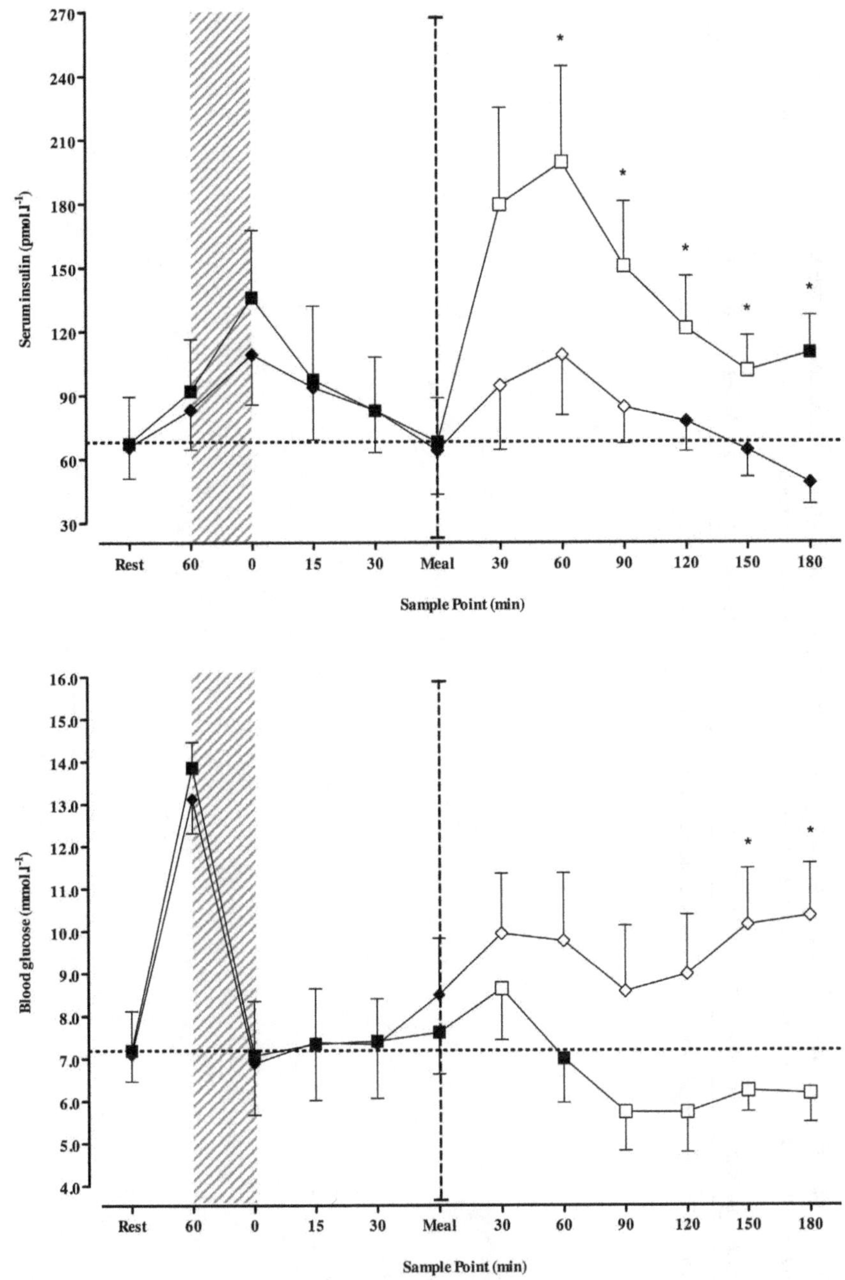

Figure 1. A–B. Time-course changes in serum insulin (A) and blood glucose (B) from rest. Full = black squares, 50% = black diamond.* indicates significantly different from Full ($p<0.05$). Transparent sample point within a condition indicates a significant difference from pre-exercise meal concentrations ($p<0.05$). Vertical dashed line break indicates post-exercise intervention. NOTE: test meal and insulin were administered immediately following rest and meal sample points.

does not augment ketonaemia in patients with type 1 diabetes. In addition, we demonstrate that inflammatory cytokines may increase with this strategy, but not above fasting concentrations, and by 180 minutes post-meal the pro-inflammatory cytokine TNF-α is lower than rest.

Patients completed an intensive bout of prolonged running exercise, running at an average speed of 9.3±0.3 km.hr^{-1} and covering a distance of 7.0±0.2 km. The respiratory exchange ratio (~0.96) exhibited by patients is typical of exercise of an intense nature [29], and reflects the predominant use of carbohydrate during exercise. Indeed, completing the exercise protocol caused a significant metabolic stress to patients, inducing large increases in blood lactate (~392%) and catecholamines (adrenaline ~287%, noradrenaline ~591%), and large decreases in blood glucose (Δ~7.6 mmol.l^{-1}). Despite subsequent reductions in glycaemia, and the administration of a second dose of rapid-acting insulin 60 minutes post-exercise, all patients under **50%** were protected from hypoglycaemia throughout their laboratory stay. As such, we demonstrate that administering a small dose of rapid-acting insulin with a carbohydrate bolus before exercise is effective in limiting pre-exercise hyperglycaemia and preventing hypoglycaemia during and immediately after exercise. Importantly, circulating insulin concentrations following exercise returned to baseline, meaning the effects of administering a pre-exercise rapid-acting insulin dose

Table 1. Counter-regulatory responses to reductions in pre- and post-exercise rapid-acting insulin dose during the experimental trials.

		Rest	60	Exercise	0	15	30	Pre-Meal	30	60	90	120	150	180	ANOVA p	
															Time	Time*Condition
Plasma Glucagon ($pg.ml^{-1}$)	Full	760±70	697±81	-	1152±99†	832±83†	698±61	710±69	1015±79†‡	1597±116†‡	1590±102†‡	1402±94†‡	1332±137†‡	1099±124†‡	<0.001	=0.006
	50%	789±85	628±85†*	-	1067±128†	854±127	815±89	609±98†	975±82†‡	1350±96†*‡	1251±97†*‡	1177±90†*‡	1085±86†*‡	889±82*‡		
Plasma Adrenaline ($nmol.l^{-1}$)	Full	0.30±0.05	0.14±0.04†	-	0.63±0.11†	0.49±0.12	0.37±0.08	0.26±0.06	0.24±0.06	0.23±0.10	0.14±0.05†	0.19±0.06	0.21±0.07	0.16±0.05†‡	<0.001	=0.808
	50%	0.30±0.07	0.21±0.05	-	0.68±0.08†	0.34±0.05	0.23±0.05	0.16±0.04	0.16±0.05	0.17±0.04	0.16±0.05	0.17±0.06	0.16±0.04	0.15±0.04		
Plasma Noradrenaline ($nmol.l^{-1}$)	Full	2.11±0.33	1.72±0.27	-	12.98±1.56†	4.76±0.69†	3.15±0.36†	2.59±0.36	2.65±0.33	2.72±0.46	2.36±0.37	2.39±0.48	2.30±0.42	2.21±0.43	<0.001	=0.407
	50%	2.25±0.34	2.17±0.32	-	13.63±1.84†	4.16±0.35†	3.34±0.25†	2.71±0.34	2.67±0.52	2.87±0.61	2.62±0.47	2.90±0.73	2.92±0.68	2.77±0.61		
Serum Cortisol ($nmol.l^{-1}$)	Full	0.23±0.04	0.22±0.03†	-	0.21±0.03†	0.25±0.03	0.22±0.03	0.18±0.02†	0.18±0.03†	0.16±0.03†‡	0.12±0.02†‡	0.12±0.03†	0.10±0.01†	0.10±0.01†	=0.019	=0.394
	50%	0.22±0.04	0.18±0.05†	-	0.20±0.03	0.24 ±0.04	0.22±0.03	0.18±0.02	0.15±0.02	0.12±0.02†	0.13±0.03†	0.11±0.02	0.09±0.01	0.07±0.01		

NOTE: Data presented as mean ± SEM. Test meal and insulin were administered immediately following rest and pre-meal sample points.
* indicates significantly different from Full ($p \leq 0.05$).
†indicates significantly different from rest.
‡indicates significantly different from pre-meal.
NOTE: Exercise commenced 60 minutes after rest.

Table 2. Metabolic responses to reductions in pre- and post-exercise rapid-acting insulin dose during the experimental trials.

		Rest	60	Exercise	0	15	30	Pre-Meal	30	60	90	120	150	180	ANOVA p Time	ANOVA p Time*Condition
Blood Lactate (mmol.l^{-1})	Full	0.38±0.14	0.72±0.15	-	3.63±0.62†	1.30±0.16†	0.93±0.11†	0.69±0.20†	0.49±0.17	0.56±0.13	0.40±0.14	0.38±0.13	0.35±0.13‡	0.37±0.13	=0.001	=0.312
	50%	0.47±0.15	0.75±0.12	-	3.60±0.43†	1.38±0.23†	0.77±0.18	0.60±0.16	0.43±0.18	0.53±0.13	0.46±0.15	0.43±0.14	0.42±0.13	0.35±0.11		
Serum NEFA (mmol.l^{-1})	Full	0.41±0.07	0.22±0.04†	-	0.24±0.04†	0.35±0.18	0.32±0.05	0.34±0.07	0.26±0.04†	0.20±0.04†‡	0.18±0.04†‡	0.26±0.04†	0.25±0.03†	0.25±0.02†	=0.019	=0.394
	50%	0.36±0.06	0.18±0.04†	-	0.17±0.02	0.26±0.05	0.15±0.04	0.24±0.06†	0.24±0.05†	0.16±0.04†	0.19±0.03†	0.33±0.03	0.39±0.05	0.44±0.05		
Serum β-OH (mmol.l^{-1})	Full	0.11±0.03	0.03±0.01†	-	0.08±0.01	0.08±0.02	0.09±0.01	0.06±0.01	0.06±0.01	0.04±0.01†	0.05±0.01	0.08±0.03	0.04±0.01†	0.04±0.01†	=0.046	=0.303
	50%	0.08±0.02	0.05±0.01†	-	0.06±0.01	0.07±0.01	0.05±0.01	0.04±0.01	0.11±0.05	0.06±0.03	0.03±0.01†	0.04±0.03†	0.04±0.03†	0.06±0.01		

NOTE: Data presented as mean ± SEM. β-OH = β-Hydroxybutyrate. Test meal and insulin were administered immediately following rest and pre-meal sample points.
* indicates significantly different from Full ($p \leq 0.05$).
† indicates significantly different from rest.
‡ indicates significantly different from pre-meal.
NOTE: Exercise commenced 60 minutes after rest.

of this size is unlikely to carry additive effects for subsequent post-exercise rapid-acting insulin administration. Therefore, reducing pre- and also post-exercise rapid-acting insulin dose is an effective strategy for preventing exercise-induced hypoglycaemia. However, preserving glycaemia consequently exposed patients under **50%** to periods of hyperglycaemia following the post-exercise meal. This finding emphasises that patients differ in their sensitivity to insulin following exercise, and as such, we advise that patients may require a smaller reduction in post-exercise rapid-acting insulin dose.

Although the majority of patients under **50%** were exposed to hyperglycaemia, β-Hydroxybutyrate concentrations following the post-exercise meal remained similar between both conditions, with values remaining less than those considered hyperketonaemic (< 1.0 mmol.l^{-1}) [6] and similar to rest. Although we applied a large reduction in rapid-acting insulin dose, serum insulin concentrations were elevated above resting and pre-meal measures under **50%** (Table 1). Despite unexplained differences in glucagon concentrations, the administration of even small amounts of rapid-acting insulin, under conditions of unchanged basal insulin dose, is likely to have raised circulating insulin concentrations to a level where β-Hydroxybutyrate production was suppressed [30], and potentially augment peripheral ketone body disposal [31]. Additionally, NEFA concentrations did not increase, likely attributable to unchanged concentrations of catecholamines, the main lipolytic stimulus [32], and cortisol [33]. Furthermore, the consumption of a large carbohydrate based meal would have helped supplement muscle and liver glycogen, reducing the energy deficit created by exercise, and limiting the appearance of catecholamines and cortisol.

We questioned whether post-exercise hyperglycaemia would exacerbate the appearance of inflammatory cytokines in our patients, indeed this may be further exacerbated if patients experienced hyperketonaemia. Hyperglycaemia associated inflammation is a major contributor to the pathogenesis of diabetes related complications [9,33], which are primarily avoided through the normalisation of glycaemic profiles [34]. Patients with type 1 diabetes exhibit chronically elevated levels of inflammatory markers at baseline [7–10,35]. Baseline measures were elevated above some of those previously reported [7,35–38], which may have resulted from patients arriving in a fasted state and with low circulating concentrations of insulin. However, comparison between studies is hampered by mixed methodologies and differing patient characteristics, indeed most studies implement glucose and/or insulin clamp procedures, and recruit children or adolescents who are usually recently diagnosed [7,35–38]. Our study population consisted of a relatively young (~24 years) group of individuals all in good glycaemic control (~7.7%/ 61 mmol.l^{-1}), exposure to inflammatory stimuli is likely to be much greater in the general diabetes population who are older, have a longer duration of diabetes, and in those with excess adiposity [10].

We witnessed only modest increases in IL-6 (~22%) and TNF-α (~45%) following exercise, which is likely due to the administration of the pre-exercise meal and concomitant insulin in our patients. The large carbohydrate bolus (1.0 g carbohydrate.kg^{-1} BM) would have helped supplement glycogen reserves [39], which may have attenuated the exercise-induced increases in IL-6 [12,40] and even completely inhibited IL-6 release from contracting skeletal muscle [40]. In addition, insulin carries anti-inflammatory properties [41], of which its administration, even in small doses, may have partially combatted the pro-inflammatory effects of TNF-α. Indeed, IL-6 concentrations were inversely related to circulation insulin concentrations. IL-6 has anti- as well

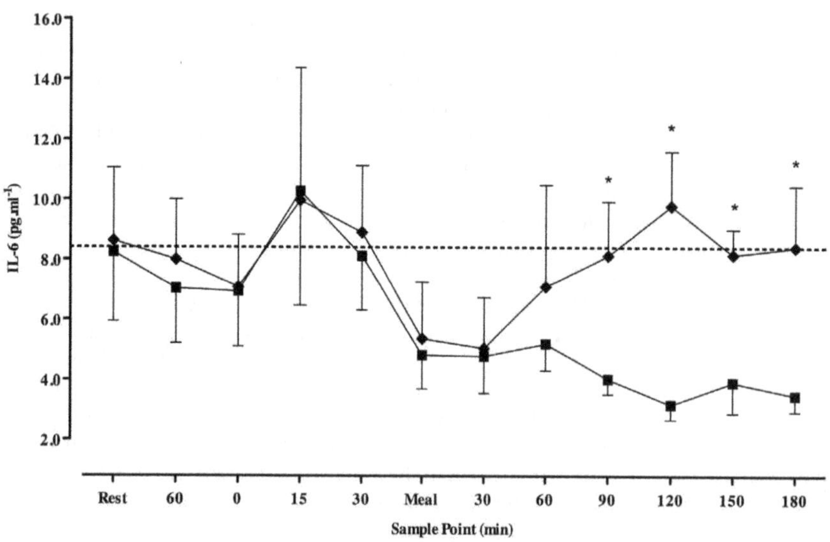

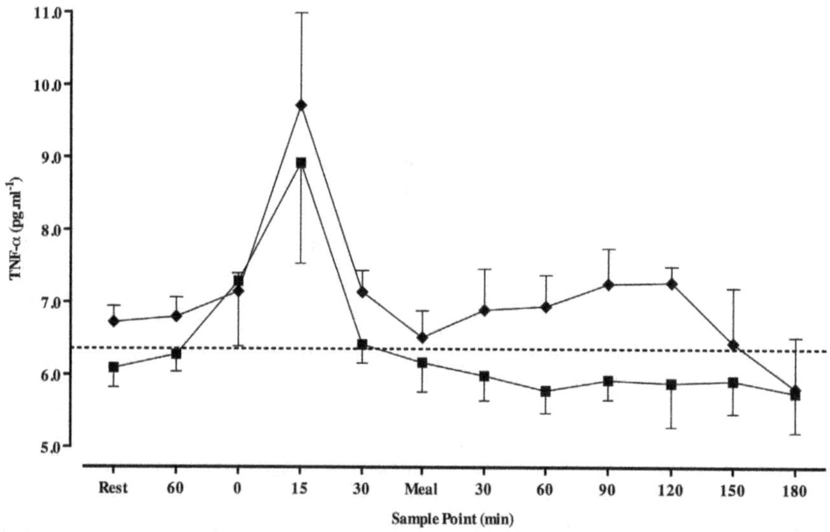

Figure 2. A–B. Time-course changes in IL-6 (A) and TNF-α (B) from rest. Full = black squares, 50% = black diamond.* indicates significantly different from Full ($p<0.05$). Transparent sample point within a condition indicates a significant difference from pre-exercise meal concentrations ($p<0.05$). Vertical dashed line break indicates post-exercise intervention. NOTE: test meal and insulin were administered immediately following rest and meal sample points.

as pro-inflammatory properties, with some studies demonstrating IL-6 to exert inhibitory effects on TNF-α. We found there to be a positive correlation between IL-6 and TNF-α. Although a relationship does not necessarily indicate cause-effect, speculatively, increases in IL-6 may indeed have been in direct response to reducing TNF-α. Irrelevant of the mechanisms at play, our data indicate that TNF-α or IL-6 are not significantly elevated above fasting concentrations, and that by 180 minutes post-meal, concentrations are lower than those following an overnight fast.

We chose IL-6 and TNF-α as our main inflammatory markers, in part, because both display the greatest quantitative change [40] and therefore have a high likelihood to yield distinct differences between our study conditions [16,20,35,37]. There is however, a known and marked inherent variability of many inflammatory markers [7,37], which reflects the remarkable metabolic complexity of that patient with type 1 diabetes in which permutations in inflammation status are variable across patients and within the same individuals overtime [7]. Indeed, some of this variability is attributed to antecedent hyperglycaemia [7,16–21,36,38], however patients in this study were kept under free-living conditions before experimentation and without correction using euglycaemic clamp procedures, and therefore likely to closely replicate the responses in patients in day-to-day life. It would be inappropriate to conclude that inflammation *per se* was unchanged in our patients, as we were only able to analyse two inflammatory cytokines within our dataset. Although TNF-α and IL-6 are readily accepted as primary markers of inflammation, future research investigating more detailed post-prandial inflammatory responses in this population is warranted.

An interesting finding was that plasma glucagon concentrations following the post-exercise meal were elevated under both conditions, and significantly greater under **Full**. Although the majority of patients under this condition experienced hypoglycaemia (BG≤3.9 mmol.l^{-1}; **50%** n = 0, **Full** n = 5), patients were treated with a corrective bolus of carbohydrate, such that blood glucose levels (group mean BG~6.6 mmol.l^{-1}) remained above the glycaemic threshold for plasma glucagon release (BG< 3.0 mmol.l^{-1}; [42]; even if an appropriate glycaemic threshold was achieved to stimulate glucagon release, it would remain a surprise to find any increase in glucagon concentrations in our patients, as its secretion under exercising and hypoglycaemic conditions is blunted in type 1 diabetes [42]. In addition, increased glucagon response to a mixed-meal stimulus has been noted previously in type 1 diabetes [43], suggestive that the α-cell secretory reserve may be unaffected by the progression of the autoimmune process [43]. Of note, the meal administered in the study by Brown et al [43], was similar in nutritional content to the post-exercise meal given to patients in our study (Carbohydrate 56 vs. 53%; Protein 21 vs. 25%, Fat 21 vs. 22%), although our meal was larger (400 kcal vs. ~660 kcal). Considering all of our patients had longstanding diabetes (length of disease ~13 years), were intensively controlled (~7.7%/61 mmol.l^{-1}), and therefore likely to have been frequently exposed to hypoglycaemia, investigation of differing types of post-exercise meal may be an important avenue to investigate as altering the composition or glycaemic index of the post-exercise meal may indeed offer more favourable glycaemic profiles by reducing the incidence of hyperglycaemia.

To conclude, heavily reducing pre- and post-exercise rapid-acting insulin dose does not induce hyperketonaemia, excessively raise inflammatory cytokines TNF-α or IL-6, or cause other metabolic or hormonal disturbances in type 1 diabetes patients treated with insulin glargine and fast-acting insulin aspart or lispro. In addition, we further highlight the importance of this strategy in preventing early-onset post-exercise hypoglycaemia. However, patients may be exposed to hyperglycaemia and are therefore encouraged to regularly monitor blood glucose concentrations after exercise, and refine these strategies such that euglycaemia can be achieved following individual exercise routines. We advise that future research investigates in more detail post-prandial inflammatory responses in this population.

Acknowledgments

The authors thank the study participants for their time, effort and commitment, and the research team at the NIHR Clinical Research Facility, Newcastle University, for their assistance. The funders had no role in study design, data collection and analysis, decision to publish, or preparation of the manuscript.

Author Contributions

Conceived and designed the experiments: MDC DJW EJS. Performed the experiments: MDC DJW. Analyzed the data: MDC DJW EJS DT RMB GD SL MR SB MW MIT. Contributed reagents/materials/analysis tools: GD SL MW MIT. Wrote the paper: MDC DJW.

References

1. Chu L, Hamilton J, Riddell MC (2011) Clinical management of the physically active patient with type 1 diabetes. Physiol Sports Med 39: 64–77.
2. West DJ, Morton RD, Bain SC, Stephens JW, Bracken RM (2010) Blood glucose responses to reductions in pre-exercise rapid-acting insulin for 24 h after running in individuals with type 1 diabetes. J Sports Sci 28: 781–788.
3. Rabasa-Lhoret R, Bourque J, Ducros F, Chiasson JL (2001) Guidelines for premeal insulin dose reduction for postprandial exercise of different intensities and durations in type 1 diabetic subjects treated intensively with a basal-bolus insulin regimen (ultralente-lispro). Diabetes Care 24: 625–630.
4. Campbell MD, Walker M, Trenell MI, Jakovljevic DG, Stevenson EJ, et al. (2013) Large Pre-and Postexercise Rapid-Acting Insulin Reductions Preserves Glycemia and Prevents Early-but Not Late-Onset Hypoglycemia in Patients With Type 1 Diabetes. Diabetes Care 36: 2217–2224.
5. Khani S, Tayek JA (2001) Cortisol increases gluconeogenesis in humans: its role in the metabolic syndrome. Clin Sci 101: 739–747.
6. Laffel L (2000) Ketone bodies: a review of physiology, pathophysiology and application of monitoring to diabetes. Diabetes Metab Rev 15: 412–426.
7. Rosa JS, Flores RL, Oliver SR, Pontello AM, Zaldivar FP, et al. (2008) Sustained IL-1α, IL-4, and IL-6 elevations following correction of hyperglycemia in children with type 1 diabetes mellitus. Pediatric Diabetes 9: 9–16.
8. Esposito K, Nappo F, Marfella R, Giugliano G, Giugliano F, et al. (2002) Inflammatory cytokine concentrations are acutely increased by hyperglycemia in humans role of oxidative stress. Circulation 106: 2067–2072.
9. Targher G, Zenari L, Bertolini L, Muggeo M, Zoppini G (2001) Elevated levels of interleukin-6 in young adults with type 1 diabetes without clinical evidence of microvascular and macrovascular complications. Diabetes Care 24: 956–957.
10. De Rekeneire N, Peila R, Ding J, Colbert LH, Visser M, et al. (2006) Diabetes, Hyperglycemia, and Inflammation in Older Individuals The Health, Aging and Body Composition study. Diabetes Care 29: 1902–1908.
11. Febbraio MA, Pedersen BK (2005) Contraction-induced myokine production and release: is skeletal muscle an endocrine organ? Exerc Sport Sci Rev 33: 114–119.
12. Stouthard J, Romijn JA, Van der Poll T, Endert E, Klein S, et al. (1995) Endocrinologic and metabolic effects of interleukin-6 in humans. Am J Physiol-Endoc Metab 268: E813–E819.
13. Karavanaki K, Kakleas K, Georga S, Bartzeliotou A, Mavropoulos G, et al. (2012) Plasma high sensitivity C-reactive protein and its relationship with cytokine levels in children with newly diagnosed type 1 diabetes and ketoacidosis. Clin Biochem 45: 1383–1388.
14. Karavanaki K, Karanika E, Georga S, Bartzeliotou A, Tsouvalas M, et al. (2011) Cytokine response to diabetic ketoacidosis (DKA) in children with type 1 diabetes (T1DM). Endocr J58: 1045.
15. Petersen AMW, Pedersen BK (2005) The anti-inflammatory effect of exercise. J App Phys 98: 1154–1162.
16. Ostrowski K, Rohde T, Asp S, Schjerling P, Pedersen BK (1999) Pro-and anti-inflammatory cytokine balance in strenuous exercise in humans. J Physiol 515: 287–291.
17. Sprenger H, Jacobs C, Nain M, Gressner A, Prinz H, et al. (1992) Enhanced release of cytokines, interleukin-2 receptors, and neopterin after long-distance running. Clin immunol and immunop 63: 188–195.
18. Drenth J, Van Uum S, Van Deuren M, Pesman GJ, Van der Ven-Jongekrijg J, et al. (1995) Endurance run increases circulating IL-6 and IL-1ra but downregulates ex vivo TNF-alpha and IL-1 beta production. J App Physiol 79: 1497–1503.
19. Nehlsen-Cannarella S, Fagoaga O, Nieman D, Henson D, Butterworth D, et al. (1997) Carbohydrate and the cytokine response to 2.5 h of running. J App Physiol 82: 1662–1667.
20. Pedersen BK, Hoffman-Goetz L (2000) Exercise and the immune system: regulation, integration, and adaptation. Physiol Rev 80: 1055–1081.
21. Nemet D, Oh Y, Kim H-S, Hill M, Cooper DM (2002) Effect of intense exercise on inflammatory cytokines and growth mediators in adolescent boys. Pediatrics 110: 681–689.
22. Tonoli C, Heyman E, Roelands B, Buyse L, Cheung SS, et al. (2012) Effects of Different Types of Acute and Chronic (Training) Exercise on Glycaemic Control in Type 1 Diabetes Mellitus: A Meta-Analysis. Sports Med 42: 1059–1080.
23. Bracken R, West D, Stephens J, Kilduff L, Luzio S, et al. (2011) Impact of pre-exercise rapid-acting insulin reductions on ketogenesis following running in Type 1 diabetes. Diabet Med 28: 218–222.
24. Diamond M, Simonson D, DeFronzo R (1989) Menstrual cyclicity has a profound effect on glucose homeostasis. Fertility and sterility 52: 204–208.

25. ACSM (2010) Clinical Exercise Testing. In: Walter R, Gordon NF, Pescatello LS, ACSM's guidelines for exercise testing and prescription. 8th ed. Baltimore: American College of Sports Medicine.
26. Dill D, Costill DL (1974) Calculation of percentage changes in volumes of blood, plasma, and red cells in dehydration. J App Physiol 37: 247–248.
27. West DJ, Stephens JW, Bain SC, Kilduff LP, Luzio S, et al. (2011) A combined insulin reduction and carbohydrate feeding strategy 30 min before running best preserves blood glucose concentration after exercise through improved fuel oxidation in type 1 diabetes mellitus. J Sports Sci 29: 279–289.
28. Hopkins W (2006) Estimating sample size for magnitude-based inferences. J Sport Sci 10: 63–70.
29. Marliss EB, Vranic M (2002) Intense Exercise Has Unique Effects on Both Insulin Release and Its Roles in Glucoregulation Implications for Diabetes. Diabetes 51: 271–283.
30. McGarry J (1996) Ellenberg and Rifkin's Diabetes Mellitus. In: Porte D, Sherwin RS, Baron A, JAMA: J Am Med Assoc. 5 ed. New York: McGraw-Hill. pp. 19–28.
31. Balasse EO, Féry F (1989) Ketone body production and disposal: effects of fasting, diabetes, and exercise. Diabetes Metab Rev 5: 247–270.
32. Kalra PR, Tigas S (2002) Regulation of lipolysis: natriuretic peptides and the development of cachexia. Int J Cardiol 85: 125–132.
33. Fowler MJ (2008) Microvascular and macrovascular complications of diabetes. Clinical Diabetes 26: 77–82.
34. Daneman D (2006) Type 1 diabetes. The Lancet 367: 847–858.
35. Galassetti P, Iwanaga K, Pontello A, Zaldivar F, Flores R, et al. (2006) Effect of prior hyperglycemia on IL-6 responses to exercise in children with type 1 diabetes. Am J Physiol-Endocrinol Metab 290: E833–E839.
36. Galassetti PR, Iwanaga K, Crisostomo M, Zaldivar FP, Larson J, et al. (2006) Inflammatory cytokine, growth factor and counterregulatory responses to exercise in children with type 1 diabetes and healthy controls. Pediatric Diabetes 7: 16–24.
37. Rosa JS, Oliver SR, Flores RL, Ngo J, Milne GL, et al. (2011) Altered inflammatory, oxidative, and metabolic responses to exercise in pediatric obesity and type 1 diabetes. Pediatric Diabetes 12: 464–472.
38. Rosa JS, Flores RL, Oliver SR, Pontello AM, Zaldivar FP, et al. (2010) Resting and exercise-induced IL-6 levels in children with Type 1 diabetes reflect hyperglycemic profiles during the previous 3 days. J App Physiol 108: 334–342.
39. Jentjens R, Jeukendrup AE (2003) Determinants of post-exercise glycogen synthesis during short-term recovery. Sports Med 33: 117–144.
40. Pedersen BK, Febbraio MA (2008) Muscle as an endocrine organ: focus on muscle-derived interleukin-6. Physioll Rev 88: 1379–1406.
41. Viardot A, Grey ST, Mackay F, Chisholm D (2007) Potential antiinflammatory role of insulin via the preferential polarization of effector T cells toward a T helper 2 phenotype. Endocrinology 148: 346–353.
42. Cryer PE (2008) The barrier of hypoglycemia in diabetes. Diabetes 57: 3169–3176.
43. Brown RJ, Sinaii N, Rother KI (2008) Too Much Glucagon, Too Little Insulin Time course of pancreatic islet dysfunction in new-onset type 1 diabetes. Diabetes Care 31: 1403–1404.

17

Intervention Effects on Adolescent Physical Activity in the Multicomponent SPACE Study: A Cluster Randomized Controlled Trial

Mette Toftager[1,2]*, Lars B. Christiansen[1,2], Annette K. Ersbøll[2], Peter L. Kristensen[1], Pernille Due[2], Jens Troelsen[1,2]

1 Institute of Sports Science and Clinical Biomechanics, University of Southern Denmark, Odense, Denmark, **2** Centre for Intervention Research in Health Promotion and Disease Prevention, National Institute of Public Health, University of Southern Denmark, Copenhagen, Denmark

Abstract

Background: Multicomponent school-based interventions have the potential to reduce the age-related decline in adolescents' physical activity (PA), yet there is not consistent evidence to guide non-curricular and school environment interventions. The aim of this study was to assess the effectiveness of a multicomponent environmental school-based intervention, designed to reduce the age-related decline in PA among adolescents.

Methods: A cluster randomized controlled trial was conducted with 7 intervention and 7 control schools. Baseline measurements were carried out in spring 2010 with 2 years of follow-up. A total of 1,348 students (11–13 years, in grade 5 and 6) enrolled in the study at baseline. The 14 schools included in the study were located in the Region of Southern Denmark. The intervention consisted of organizational and physical changes in the school environment with a total of 11 intervention components. The primary outcome measure was overall PA (cpm, counts per minute) and was supported by analyses of time spent in MVPA, and time spent sedentary. Furthermore, a secondary outcome measure was PA in school time and during recess. PA was measured using accelerometer (Actigraph GT3X).

Results: A total of 797 students completed the trial and had valid accelerometer data. No significant difference was found for overall PA with an adjusted difference of −19.1 cpm (95% CI: −93, 53) or for school time activity with an adjusted difference of 6 cpm (95% CI: −73, 85). A sensitivity analysis revealed a positive significant intervention effect of PA in recess with an adjusted difference of 95 cpm.

Conclusions: No evidence was found of the overall effect of a non-curricular multicomponent school-based intervention on PA among Danish adolescents. The intervention was positively associated with PA during school time and recess, however, with small estimates. Lack of effect on overall PA could be due to both program theory and different degrees of implementation.

Trial Registration: www.Controlled-Trials.com ISRCTN79122411

Editor: Marc A Adams, Arizona State University, United States of America

Funding: Trygfonden supported the SPACE study. The SPACE study is part of the Centre for Intervention Research in Health Promotion and Disease prevention. The funders had no role in study design, data collection and analysis, decision to publish, or preparation of the manuscript.

Competing Interests: The authors have declared that no competing interests exist.

* E-mail: mtoftager@health.sdu.dk

Introduction

Adolescence is a period of physical activity (PA) decline [1,2]. As young people spend a large proportion of their waking hours at school, schools have long been recognized as potentially effective settings for public health initiatives including PA interventions [3,4]. Studies in school-based PA interventions have reported varying results and there is still a need for high quality and systematic studies among adolescents [3,5–7]. The development of multicomponent interventions (interventions with several intervention components), originates from principles of social ecological models to behavior change, which state that as health behavior is influenced at multiple levels (individual, social, environmental and policy levels), so should interventions in order to maximize effectiveness [8]. Several studies have used the social ecological framework for the design of PA interventions [6,9–12]. The multicomponent intervention study *SPACE for physical activity* has likewise been developed based on a social ecological framework [12]. The overall purpose of the SPACE study was to design, develop, document and assess a comprehensive intervention in schools to promote everyday PA among adolescents. The intervention consisted primarily of non-curricular and environmental components.

The purpose of the current study was to assess the effectiveness of the intervention in reducing the decline in PA among students in the period from grade 5 and 6 (11–13 years) to grade 7 and 8

(13–15 years). The effect of the intervention was estimated with regards to overall PA as well as moderate and vigorous PA (MVPA) and sedentary time. Furthermore, the effect on PA in school time and during recess was investigated.

Methods

Study design, setting and participants

The SPACE study used a cluster randomized controlled study design. In 2009, all municipalities in the Region of Southern Denmark were invited to participate in the SPACE study. Five municipalities out of 22 accepted the invitation and were asked to enroll public schools that contained grade 8. A total of 28 schools were recommended or deemed eligible by the municipalities. Among the proposed schools, the project group excluded schools if: a) they were placed in the countryside and had more than 50% of all students living further than 2 km Euclidian distance from the school, and b) the majority of all students were non-native Danish. The research team excluded five schools based on the above-mentioned criteria. This resulted in the enrolment of 23 schools in the five municipalities. The audit tool consisted of a total of eight school characteristics comprising four objective and four subjective characteristics of the 23 schools. The objective characteristics were: 1) Euclidian distance from residence to school for grades 5 and 6, 2) area household income, 3) area education level, and 4) area ethnicity distribution. The information was obtained from Statistics Denmark and by use of a Geographic Information System (GIS). The subjective information, which was based on interviews with municipality consultants and managing school personnel at each school site, consisted of the following variables: 1) school district urbanicity, 2) condition and characteristics of school outdoor areas, 3) school health policy, and 4) level of active transport in the local area. After meetings with schools and visits to the school sites, two schools declined to participate in the project, resulting in 21 eligible schools. A Spearman rank correlation analysis was conducted of the standardized values of the eight variables between the 21 schools to identify the best matches. Based on this 14 schools were matched into 7 pairs and randomized to an intervention or a control group.

Due to the limited number of schools, a matched pair design was applied to optimize the randomization. In order to increase power an unmatched analysis of the matched data was adopted. Diehr et al [13] recommend that for 3–9 pairs, either to use an unmatched design and unmatched analysis or a matched design and unmatched analysis. Matching is helpful in balancing important characteristics between intervention and control groups [13].

A total of 1,348 adolescents in grade 5 and 6 (11–13 years old, mean age 12.5 years, 48.4% girls) entered the study (Figure 1). Further information on the enrolment procedure and the study design has been described in detail elsewhere [14].

Estimation of sample size

Sample size calculations were performed prior to the study. Conventional levels of statistical power (0.8), level of significance (0.05) and a two-sided test were used. The minimum detectable effect size between groups was determined at 60 counts per minute, representing an approximate 10% difference in the outcome measure at follow-up. We used data from the Danish part of the European Youth Heart Study (EYHS) [15] to estimate the variability in the change in physical activity from baseline to follow-up. Data from the EYHS was also used to estimate the between school variation in physical activity in order to take into account the clustering within schools (ICC = 0.011). The between school variation was estimated while controlling for most of the school matching variables described above. All analyses were performed with statistical software STATA v10 using the modules Sampsi and Sampclus. The calculations showed that a minimum of 12 schools (6 control and 6 intervention schools) were required, based on an average number of 100 students per school.

Ethical approval

The Danish National Committee on Health Research Ethics reviewed the study protocol and concluded that formal ethical approval was not required. The study was registered and listed in the Danish Data Protection Agency (reference number: 2009-41-3628) and registered in The Current Controlled Trials (ISRCTN79122411, http://www.controlled-trials.com/ISRCTN79122411). Personalized written information about the SPACE study was distributed to parents and students. Parents of the participating adolescents received a passive informed consent form that explained the nature and procedures of the study. Both adolescents and parents were informed that it was possible to withdraw at any stage of the study. This procedure has been found to be ethically appropriate in low-risk research in adolescents [16].

Intervention

The intervention consisted of 11 intervention components changing the physical and organizational environment of the schools. The multicomponent intervention was developed according to social ecological models of behavioural change [8,10] and constructed in accordance with existing knowledge-based research and practical experiences from Danish school settings [17]. A detailed written description of the intervention components was delivered to all participating schools and included four physical environment changes and seven organizational environment changes as described in Table 1. The physical environment changes required included the following components: 1) upgrade existing outdoor areas at the school for PA, including unfixed equipment, 2) develop and build playgrounds specially designed for adolescents: play spots, 3) improve safety for active transport to and from school, 4) establish an after school fitness program. The organizational environment changes included: 5) formulate and implement school PA policy, 6) educate teachers as "kick-starters", who facilitate and motivate PA during recess, 7) establish school play patrol: older students were trained to initiate play and games for minors during school recess, 8) mandatory outdoor recess and/or free access to gym/sports hall, 9) school traffic patrol: older students helped minors cross the streets near the school, 10) educate and train students in safe cycling, and finally 11) school project/theme week once a year focusing on learning about and doing PA during school lessons. Further details of the intervention components are described in the study design protocol [14] and at the project website [18].

Implementation

The implementation of the intervention began in autumn 2010. All intervention schools upgraded the outdoor areas (costing €10,000–20,000) and established play spots (costing €65,000–250,000). Furthermore, as documented in the process evaluation [17], PA policy, kick-starters, mandatory outdoor recess/open sports hall, and school theme week were implemented in all intervention schools. The school play patrol was already implemented at two schools prior to involvement in the intervention. School traffic patrol was already implemented in four of the schools. In the remaining three schools it was not relevant because traffic authorities have ranked the access to the schools as safe. Cyclist education was already implemented at all seven schools,

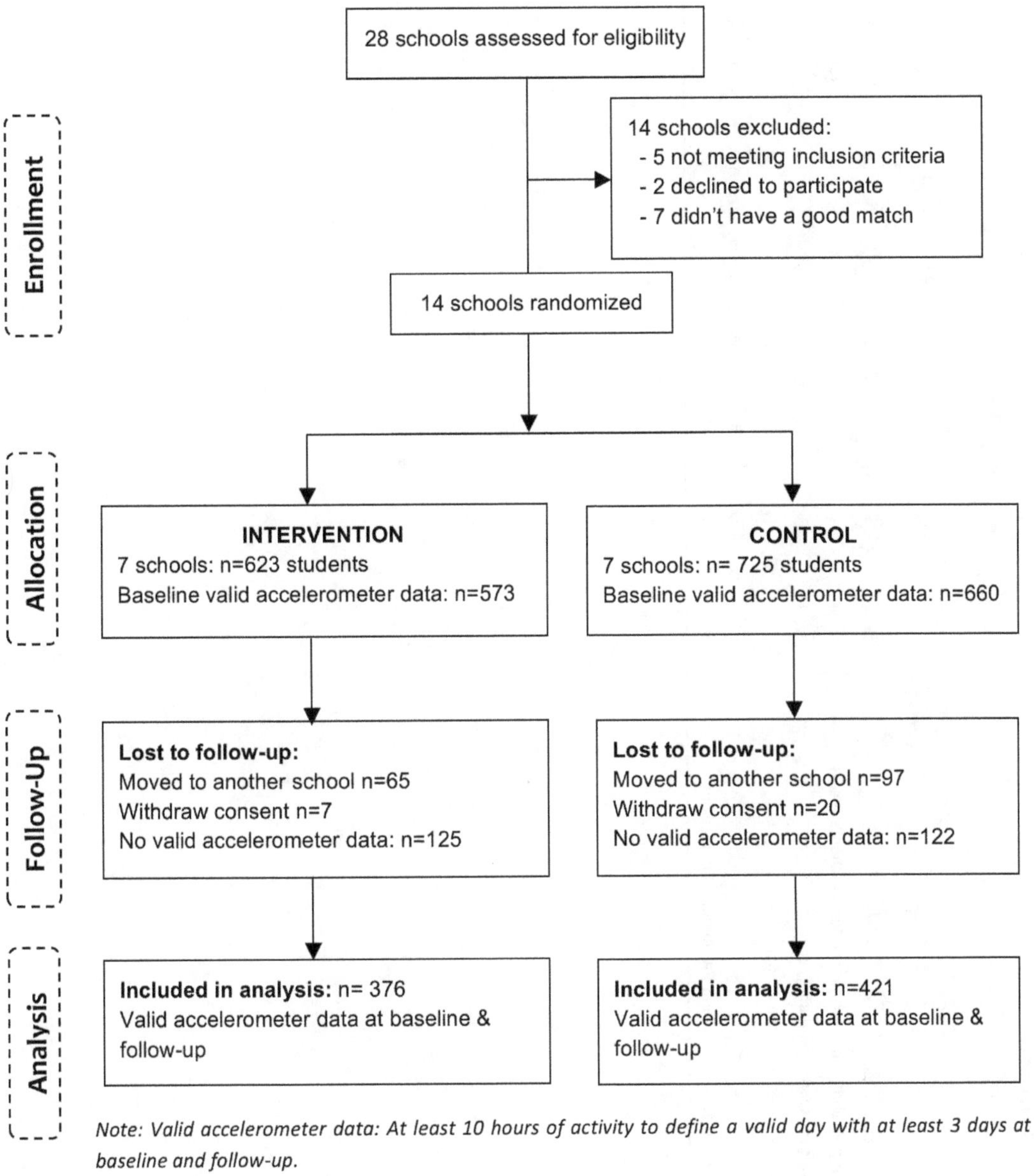

Figure 1. Flow diagram of participants.

and did not directly change, apart from being included in the school's PA policy. Improvement of cycling infrastructure was partly met at two schools, but lack of financial support made it impossible to implement this component in the remaining five schools. The organization of the after school fitness program was implemented in two local school areas. Lack of voluntary instructors made the component impossible to implement in the other five areas (Table 1).

Data collection

Baseline measurements were obtained in spring (April to June) 2010 among all students in grade 5 and 6 in seven intervention and seven control schools, with follow-up measurements in spring 2012. PA was objectively assessed among all students using accelerometers (Actigraph GT3X). Sex and age were obtained through school records. The parental income was obtained through Statistics Denmark using the Danish Civil Registration System, which monitors individual level information such as address and income [19,20]. The income was dichotomized as above or below the relative poverty line using 50% of median household income as the threshold [21]. Similarly, parents' ethnicity (both born in Denmark) was obtained through the Danish Civil Registration System. The adolescents' height and weight were objectively measured by the research team using standard anthropometric procedures. Overweight was defined using sex and age specific BMI cut points relative to 25 kg/m^2 for adults [22].

Accelerometer data reduction

The adolescents were instructed to wear the accelerometers all waking hours for seven consecutive days except when doing water activities. The accelerometers were downloaded using Actilife (Actigraph) and analyzed by the software program Propero (University of Southern Denmark). Data were analyzed using 30

Table 1. Intervention components and implementation.

Intervention components		Implementation in intervention schools						
		1i	2i	3i	4i	5i	6i	7i
Physical environment changes								
1	Upgrade existing outdoor areas at the school for PA including unfixed equipment	+	+	+	+	+	+	+
2	Develop and build specially designed playgrounds for adolescents: Play spots	+	+	+	+	+	+	+
3	Improve safety for active transport to/from school			(+)		+	+	
4	Establish an after school fitness program			+		+		
Organizational environment changes								
5	Formulate and implement school PA policy	+	+	+	+	+	+	+
6	Educate teachers as "kick-starters", who facilitate and motivate PA during recess	+	+	+	+	+	+	+
7	Implement school's play patrol: older students trained to initiate play and games for minors during school's recess	+	+	(+)	+	+	+	(+)
8	Establish mandatory outdoor recess and/or free access to school gym/sports hall during recess	+	+	+	+	+	+	+
9	Establish school's traffic patrol: older students help minors cross the streets near the school		(+)	(+)	(+)		(+)	
10	Educate and train students in safe cycling	(+)	(+)	(+)	(+)	(+)	(+)	(+)
11	Implement school project/theme week once a year focus on learning about and doing PA during school lessons	+	+	+	+	+	+	+

+ Implemented in intervention period, (+) Implemented before intervention start.

seconds of epoch, and activity for all 24 hours was included. Strings of 60 minutes or more of consecutive zeroes, allowing for two epoch periods of non-zero interruptions, were interpreted to represent non-wear time and were excluded from each individual recording [23]. Adolescents with valid accelerometer data i.e. at least 3 days with at least 10 hours (600 min) of activity recorded per day, at both baseline and follow-up were included in this study (n = 797). Data were aggregated at the individual level as mean measures on weekdays and weekend days. The average number of minutes per day that the participants wore the accelerometer and the number of activity counts per minute (cpm) were calculated. To investigate time in different PA intensities the Evenson activity cut points were used [24]. These cut points have been recommended and validated in previous studies [25]. Sedentary time (≤100 cpm) and MVPA (≥2296 cpm) were expressed as minutes per day of accelerometer activity. Information on schools' timetables and periods of recess with exact bell times was obtained from each of the participating schools and merged with the accelerometer data.

Statistical analyses

Lost to follow-up analyses were performed for baseline outcome measures and background characteristics using logistic (binary outcome such as sex) and linear (continuous outcome such as age) regression models for each of the background variables (sex, age, BMI, weight status, household income and parents ethnicity) and for each of the outcome measures on PA and sedentary time. Lost-to-follow status was included as exposure. Clustering of students within schools was accounted for by including schools as a random effect in the analyses.

When estimating effects multilevel linear mixed models were used taking into account clustering of students within classes and classes within schools. The primary outcome measure was overall PA (cpm) and was supported by analyses of time spent in MVPA, and time spent sedentary. Furthermore, a secondary outcome measure was PA in school time and during recess. The outcome measure at follow-up was used as the dependent variable and the intervention condition was the explanatory variable. Analyses were adjusted for differences in baseline PA, sex and age at baseline. The primary outcome measures were derived for weekdays and weekend days, whereas the secondary outcome measures were only derived for weekdays. Students were measured for seven consecutive days, five weekdays and two weekend days. In the analyses of overall PA a random effect for student was included with an aggregated measure for weekdays and an aggregated measure for weekends. Therefore, for each student we had two observations. The random effect of school and classes within schools were included in the primary and secondary analyses. Furthermore, the random effect of students within classes and schools was included in the primary analyses. The primary analyses were also adjusted for differences in weekday/weekend day. Figure 2 shows the regression model for the primary outcome. We used the intention to treat principle in that it analyses the individuals in the groups to which they were originally assigned [26].

Effect modification was explored for sex, parental income, weight and PA at baseline by adding one interaction term at a time in the multilevel model. Residual plots were conducted to evaluate the model assumptions (i.e. normal distribution of residuals and equal variances). When model assumptions were not met outcome variables were analyzed using a log-transformation. When no differences in the effect of intervention and p-values were seen, results were reported without the log-transformation. When log-transformation of the outcome was necessary (due to lack of fulfilled model assumptions), the intervention effect was estimated as the difference between the back-transformed least square mean estimates of log(PA) for the intervention and control groups (all other effects in the model than intervention were kept at the mean value). Due to the use of log-transformation, confidence intervals cannot be estimated for the difference in PA between the intervention and control groups [27].

To interpret the variation between schools, classes within schools and students within classes and schools, intraclass correlation coefficients (ICC) were calculated.

Sensitivity analyses were conducted with at least one valid accelerometer day as the inclusion criteria. There were only minor differences in the results, and results based on the three days inclusion criterion are reported.

Finally, descriptive analyses of PA (cpm) at each school were reported to illustrate the variance between schools. One school (school c7 in Figure 3) had a markedly higher PA level at follow-up compared to the other schools. Information from the students and the school staff showed that many students from this school had attended an outdoor local music festival in the same week of PA measurement, which was a plausible explanation for the very high level of activity. Based on this it was decided to conduct a sensitivity analysis, excluding the specific school from the analysis.

Data were analyzed by Stata/SE, version 12. A 5% significance level was used.

The protocol for this trial and supporting CONSORT checklist are available as supporting information; see Checklist S1 and Protocol S1.

Results

Participants

A total of 1,348 students entered the study of which 1,233 (91%) provided valid accelerometer data at baseline (Figure 1). Out of the participating adolescents at baseline 13% (n = 162) had moved to another school at follow-up, and 2% (n = 27) withdrew consent. A total of 797 adolescents (65%) had at least three days of valid accelerometer data at baseline and follow up and were included in the follow-up analyses. Average daily accelerometer wear time was 14 hours and number of valid days was 6.6 in both the intervention and control group. Average BMI was 18.7 kg/m^2 and the proportion of overweight was 11.7% and 13.8% in intervention and control group, respectively. Most parents (>90%) were born in Denmark and 13% had a low household income (Table 2). There were on average 4.8 classes per school with a minimum of 4 and a maximum of 6 classes. There were on average 11.2 students in each class with valid data at both baseline and follow-up with a minimum of 3 and a maximum of 20 students (data not shown).

Lost to follow-up

The differences between students included in analyses and students lost to follow-up are shown in Table 3. The lost to follow-up group was defined as students who moved to another school, withdrew their consent or had missing data at baseline or follow-up accelerometer measurements (Figure 1). The lost to follow-up group consisted of fewer girls (42.1% vs. 52.8%), was a little older (12.7 years vs. 12.5 years), was more likely to have a higher BMI (19.2 vs. 18.8), and more likely to be from low economic background (23.0% vs. 14.1%) at baseline compared to adolescents included in the analysis. Regarding the outcome measures, the lost to follow-up group had a higher level of PA in school time (581 vs 547cpm) (Table 3). No significant differences were

$$y_{ijklmn} = \mu + \beta_1 X_{1ijklmn} + \beta_2 X_{2ijklmn} + A_i + B_j + C_k + \vartheta_{l(j)} + \omega_{m(jl)} + \gamma_{n(jlm)} + \varepsilon_{ijklmn}$$

where

y_{ijklmn} is physical activity (PA) for student, n in school-class, *m* and school, *l*

μ is the intercept

A_i is the effect of sex, *i*=male, female

B_j is the effect of intervention, *j*=yes, no

C_k is the effect of day in the week, *k*=weekday, weekend day

$\vartheta_{l(j)}$ is the random effect of school, *l* within intervention, *j*

$\omega_{m(jl)}$ is the random effect of school-class, *m* within school, *l* and within intervention, *j*

$\gamma_{n(jlm)}$ is the random effect of student, *n* within school-class, *m* within school, *l* and within intervention, *j*

ε_{ijklmn} is the residual random error

Figure 2. Regression model for the primary outcome, physical activity (cpm).

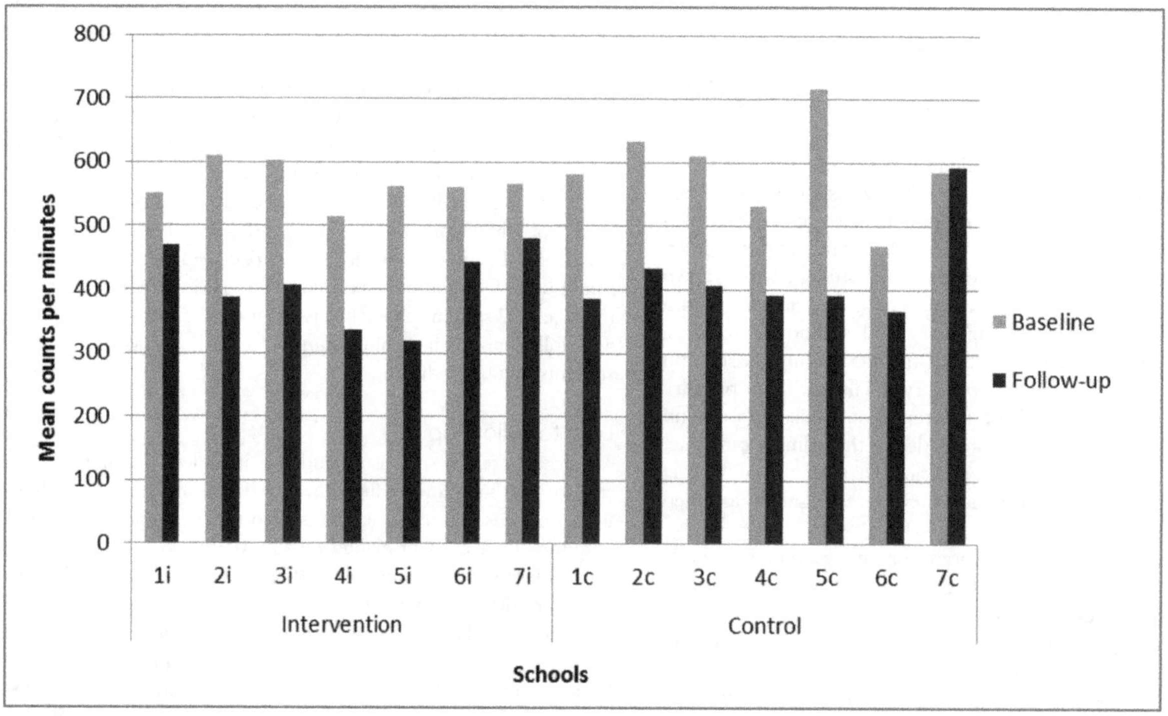

Figure 3. Physical activity (cpm) in the intervention (n = 376) and control (n = 421) schools at baseline and follow-up.

Table 2. Baseline characteristics of participants.

	Intervention (n = 376)	Control (n = 421)
Girls, %	51.3	47.9
Age, years	12.5 (0.63)	12.5 (0.61)
BMI, kg/m^2	18.7 (2.6)	18.6 (3.0)
Overweight[a], %	11.7	13.8
Low household income[b], %	13.0	13.3
Parents' native Danish[c], %	91.2	93.1
Daily accelerometer wear time, hours	14.2 (1.10)	14.0 (1.02)
Number of valid accelerometer days	6.7 (1.25)	6.6 (1.11)

M(SD) unless otherwise stated. N = 797
[a]*Sex and age standardized cut points [22].* [b]*Household income lower than 50% of the sample median income.* [c]*Both parents native Danish. n varies due to different data sources*

observed between the intervention and control group among individuals lost to follow-up (data not shown).

Physical activity level

Table 4 shows PA in the intervention and control group at baseline and follow-up and the adjusted intervention effect. The 2-year follow-up time resulted in an average decrease in PA for all PA outcome measures. For overall PA, the crude decrease during the 2-year period was 157 cpm in the intervention group and 162 cpm in the control group. Time spent in MVPA was 57 minutes/day at baseline and declined to 44 minutes and 48 minutes in the intervention and control group, respectively. Sedentary time increased in both groups with 1 hour (daily accelerometer wear time remained the same at baseline and follow-up, approx. 14 hours). Adjusted for baseline values of sex, age, weekend/weekdays and clustering, the difference between intervention and control was −19 cpm of overall PA (95% CI: −93, 53), -3 minutes/day in MVPA (95% CI: −15, 8), and for sedentary time the adjusted effect was zero (95% CI: −20, 22).

Stratifying the analyses by weekdays and weekend days showed lower PA at weekends compared to weekdays, especially at follow-up. PA in school time declined with 141 cpm in intervention group and 138 cpm in the control group, and no significant intervention effect was found (6 cpm, 95% CI: −73, 85). Recess PA for the intervention group declined from an average of 1005 cpm at baseline to 662 cpm at follow-up, and the control group PA declined from 929 cpm to 617 cpm, and no significant intervention effect was found (19 cpm, 95% CI: −156, 195) (Table 4). No significant interactions were seen between intervention and sex, parental income, weight and PA at baseline.

The intervention effect was further explored by analyses stratified by sex, household income, overweight and PA level at baseline. No effect of the intervention was seen in these analyses. In general, boys were more active than girls, and overweight adolescents less active than normal weight adolescents. The intervention did not change this pattern from baseline to follow-up (data not shown).

Variation in PA between schools was explored and revealed considerable differences across schools during the 2-year study period (Figure 3). The biggest difference was seen in school 5i and 5c, with a 45% decline in average PA level (cpm). The smallest decline (15%) was observed for the two intervention schools, 1i

Table 3. Baseline characteristics individuals lost to follow-up and with complete data.

	Lost to follow-up or missing data (n = 551)	Complete data (n = 797)	p-value
Girls, %	42.1 (38.0, 46.3)	52.8 (49.4, 56.3)	<0.001
Age, years	12.7 (12.6, 12.8)	12.5 (12.5, 12.6)	<0.001
BMI, kg/m^2	19.2 (18.8, 19.6)	18.8 (18.4, 19.1)	0.008
Overweight[a], %	16.7 (12.6, 20.7)	13.8 (10.2, 17.5)	0.160
Low household income[b], %	23.0 (18.7, 27.3)	14.1 (10.2, 18.0)	<0.001
Parents' native Danish[c], %	89.9 (84.9, 94.9)	90.5 (85.7, 95,3)	0.692
Overall PA, cpm	574.7 (543.2, 606.2)	582.1 (553.5, 610.7)	0.595
Time in MVPA/day, min	60.1 (56.7, 63.4)	57.5 (54.5, 60.5)	0.087
Time in sedentary activity/day, min	511.7 (504.6, 518.7)	509.0 (503.7, 514.6)	0.577
School time PA, cpm	581.1 (532.9, 629.2)	547.5 (500.6, 594.4)	0.003
PA in recess, cpm	1032.6 (901.3, 1163.9)	976.5 (848.8, 1104.3)	0.078

M (CI 95%) unless otherwise stated.
Based on a regression model adjusted for cluster on school level.
PA: physical activity. MVPA: moderate to vigorous physical activity. Cpm: counts per minute
[a]*Sex and age standardized cut points [22].* [b]*Household income lower than 50% of the sample median income.* [c]*Both parents native Danish*

Table 4. PA in the intervention (n = 376) and control (n = 421) group at baseline and follow-up.

	Baseline	Follow-up	Crude difference within groups	Adjusted difference between groups	p-value	ICC
	M (SD)	*M (SD)*		*(95% CI)*		
Overall PA, cpm						
Intervention	566 (221)	408 (167)	−158	−19.1 (−92.6, 53.1)[a]	0.591	0.09 (school)
Control	596 (252)	433 (206)	−163			0.11 (class)
						0.42 (student)
MVPA time, min/day						
Intervention	57 (24)	44 (23)	−13	−3.3 (−15.4, 8.7)[a]	0.587	0.15 (school)
Control	57 (24)	48 (27)	-9			0.17 (class)
						0.32 (student)
Sedentary time, min/day						
Intervention	515 (81)	575 (88)	60	0.1 (−20.0, 21.7)[a]	0.938	0.02 (school)
Control	503 (100)	565 (106)	62			0.04 (class)
						0.35 (student)
Weekday PA, cpm						
Intervention	574 (222)	422 (173)	−152	−8.4 (−67.2, 50.3)[b]	0.782	0.08 (school)
Control	601 (250)	439 (203)	−162			0.13 (class)
Weekend PA, cpm						
Intervention	555 (357)	345 (225)	−210	−40.3 (−141.3, 60.7)[b]	0.433	0.11 (school)
Control	596 (406)	417 (313)	−179			0.12 (class)
School time PA, cpm						
Intervention	554 (221)	413 (187)	−141	5.8 (−73.1 84.7)[b]	0.886	0.15 (school)
Control	533 (196)	395 (202)	−138			0.29 (class)
Recess PA, cpm						
Intervention	1005 (546)	662 (402)	−342	19.2 (−156.3,194.7)[b]	0.834	0.11 (school)
Control	929 (650)	617 (507)	−311			0.27 (class)

[a]*Effect analyses adjusted for baseline PA, sex, age, weekend/weekdays. School, class and student were included as random effects to account for clustering.* [b]*Effect analyses adjusted for baseline PA, sex, age. School and class included as random effects to account for clustering. PA: physical activity, MVPA: moderate and vigorous physical activity. Cpm: counts per minute, ICC: Intraclass correlation*

and 7i. The control school 7c increased PA from baseline to follow-up most likely due to a local music festival (Figure 3). A sensitivity analysis investigating the intervention effect, when excluding school 7c showed positive intervention effects for all outcomes (non-significant for most parts). For overall PA, the effect was 12 cpm (95% CI: −35, 60) and for school time PA the effect was 29 cpm (95% CI: −43, 101). A significant effect for PA in recess was observed ($p = 0.046$) with an estimated difference at 95 cpm (Table 5).

Discussion

The aim of this study was to investigate whether an environmental non-curricular intervention in the school setting was able to change the level of PA in Danish adolescents. The overall effect evaluation showed no significant intervention effect. Lack of effect could be due to the design of the intervention, lack of effect in single intervention components, and the implementation of the intervention components. The intervention package in the SPACE study consisted of 11 intervention components, combining physical environment changes with supportive organizational changes. The intervention could be categorized as a complex intervention, with regards to both the number of intervention components and the diverse contents and processes of developing and implementing each of the components. The implementation of several components turned out to be a challenging task for some schools, mainly due to economic reasons. The most successfully implemented intervention components in the SPACE study aimed at increasing PA in recess (e.g. kick-starters, mandatory outdoor recess/open sports hall, upgrading school outdoor areas and establishing Play spots). This seems to be reflected by the positive (but non-significant) intervention effect estimates for PA in school time and recess in the complete case analysis. In the sensitivity analysis, a significant and relative high estimate of 95 cpm was obtained for PA in recess.

The intervention components in the SPACE study were primarily non-curricular but had focus on PA in several arenas. It could be argued that interventions with a more mandatory structure might be more effective on improving the frequency, intensity and duration of PA, e.g. physical education and other curricular interventions as shown in other studies. For example, Kriemler et al concluded that a Swiss school-based multicomponent intervention with compulsory elements improved MVPA in school with 13 min/day and total MVPA with 11 min/day [28].

There seems to be general consensus in recent published reviews and studies on school-based interventions that multicomponent approaches are the most effective way of increasing PA levels in

Table 5. Sensitivity analysis, school c7 excluded.

	Baseline	Follow-up	Crude difference within groups	Adjusted difference between groups	p-value	ICC
	M (SD)	*M (SD)*		*(95% CI)*		
Overall PA, cpm						
Intervention	566 (221)	408 (167)	−158	12.3 (−34.9, 59.5)[a]	0.611	0.03 (school)
Control	598 (247)	400 (191)	−198			0.05 (class)
						0.42 (student)
MVPA time, min/day						
Intervention	57 (24)	44 (23)	−13	2.2 (−4.2, 8.6)[a]	0.497	0.04 (school)
Control	57 (24)	42 (21)	−15			0.07 (class)
						0.26 (student)
Sedentary time, min/day						
Intervention	515 (81)	575 (88)	60	−6.0 (−20.3, 8.3)[a]	0.413	0.01 (school)
Control	501 (70)	584 (77)	83			0.02 (class)
						0.31 (student)
Weekday PA, cpm						
Intervention	574 (222)	422 (173)	−152	16.8 (−24.0, 57.6)[b]	0.421	0.02 (school)
Control	601 (235)	410 (193)	−191			0.07 (class)
Weekend PA, cpm						
Intervention	555 (357)	345 (225)	−210	2.0 (−62.6, 66.7)[b]	0.952	0.03 (school)
Control	606 (424)	366 (290)	−240			0.03 (class)
School time PA, cpm						
Intervention	554 (221)	413 (187)	−141	28.6 (−43.4, 100.7)[b]	0.436	0.11 (school)
Control	552 (200)	370 (189)	−182			0.27 (class)
Recess PA, cpm						
Intervention	1005 (546)	662 (402)	−343	95.0*[b]	0.046	0.04 (school)
Control	967 (550)	584 (524)	−383			0.20 (class)

PA in the intervention (n = 376) and control (n = 344) group at baseline and follow-up.
*[a]Effect analyses adjusted for baseline PA, sex, age, weekend/weekdays. School, class and student were included as random effects to account for clustering. [b]Effect analyses adjusted for baseline PA, sex, age. School and class included as random effects to account for clustering.*Back-transformed estimate based on analysis of log-transformed outcome. Due to log-transformation, no confidence interval is calculated. PA: physical activity, MVPA: moderate and vigorous physical activity. Cpm: counts per minute, ICC: Intraclass correlation.*

adolescents [3,5]. In the SPACE study, no overall effect was achieved despite the fact that the study included a large number of components, raising the question that maybe the intervention had too many components and was too complex to implement. This could however also be more related to the content of the intervention components, and not because of the multi-stringed intervention package itself. A possible explanation for the no overall effect could be that the content of some of the intervention components in practice turned out to be more attractive for younger students (grade 3–5) instead of older students (grade 7–8) as intended. This was indicated in qualitative research on the SPACE study, which also showed that it is a challenge to activate adolescents in this age group. Especially the girls perceived several barriers for being physically active, primarily related to their attitude to childish behavior and being sweaty. The analyses of PA in recess also showed that boys in general were more active than girls, which indicate that boys and girls may experience recess in different ways. Boys view recess as an opportunity to play competitive games, while girls may view recess as an opportunity to socialize with friends [17]. This pattern has been found in other studies too [29].

Another possible explanation for not finding an effect could be that PA behavior, like healthy eating habits, are established earlier in childhood and are relatively resistant to changes. Recent successful multicomponent RCT intervention studies that have used accelerometry, have in general focused on younger age groups than in the SPACE study, e.g. the Swiss KISS study [28] and the Norwegian HEIA study [30]. Thus, it can be argued that interventions to increase PA should begin before adolescence [31]. Furthermore, it could be suggested that involvement of the family/parents should play a more significant role of the intervention, as shown effective in other studies [32]. Social network and peer influence in adolescents play an important role for health behavior. Several of the intervention components were developed with a specific focus on the aspect of social relations. The play spots were designed to encourage social interaction among the adolescents as a local "hangout spot", also after school hours, and the kick-starters initiated team play and activities in recess. The play patrol highlighted the importance of role models, with older students initiating play and games for minors during recess. Nonetheless, it is possible that the intervention could have succeeded with more focus on the social relational environment.

The non-effect for overall PA found in this study is in line with findings from a recent meta-analysis of studies that examined 30 interventions aimed at promoting PA in children. The results indicate a small to negligible pooled effect on total time spent in MVPA (4 minutes a day). The meta-analysis differs from previous systematic reviews with inclusion of only accelerometry as objective measurements of PA [7].

At baseline a high participation rate was obtained with 91% (n = 1,233) of eligible students contributing with valid accelerometer data for at least three days. At follow-up the participation rate dropped to 65% (n = 797) of those participating at baseline. In large-scale school-based interventions a certain dropout rate is expected. Efforts were done to increase participation rate at both baseline and follow-up, e.g. passive informed consent procedure was used and text messages to remind of wearing the accelerometer were sent to students/parents if they signed up for it. To explore if the definitions of lost to follow-up affected the results, the analyses were repeated excluding students who moved to another school (n = 162), and for participants with at least one valid day (n = 965). This did not change the results significantly.

To investigate if the accelerometer data reduction criterion, of at least three valid days had an impact on the effect results, a sensitivity analysis was conducted including all participants with at least one valid day of accelerometer data. This did not change the results of the study, but it did improve the participation rate considerably to 76% (n = 965). Using at least one valid accelerometer day as inclusion criterion thus increased the sample size and statistical power, however, very few studies are reported based on only one valid day. Therefore, to compare with other studies and to increase the validity of the study, the three valid day criterion was used [33].

Strengths and limitations

A strong aspect of this study is the cluster randomized controlled design and the large sample size. PA was measured objectively and both overall PA and school time PA was assessed. Furthermore, the 2-year follow-up period is considered long, compared to most other intervention studies reported [3,5].

Limitations of the study relate to the fact that the intervention was implemented with varying degree in the intervention schools. On the other hand, it could be stated that the results from this study reflect the real-life school setting.

The students lost to follow-up were significantly different from those included on several variables. In general, the lost to follow-up group consisted of fewer girls, was a little older, more likely to be from low socioeconomic background and was more likely to have a high BMI at baseline compared to adolescents included in analyses. Thus, we are unable to rule out that the lost to follow-up group may well have benefited from the intervention.

The majority of students at the schools involved were native Danes and all lived in the same region of Southern Denmark. Although the schools and students included in the study may not be representative of the Danish population of schools and students, the lack of association might be valid for the Danish students in general.

The SPACE study fulfils the intention to treat principles in that it analyses the individuals in the groups to which they were originally assigned. The most important reason for conducting intention to treat analyses is that it preserves the randomization, and thus is a defense against bias [26]. For example, there were ten students who moved to another SPACE school in the period from baseline to follow-up. They were all categorized as belonging to the group they were randomized to initially. Furthermore, the intervention effect was analyzed with no regards to implementation status, and not as a per protocol analysis where a trial is evaluated with regards to adherence to the study protocol [34,35].

Despite the benefits of using accelerometers to assess PA, some limitations should also be addressed, such as the problem of adequately measuring cycling activity. In Denmark, cycling is very common as part of daily active transport. Therefore, this aspect of the SPACE study was evaluated using self-reported measures. Another issue is that accelerometers may be impractical to wear during contact sport. Participants can forget to put the sensor on or choose not to wear it because of concerns related to appearance. Furthermore, shortcomings are that accelerometers do not capture swimming, weight bearing activities (e.g. weight training or stair climbing) and there is a risk of 'leveling-off' when running at a high speed. Because of these issues, accelerometers may underestimate PA in adolescents [36]. Despite these limitations, there are still several good reasons for using accelerometers in intervention research compared to self-reported measures. An important aspect is that it is very difficult to measure a specific change in PA with a self-reported measure due to a risk of recall bias and because the details with regards to overall duration, frequency and intensity are difficult to capture in a simple questionnaire [37].

Measurement of PA, as done in the SPACE study, will always be a snapshot of the adolescents' PA behavior, and despite efforts to account for schools to have a "usual" week in the data collection period, external factors, such as a local music festival, can have substantial impact on the results.

Future studies

Future intervention studies should aim at designing an intervention that builds on the experiences from the SPACE study. Especially the organizational intervention components, for example the kick-starter initiative proved to be a success, according to interview with school staff. The building of play spots and upgrading of school outdoor areas were relatively expensive, and the attempts to improve the physical environment for active transport demanded a high degree of political involvement and support, and such projects take a long time from proposal to implementation, and are therefore not easy to implement nationwide. Finally, and important to mention, the design of the build environment for promotion of PA and active transport in Denmark seems in general rather good compared to many other countries.

Qualitative findings from the process and anthropological part of the SPACE study have been useful in the discussion of the reasons for the lack of effect. The qualitative data collection was conducted after the implementation, and future studies should consider incorporating qualitative work also before the planning and implementation of the intervention in an effort to ensure that the intervention reaches the desired target group and is filling the most important gaps.

Conducting randomized controlled trials in a real life setting is challenging, time consuming and expensive. There are many stakeholders, and many issues should be taken into consideration. Therefore, a solution for researchers could also be focusing on evaluating the effect of natural experiments, for example where planned improvements of the physical environment around schools are accompanied by supportive organizational interventions.

Conclusions

No evidence was found of the overall effect of a non-curricular multicomponent school-based intervention on PA among Danish adolescents. Lack of effect on overall PA could be due to both program theory and different degrees of implementation. The intervention was positively associated with PA during school time and recess, however with small and non-significant estimates. A sensitivity analysis revealed a significant intervention effect of 95 cpm in recess.

Acknowledgments

The SPACE study is part of the Centre for Intervention Research in Health Promotion and Disease prevention. TrygFonden supported the SPACE study. Jan Brønd, University of Southern Denmark, developed the accelerometer software program, Propero used for data processing.

We thank the participating schools, their teachers and students, field staff who assisted in data collection, and others involved in the project.

Author Contributions

Conceived and designed the experiments: MT LBC PLK JT. Analyzed the data: MT AKE. Wrote the paper: MT LBC PD PLK AKE JT.

References

1. Nader PR, Bradley RH, Houts RM, McRitchie SL, O'Brien M (2008) Moderate-to-vigorous physical activity from ages 9 to 15 years. JAMA 300: 295–305.
2. Dumith SC, Gigante DP, Domingues MR, Kohl HW 3rd (2011) Physical activity change during adolescence: a systematic review and a pooled analysis. Int J Epidemiol 40: 685–698.
3. Dobbins M, Husson H, DeCorby K, LaRocca RL (2013) School-based physical activity programs for promoting physical activity and fitness in children and adolescents aged 6 to 18. Cochrane Database Syst Rev 2: CD007651.
4. Harold WK III, Cook HD (2013) Educating the Student Body: Taking Physical Activity and Physical Education to School: The National Academies Press.
5. Kriemler S, Meyer U, Martin E, van Sluijs EM, Andersen LB, et al. (2011) Effect of school-based interventions on physical activity and fitness in children and adolescents: a review of reviews and systematic update. British Journal of Sports Medicine 45: 923–930.
6. van Sluijs EM, McMinn AM, Griffin SJ (2007) Effectiveness of interventions to promote physical activity in children and adolescents: systematic review of controlled trials. BMJ 335: 703.
7. Metcalf B, Henley W, Wilkin T (2012) Effectiveness of intervention on physical activity of children: systematic review and meta-analysis of controlled trials with objectively measured outcomes (EarlyBird 54). BMJ 345: e5888.
8. Sallis JFON, Fisher EB (2008) Ecological models of health behaviour; Glanz K RB, Viswanath K, editor. San-Fransisco: Jossey-Bass.
9. Giles-Corti B, Timperio A, Bull F, Pikora T (2005) Understanding Physical Activity Environmental Correlates: Increased Specificity for Ecological Models. Exercise and Sports Science and Reviews 33: 175–181.
10. King AC (2002) Theoretical Approaches to the Promotion of Physical Activity. Forging a Transdisciplinary Paradigm. American Journal of Preventive Medicine 23.
11. Pate RR, Saunders R, Dishman RK, Addy C, Dowda M, et al. (2007) Long-term effects of a physical activity intervention in high school girls. American Journal of Preventive Medicine 33: 276–280.
12. Sallis JF, Cervero RB, Ascher W, Henderson KA, Kraft MK, et al. (2006) An ecological approach to creating active living communities. Annual Review of Public Health 27: 297–322.
13. Diehr P, Martin DC, Koepsell T, Cheadle A (1995) Breaking the matches in a paired t-test for community interventions when the number of pairs is small. Stat Med 14: 1491–1504.
14. Toftager M, Christiansen LB, Kristensen PL, Troelsen J (2011) SPACE for physical activity -a multicomponent intervention study: study design and baseline findings from a cluster randomized controlled trial. BMC Public Health 11: 777.
15. Riddoch CJ, Andersen LB, Wedderkopp N, Harro M, Klasson-Heggebo L, et al. (2004) Physical activity levels and patterns of 9-and 15-yr-old European children. Med Sci Sports Exerc 36: 86–92.
16. Santelli JS, Smith Rogers A, Rosenfeld WD, DuRant RH, Dubler N, et al. (2003) Guidelines for adolescent health research. A position paper of the Society for Adolescent Medicine. J Adolesc Health 33: 396–409.
17. Troelsen J, Brøcker A, Ballegaard SA, Grøn L, Olesen E, et al. (2013) SPACE - rum til fysisk aktivitet. Organisatorisk evaluering og brugerperspektiv på en helhedsorienteret, forebyggende indsats for børn og unge. Odense, Denmark: Center for intervention research, University of Southern Denmark.
18. Centre for Intervention Research in Health Promotion website. Available: www.cirhp.dk. Accessed 2014 April 4. Intervention components in the SPACE study.
19. Pedersen CB (2011) The Danish Civil Registration System. Scandinavian Journal of Public Health 39: 22–25.
20. Baadsgaard M, Quitzau J (2011) Danish registers on personal income and transfer payments. Scandinavian Journal of Public Health 39: 103–105.
21. Hagenaars AJM, van Praag BMS (1985) A synthesis of poverty line definitions. Review of Income and Wealth 31: 139–154.
22. Cole TJ, Bellizzi MC, Flegal KM, Dietz WH (2000) Establishing a standard definition for child overweight and obesity worldwide: international survey. BMJ 320: 1240–1243.
23. Sherar LB, Griew P, Esliger DW, Cooper AR, Ekelund U, et al. (2011) International children's accelerometry database (ICAD): design and methods. BMC Public Health 11: 485.
24. Evenson KR, Catellier DJ, Gill K, Ondrak KS, McMurray RG (2008) Calibration of two objective measures of physical activity for children. J Sports Sci 26: 1557–1565.
25. Trost SG, Loprinzi PD, Moore R, Pfeiffer KA (2011) Comparison of accelerometer cut points for predicting activity intensity in youth. Med Sci Sports Exerc 43: 1360–1368.
26. White IR, Horton NJ, Carpenter J, Pocock SJ (2011) Strategy for intention to treat analysis in randomised trials with missing outcome data. BMJ 342: d40.
27. Bland JM, Altman DG (1996) The use of transformation when comparing two means. BMJ 312: 1153.
28. Kriemler S, Zahner L, Schindler C, Meyer U, Hartmann T, et al. (2010) Effect of school based physical activity programme (KISS) on fitness and adiposity in primary schoolchildren: cluster randomised controlled trial. BMJ 340: c785.
29. Ridgers ND, Salmon J, Parrish A-M, Stanley RM, Okely AD (2012) Physical Activity During School Recess: A Systematic Review. American Journal of Preventive Medicine 43: 320–328.
30. Grydeland M, Bergh IH, Bjelland M, Lien N, Andersen LF, et al. (2013) Intervention effects on physical activity: the HEIA study - a cluster randomized controlled trial. International Journal of Behavioral Nutrition and Physical Activity 10: 17.
31. Kahn JA, Huang B, Gillman MW, Field AE, Austin SB, et al. (2008) Patterns and determinants of physical activity in U.S. adolescents. J Adolesc Health 42: 369–377.
32. Kriemler S, Meyer U, Martin E, van Sluijs EM, Andersen LB, et al. (2011) Effect of school-based interventions on physical activity and fitness in children and adolescents: a review of reviews and systematic update. Br J Sports Med 45: 923–930.
33. Cain KL, Geremia Carrie M (2012) Accelerometer Data Collection and Scoring Manual For Adult & Senior Studies. San Diego State University, San Diego, CA.
34. Gupta SK (2011) Intention-to-treat concept: A review. Perspect Clin Res 2: 109–112.
35. Abraha I, Montedori A (2010) Modified intention to treat reporting in randomised controlled trials: systematic review. BMJ 340.
36. Trost SG (2007) State of the Art Reviews: Measurement of Physical Activity in Children and Adolescents. American Journal of Lifestyle Medicine 1: 299–314.
37. Corder K, Ekelund U, Steele RM, Wareham NJ, Brage S (2008) Assessment of physical activity in youth. Journal of Applied Physiology 105: 977–987.

18

Neurological Assessment and Its Relationship to CSF Biomarkers in Amateur Boxers

Sanna Neselius[1,2]*, Helena Brisby[1,2], Jan Marcusson[3,4], Henrik Zetterberg[5,6,7], Kaj Blennow[5,6], Thomas Karlsson[8,9]

1 Department of Orthopaedics, Sahlgrenska University Hospital, Gothenburg, Sweden, **2** Institute for Clinical Sciences, the Sahlgrenska Academy at the University of Gothenburg, Gothenburg, Sweden, **3** Geriatric Section, University Hospital in Linköping, Linköping, Sweden, **4** Institution of Clinical and Experimental Medicine, Linköping University, Linköping, Sweden, **5** Clinical Neurochemistry Laboratory, Sahlgrenska University Hospital, Mölndal, Sweden, **6** Institute of Neuroscience and Physiology, Department of Psychiatry and Neurochemistry, the Sahlgrenska Academy at the University of Gothenburg, Gothenburg, Sweden, **7** UCL Institute of Neurology, Queen Square, London, United Kingdom, **8** Disability Research, Department of Behavioral Sciences and Learning, Linköping University, Linköping, Sweden, **9** Linnaeus Centre HEAD, Linköping University, Linköping, Sweden

Abstract

Background: Mild traumatic brain injury (TBI) or concussion is common in many sports. Today, neuropsychological evaluation is recommended in the monitoring of a concussion and in return-to-play considerations. To investigate the sensitivity of neuropsychological assessment, we tested amateur boxers post bout and compared with controls. Further the relationship between neuropsychological test results and brain injury biomarkers in the cerebrospinal fluid (CSF) were investigated.

Method: Thirty amateur boxers on high elite level with a minimum of 45 bouts and 25 non-boxing matched controls were included. Memory tests (Rey Osterrieth Complex Figure, Listening Span, Digit Span, Controlled Word Association Test, and computerized testing of episodic memory), tests of processing speed and executive functions (Trail Making, Reaction Time, and Finger Tapping) were performed and related to previously published CSF biomarker results for the axonal injury marker neurofilament light (NFL).

Results: The neurological assessment showed no significant differences between boxers and controls, although elevated CSF NFL, as a sign of axonal injury, was detected in about 80% of the boxers 1–6 days post bout. The investigation of the relationship between neuropsychological evaluation and CSF NFL concentrations revealed that boxers with persisting NFL concentration elevation after at least 14 days resting time post bout, had a significantly poorer performance on Trail Making A ($p = 0.041$) and Simple Reaction Time ($p = 0.042$) compared to other boxers.

Conclusion: This is the first study showing traumatic axonal brain injury can be present without measureable cognitive impairment. The repetitive, subconcussive head trauma in amateur boxing causes axonal injury that can be detected with analysis of CSF NFL, but is not sufficient to produce impairment in memory tests, tests of processing speed, or executive functions. The association of prolonged CSF NFL increase in boxers with impairment of processing speed is an interesting observation, which needs to be verified in larger studies.

Editor: Sonia Brucki, University Of São Paulo, Brazil

Funding: This work was supported by ALF Grants, County Council of Västra Götaland, Sweden; Gothenburg Medical Society, Sweden; and ALF Grants, County Council of Östergötland. The funders had no role in study design, data collection and analysis, decision to publish, or preparation of the manuscript.

Competing Interests: The authors have declared that no competing interests exist.

* E-mail: sanna.neselius@vgregion.se

Introduction

Mild traumatic brain injury (TBI) or concussion is defined as a complex pathophysiologic process affecting the brain, induced by traumatic biomechanical forces with or without loss of consciousness [1]. They represent 80–90% of all traumatic brain injuries [1] and account for between 5.8–8.9% of all athlete injuries among United States high school and collegiate athletes [2]. It is also worth pointing out that most athletes experiencing a concussion, up to 70%, do not seek medical attention [3]. Since concussion is now recognized as an increasing and serious health problem in many sports, it has gained increased attention among medical professionals, scientists, sport organizations as well as athletes.

A TBI causes axonal and glial damage, which disturbs the cerebral physiology, and makes the brain more vulnerable for additional concussions. The primary neuropathology of mild TBI is a diffuse axonal injury (DAI) [4,5]. It is caused by shearing of fragile axons, due to acceleration and deceleration forces during the trauma [6]. The DAI inflicted by a mild TBI, causes predominantly cell dysfunction, rather than cell death [7]. A boxer can receive a mild TBI due to a knockout punch. The knockout frequency in modern amateur boxing is very low, in average 0.7% [8], however, it is known that also the repetitive subconcussive trauma in boxing causes axonal injury [9–12].

Neuropsychological Evaluation of Mild Traumatic Brain Injury

Neuropsychological evaluation has been advocated as the most sensitive tool for early detection of central nervous system pathology and numerous studies have shown that both traditional and computerized neuropsychological tests (emphasizing mental processing efficiency and speed) are sensitive for the acute cognitive impairment after a mild TBI up to 10 days post injury [13–16]. Also in studies where patients with mild TBI have been followed for longer time periods have concluded that neuropsychological assessment in mild TBI are of clinical value and contributes with significant information in the evaluation, in combination with symptom and physical assessment [17,18]. In a meta-analysis of neuropsychological outcome after a single mild TBI, the largest impairment was seen in verbal, visual and working memory (attention, concentration, processing speed) up to 30 days post trauma [17]. However, the largest effect was observed during the first seven days and no neuropsychological changes were detectable after three months [17]. In a study on 698 jockeys decrements in high-level executive/attentional functioning after multiple concussions, persisting more than three months post trauma, were seen [18]. Younger athletes were here found to be more vulnerable to concussions than adults.

For amateur boxing there is a recently published study showing cognitive impairment, after self-reported concussions (knockouts), when compared to controls [19]. Here, cognitive recovery occurred within a week. In this study the computerized test Automated Neuropsychological Assessment Metrics (ANAM) [20] was administered and the study objects in the boxer group were tested at baseline and post injury and thereafter compared to a group of baseline tested boxers without concussion. However, to our knowledge, no neuropsychological assessment has been able to show any pathology caused by the repetitive subconcussive trauma in amateur boxing [21–23], indicating that there are no cognitive tests that are sensitive enough to detect small axonal injuries.

Neuropsychological Tests used in the Diagnosis and Monitoring of TBI

Episodic memory. The Rey-Osterrieth Complex Figure (ROCF) Test is commonly used to test episodic memory and visuospatial skills [24]. It correlates with the Trail Making test and Wechsler Adult Intelligence Scale – Revised (WAIS-R) [25]. A study comparing subjects with traumatic brain injury (TBI) and patients with Alzheimer's disease (AD) showed that the TBI subjects did not have any dysfunctions in copying the figure, only with recall, but the AD subjects had dysfunctions both with copying and recall [26]. There are also computerized possibilities, for example testing made by a model from Tulving [27], to evaluate episodic memory.

Episodic memory after severe TBI has been shown to be impaired initially [28], but no long-term consequences have been seen after mild to moderate traumatic brain injury [29].

Language and semantic memory. Vocabulary intervention is part of the WAIS-R and related to level of education and is critical for studies where educational background may interfere with neuropsychological results [30].

Controlled Oral Word Association Test (COWAT) is a part of the Multilingual Aphasia Examination and provides a measure of word retrieval and word fluency [31,32]. A study on 96 athletes suffering from a sport-related concussion did not reveal significant difference with controls [33], but in mild cognitive impairment (preclinical stage of AD), impairment was seen compared to controls [34].

Working memory. Listening span Test has been used extensively in our laboratories [35] and measures complex, executive aspects of working memory that are related to short-term memory capacity [36,37]. It is impaired in preclinical stages of AD [38] but seems not to be affected by sport-related concussions [39]. **Digit Span Test** is part of the Wechsler Adult Intelligence Scale – Revised (WAIS-R) and addresses short-term auditory memory that is part of the working memory [30]. It can be used to monitor less effortful attention skills, in contrast to the Listening Span task, that involves effortful working memory and attention skills. Typically, performance on the Digit Span task is relatively insensitive to effects of mild TBI [40]. However, it ascertains that participants master necessary attention skills in order to allow meaningful interpretation of other neuropsychological data.

Processing speed and executive functions. Trail Making Test is used for assessing processing speed, attention and executive functioning [41]. There is ample evidence that it can detect brain damage and predict long-term outcomes after traumatic brain injury [42–44]. **Reaction time Test** is sensitive to the effects of mild TBI [45].

Previous studies have reported that **Finger tapping Test** is impaired after a mild TBI [46,47] and that boxers show a reduced performance compared to controls [48].

Evaluation of Biomarkers in Cerebrospinal Fluid and Blood in this Cohort of Boxers

We have previously shown that amateur boxing causes elevation of brain injury biomarkers in blood and CSF [9–11]. CSF Neurofilament Light Protein (NFL), a marker of axonal injury, was shown to be the most sensitive biomarker and to correlate with the amount of injury [9]. NFL levels were elevated in 77% of the boxers 1–6 days after a bout as a sign of mild TBI, when compared to matched controls. After a rest period of at least 14 days, the levels were still elevated in 46% of the boxers [9].

Aim of the Study

The primary aim of the study was to investigate if neurological assessment can detect cognitive impairment caused by subconcussive trauma in amateur boxing and if possible deficits are related to specific cognitive domains. Secondly, as the first study, we sought to investigate the relationship between neuropsychological evaluation and CSF NFL, previously analyzed in the same cohort [9].

Method

Study Population

The study was designed as a prospective prognostic follow-up study. Thirty Olympic boxers competing at high national and/or international level were compared to 25 healthy, age-matched controls. All boxers had completed at least 45 bouts. This inclusion criterion was based on the regulation of the National Boxing Federation demanding an examination including magnetic resonance imaging (MRI), computer tomography (CT) or electroencephalography (EEG) every 50 bouts. The controls consisted of friends or relatives to the boxers, aiming to make certain the enrolment of controls with similar social background and education level similar to the boxers. Exclusion criteria included performance at elite level in sports where head trauma frequently occurs, such a soccer, ice hockey and martial arts. On the same cohort results from biomarker analysis in blood and CSF have been previously published [9–11].

Ethical Approval

The regional ethical review board at Linköping Health University, Sweden approved the study. Written informed consent was obtained from all participants.

Magnetic Resonance Imaging

Magnetic resonance imaging (MRI) of the brain was performed in all participants without any structural injuries (haemorrhages, subdural haematomas) or other major findings observed.

Questionnaire Design

All participants filled in a questionnaire about medical history, medication, education, present occupation, information about previous concussions and quantification of alcohol and drug intake. Previous sports career was reported to identify those who had trained in sports with risk of TBI. The questionnaire included a 10-question symptom evaluation of head and neck injuries based on a previous study [49]. The number of symptoms that had worsened over the last 5–10 years was combined in a score. The boxers reported about their boxing career; fighting record, number of knock-out losses, number of Referee Stopping Contest losses due to several hard punches to Head (RSC-H), present weight class, duration of career, age at career start and age at first bout [49,50]. Boxers gave an account for total amount of bouts the last week prior testing (1–3 bouts) and estimated these bouts as easy (1), intermediate (2) or tough (3). Three boxing experts independently (without knowledge of any results) graded the boxers considering head trauma during total boxing career, 1 to 5 (Type 1 is a boxer that has a low risk to receive blows to the head, according to boxing style, skills and the skills of the opponents. Type 5 is a boxer with high risk to receive repeated blows to the head). The total amount of bouts the last week before test A, the boxers own grading of the bouts and the mean of the expert grading were combined in a score named "Boxing Exposure". The aim was to calculate the total mild TBI risk prior testing.

Neurological Examination

All participants underwent a neurological examination by the same physician [51]. The neurological examination protocol included anamnestic questions about concussion symptoms, a general somatic status (general condition, examination of mouth and throat, heart, blood pressure, abdominal palpation, peripheral circulation and skin status) and a neurological status (GCS, orientation, alertness, speech function, cranial nerves 1–12, motor skills, balance testing, coordination, gate, sensibility testing and testing of reflexes).

Neuropsychological Assessment

The cognitive testing was administered at 1–6 days after the last bout (in average 2 days after bout), prior to, but at the same day as CSF and blood tests (test A) [9]. The cognitive testing was performed in a quiet room without distraction at the university hospital at daytime. The same examiner administrated all the tests following a standardized procedure. The duration for the assessment was approximately 60 minutes. A blinded experienced neuropsychologist analyzed the results. Following parts in presented order constituted the test:

1. Rey osterrieth complex figure test, part 1. Part one involved the untimed reproduction of a complex figure [24].

2. Vocabulary test. The task involved the explanation of the meaning of words, ranging from common to less well-known items.

3. Controlled Oral Word Association Test (COWAT). Participants were asked to generate as many words as possible that begins with a given letter, (i.e. F, A OR S, excluding proper names, numbers or words with different tenses or endings). Sixty seconds was allowed for each letter. The dependent variable was the total number of correct words produced, minus any repetitions [24].

4. Listening span test. The participants listened to a set of sentences, half of which were semantically correct and the other half incorrect. Participants were instructed to report whether each sentence was correct or not and to remember the last word in each sentence. This procedure was repeated for two to five sentences. After the sentences had been presented, the participants were asked to recall all the target words in correct order. The task was repeated five times at each level of difficulty [52].

5. Rey osterrieth complex figure test, part 2. The second part of the ROCF was included after the Listening Span Test and involved the reproduction (i.e., delayed recall) of the complex figure 30 minutes after the first presentation.

6. Computerized testing: episodic memory – part one. This test was computerized and constructed by a model from Tulving [27]. Two consecutive lists, one visual and one auditory list containing 36 words each were presented. The visual list was presented on a computer screen and the other list was presented auditory from computer. All words were presented once with interstimulus interval of 2.0 s. Presentation of the words was randomized. After the presentation of the two lists the participants were informed that the test would occur at a later point.

7. Digit span. Participants were presented with series of numbers, starting with three (for example 3–4–8). There were two series in each level and in total seven levels. The task was to immediately repeat the numbers back. When doing this successfully, the participants were allowed to continue to next level.

8. Trail making test, A and B. In trail A the participant was instructed to trace a line that connects circled numbers in consecutive order. In trail B the task was to trace a line by alternating circled numbers and circled letters in consecutive order (1–A–2–B–3–C, and so on) [53].

9. Computerized testing: simple and complex reaction time. The test was computerized and constructed by a standardized model [54]. In our version of the task, participants were presented with one of two geometrical figures (a circle or a triangle). The size of the stimuli was approximately 80×80 mm. In the condition involving simple reaction time, participants were instructed to respond as quickly as possible whenever the circle appeared on the screen. Complex reaction time required participants to respond with right index finger to the circle and left index finger to the triangle. Each stimulus was presented for 100 msec. A randomly varying interstimulus interval (ISI) was used, ranging between 300 and 5000 msec. The measurement was based on 40 repetitions of each condition. Individual mean values for the simple and complex reaction time were calculated and the difference between complex and simple reaction time used in the further analysis of the results.

10. Computerized testing: Finger Tapping. The task is a modified version of the Halstead-Reitan Finger Tapping (or Oscillation) Test [55,56].

The participants were asked to keep their right hand palm down; fingers extended, and rest the index finger on a designated key (the space bar) on a computer keyboard. The participants were instructed to press the key as many times and as fast as possible until a brief pause was introduced. The entire session consisted of five consecutive trials of 15 seconds each with a 15 second rest in between trials. We used the pace (= mean number of finger taps across trials) in our further analyses.

11. Computerized testing: episodic memory – part two. Following the part one of the Episodic Memory task, a self-paced, computerized, yes-no recognition test took place. In this test, the words from the two previous word lists were presented, together with distracting words. That is, half the target words were previously listed in the free recall task, half of the target words were uncontaminated by previous attempts at free recall.

Along with the presentation of each word, the participants were asked whether the word had occurred in the previous study lists. When an affirmative answer was given, the subject was also asked to decide if the recognition was accompanied by recollection. If a yes response was connected to an explicit recollection from the presentation earlier, the subject was asked to provide a remember response. The participants were informed that recollections could be associations that took place during the previous presentation, feelings or thoughts that linked the affirmative recognition decision to the previous presentation of the specific word. On the other hand, if the yes-response was not associated with a specific memory (i.e., the decision was based upon another criteria than explicit recollection, such as familiarity or ease of perceptual fluency), the subject was asked to provide a know response. Written instructions explaining the nature of the recollection classification task (including particular examples) were presented on the computer screen during the recognition test. In addition, the experimenter provided additional examples and explanations when the subject found the distinction between knowing and remembering difficult to use.

When the word recognition task was completed followed another word recognition task, also a self-paced computerized, yes-no recognition test. In this test, the participant was asked to discriminate and identify earlier presented audile words among earlier visual presented words and fifteen new distracters. Along with the presentation of each word, the participant was asked to decide whether the word had occurred in the previous study lists as audile stimuli. When an affirmative answer was given, the subject was also asked to decide if the recognition was accompanied by recollection. If a yes response was connected with an explicit recollection from the presentation earlier on, the subject was asked to provide a remember response. On the other hand, if the yes-response was not associated with a specific memory (i.e., the decision was based upon another criteria than explicit recollection, such as familiarity or ease of perceptual fluency), the subject was asked to provide a know response. Also in this task written instructions explaining the nature of the recollection classification task (including particular examples) were presented on the computer screen during the recognition test.

Investigation of Relationship between Neurological Assessment and CSF NFL

Boxers with NFL concentrations elevated more than 2 SD above the control mean, were considered to have abnormal levels.

Statistics

Statistical analysis was carried out with IBM SPSS Statistics 21.0. Comparisons between groups were performed using the non-parametric Mann-Whitney U-test, due to sample sizes and since some of variables had skewed distributed data, following an initial MANOVA (multivariate analysis of variance). When variables did not meet criteria for conventional MANOVA procedures, the initial MANOVA was carried out on ranked results [57].

Results

Questionnaire Design and Neurological Examination

The questionnaire about medical and social history and the 10-question survey were similar between boxers and controls [9]. None of the boxers suffered from loss of consciousness during their last bout before test A. Only one of the boxers reported concussion related symptoms after the bout (in this case headache) at the clinical examination, but the medical and neurological examination was normal in all subjects, GCS 15.

Neuropsychological Assessment

Criteria for statistical significance was not reached with an initial MANOVA encompassing neuropsychological results, except for the tests Rey-Osterrieth Figure - part two and Auditory Know HR ($F(14,40) = 1.04$, $p = 0.44$). These two did not fulfill criteria for the use of conventional MANOVA. MANOVA of ranked data failed to disclose a statistically significant effect ($L(2) = 0.11$, $p = 0.74$). Univariate results are shown in Table 1.

Episodic, language, semantic and working memory. The scoring in the Rey-Osterrieth Figure Test was made according to established criteria developed by David Loring [58]. Nor the Rey-Osterrieth Figure test or "the delay and episodic memory computer task" revealed any impairment in the boxers compared to controls. In one condition (Visual – Remember HR) the boxers presented with a larger proportion of 'know' responses ($p = 0.02$) than the control group (Table 1).

The test parameters Vocabulary and COWAT showed no differences between the groups (Table 1).

Digit Span and Listening Span were used to assess working memory. No differences were seen in Digit Span but the boxers performed better than the matched controls in the Listening Span Task ($p = 0.049$, Table 1).

Processing speed and executive functions. Trail Making, Reaction Time and Finger Tapping were used to evaluate processing speed and executive functions. No differences between the groups were detected in any of those tests.

Visuospatial ability: rey-osterrieth figure test, part one. Performance on ROCF was similar in boxers and controls (Table 1).

Investigation of Relationship between Neuropsychological Assessment and CSF NFL

Criteria for statistical significance was not reached with an initial MANOVA encompassing neuropsychological results, except for the tests Trail Making B and Simple Reaction Time. ($F(14) = 1.4$, $p = 0.26$). These two did not fulfill criteria for the use of conventional MANOVA. MANOVA of ranked data indicated a statistically significant effect ($L(2) = 5.4$, $p = 0.02$). Univariate results are shown in Table 2.

Differences in the neuropsychological test results were seen between boxers with abnormal, as compared to normal, CSF NFL at test B (follow-up sample after rest from boxing). Boxers with prolonged NFL elevation had deficits regarding Trail Making A ($p = 0.041$) and simple reaction time ($p = 0.042$) (table 2). Comparisons for NFL in closer relation to bout (test A) revealed no statistical significances.

Discussion

None of the neuropsychological assessment tools could reveal any impairment in the boxers, when compared to controls, although our test battery included attention, processing speed, working memory and visual learning; all the areas where

Table 1. Results of the neuropsychological assessment for boxers vs. controls.

TEST	BOXERS N = 30 Mean (range) SD	CONTROLS N = 25 Mean (range) SD	P-value Boxers vs. Controls
ROCF[1]			
Copy (max 36)	33.6 (8.0–36) 6.6	35.3 (31–36) 1.2	0.78
Delay (max 36)	17.9 (1–31) 8.3	19.1 (6.5–34) 8.0	0.71
VOCABULARY[2] (max 70)	31.9 (16–60) 11.3	30.5 (15–46) 9.5	0.61
COWAT[3]	36.9 (18–54) 10.7	37.6 (15–53) 9.2	0.91
DIGIT SPAN[4] (max 14)	7.1 (3–11) 2.0	6.5 (4–12) 2.0	0.13
LISTENING SPAN[5] (max 38)	14.3 (1–33) 7.6	10.6 (2–29) 6.6	**0.05**
TRAILMAKING[6]			
Part A, (s)	29.9 (15–75) 13.0	29.2 (17–51) 8.9	0.68
Part B, (s)	80.5 (40–240) 39.6	81.3 (41–210) 34.3	0.61
REACTION TIME[7]			
Simple (msec)	323.3 (233–951) 131.1	297.4 (229–652) 80.6	0.37
Difference (complex-simple, msec)	245.4 (−248–3088) 549.0	203.8 (49–506) 119.6	0.31
FINGER TAPPING[8]			
Dominant Hand	52.2 (range) 10.8	52.8 (range) 16.0	0.94
Non-Dominant Hand	58.2 (range) 14.7	57.1 (range) 17.6	0.68
EPISODIC MEMORY[9]			
Auditory – Remember HR	0.41 (0.04–0.86) 0.24	0.35 (0.04–0.77) 0.27	0.22
Auditory – Know HR	0.18 (0.04–0.68) 0.18	0.24 (0.04–0.77) 0.24	0.95
Visual – Remember HR	0.31 (0.04–0.77) 0.24	0.18 (0.04–0.68) 0.16	**0.02**
Visual – Know HR	0.16 (0.04–0.86) 0.16	0.15 (0.04–0.5.) 0.13	0.33

The boxers performed significantly better than the controls in the Listening Span and Visual – Remember HR tests (p = 0.05 and 0.02 respectively). No other significant differences were seen between the groups.

[1]*ROCF: Rey Osterrieth Complex Figure Test.*

[2]*Vocabulary: 35 words were presented and for each word 0,1 or 2 points were assigned.*

[3]*COWAT (Controlled Word Association Test): Participants were asked to generate as many words as possible that begins with the given letters F, A and S. Sixty seconds were allowed for each letter. One point per word was received.*

[4]*Digit Span: Participants were presented with series of numbers, starting with three (for example 3–4–8). There were two series in each level and in total seven levels. The task was to immediately repeat the numbers back. When doing this successfully, the participants were given a longer serie of numbers.*

[5]*Listening Span: A mixed lists of digits and letters were read aloud to the participants and they were asked to recall this list in correct numeric and alphabetic order.*

[6]*Trail Making: In trail A the participant is instructed to trace a line that connects circled numbers in consecutive order. In trail B the task is to trace a line by alternating circled numbers and circled letters in consecutive order. Time is measured in seconds(s).*

[7]*Reaction time: a) Simple reaction time: Participants were instructed to respond as quickly as possible whenever the circle appeared on the screen. Complex reaction time: Required participants to respond with right hand to the circle and left hand to the triangle. Difference = Complex−Simple reaction time.*

[8]*Finger Tapping. In total five trials with 15 s pauses between the trials. The participants were asked to press the space board with their index finger on the computer keyboard as many times as possible for 15 s, alternating dominate and non-dominant hand. The mean value was calculated.*

[9]*Propotional values (range 0.04–0.96). There are 30 words respectively in the auditory and visual conditions. The proportion of correct recognition hit rates (HR) is presented.*

impairment after mild TBI has been previously demonstrated [59]. The performance in some of the boxers was very poor, but similar results were also found among controls. In most tasks the performance was identical or slightly in favor for the boxers.

We have previously in the same cohort of boxers been able to show that the repetitive subconcussive trauma in amateur boxing causes axonal injury detectable by CSF biomarkers [9,11]. This is the first study to investigate the relationship between neuropsychological evaluation and CSF NFL (an axonal injury biomarker [9,12]), and the results were quite interesting.

Amateur boxers still having increased CSF NFL concentrations after a rest period of at least 14 days, had significantly worse performance on two (out of four) tasks involving processing speed responses, Trail Making part A ($p = 0.04$) and Simple Reaction Time ($p = 0.04$), compared to the other boxers. The boxers with prolonged elevation of CSF NFL had most likely received more punches during bout leading to greater degree of axonal injury, compared to the other boxers [9,12]. Another interpretation is that these boxers may suffer from ongoing neurodegeneration. This interpretation may be speculative but in our mind not irrelevant in the light of recent data on progressive neurodegeneration following repeated concussions [60]. The association of CSF NFL with speed measures gives a functional correlate to the CSF biomarker findings and calls for further investigations with repeated CSF samplings and long-term clinical and neuropsychological follow-up within this group.

Our study has some limitations: First, the absence of baseline neuropsychological assessment before bouts may make it hard to determine if the test scores reflect the actual boxing bout. Second, since several statistical tests were performed, there is a risk of type I errors, why the observed relationship between processing speed and prolonged increase in CSF NFL concentration need to be repeated in independent studies before stronger conclusions can be drawn. Whether baseline testing has greater diagnostic accuracy

Table 2. Investigation of relationship between neurological assessment and neurofilament light (NFL) in the cerebrospinal fluid (CSF).

TEST	ELEVATED NFL(B) N = 12 Mean (range) SD	NORMAL NFL(B) N = 14 Mean (range) SD	P-value Elevated vs. normal
ROCF[1]			
Copy (max 36)	32.1 (8–36) 9.1	35.5 (4–32) 1.1	0.80
Delay (max 36)	18.0 (3.5–31) 9.5	171 (1–31) 7.7	0.67
VOCABULARY[2] (max 70)	28.4 (16–47) 11.5	34.3 (17–60) 11.4	0.16
COWAT[3]	32.2 (18–48) 11.2	39.3 (19–54) 11.4	0.09
DIGIT SPAN[4] (max 14)	6.8 (4–10) 2.1	7.3 (3–11) 2.0	0.40
LISTENING SPAN[5] (max 38)	12.8 (1–21) 6.1	15.4 (6–33) 8.3	0.56
TRAIL MAKING[6]			
Part A, (s)	35.8 (20–75) 15.7	26.2 (15–55) 9.9	**0.04**
Part B, (s)	98.7 (43–240) 54.7	69.0 (45–100) 18.1	0.18
REACTION TIME[7]			
Simple (msec)	371.1 (259.6–956.8) 191.3	285.1 (242.0–361.6)	**0.04**
Difference (complex-simple, msec)	126.2 (−248.0–388.0) 161.7	349.6 (92.7–3087.9) 733.3	0.84
FINGER TAPPING[8]			
Dominant Hand	48.3 (36.6–67.2) 9.1	45.4 (29.1–61.3) 11.5	0.59
Non-Dominant Hand	55.7 (41.2–70.2) 9.4	49.2 (31.3–70.4) 11.4	0.17
EPISODIC MEMORY[9]			
Auditory - Remember HR	0.42 (0.05–0.95) 0.32	0.50 (0.14–0.77) 0.20	0.34
Auditory - Know HR	0.26 (0.05–0.86) 0.29	0.20 (0.05–0.59) 0.14	0.96
Visual - Remember HR	0.50 (0.05–0.86) 0.28	0.43 (0.05–0.86) 0.19	0.52
Visual - Know HR	0.17 (0.05–0.41) 0.14	0.24 (0.05–0.68) 0.19	0.39

NFL in the cerebrospinal fluid has been analyzed in the same cohort of boxers and the results are previously published [9]. After a boxing bout, cerebrospinal fluid was collected at two occasions, first 1–6 days (test A) after bout and then after a rest period of at least 14 days (test B). 23 of 30 boxers had elevated concentrations of the axonal injury biomarker NFL at test A. At follow up, 4 of the boxers were lost, 12 of 26 (46%) boxers still hade elevated concentrations and these had significantly lesser performance on Trail Making A ($p = 0.041$) and Simple Reaction Time ($p = 0.042$) compared to the other boxers.

[1] *ROCF: Rey Osterrieth Complex Figure Test.*

[2] *Vocabulary: 35 words were presented and for each word 0,1 or 2 points were assigned.*

[3] *COWAT (Controlled Word Association Test): Participants were asked to generate as many words as possible that begin with the given letters F, A and S. Sixty seconds were allowed for each letter. One point per word was received.*

[4] *Digit Span: Participants were presented with series of numbers, starting with three (for example 3–4–8). There were two series in each level and in total seven levels. The task was to immediately repeat the numbers back. When doing this successfully, the participants were given a longer serie of numbers.*

[5] *Listening Span: A mixed lists of digits and letters were read aloud to the participants and they were asked to recall this list in correct numeric and alphabetic order.*

[6] *Trail Making: In trail A the participant is instructed to trace a line that connects circled numbers in consecutive order. In trail B the task is to trace a line by alternating circled numbers and circled letters in consecutive order. Time is measured in seconds(s).*

[7] *Reaction time: a) Simple reaction time: Participants were instructed to respond as quickly as possible whenever the circle appeared on the screen. Complex reaction time: Required participants to respond with right hand to the circle and left hand to the triangle. Difference = Complex−Simple reaction time.*

[8] *Finger Tapping. In total five trials with 15 s rests between the trials. The participants were asked to press the space board with their index finger on the computer keyboard as many times as possible for 15 s, alternating dominate and non-dominant hand. The mean value was calculated.*

[9] *Proportional values (range 0.04–0.96). The number of words in the auditory and visual conditions was 30 respectively. The correct recognition hit rates (HR) are presented.*

than post concussion assessment alone still remains to be determined [61], since also the test-retest reliability must be taken into account [62] and findings further suggest that post injury neuropsychological test data are robust and may not require baseline testing, as long as there exist appropriate, well-developed normative data [63]. However, traditional test norms are based upon quota sampling, the recruitment of a normative sample reflecting the demographic properties of the national census. A problem in investigations involving clinical patients, ethnical minorities, or groups with special skills (such as the athletes in our study) is that these populations often do not reflect the national census in crucial aspects. Hence, census-based norms may bias the interpretation of results in unpredictable ways. In our study, such a method would have overestimated the effects of boxing upon language and possibly episodic memory. Over the years, several different methods for correcting recruitment bias have been suggested [64]. We tried to cope with this problem by recruiting a group of scrupulously matched controls. It should be noted, that this approach in the future should be supplemented with norms derived from meta-analyses of boxer studies. Using Monte Carlo simulation, census-based norms can then be adjusted to reflect recruitment bias. Such a necessary enterprise requires the publication of a larger number of studies than currently available.

The clinical value and validity of neuropsychological assessment in the diagnosis and monitoring of mild TBI has been under discussion. Until now, neuropsychological evaluation has been advocated as the most sensitive tool for detecting early neurological pathology, but our results indicate that without baseline testing and in absence of clinical symptoms, neuropsychological assessment cannot detect the small axonal injuries caused by the repetitive subconcussive trauma in boxing. However, specific test of processing speed and executive functions may indicate protracted or delayed injury and may hold promise as markers for more severe trauma. The clinical relevance of elevated CSF NFL without clinical symptoms or without cognitive impairment can be discussed, but earlier studies have shown that concussion increases the risk for additional concussions [51], that at least 12% of the athletes with fatal sport-related intracerebral bleeding have suffered from a concussion within 4 weeks prior to the injury [65] and that sport-related concussion is associated with long-term effects in form of chronic traumatic encephalopathy [60]. The results of these studies indicate that the risk for complications increases if athletes return to sport before the traumatic brain injury has healed and that it today is difficult to decide correctly when that is the case. Just as in fracture healing, absence of clinical symptoms might not be equivalent with absence of/healed traumatic brain injury, why more sensitive analysis tools, such as analysis of CSF brain injury biomarkers, might be helpful for the clinician.

In the future, it would be valuable also investigate the relationship between CSF NFL and some of the established neuropsychological computerized concussion batteries of today (Immediate Postconcussion Assessment and Cognitive Testing (ImPACT), Axon Sports, the Automated Neuropsychological Assessment Metrics (ANAM), Headminder (ImPACT Applications, Inc; Axon Sports, LLC)) in concussed athletes.

Conclusion

This is to our knowledge the first study showing traumatic axonal brain injury can be present without measureable cognitive impairment. Absence of clinical symptoms/cognitive impairment after concussion does not seem to be equivalent to absence of brain injury. Our conclusion is that assessment of memory tests, tests of processing speed or executive functions, cannot detect the small axonal injuries that can be diagnosed with CSF NFL analysis in amateur boxing. However, these modalities can provide complementary information and link CSF biomarker results to functional outcome.

Acknowledgments

The authors want to thank Lisbeth Hjälle for her helpful assistance with this study.

Author Contributions

Conceived and designed the experiments: SN TK JM. Performed the experiments: SN. Analyzed the data: SN HB JM HZ KB TK. Contributed reagents/materials/analysis tools: SN TK KB HZ. Wrote the paper: SN HB JM KB HZ TK.

References

1. McCrory P, Meeuwisse WH, Aubry M, Cantu B, Dvorak J, et al. (2013) Consensus statement on concussion in sport: the 4th International Conference on Concussion in Sport held in Zurich, November 2012. British journal of sports medicine 47: 250–258.
2. Gessel LM, Fields SK, Collins CL, Dick RW, Comstock RD (2007) Concussions among United States high school and collegiate athletes. Journal of athletic training 42: 495–503.
3. McCrea M, Hammeke T, Olsen G, Leo P, Guskiewicz K (2004) Unreported concussion in high school football players: implications for prevention. Clin J Sport Med 14: 13–17.
4. Iverson GL (2005) Outcome from mild traumatic brain injury. Current opinion in psychiatry 18: 301–317.
5. Meythaler JM, Peduzzi JD, Eleftheriou E, Novack TA (2001) Current concepts: diffuse axonal injury-associated traumatic brain injury. Archives of physical medicine and rehabilitation 82: 1461–1471.
6. Browne KD, Chen XH, Meaney DF, Smith DH (2011) Mild traumatic brain injury and diffuse axonal injury in swine. Journal of neurotrauma 28: 1747–1755.
7. Kirov II, Tal A, Babb JS, Lui YW, Grossman RI, et al. (2013) Diffuse axonal injury in mild traumatic brain injury: a 3D multivoxel proton MR spectroscopy study. Journal of neurology 260: 242–252.
8. Bianco M, Loosemore M, Daniele G, Palmieri V, Faina M, et al. (2013) Amateur boxing in the last 59 years. Impact of rules changes on the type of verdicts recorded and implications on boxers' health. British journal of sports medicine 47: 452–457.
9. Neselius S, Brisby H, Theodorsson A, Blennow K, Zetterberg H, et al. (2012) CSF-biomarkers in Olympic boxing: diagnosis and effects of repetitive head trauma. PloS one 7: e33606.
10. Neselius S, Zetterberg H, Blennow K, Randall J, Wilson D, et al. (2013) Olympic boxing is associated with elevated levels of the neuronal protein tau in plasma. Brain injury: [BI] 27: 425–433.
11. Neselius S, Zetterberg H, Blennow K, Marcusson J, Brisby H (2013) Increased CSF Levels of Phosphorylated Neurofilament Heavy Protein following Bout in Amateur Boxers. PLOS one 8: e81249.
12. Zetterberg H, Hietala MA, Jonsson M, Andreasen N, Styrud E, et al. (2006) Neurochemical aftermath of amateur boxing. Arch Neurol 63: 1277–1280.
13. Collins MW, Grindel SH, Lovell MR, Dede DE, Moser DJ, et al. (1999) Relationship between concussion and neuropsychological performance in college football players. JAMA: the journal of the American Medical Association 282: 964–970.
14. Hinton-Bayre AD, Geffen G (2002) Severity of sports-related concussion and neuropsychological test performance. Neurology 59: 1068–1070.
15. Macciocchi SN, Barth JT, Alves W, Rimel RW, Jane JA (1996) Neuropsychological functioning and recovery after mild head injury in collegiate athletes. Neurosurgery 39: 510–514.
16. Echemendia RJ, Putukian M, Mackin RS, Julian L, Shoss N (2001) Neuropsychological test performance prior to and following sports-related mild traumatic brain injury. Clinical journal of sport medicine: official journal of the Canadian Academy of Sport Medicine 11: 23–31.
17. Rohling ML, Binder LM, Demakis GJ, Larrabee GJ, Ploetz DM, et al. (2011) A meta-analysis of neuropsychological outcome after mild traumatic brain injury: re-analyses and reconsiderations of Binder, et al. (1997), Frencham, et al. (2005), and Pertab, et al. (2009). The Clinical neuropsychologist 25: 608–623.
18. Wall SE, Williams WH, Cartwright-Hatton S, Kelly TP, Murray J, et al. (2006) Neuropsychological dysfunction following repeat concussions in jockeys. Journal of neurology, neurosurgery, and psychiatry 77: 518–520.
19. Bleiberg J, Cernich AN, Cameron K, Sun W, Peck K, et al. (2004) Duration of cognitive impairment after sports concussion. Neurosurgery 54: 1073–1078; discussion 1078–1080.
20. Bleiberg J, Kane RL, Reeves DL, Garmoe WS, Halpern E (2000) Factor analysis of computerized and traditional tests used in mild brain injury research. The Clinical neuropsychologist 14: 287–294.
21. Butler RJ (1994) Neuropsychological investigation of amateur boxers. British journal of sports medicine 28: 187–190.
22. Heilbronner RL, Bush SS, Ravdin LD, Barth JT, Iverson GL, et al. (2009) Neuropsychological consequences of boxing and recommendations to improve safety: a National Academy of Neuropsychology education paper. Archives of clinical neuropsychology: the official journal of the National Academy of Neuropsychologists 24: 11–19.
23. Porter MD (2003) A 9-year controlled prospective neuropsychologic assessment of amateur boxing. Clinical journal of sport medicine: official journal of the Canadian Academy of Sport Medicine 13: 339–352.
24. Lezak MD (1984) Neuropsychological assessment in behavioral toxicology–developing techniques and interpretative issues. Scandinavian journal of work, environment & health 10 Suppl 1: 25–29.
25. Cornell DG, Roberts M, Oram G (1997) The Ray-Osterrieth Complex Figure Test as a neuropsychological measure in criminal offenders. Arch Clin Neuropsychol 12: 47–56.
26. Bigler ED, Rosa L, Schultz F, Hall S, Harris J (1989) Rey-Auditory Verbal Learning and Rey-Osterrieth Complex Figure Design performance in Alzheimer's disease and closed head injury. Journal of clinical psychology 45: 277–280.
27. Tulving E (1985) Memory and consciousness. Canadian Psychologist 25: 1–12.
28. Wright MJ, Schmitter-Edgecombe M, Woo E (2010) Verbal memory impairment in severe closed head injury: the role of encoding and consolidation. Journal of clinical and experimental neuropsychology 32: 728–736.
29. Himanen L, Portin R, Isoniemi H, Helenius H, Kurki T, et al. (2006) Longitudinal cognitive changes in traumatic brain injury: a 30-year follow-up study. Neurology 66: 187–192.
30. Wechsler D (1981) Wechsler Adult Intelligence Scale – Revised. Psychological Corporation, New York.

31. Benton AL, Hamsher Kd, Sivan AB (1994) Multilingual aphasia examination. Iowa City: AJA Associates, Inc.
32. Ross TP (2003) The reliability of cluster and switch scores for the Controlled Oral Word Association Test. Archives of clinical neuropsychology: the official journal of the National Academy of Neuropsychologists 18: 153–164.
33. Baillargeon A, Lassonde M, Leclerc S, Ellemberg D (2012) Neuropsychological and neurophysiological assessment of sport concussion in children, adolescents and adults. Brain injury: [BI] 26: 211–220.
34. Malek-Ahmadi M, Small BJ, Raj A (2011) The diagnostic value of controlled oral word association test-FAS and category fluency in single-domain amnestic mild cognitive impairment. Dementia and geriatric cognitive disorders 32: 235–240.
35. Malm J, Kristensen B, Karlsson T, Carlberg B, Fagerlund M, et al. (1998) Cognitive impairment in young adults with infratentorial infarcts. Neurology 51: 433–440.
36. Haut MW, Kuwabara H, Leach S, Arias RG (2000) Neural activation during performance of number-letter sequencing. Applied neuropsychology 7: 237–242.
37. Kane MJ, Engle RW (2002) The role of prefrontal cortex in working-memory capacity, executive attention, and general fluid intelligence: an individual-differences perspective. Psychonomic bulletin & review 9: 637–671.
38. Rosen VM, Bergeson JL, Putnam K, Harwell A, Sunderland T (2002) Working memory and apolipoprotein E: what's the connection? Neuropsychologia 40: 2226–2233.
39. Mayers LB, Redick TS, Chiffriller SH, Simone AN, Terraforte KR (2011) Working memory capacity among collegiate student athletes: effects of sport-related head contacts, concussions, and working memory demands. Journal of clinical and experimental neuropsychology 33: 532–537.
40. Vallat-Azouvi C, Weber T, Legrand L, Azouvi P (2007) Working memory after severe traumatic brain injury. Journal of the International Neuropsychological Society: JINS 13: 770–780.
41. Reitan RM, Wolfson D (1992) Neuropsychological evaluation of older children. Tucson, AZ: Neuropsychology Press.
42. Atchison TB, Sander AM, Struchen MA, High WM Jr, Roebuck TM, et al. (2004) Relationship between neuropsychological test performance and productivity at 1-year following traumatic brain injury. The Clinical neuropsychologist 18: 249–265.
43. Lange RT, Iverson GL, Zakrzewski MJ, Ethel-King PE, Franzen MD (2005) Interpreting the trail making test following traumatic brain injury: comparison of traditional time scores and derived indices. Journal of clinical and experimental neuropsychology 27: 897–906.
44. Perianez JA, Rios-Lago M, Rodriguez-Sanchez JM, Adrover-Roig D, Sanchez-Cubillo I, et al. (2007) Trail Making Test in traumatic brain injury, schizophrenia, and normal ageing: sample comparisons and normative data. Archives of clinical neuropsychology: the official journal of the National Academy of Neuropsychologists 22: 433–447.
45. Kontos AP, Covassin T, Elbin RJ, Parker T (2012) Depression and Neurocognitive Performance After Concussion Among Male and Female High School and Collegiate Athletes. Archives of physical medicine and rehabilitation 93(10): 1751–1756.
46. Haaland KY, Temkin N, Randahl G, Dikmen S (1994) Recovery of simple motor skills after head injury. Journal of clinical and experimental neuropsychology 16: 448–456.
47. Prigatano GP, Borgaro SR (2003) Qualitative features of finger movement during the Halstead finger oscillation test following traumatic brain injury. Journal of the International Neuropsychological Society: JINS 9: 128–133.
48. Murelius O, Haglund Y (1991) Does Swedish amateur boxing lead to chronic brain damage? 4. A retrospective neuropsychological study. Acta Neurol Scand 83: 9–13.
49. Jordan BD (1996) Acute and chronic brain injury in United States National Team Soccer Players. Am J Sports Med 24: 704–705.
50. Kaste M, Kuurne T, Vilkki J, Katevuo K, Sainio K, et al. (1982) Is chronic brain damage in boxing a hazard of the past? Lancet 2: 1186–1188.
51. Guskiewicz KM, McCrea M, Marshall SW, Cantu RC, Randolph C, et al. (2003) Cumulative effects associated with recurrent concussion in collegiate football players: the NCAA Concussion Study. JAMA 290: 2549–2555.
52. Daneman M, Carpenter PA (1980) Individual differences in working memory and reading. Journal of Verbal Learning and Verbal Behavior 4: 450–466.
53. Reitan RM (1994) Ward Halstead's contributions to neuropsychology and the Halstead-Reitan Neuropsychological Test Battery. Journal of clinical psychology 50: 47–70.
54. Hannay HJ (1986) Experimental techniques in human neuropsychology. New York: Oxford University Press.
55. Spreen O, Strauss E (1998) A Compendium of neuropsychological tests: Administration, norms, and commentary, 2nd ed. New York: Oxford University Press.
56. Halstead WC (1947) Brain and Intelligence. A Quantitative Study of the Frontal Lobes. Chicago, IL: University of Chicago Press.
57. Thomas JR, Nelson JK, Thomas KT (1999) A generalized rank-order method for nonparametric analysis of data from exercise science: a tutorial. Res Q Exerc Sport 70: 11–23.
58. Loring DW, Bauer RM (1990) Testing the limits: cautions and concerns regarding the new Wechsler IQ and Memory scales. Neurology 74: 685–690.
59. Maruff P, Thomas E, Cysique L, Brew B, Collie A, et al. (2009) Validity of the CogState brief battery: relationship to standardized tests and sensitivity to cognitive impairment in mild traumatic brain injury, schizophrenia, and AIDS dementia complex. Archives of clinical neuropsychology: the official journal of the National Academy of Neuropsychologists 24: 165–178.
60. McKee AC, Stern RA, Nowinski CJ, Stein TD, Alvarez VE, et al. (2013) The spectrum of disease in chronic traumatic encephalopathy. Brain: a journal of neurology 136: 43–64.
61. Randolph C, Kirkwood MW (2009) What are the real risks of sport-related concussion, and are they modifiable? Journal of the International Neuropsychological Society: JINS 15: 512–520.
62. Comper P, Hutchison M, Magrys S, Mainwaring L, Richards D (2010) Evaluating the methodological quality of sports neuropsychology concussion research: a systematic review. Brain injury: [BI] 24: 1257–1271.
63. Echemendia RJ, Bruce JM, Bailey CM, Sanders JF, Arnett P, et al. (2012) The utility of post-concussion neuropsychological data in identifying cognitive change following sports-related MTBI in the absence of baseline data. The Clinical neuropsychologist 26: 1077–1091.
64. Mitrushina M, Boone K, D'Elia L (2005) Handbook of normative data for neuropsuchological assessment. New York: Oxford University Press.
65. Thomas M, Haas TS, Doerer JJ, Hodges JS, Aicher BO, et al. (2011) Epidemiology of sudden death in young, competitive athletes due to blunt trauma. Pediatrics 128: e1–8.

Cardiac Repolarization and Autonomic Regulation during Short-Term Cold Exposure in Hypertensive Men

Heidi Hintsala[1,2], Tuomas V. Kenttä[2,3], Mikko Tulppo[4,13], Antti Kiviniemi[4], Heikki V. Huikuri[2,3], Matti Mäntysaari[5], Sirkka Keinänen-Kiukaannemi[5,6], Risto Bloigu[7], Karl-Heinz Herzig[8,9], Riitta Antikainen[2,5,10], Hannu Rintamäki[8,11], Jouni J. K. Jaakkola[1,2,5,12], Tiina M. Ikäheimo[1,2,5]*

1 Center for Environmental and Respiratory Health Research, University of Oulu, Oulu, Finland, **2** Medical Research Center Oulu, Oulu University Hospital and University of Oulu, Oulu, Finland, **3** Institute of Clinical Medicine, Department of Internal Medicine, University of Oulu, Oulu, Finland, **4** Department of Exercise and Medical Physiology, Verve Research, Oulu, Finland, **5** Institute of Health Sciences, University of Oulu, Oulu, Finland, **6** Unit of General Practice, Oulu University Hospital, Oulu, Finland, **7** Medical Informatics and Statistics Research Group, University of Oulu, Oulu, Finland, **8** Institute of Biomedicine, Department of Physiology and Biocenter of Oulu, University of Oulu, Oulu, Finland, **9** Department of Psychiatry, Kuopio University Hospital, Kuopio, Finland, **10** Oulu City Hospital, Oulu, Finland, **11** Finnish Institute of Occupational Health, Oulu, Finland, **12** Department of Medicine, Oulu University Hospital, Oulu, Finland, **13** Department of Applied Science, London South Bank University, London, England

Abstract

Objectives: The aim of our study was to assess the effect of short-term cold exposure, typical in subarctic climate, on cardiac electrical function among untreated middle-aged hypertensive men.

Methods: We conducted a population-based recruitment of 51 hypertensive men and a control group of 32 men without hypertension (age 55–65 years) who underwent whole-body cold exposure (15 min exposure to temperature −10°C, wind 3 m/s, winter clothes). Conduction times and amplitudes, vectorcardiography, arrhythmias, and heart rate variability (autonomic nervous function) were assessed.

Results: Short-term cold exposure increased T-peak to T-end interval from 67 to 72 ms ($p<0.001$) and 71 to 75 ms ($p<0.001$) and T-wave amplitude from 0.12 to 0.14 mV ($p<0.001$) and from 0.17 to 0.21 mV ($p<0.001$), while QTc interval was shortened from 408 to 398 ms ($p<0.001$) and from 410 to 401 ms ($p<0.001$) among hypertensive men and controls, respectively. Cold exposure increased both low (from 390 to 630 ms^2 ($p<0.001$) and 380 to 700 ms^2 ($p<0.001$), respectively) and high frequency heart rate variability (from 90 to 190 ms^2 ($p<0.001$) and 150 to 300 ms^2 ($p<0.001$), respectively), while low-to-high frequency-ratio was reduced. In addition, the frequency of ventricular ectopic beats increased slightly during cold exposure. The cold induced changes were similar between untreated hypertensive men and controls.

Conclusions: Short-term cold exposure with moderate facial and mild whole body cooling resulted in prolongation of T-peak to T-end interval and higher T-wave amplitude while QTc interval was shortened. These changes of ventricular repolarization may have resulted from altered cardiac autonomic regulation and were unaffected by untreated hypertension.

Trial Registration: ClinicalTrials.gov NCT02007031

Editor: Larisa G. Tereshchenko, Johns Hopkins University SOM, United States of America

Funding: The study was funded through grants from the National Institute for Health and Welfare as well as Paavo Nurmi, Emil Aaltonen and Ida Montin Foundations. The funders had no role in study design, data collection and analysis, decision to publish, or preparation of the manuscript.

Competing Interests: The authors have declared that no competing interests exist.

* Email: tiina.ikaheimo@oulu.fi

Introduction

Wintertime is associated with increased morbidity and mortality and a majority of this is related to cardiovascular causes [1,2], such as myocardial infarctions [3], ruptures/dissection of aortic aneurysms [4], heart failures [5], as well as strokes [6]. Also ventricular arrhythmias [7] and sudden cardiac death [8] exhibit seasonal changes among cardiac patients, with higher occurrence during cold season.

Whole body exposure to cold and the resulting superficial cooling activates the sympathetic nervous system [9] that increases heart rate (HR) and constricts peripheral vasculature reducing heat loss from human to the environment. Sympathetic activation in general may produce altered cardiac function involving a higher risk of arrhythmias and cardiac events [10]. Facial cooling, on the other hand, is known to increase the vagal tone through the trigeminal nerve stimulation with a decrease in HR [11]. This may serve as a protective cardiovascular effect. However, for instance during whole body cold water immersion [12] or facial cooling [13] a co-activation of sympathetic and parasympathetic nervous system is observed. This causes conflicting inotropic and chronotropic drives to the heart (autonomic conflict) which may have an additional arrhythmogenic effect over the sympathetic activation alone [12,13].

At present, the effects of short-term cold exposure with only superficial cooling on cardiac electrical function are not well known. Previous studies using pronounced whole-body cooling and hypothermia have detected electrocardiographic (ECG) manifestations such as the J (Osborne) waves, interval prolongation, T-wave abnormalities, and atrial and ventricular arrhythmias [12,14,15]. Furthermore, exercise in a cold environment induces pronounced cardiac symptoms in patients with cardiac disease [16,17] and impairs post exercise cardiovagal regulation among healthy subjects [18].

Cold-induced arrhythmias might be pronounced in patients with hypertension in which sympathetic nervous system is already overactive [19]. Hypertension itself is a risk factor for arrhythmias, such as atrial fibrillation [20]. In addition, both short [21,22] and long term [23] exposure to cold elevate blood pressure (BP) mainly as a result of the increased sympathetic activity. Hence, this augmented sympathetic drive could further aggravate the course of hypertension and increase the risk for arrhythmias and associated adverse health events. However, no previous studies explored the effect of cold exposure to cardiac electrical function among hypertensive subjects.

The objective of the present study was to assess the effects of short-term cold exposure similar to everyday winter circumstances on cardiac electrical function, incident arrhythmias, and the autonomic nervous system among subjects with untreated hypertension. We hypothesized that, compared to a warm environment, a cold exposure would increase sympathetic drive and induce electrophysiological changes known to be associated with arrhythmias. We also expected these changes to be pronounced among subjects with hypertension. The primary outcome measure of the study was ECG and vectorcardiographic features and secondary measure arrhythmias. The information of how cold exposure affects cardiac electrical function is relevant for medical professionals involved with treating cardiovascular diseases.

Materials and Methods

Subjects

We conducted a population-based recruitment (Figure 1) from April to November in 2011 which has been previously described in detail [21]. Briefly, men aged 55–65 years were randomly chosen from the population register in Oulu, Finland (65°N, 25°E), interviewed for eligibility and performed home BP measurements according to the recommendations of the European Society of Hypertension [24]. According to the sample size estimation and power analysis (G-Power 3.1.0) we estimated to detect statistically significant differences in brachial BP between a warm and cold environment [Power (1-β err prob), 0.9, Cohen's effect size 0.8, α err prob 0.05] in 23 participants. We aimed at a 2:1 ratio of hypertensive men and control subjects for possible subgroup analyses among hypertensive, i.e. 46 hypertensive and 23 men in control group in final data-analyses. Based on the home BP measurements 83 subjects were enrolled into the study: 51 hypertensive men (the mean of 28 systolic BP measurements $\geq$ 135 and/or the mean of 28 diastolic measurements BP $\geq$ 85 mmHg) and 32 controls (the mean of 28 systolic/diastolic BP measurements <135/85 mmHg) (Table 1). The exclusion criteria of the study were presence of coronary heart disease or respiratory disease, use of antihypertensive drugs for any indication, an average home BP $\geq$175/105 mm Hg, no home BP measurements, inadequate data quality in the laboratory measurements (n = 1), and having a respiratory infection a week before exposure measurements. The other clinical characteristics did not differ among the groups except of 4 subjects had type 2 diabetes in the hypertensive group, and the hypertensive men had higher weight, body-mass index (BMI), and fat percentage. The study was approved by the ethics committee of Oulu University Hospital and all participants of the study gave written informed consent. The protocol for this trial and supporting Trend checklist are available as supporting information; see Checklist S1, Protocol S1, and Protocol S2. The trial was not registered prospectively because this observational controlled study does not any involve any clinical intervention. The authors confirm that all ongoing and related trials for this intervention are registered.

Experimental Protocol

The experimental measurements were performed from August to November 2011 before the start of the cold season by trained professionals. The experiments began with a short introduction of the measurement protocol and visit to the climatic chamber. Height was measured. Body composition was assessed by bioelectrical impedance analysis (InBody 720 Biospace Ltd, Korea) and physical fitness was measured while resting with the Polar Own Index Fit Test (Polar S610, Polar, Finland). After the measurements the study subjects were equipped with thermistors (skin temperature), ECG electrodes, and a cuff for measuring brachial BP and dressed with winter clothing (ca. 2 clo during cold exposure and 1.6 clo during baseline and recovery measurements [25]). The exposure protocol consisted of three consecutive 15 minutes phases: baseline, cold exposure, and recovery period in baseline conditions. The subjects were exposed to cold in a wind tunnel (air temperature $T_a = -10$°C, air velocity $V_a = 3$ m/s, and relative air humidity $H_a = 50$%) adjacent to a climatic chamber in which baseline and recovery measurements were performed ($T_a = 18$°C, $V_a < 0.2$ m/s, $H_a = 30$%). All measurements were performed during the office hours.

Digital ECG Recordings

Derived 12-lead ECG recordings (Medilog AR12, Huntleigh Healthcare, Austria) were performed in order to measure the electrical function of the heart throughout the experiment. Recordings were made using 16 bit amplitude resolution and 256 Hz sampling rate.

ECG and Vectorcardiographic Features

The signal processing and analysis were carried out with custom-made software written in Matlab (MathWorks, inc., Natick, MA, USA). Baseline wander was removed with cubic spline interpolation and high-frequency noise was suppressed with a bidirectional 40 Hz low-pass filter. Ectopic and abnormally shaped beats were removed from the analysis. Beats were considered ectopic if the preceding RR interval differed by more than 20% from the last valid RR interval. Beats with deviating morphology were identified with template matching. The template was updated with each accepted beat and the threshold for acceptance was 95% match. Subsequently, the signal was resampled from 256 Hz to 512 Hz in order to improve the morphological alignment of the beats. All beats were aligned in each of the leads based on cross-correlation (time alignment between the leads was not changed). The aligned beats were then

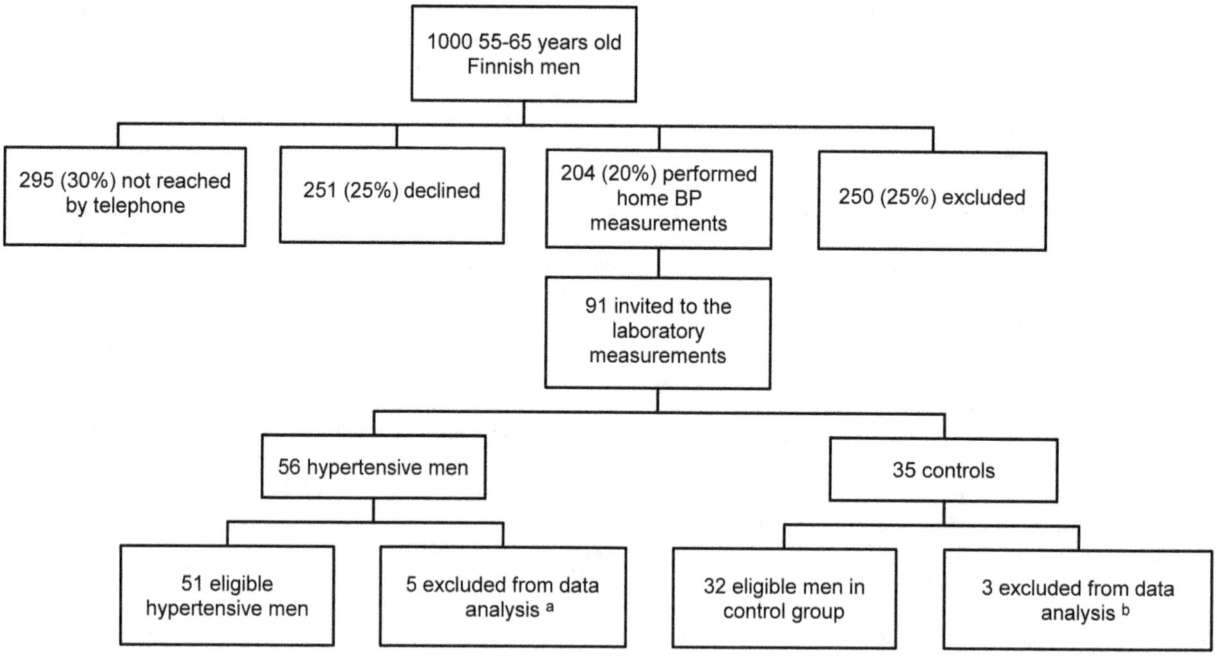

Figure 1. The recruitment procedure. BP, blood pressure. [a] Four subjects excluded for the usage of BP medication and one for inadequate data quality.[b] One subject excluded for the usage of BP medication and two did not perform cold exposure for safety reasons.

filtered with a ten-beat wide sliding window in order to produce representative median beats for each cardiac cycle and to suppress the noise within the beats.

Three representative median beats were taken five minutes apart from each other, starting from the beginning of each phase, i.e. baseline, cold and recovery phases. In order to assure the accuracy of the interval measurements, these samples were analyzed manually by a trained operator, who identified the P-wave onset, QRS boundaries, T-wave peak and T-wave offset from each of the 12 leads for each sample. Subsequently, PR, QRS, QT and T-peak to T-end intervals were calculated in leads II and V5. QT interval was corrected for HR with nomogram method (QTc) [26]. Left ventricular hypertrophy (LVH) was evaluated by Sokolow-Lyon voltage criteria. LVH was defined as a sum of S amplitude in lead V1 and R amplitude in lead V5 or V6 (lead with higher amplitude was chosen) $\geq$3.5 mV.

Mean spatial QRS-T angle and maximum T-wave amplitude were calculated in a beat-to-beat manner. For this purpose, the QRS boundaries, T-wave peak and T-wave offset were located automatically for each beat. The QRS onset and offset detection was based on the method described by Daskalov and Cristov [27], utilizing the morphology of the ECG in the determination of the QRS boundaries. T-wave offset was defined as the intersection of the isoelectric line and a line fitted by least squares to the

Table 1. Characteristics of the study group.

Variable	Hypertensive, N = 51	Controls, N = 32	P-values
Age, years	60±3	60±3	p = 0.90
Height, cm	177±6	176±6	p = 0.89
Weight, kg	84±9	79±11	p = 0.02
BMI, kg/m^2	27±3	25±3	p = 0.01
BF, %	25±6	21±6	p = 0.01
SBP, mmHg	143±9	120±8	-
DBP, mmHg	86±6	73±6	-
Sokolow-Lyon index, mV	1.8±0.6	1.9±0.6	p = 0.51
Estimated VO2max, ml/kg/min	37±6	38±7	p = 0.19
Diabetes mellitus, n	4	0	-
Ever smoker, n	28	20	p = 0.56
Alcohol consumption ≥1 time/month, n	35	25	p = 0.42

Continuous variables are presented as mean values ± standard deviation, categorical variables as number of cases. BMI, body mass index; BF, body fat percentage; SBP, systolic blood pressure in home measurements; DBP, diastolic blood pressure in home measurements; estimated VO2max, indirectly estimated maximal oxygen uptake; and Sokolow-Lyon index, estimate of left ventricular hypertrophy.

maximum slope of the T-wave. Isoelectric line was defined as the mean amplitude of the preceding and following TP intervals. The maximum amplitude between QRS offset and T-wave offset was taken as the T-wave peak (minimum T-wave amplitude if inverted T-wave was observed).

Mean QRS and T axes were calculated from the orthogonal X, Y and Z leads, which were reconstructed from the 12-lead ECG samples with inverse-Dower matrix [28]. The mean spatial axes were based on the position vectors defined by the areas of the QRS and T-wave loops in the X, Y and Z leads and the mean spatial QRS-T angle was defined as the angle between these axes. Additionally, the maximum T-wave amplitude was calculated from leads V5 and II. However, instead of lead V5, lead V4 or V6 (which ever had the highest amplitude of T-wave) was used if the amplitude in V5 was below 0.15 mV.

Arrhythmias

We also analyzed the frequency of single ventricular and atrial ectopic beats. Automatic detection of ectopic beats was performed from baseline, cold exposure, and recovery ECG recordings with Medilog Darwin Holter Analyses software version V1.13.4 (TOM Medical Handels Gmbh, Austria). Automatic detection of ectopic beats was based on Medilog ADAPT algorithm [29]. Prematurity threshold was set to 15% compared to three normal preceding beats. Detected ectopic beats were confirmed with visual inspection by trained health care professionals.

Heart Rate Variability

Heart rate variability (HRV) analyses were performed in time and frequency domain as described previously [30] (Hearts 8, Heart Signal Co., Oulu, Finland) to assess activity of the autonomic nervous system. Artifacts and ectopic beats were removed and replaced with the local average. Linear de-trending was applied in measured RR interval data. Fast Fourier transform was applied to estimate the power spectral densities of the RR interval variability. Low (LF, 0.04–0.15 Hz) and high frequency power (HF, 0.15–0.40 Hz) of RR interval oscillations were quantified. The ratio between LF and HF powers (LF/HF-ratio) was also analyzed. The power spectral components of HRV were computed in 5 min periods and then averaged over each 15 min phase, i.e. baseline, cold, and recovery. To analyze the overall HRV, we computed the standard deviation of all normal RR intervals (SDNN) in time domain for each 15 minutes phase.

Blood Pressure

Brachial BP was measured with the use of oscillometric sphygmomanometry (Schiller BP 200 Plus, Schiller, Switzerland) at 3-minute intervals during baseline, cold exposure, and recovery measurements. The arm of the subject was supported and the position of the cuff was at the level of the heart.

Skin Temperatures and Thermal Sensations

Skin temperature was measured continuously with the use of thermistors (NTC DC95, Digi-Key, Thief River Falls, MN, USA) and data was recorded at 12 s intervals with an eight channel temperature data logger (SmartReaderPlus, Acr Systems Inc., BC, Canada). The thermistors were placed on the middle finger, back of the hand, shoulder blade, and cheek. Thermal perception for the whole body and face was assessed using subjective judgement scales [31].

Statistical Methods

Subject characteristics between study groups were compared with independent t–test for continuous variables and chi-square test for categorical variables. Sensitivity analyses were conducted separately for BMI, weight, fat percentage and chronic diseases. Due to lack of effect to the results these were ignored in further analyses. Means between baseline, cold, and recovery as well as study groups were compared by 2-way repeated measures ANOVA and contrast tests. Parameters with non-Gaussian distribution were transformed into natural logarithm. In addition, we executed linear regression analyses to evaluate the rate-dependency (HR changes) of T-wave amplitude change. The results are expressed as means and their standard deviations (SD) or 95% confidence intervals (CI). Statistical analyses were performed with IBM SPSS for Windows version 19 (IBM Corp. Released 2010, Armonk, NY, USA) and significance was set at $p < 0.05$.

Results

Thermoregulatory Responses

The employed cold exposure involved facial cooling which could be demonstrated as a rapid (30°C to 21°C in 2 min) and robust (30°C to 15°C in 10 min) reduction in skin temperature of the cheek. In general, the winter clothing slowed down or even prevented superficial cooling of most areas of the body, as demonstrated by the only slightly lowered shoulder blade temperature (baseline 34°C vs. cold 31°C). Finger temperatures decreased by 3–4°C in the cold (26°C to 22°C). Skin temperatures on cheek and finger remained 4–7°C lower 10–15 minutes after the exposure compared to baseline measurements both in hypertensive men and controls. Skin temperature responses during baseline, cold exposure and the recovery measurements did not differ between hypertensive men and control group. Thermal perceptions (median) of the whole body and face were neutral during baseline and recovery measurements and cool during cold exposure in both study groups.

Cold exposure, ECG, HRV, BP, and arrhythmias

The detected changes in T-wave amplitude, T-peak to T-end interval, QTc, and HR are depicted in Figure 2. Cold exposure resulted in higher maximum T-wave amplitude compared to baseline in both hypertensive and control subjects in leads II and V5 (Table 2, Figure 2). We also examined the HR dependency of this parameter and estimated the following regression equation: T-wave amplitude change = 48.370+0.426 * RR change (adjusted $R^2 = 0.296$, $p<0.001$). QRS-T angle and QTc interval decreased during cold exposure in both groups (Table 2). T-peak to T-end interval increased in lead II (Figure 2), but remained constant in lead V5. An example ECG presenting changes in cardiac repolarization during cold exposure is depicted in Figure 3. PR and QRS intervals were mainly unaltered. Cold exposure increased systolic (26–27 mmHg) and diastolic BP (12 mmHg) both among hypertensive and control subjects. Cold induced ECG changes did not return to the baseline level during 15 minutes recovery follow-up after the exposure (Table 2). Cold exposure increased the frequency of ventricular, but not atrial ectopic beats (Table 2). In all phases, frequency of ectopic beats was low in both study groups.

When examining the HRV parameters, cold exposure increased both LF (60–80%) and HF (100–110%) components of HRV, as well as SDNN (25%) in both hypertensive and control subjects (Table 2). LF/HF-ratio and HR decreased during cold exposure in

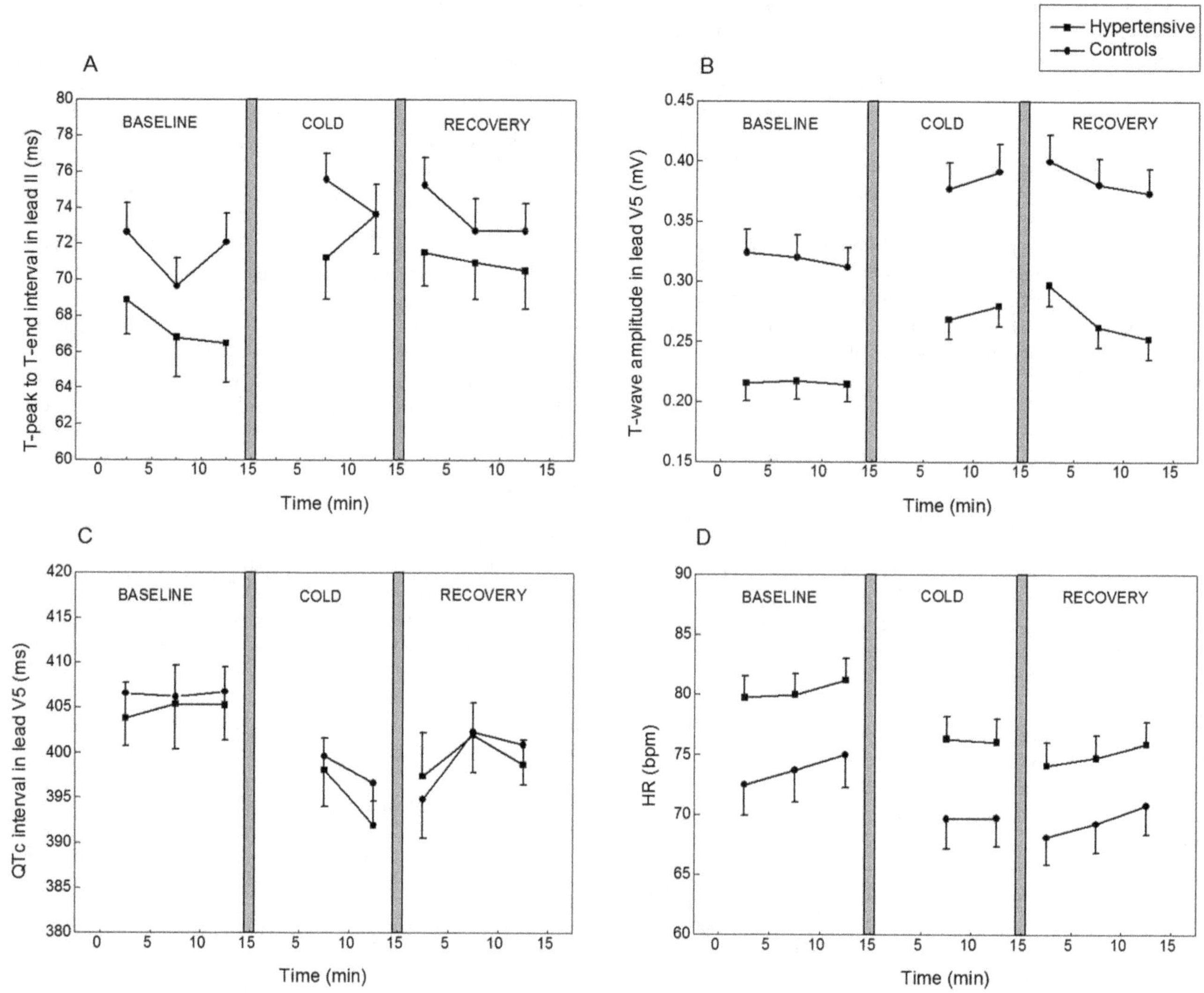

Figure 2. ECG changes during cold exposure. T-peak to T-end interval in lead II (A), T-wave amplitude in lead V5 (B), QTc in lead V5 (C), and HR (D) of hypertensive men (N = 51) and controls (N = 32) before (baseline), during, and after (recovery) cold exposure. Values represent means and standard error of the means.

both groups. HRV parameters did not return to the baseline level during 15 minutes recovery follow-up after cold exposure.

Hypertension, ECG, HRV, BP, and arrhythmias

There were no differences in ECG parameters or arrhythmias between the study groups, except for T-wave amplitude which was ca. 0.1 mV higher in controls compared with hypertensive men during all phases ($p<0.001$) and for unadjusted QT ($p<0.05$). HR was lower (6–7 beats) and LF/HF-ratio higher among hypertensive compared to control subjects. Otherwise, there were no differences in the HRV parameters between the study groups. Hypertensive subject had a higher SBP and DBP compared to controls during all phases ($p<0.001$), as expected.

Cold, hypertension and changes in ECG, HRV, BP, and arrhythmias

All cold induced changes were comparable among hypertensive men and controls (no time×group effect).

Discussion

The present study is the first to assess cardiac electrical activity, cardiovascular autonomic regulation, and arrhythmias in hypertensive middle-aged men during cold exposure similar to everyday winter circumstances in a subarctic climate. We observed that cold exposure slightly increased T-peak to T-end interval, T-wave amplitude and decreased QTc interval reflecting changes in ventricular repolarization. Simultaneously an autonomic co-activation with increased sympathetic and parasympathetic activity during the cold exposure was observed. The frequency of ventricular ectopic beats increased slightly in the cold. These cold-related responses were similar in hypertensive and control subjects.

According to our results, short-term cold exposure not involving substantial whole body cooling increased T-peak to T-end interval in lead II, reflecting prolongation of cardiac repolarization. The observed increase in T-wave amplitude, on the other hand, may indicate dispersion in duration of action potentials [32]. In addition, cold exposure had no effect on QT interval despite a

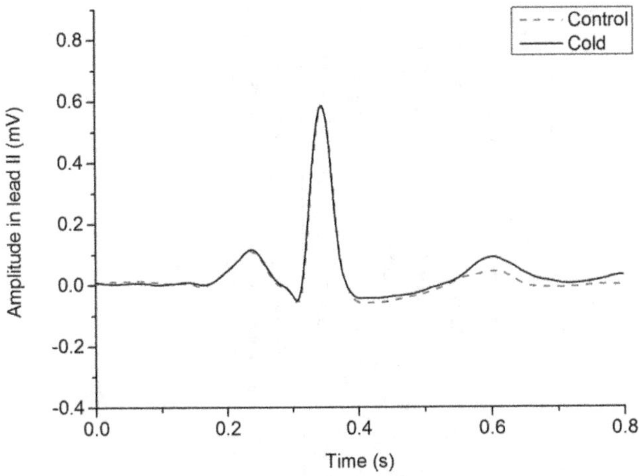

Figure 3. Example ECG presenting changes in cardiac repolarization. Figure presents a median ECG from 10 consecutive beats as an example of changes in T-wave in lead II before (baseline), during, and after (recovery) cold exposure. Cold exposure increased T-peak to T-end interval and T-wave amplitude.

reduction in HR. The frequency of ventricular ectopic beats was slightly increased during cold exposure, which may reflect the observed cardiac electrical changes.

Previous experimental or clinical studies examining the effects of cold on cardiac electrical function have involved intense whole-body exposures, such as hypothermia [14,15,33] and immersion to cold water [12] or employed exercise in cold [16–18]. These studies have shown several different effects on ECG, such as atrial [12,14,15,33] and ventricular [15,33] arrhythmias, interval prolongation [14,15,33], T-wave abnormalities [14,15], Osborne waves [14,15,33], and pronounced ST-depression during exercise among cardiac patients [16], depending on cold exposure duration and its intensity. Only a few studies have examined cardiac electrical activity under superficial or local cold exposure, such as facial cooling with [34] or without breath holding [13].

The observed changes in our study in cardiac electrophysiology during cold exposure are based on current knowledge caused by an altered autonomic nervous system activity [9,12,13,18,35]. This altered autonomic regulation persisted throughout the 15 minutes recovery period. One plausible reason for this could be lowered skin temperatures at recovery, which could have provided a continuing parasympathetic and sympathetic stimulus. Also, irrespective of skin temperature, the autonomic nervous system regulation may not recover immediately after the cessation of stressor. The applied cold exposure increased sympathetic activity [9], as demonstrated by the increased peripheral BP and cardiac work [21]. Furthermore, the spectral analysis of HRV showed that both LF and HF increased while HR decreased as a sign of parasympathetic activation during cold exposure. Sympathetic stimulation increases T-peak to T-end interval in limb leads [36]. Sympathetic stimulation results in either inverted or positive T-wave depending on the stimulated area [37,38]. Sympathetic activation also increases risk of arrhythmias [10]. The observed shortened cold-related QTc interval with reduced HR but unaltered QT interval in the present study probably reflects the simultaneous effects of increased vagal and sympathetic activity [35,39].

Sympathovagal co-activation of autonomic nervous system is a regulatory process but could cause conflicting pressures on the heart and may partially explain the observed increases in T-peak to T-end interval, T-wave amplitude, and ventricular arrhythmias. Such co-activation has been previously described in association with stimuli, like facial cooling [13], during cold water immersion involving breath holding [12], as well as during the recovery phase of exercise [40]. The co-activation of the sympathetic and vagal outflow changes HR dynamics from more fractal to random HR organization [13] and could predispose to arrhythmias [12,41].

Hypertension is related to increased sympathetic activity [19,42] and is a risk factor of cardiac events such as arrhythmia [20] and ischemic changes [20,43]. In our study, untreated hypertensive men had higher HR and LF/HF- ratio and lower T-wave amplitude compared to controls in both warm and cold conditions, consistent with previous non-cold related studies [44,45] and indicating elevated sympathetic activity in hypertension. Sympathetic hyperactivity combined with the cold stressor could potentate adverse ECG changes during cold exposure. Contrary to our hypothesis, we did not observe major differences in cardiac responses to cold exposure between hypertensive men and controls. The lack of major ECG changes may be due to a short disease history among the untreated hypertensive subjects in our study. It is possible that in persons whose cardiovascular disease is at a more advanced stage, disturbed circulatory adjustments or compromised cardiac oxygen supply could lead to aggravated cardiovascular responses and impaired cardiac function.

ECG parameters are commonly rate-dependent [46], and some of the observed changes in our study could be explained by slightly decreased HR in the cold. According to the linear regression model less than one third of the observed change in T-wave amplitude could be explained by change in HR in our study, i.e. most of the change is related to other factors. T-peak to T-end interval has been presented to have minor or no connection with HR [46]. In contrast, QT interval is known to be strongly dependent of HR [46] and rate dependency of it varies with altered autonomic function [35,39]. QRS-T angle decreased with decreasing HR in our study, consistent with a previous study assessing rate-dependency of QRS-T-angle during exercise test [47].

Strengths and limitations

The strength of our study is that all subjects were drawn from the general population and thus the results reflect typical cardiovascular response to cold among untreated middle aged hypertensive men and men without hypertension. Furthermore, we were able to produce a strictly controlled and equal cold exposure to all subjects. Hence, we consider that our results have public health implications due to the population-based sample and the utilized cold exposure which was similar to everyday winter circumstances in a cold climate.

Performing a randomized controlled trial would have reduced possible bias related to anticipation caused by measurements. However, we emphasized familiarization and reduction of stress of all participants caused by the experimental conditions. Another limitation of our study was that some of the study participants had other chronic diseases in addition to hypertension. However, we conducted sensitivity analyses by excluding the participants with these chronic diseases, but did not detect any effects on the main results. Also, despite the population based recruitment, some selection may still occur through non-participation. We do not have information of the characteristics of the subjects declining to participate in the study.

Table 2. Cardiovascular responses to cold exposure among hypertensive men and control group.

Variable	Hypertensive, N = 51				Controls, N = 32			
	Baseline (Mean±SD)	Cold Exposure (Mean±SD)	Recovery (Mean±SD)	Effect of cold exposure (Mean, 95% CI)	Baseline (Mean±SD)	Cold Exposure (Mean±SD)	Recovery (Mean±SD)	Effect of cold exposure (Mean, 95% CI)
HR, bpm†	80±13	77±14*	75±13*	−3 (−5 to −2)	73±15	70±14*	69±13*	−4 (−6 to −1)
T-peak (II), mV†	0.12±0.06	0.14±0.06*	0.14±0.07*	0.03 (0.02 to 0.03)	0.17±0.06	0.21±0.07*	0.21±0.07*	0.04 (0.02 to 0.05)
TpTe (II), ms	67±14	72±16*	71±13*	5 (3 to 7)	71±8	75±8*	74±8*	3 (0 to 6)
QT (II), ms†	368±27	366±30	369±31	−1 (−4 to 2)	381±31	382±30	383±29	1 (−4 to 6)
QTc (II), ms	408±27	398±19*	402±24*	−10 (−16 to −5)	410±31	401±28*	403±24*	−10 (−13 to −6)
PR (II), ms	153±17	154±20	153±19	2 (0 to 3)	155±22	156±20	155±23	2 (−3 to 7)
QRS (II), ms†	97±12	96±13*	97±13	0 (−2 to 1)	92±9	90±9*	91±9	1 (−1 to 2)
T-peak (V5), mV†	0.22±0.11	0.27±0.12*	0.27±0.12*	0.06 (0.05 to 0.07)	0.32±0.10	0.38±0.13*	0.38±0.12*	0.07 (0.04 to 0.09)
TpTe (V5), ms	80±15	81±12	82±13	1 (−2 to 3)	80±13	80±9	80±9	0 (−4 to 3)
QT (V5), ms†	365±27	364±31	367±30	−1 (−4 to 2)	377±31	379±29	379±29	2 (−3 to 7)
QTc (V5), ms	405±27	395±20*	399±23*	−10 (−16 to −4)	406±32	398±28*	400±25*	−8 (−12 to −5)
PR (V5), ms	152±17	154±17	153±18	2 (0 to 3)	154±22	156±21	153±24	2 (−3 to 7)
QRS (V5), ms	90±13	90±14	91±13	0 (−2 to 1)	89±10	90±10	89±10	1 (−1 to 2)
QRS-T angle, °	56±48	48±47*	48±46*	−7 (−2 to −12)	41±48	37±46*	39±47*	−3 (−6 to −1)
VEB, count/15 min	1.3±4.0	1.8±4.2*	1.4±3.9	0.5 (0.0 to 1.0)	0.4±0.9	0.7±1.6*	0.3±0.9	0.3 (−0.2 to 0.7)
AEB, count/15 min	0.6±2.7	0.7±3.9	0.5±2.7	0.2 (−0.4 to 0.7)	0.1±0.4	0.1±0.2	0.1±0.3	−0.1 (−0.2 to 0.1)
VEB2, count/15 min	2.3±5.2	3.2±5.3*	2.5±5.1	1.0 (0.0 to 1.9)	0.9±1.3	1.6±2.1*	0.8±1.3	0.7 (−0.5 to 1.9)
AEB2, count/15 min	1.0±3.7	1.3±5.2	0.9±3.6	0.3 (−0.7 to 1.3)	0.3±0.6	0.2±0.4	0.2±0.4	−0.2 (−0.6 to 0.3)
Systolic BP, mmHg†	148±13	175±16*	153±13*	27 (24 to 30)	126±13	152±14*	133±12*	26 (21 to 30)
Diastolic BP, mmHg†	92±10	104±10*	94±9*	12 (10 to 14)	79±10	91±10*	83±8*	12 (10 to 14)
LF RR, ms²	390±420	630±600*	550±480*	240 (120 to 360)	380±290	700±650*	580±500*	320 (140 to 500)
HF RR, ms²	90±110	190±220*	150±160*	100 (60 to 150)	150±200	300±370*	220±220*	150 (50 to 250)
LF/HF-ratio†	6.4±4.8	4.6±2.9*	5.2±4.2*	−1.9 (−3.0 to −0.7)	4.3±3.2	3.4±1.8*	4.0±3.2*	−0.9 (−2.0 to 0.2)
SDNN RR, ms²	32±12	40±16*	39±16*	8 (6 to 11)	33±12	41±8*	43±18*	8 (3 to 13)

Values are group means over each phase (baseline, cold, and recovery) ± standard deviations (SD). Effect of cold exposure: mean of intra-individual differences between "Cold exposure" and "Baseline" with 95% confidence intervals (95% CI). HR, heart rate; T-peak, T-wave amplitude; TpTe, T-peak to T-end interval; QT, QT-interval; QTc, QT adjusted to HR; PR, and QRS, corresponding intervals on ECG; QRS-T angle, spatial angle between QRS and T; VEB, ventricular and AEB, atrial ectopic beats; VEB2, ventricular and AEB2, atrial ectopic beats for those who had ectopic beats during the measurements (n = 28 hypertensive and 13 controls); BP, blood pressure; LF, low frequency; HF, high frequency; LF/HF, the ratio of LF and HF; SDNN, standard deviation of all normal RR intervals; .

* $p<0.05$ vs. baseline (time),

† $p>0.05$ vs. hypertensive (group).

There were no significant difference in responses to cold between hypertensive men and controls (no time×group effect).

Conclusions

In conclusion, our results demonstrate that moderate short-term whole body cold exposure commonly occurring in everyday life [48] results in altered cardiac repolarization among middle-aged men. Rather than being of clinical importance, the detected changes may be physiological responses to short-term cold exposure. Furthermore, as compared to the control group, the untreated hypertensive men are not more susceptible to cold induced changes in cardiac electrical function. However, the detected cold effects could be more substantial with more intense cold exposure or among patients with cardiac disease. Future studies are warranted to examine cardiac electrical function during cold exposure among persons with advanced cardiovascular diseases.

Acknowledgments

The authors wish to thank Saana Rautakoski, Henna Hyrkäs, Jukka Jauhiainen, Heta Helakari, Arno Kandelberg, and Jaakko Takkunen for their great help in the collection of the data.

Author Contributions

Conceived and designed the experiments: HH TVK MT AK HVH MM SKK KHH RA HR JJKJ TMI. Performed the experiments: HH MT AK HR JJKJ TMI. Analyzed the data: HH TVK MT AK HVH RB HR JJKJ TMI. Wrote the paper: HH TVK MT AK HVH MM SKK RB KHH RA HR JJKJ TMI.

References

1. The Eurowinter Group (1997) Cold exposure and winter mortality from ischaemic heart disease, cerebrovascular disease, respiratory disease, and all causes in warm and cold regions of Europe. The Eurowinter Group. Lancet 349: 1341–1346.
2. Fares A (2013) Winter cardiovascular diseases phenomenon. N Am J Med Sci 5: 266–279.
3. Manfredini R, Manfredini F, Boari B, Bergami E, Mari E, et al. (2009) Seasonal and weekly patterns of hospital admissions for nonfatal and fatal myocardial infarction. Am J Emerg Med 27: 1097–1103.
4. Mehta RH, Manfredini R, Hassan F, Sechtem U, Bossone E, et al. (2002) International Registry of Acute Aortic Dissection (IRAD) Investigators (2002) Chronobiological patterns of acute aortic dissection. Circulation 106: 1110–1115.
5. Gallerani M, Boari B, Manfredini F, Manfredini R (2011) Seasonal variation in heart failure hospitalization. Clin Cardiol 34: 389–394.
6. Palm F, Dos Santos M, Urbanek C, Greulich M, Zimmer K, et al. (2013) Stroke seasonality associations with subtype, etiology and laboratory results in the ludwigshafen stroke study (LuSSt). Eur J Epidemiol 28: 373–381.
7. Anand K, Aryana A, Cloutier D, Hee T, Esterbrooks D, et al. (2007) Circadian, daily, and seasonal distributions of ventricular tachyarrhythmias in patients with implantable cardioverter-defibrillators. Am J Cardiol 100: 1134–1138.
8. Page RL, Zipes DP, Powell JL, Luceri RM, Gold MR, et al. (2004) Seasonal variation of mortality in the antiarrhythmics versus implantable defibrillators (AVID) study registry. Heart Rhythm 1: 435–440.
9. Leppäluoto J, Pääkkönen T, Korhonen I, Hassi J (2005) Pituitary and autonomic responses to cold exposures in man. Acta Physiol Scand 184: 255–264.
10. Vaseghi M, Shivkumar K (2008) The role of the autonomic nervous system in sudden cardiac death. Prog Cardiovasc Dis 50: 404–419.
11. Khurana RK, Wu R (2006) The cold face test: A non-baroreflex mediated test of cardiac vagal function. Clin Auton Res 16: 202–207.
12. Shattock MJ, Tipton MJ (2012) 'Autonomic conflict': A different way to die during cold water immersion? J Physiol (Lond) 590: 3219–3230.
13. Tulppo MP, Kiviniemi AM, Hautala AJ, Kallio M, Seppänen T, et al. (2005) Physiological background of the loss of fractal heart rate dynamics. Circulation 112: 314–319.
14. Aslam AF, Aslam AK, Vasavada BC, Khan IA (2006) Hypothermia: Evaluation, electrocardiographic manifestations, and management. Am J Med 119: 297–301.
15. De Souza D, Riera AR, Bombig MT, Francisco YA, Brollo L, et al. (2007) Electrocardiographic changes by accidental hypothermia in an urban and a tropical region. J Electrocardiol 40: 47–52.
16. Backman C, Linderholm H (1991) Reaction of patients with effort angina to cold exposure during exercise. Arctic Med Res Suppl: 526–528.
17. Schmid JP, Morger C, Noveanu M, Binder RK, Anderegg M, et al. (2009) Haemodynamic and arrhythmic effects of moderately cold (22 degrees C) water immersion and swimming in patients with stable coronary artery disease and heart failure. Eur J Heart Fail 11: 903–909.
18. Sanchez-Gonzalez MA, Figueroa A (2013) Cold exposure attenuates post exercise cardiovagal reactivation and sympathetic withdrawal. Auton Neurosci 176: 95–97.
19. Parati G, Esler M (2012) The human sympathetic nervous system: Its relevance in hypertension and heart failure. Eur Heart J 33: 1058–1066.
20. Manolis AJ, Rosei EA, Coca A, Cifkova R, Erdine SE, et al. (2012) Hypertension and atrial fibrillation: Diagnostic approach, prevention and treatment. position paper of the working group 'hypertension arrhythmias and thrombosis' of the european society of hypertension. J Hypertens 30: 239–252.
21. Hintsala H, Kandelberg A, Herzig KH, Rintamäki H, Mäntysaari M, et al. (2014) Central aortic blood pressure of hypertensive men during short-term cold exposure. Am J Hypertens 27(5):656–664.
22. Komulainen S, Tähtinen T, Rintamäki H, Virokannas H, Keinänen-Kiukaanniemi S (2000) Blood pressure responses to whole-body cold exposure: Effect of carvedilol. Eur J Clin Pharmacol 56: 637–642.
23. Barnett AG, Sans S, Salomaa V, Kuulasmaa K, Dobson AJ, et al. (2007) The effect of temperature on systolic blood pressure. Blood Press Monit 12: 195–203.
24. Parati G, Stergiou GS, Asmar R, Bilo G, de Leeuw P, et al. (2008) European society of hypertension guidelines for blood pressure monitoring at home: A summary report of the second international consensus conference on home blood pressure monitoring. J Hypertens 26: 1505–1526.
25. ISO 9920 (2007) Ergonomics of the thermal environment - estimation of thermal insulation and water vapour resistance of a clothing ensemble.
26. Karjalainen J, Viitasalo M, Mänttäri M, Manninen V (1994) Relation between QT intervals and heart rates from 40 to 120 beats/min in rest electrocardiograms of men and a simple method to adjust QT interval values. J Am Coll Cardiol 23: 1547–1553.
27. Daskalov IK, Christov II (1999) Electrocardiogram signal preprocessing for automatic detection of QRS boundaries. Med Eng Phys 21: 37–44.
28. Edenbrandt L, Pahlm O (1988) Vectorcardiogram synthesized from a 12-lead ECG: Superiority of the inverse dower matrix. J Electrocardiol 21: 361–367.
29. Pardey J, Jouravleva S (2004) The next-generation holter revolution: From "analyse, edit, print" to "analyse, print". Computers in cardiology 31: 373–376.
30. Huikuri HV, Valkama JO, Airaksinen KE, Seppänen T, Kessler KM, et al. (1993) Frequency domain measures of heart rate variability before the onset of nonsustained and sustained ventricular tachycardia in patients with coronary artery disease. Circulation 87: 1220–1228.
31. ISO 10551 (1995) Ergonomics of the thermal environment - assessment of the influence of the thermal environment using subjective judgement scales.
32. Bernardo D, Murray A (2000) Explaining the T-wave shape in the ECG. Nature 403: 40.
33. Mattu A, Brady WJ, Perron AD (2002) Electrocardiographic manifestations of hypothermia. Am J Emerg Med 20: 314–326.
34. Wierzba T, Musial P, Cwikalowska H (2011) Variable profile of individual heart rate responses to cold water immersion apnea in healthy late adolescent men. - Georgian Med News 196–197:28–38.
35. Sundaram S, Carnethon M, Polito K, Kadish AH, Goldberger JJ (2008) Autonomic effects on QT-RR interval dynamics after exercise. Am J Physiol Heart Circ Physiol 294: H490–H497.
36. Vaseghi M, Yamakawa K, Sinha A, So E, Zhou W, et al. (2013) Modulation of regional dispersion of repolarization and T-peak to T-end interval by right and left stellate ganglia. - Am J Physiol Heart Circ Physiol: 305(7):H1020–H1030
37. Kralios FA, Martin L, Burgess MJ, Millar K (1975) Local ventricular repolarization changes due to sympathetic nerve-branch stimulation. Am J Physiol 228: 1621–1626.
38. Conrath CE, Opthof T (2006) Ventricular repolarization: An overview of (patho)physiology, sympathetic effects and genetic aspects. Prog Biophys Mol Biol 92: 269–307.
39. Arai K, Nakagawa Y, Iwata T, Horiguchi H, Murata K (2013) Relationships between QT interval and heart rate variability at rest and the covariates in healthy young adults. Auton Neurosci 173: 53–57.
40. Tulppo MP, Kiviniemi AM, Hautala AJ, Kallio M, Seppänen T, et al. (2011) Sympatho-vagal interaction in the recovery phase of exercise. Clin Physiol Funct Imaging 31: 272–281.

41. Chen PS, Tan AY (2007) Autonomic nerve activity and atrial fibrillation. Heart Rhythm 4: S61–S64.
42. Grassi G (2010) Sympathetic neural activity in hypertension and related diseases. Am J Hypertens 23: 1052–1060.
43. Murphy BP, Stanton T, Dunn FG (2009) Hypertension and myocardial ischemia. Med Clin North Am 93: 681–695.
44. Wu JS, Lu FH, Yang YC, Lin TS, Chen JJ, et al. (2008) Epidemiological study on the effect of pre-hypertension and family history of hypertension on cardiac autonomic function. J Am Coll Cardiol 51: 1896–1901.
45. Dilaveris P, Gialafos E, Poloniecki J, Hnatkova K, Richter D, et al. (2000) Changes of the T-wave amplitude and angle: An early marker of altered ventricular repolarization in hypertension. Clin Cardiol 23: 600–606.
46. Andersen MP, Xue JQ, Graff C, Kanters JK, Toft E, et al. (2008) New descriptors of T-wave morphology are independent of heart rate. J Electrocardiol 41: 557–561.
47. Kenttä T, Karsikas M, Kiviniemi A, Tulppo M, Seppänen T, et al. (2010) Dynamics and rate-dependence of the spatial angle between ventricular depolarization and repolarization wave fronts during exercise ECG. Ann Noninvasive Electrocardiol 15: 264–275.
48. Mäkinen TM, Raatikka VP, Rytkönen M, Jokelainen J, Rintamäki H, et al. (2006) Factors affecting outdoor exposure in winter: Population-based study. Int J Biometeorol 51: 27–36.

Efficacy and Safety of Tai Chi for Parkinson's Disease: A Systematic Review and Meta-Analysis of Randomized Controlled Trials

Xiaojia Ni[1,2], Shaonan Liu[3], Fuchang Lu[2], Xiaogeng Shi[4], Xinfeng Guo[3]*

1 Research and Development Department of New Drugs, Guangdong Provincial Hospital of Chinese Medicine, Guangzhou, Guangdong Province, China, 2 The Second College of Clinical Medicine, Guangzhou University of Chinese Medicine, Guangzhou, Guangdong Province, China, 3 Key Unit of Methodology in Clinical Research, Guangdong Provincial Hospital of Chinese Medicine, Guangzhou, Guangdong Province, China, 4 Department of Neurology, Guangdong Provincial Hospital of Chinese Medicine, Guangzhou, Guangdong Province, China

Abstract

Background and Objective: In Parkinson's disease (PD), wearing off and side effects of long-term medication and complications pose challenges for neurologists. Although Tai Chi is beneficial for many illnesses, its efficacy for PD remains uncertain. The purpose of this review was to evaluate the efficacy and safety of Tai Chi for PD.

Methods: Randomized controlled trials (RCTs) of Tai Chi for PD were electronically searched by the end of December 2013 and identified by two independent reviewers. The tool from the Cochrane Handbook 5.1 was used to assess the risk of bias. A standard meta-analysis was performed using RevMan 5.2 software.

Results: Ten trials with PD of mild-to-moderate severity were included in the review, and nine trials (n = 409) were included in the meta-analysis. The risk of bias was generally high in the blinding of participants and personnel. Improvements in the Unified Parkinson's Disease Rating Scale Part III (mean difference (MD) −4.34, 95% confidence interval (CI) −6.67−−2.01), Berg Balance Scale (MD: 4.25, 95% CI: 2.83–5.66), functional reach test (MD: 3.89, 95% CI: 1.73–6.04), Timed Up and Go test (MD: −0.75, 95% CI: −1.30−−0.21), stride length (standardized MD: 0.56, 95% CI: 0.03–1.09), health-related quality of life (standardized MD: −1.10, 95% CI: −1.81−−0.39) and reduction of falls were greater after interventions with Tai Chi plus medication. Satisfaction and safety were high. Intervention with Tai Chi alone was more effective for only a few balance and mobility outcomes.

Conclusions: Tai Chi performed with medication resulted in promising gains in mobility and balance, and it was safe and popular among PD patients at an early stage of the disease. This provides a new evidence for PD management. More RCTs with larger sample size that carefully address blinding and prudently select outcomes are needed.

PROSPERO registration number CRD42013004989.

Editor: Antony Bayer, Cardiff University, United Kingdom

Funding: This study was supported by Joint Special Project of Guangdong Provincial Department of Science and Technology-Guangdong Provincial Academy of Chinese Medical Sciences: Construction and Application of Evidence-Based Knowledge Management System for Traditional Chinese Medicine (No. 2012A032500009), China. http://pro.gdstc.gov.cn/stms/main.jsp The funders had no role in study design, data collection and analysis, decision to publish, or preparation of the manuscript.

Competing Interests: The authors have declared that no competing interests exist.

* E-mail: drguoxinfeng@163.com

Introduction

Parkinson's disease (PD) is a progressive neurodegenerative disorder characterized by static tremor, rigidity, bradykinesia and postural disturbance [1] with a crude incidence rate of 4.5 to 19 per 100,000 people globally [2]. It afflicts 1.7% of the Chinese population >65 years old, a similar prevalence to that reported in developed countries [3]. The management of PD is complex and individualized. Levodopa replacement therapy and various other drug combinations achieve gains in the early stage of the disease, especially in motor impairments [4]. However, with the progress of the disease and wearing off of the medication, long-term side effect involving symptom fluctuation, dyskinesia and psychiatric comorbidity [5] is a great challenge for neurologists. Infusion therapy [6] and functional surgery such as deep brain stimulation [7] have emerged to address the unsolved problems induced by classical medications, yet their efficacy and safety require further validation. In addition to the major motor symptoms caused by PD, patients experience complications including insomnia, excessive daytime sleepiness, autonomic dysfunction, dementia and depression that are typically tackled by combined drug therapy with unknown risks [8].

Increasing evidence is being found that physiotherapy can benefit PD patients [9]. Tai Chi is a balance-based exercise guided by the yin-yang theory of traditional Chinese medicine that combines deep-breath relaxation and slow and gentle movements with awareness [10]. Tai Chi has been reported to reduce the incidence of falls in an elderly population [11], decrease blood pressure [12], improve lung [13] and cardiac [14] functions, alleviate menopausal osteoporosis [15], relieve psychological dysfunction [16], insomnia [17] and low back pain [18], rehabilitate post-stroke syndromes [19], and slow the progression of rheumatic illness [20,21] and dementia [22]. In light of these gains, Tai Chi shows potential to help both the motor dysfunction and non-motor complications of PD. However, the clinical benefit of Tai Chi in PD remains uncertain due to different study designs, small sample size and inconsistent methodological quality of the published clinical studies. Some trials even pose contradictory results for the same outcome [23].

A systematic review aims to minimize bias and providing more reliable findings by using explicit and systematic method [24,25]. Also, a meta-analysis adds to the review can increase power of testing, improve precision of estimated effect, settle controversies and answer clinical question not posed by the individual studies [26]. To identity whether Tai Chi safely benefits PD patients, we performed a systematic review and meta-analysis of randomized controlled trials (RCTs) of Tai Chi for PD.

Methods

1. Protocol and registration

The study was prospectively registered and the protocol was specified in advance and documented in the PROSPERO database with the number CRD42013004989.

2. Eligibility

Eligible studies were RCTs without restriction of publication language, date or status. Participants of any age, gender and ethnic group were clinically diagnosed as PD in any stage. Tai Chi was practiced alone or in combination with conventional medication, compared to other exercise with or without conventional medication, medication alone, placebo, or no intervention. Intervention duration and length of follow up were not restricted.

The primary outcome was the global scores of Unified Parkinson's Disease Rating Scale Part III (UPDRS III). The UPDRS III is a 14-item instrument that integrates all aspects of motor symptoms caused by PD, and the score ranges from 0 to 56, with lower values indicating less motor disability [27]. Secondary outcomes were: 1) balance and mobility function assessed using the Berg Balance Scale (BBS), the functional reach test (FRT) or the Timed Up and Go test (TUG); 2) health-related quality of life (HRQOL) assessed using the Parkinson's Disease Questionairre-39 (PDQ-39) or the PDQ-39 Summary Index (PDQ-39SI); 3) gait, including velocity and stride length; 4) falls; 5) post-program survey (PPS); and 6) adverse events (AE). The studies finally included should have at least one of these outcomes.

3. Information source and search strategy

A systematic search, as recommend by the PRISMA statement [28], was performed in online databases, including PubMed (from 1966), Embase (from 1985), the Cochrane Library, the Chinese Biomedical Database (from 1979), the China National Knowledge Infrastructure (from 1915), VIP Journal Integration Platform (from 1989), Wanfang Med Online (from 1982), and the Japan Medical Abstracts Society using the following search terms: Tai Chi, Tai Ji, T'ai Chi, Taijiquan, Parkinson disease, Parkinson's disease, Primary Parkinsonism and Paralysis Agitans. The websites of ClinicalTrials.gov and the Chinese Clinical Trial Registry were also searched to identify unpublished clinical trials. In addition, a search was performed in Google Scholar to find reports from other sources. The final search was performed on December 31, 2013. The search strategy is specified in the appendix.

4. Study selection and data collection

Two authors (Xiaojia Ni and Fuchang Lu) independently identified and selected studies in a standardized manner. The primary search was carried out in all information sources and was followed by duplication screening. Abstracts and full texts were then reviewed for eligibility criteria. The decision on which studies to include in qualitative and quantitative synthesis was made according to the type of outcome data reported. Disagreement was resolved by a third author (Shaonan Liu).

Two authors (Xiaojia Ni and Fuchang Lu) independently extracted the following information from the included trials and entered it into an Excel spreadsheet: (1) study design and number of patients; (2) baseline patient characteristics (age, gender, disease stage or severity and disease history); (3) intervention and control (type, dose, duration, frequency and any medication); (4) outcomes; (5) length and frequency of follow up; and (6) AE. Duplicate publications were carefully detected and incomplete information was dealt with by contacting the investigators for further data. Disagreements were resolved by discussion or by consulting a third author (Shaonan Liu).

5. Risk of bias assessment

Two authors (Xiaojia Ni and Shaonan Liu) independently assessed the risk of bias in individual studies using the Cochrane Collaboration tool [29]. When necessary, information contained in the published articles was supplemented by the published protocol, registration records or by contacting the corresponding authors. Any discrepancy was resolved by another author (Xinfeng Guo). The assessment of blinding was made based on different groups of outcomes, including: 1) clinician-reported outcomes (UPDRS III, BBS, FRT, TUG, gait velocity and stride length), 2) subjective patient-reported outcomes (PDQ-39, PDQ-39SI and PPS,), and 3) objective patient-reported outcome (falls). Seven aspects were evaluated, as follows: (1) random sequence generation, (2) allocation concealment, (3) blinding of participants and personnel (healthcare providers), (4) blinding of outcome assessment, (5) incomplete outcome data, (6) selective reporting and (7) other bias. Judgments were categorized as 'low risk of bias', 'high risk of bias', or 'unclear risk of bias'. According to our knowledge of Tai Chi and experience of clinical research, other bias was assessed and judgment was made as 'high risk of bias' if control group lacking validation, unreliable randomization, or insufficient sample size occurred.

6. Data synthesis and analysis

Dichotomous data were presented as relative risk (RR) with 95% confidence interval (CI) and continuous outcomes were presented as mean difference (MD) between intervention and control groups with 95% CI. HRQOL and gait outcomes are presented as standardized MD (SMD) because the scales or units were not consistent across studies.

In studies with multiple groups, the 'shared' group was evenly divided into two or more groups with smaller sample size, and two or more (reasonably independent) comparisons were performed. For dichotomous outcomes, both the number of events and the total number of patients were divided. For continuous outcomes, only the total number of participants was divided and the mean and standard deviation was left unchanged.

Review Manager software (RevMan, Version 5.2, Copenhagen: The Nordic Cochrane Centre, The Cochrane Collaboration,

2012) was used for data analysis. Heterogeneity between trials was detected using a chi-square test. For studies with good homogeneity ($P>0.10$, $I_2<40\%$), a fixed model was used for the meta-analysis. For all other studies, a random model was used and particular care was taken when interpreting the results. Subgroup analysis was used to compare the effect of Tai Chi with medications to medications alone, and the effect of Tai Chi alone to no intervention. Publication bias was assessed by funnel plot analysis if the group included more than ten trials.

Results

1. Study identification

A total of ten articles [30–39] were included in the review. One article [33] reported two different RCTs and two articles [32,34] reported different outcomes for the same trial. Eight articles [30–35,38–39] were published in English and two [36,37] were published in Chinese. The flow diagram of search and identification is shown in Figure 1.

2. Study characteristics

All trials included were randomized, parallel, controlled clinical trials with blinded assessment. Only two studies [32,34,36] were conducted in multiple centers. A total of 470 patients with PD of mild-to-moderate severity (evaluated using Hoehn and Yahr stage) were studied in the review. Seven trials [30–32,34,36–39] used stable medications (e.g., levodopa) as part of the basic treatment and the others [33,35] did not report the pharmacologic therapy. One trial [32,34] performed a 3 month post-intervention follow up to assess the maintenance of intervention gains while the other trials only conducted testing immediately after the intervention. One trial [38] was excluded from the quantitative analysis due to a lack of important outcome data. The details of study characteristics are provided in Tables 1 and 2.

3. Risk of bias

The protocol was registered and published for only one trial [32,34]. For the other nine trials [30–31,33,35–39], the risk of bias was assessed according to the methods section of the published article. Six trials [32,34–39] reported the method of randomization sequence generation, which included computer generation, randomization number table, coin toss and drawing of lots. Five trials [30,31,35–37] lacked detailed descriptions on whether allocation concealment was performed or not while two trials [38,39] did not use allocation concealment judged by the articles and authors' responses. None of the trials blinded the participants

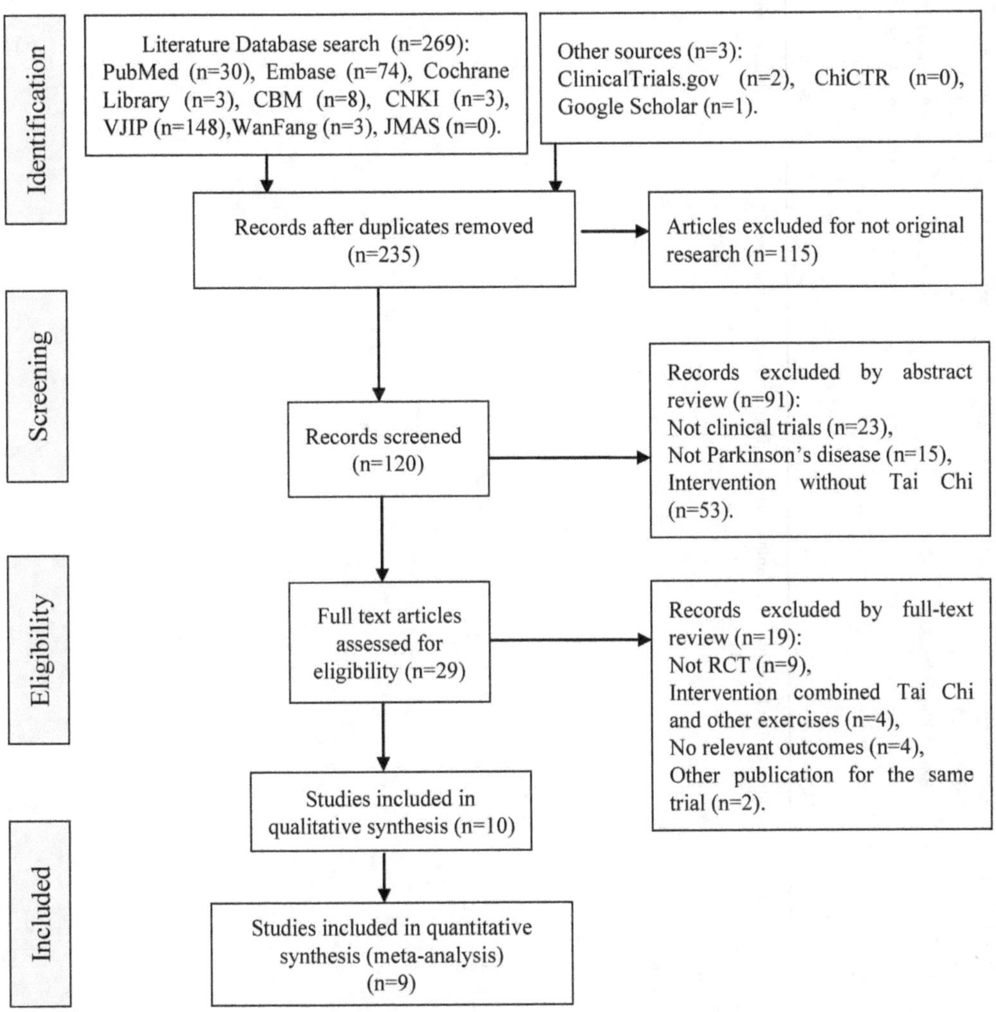

Figure 1. Flow diagram of study selection and identification. The total number of articles and studies differs because one article reported two independent trials and two articles reported different outcomes for the same trial.

Table 1. Characteristics of the participants in the included studies.

Source	Location	Number of centers	Number of patients	Gender (M/F)	Age (years)	Disease severity (H & Y scale stage)	Disease duration (years)
Choi HJ 2013 [30]	Seoul, Republic Korea	1	20	/	60.81±7.6/65.54±6.8	1.6±0.6/1.8±0.3	5.2±2.7/5.2±2.7
Nocera JR 2013 [32]	Georgia, USA	1	21	11/10	66±11/65±7	2–3/2–3	8.08±5.42/6.83±1.83
Amano S 2013 (project 1) [33]	Georgia, USA	1	21	14/7	64±13/68±7	2.3±0.4/2.2±0.4	7±7/12±7
Amano S 2013 (project 2) [33]	Florida, USA	1	24	14/10	66±11/66±7	2.4±0.6/2.4±0.4	8±5/5±3
Li F 2012 [34] and Li F 2013 [32]	Oregon, USA	4	195	122/73	68±9/69±8[a]/69±9[b]	2.5	8±9/8±9/6±5
Gladfelter BA 2011 [35]	Indiana, USA	1	17	12/5	72±8.52	2.4±0.87	5.88±3.48
Zhu Y 2011 [36]	Taipei and Shanghai, China	2	38	23/17	63.35±8.72/64.83±9.29	1–2	2.27±1.95/2.78±2.29
Li JX 2011 [37]	Taipei, China	1	47	22/25	68.28±6.62/67.13±6.73	2.5–3	5.62±3.94/5.71±30.79
Hackney ME 2009 [38]	St. Louis, USA	1	61	45/16	64.9±2.3/66.8±2.4[c]/68.2±1.4[d]/ 66.5±2.8[e]	2.0±0.1/2.0±0.2/2.1±0.1/2.2±0.2	8.7±1.3/9.2±1.4/6.9±1.3/ 5.9±1.0
Hackney ME 2008 [39]	St. Louis, USA	1	26	21/5	64.9±8.3/62.6±10.2	2.0/2.0	8.7±4.7/5.5±3.3

Notes: Sources are stated as first author and publication year. Continuous data describing age, disease severity and disease duration are presented as mean ± SD or median or range. H & Y is for Hoehn and Yahr.
[a]Resistance exercise.
[b]Stretching.
[c]Waltz with Foxtrot.
[d]Tango.
[e]No intervention.

Table 2. Characteristics of the included studies.

Source	Intervention	Control	Outcomes
Choi HJ 2013 [30]	Tai Chi: 50 min/session, three times a week for 12 weeks with stable medication	Stable medication alone	UPDRS, OLS,TUG,TS,SMW, RTLS
Nocera JR 2013 [31]	Tai Chi: Short forms of Yang-style movements, 60 min/session, three times a week for 16 weeks with stable medication.	Stable medication alone	DSB-WMS, LVF, CVF, SCWT, Trail A-B, Tinetti's FE, PDQ-39
Amano S 2013 (project 1) [33]	Tai Chi: Eight Yang-style movements, 60 min/ session, twice a week for 16 weeks	Qigong	Gait initiation, gait performance (cadence, gait velocity, step length, step duration, swing time, double-limb support time, gait asymmetry), UPDRS III.
Amano S 2013 (project 2) [33]	Tai Chi: Eight Yang-style movements, 60 min/ session, three times a week for 16 weeks.	No intervention	
Li F 2012 [34] and Li F 2013 [32]	Tailored Tai Chi: Six movements integrated nto an eight-form routine, 60 min/session, twice a week for 24 weeks with stable medication.	a. Resistance training with stable medication. b. Stretching with stable medication	Postural stability (maximum excursion, directional control), gait performance (stride length, gait velocity), peak knee extension and knee flexion torque, FRT, TUG, UPDRS III, falls; short version of PDQ-39 (PDQ-8),VPS, UPDRS-ME, 50-foot speed walk test, continuing exercise measure
Gladfelter BA 2011 [35]	Tai Chi: Short forms of Yang-style movements, 60 min/session, once a week for 12 weeks.	Routine physical exercise	BBS, FRT, TUG, PDQ-39, falls, PPS.
Zhu Y 2011 [36]	Tai Chi: 24 movements of national standard, 30–45 min/session, twice a day, five times a week for 4 weeks, with Madopar	Walking exercise with Madopar	UPDRS III, BBS.
Li JX 2011 [37]	Tai Chi (24 movements of national standard, 30–45 minutes/session, twice a day, 5 times a week for 8 weeks) with Madopar	Walking exercise with Madopar	UPDRS III, BBS, PDQ-39SI.
Hackney ME 2009 [38]	Tai Chi: Short forms of Yang-style movements, 60 min/session, twice a week for 13 weeks with stable medication.	a. Waltz with Foxtrot. b. Tango. c. No intervention. All groups received stable medication	PDQ-39 and PDQ-39SI
Hackney ME 2008 [39]	Tai Chi (short forms of Yang-style, 60 minutes/ session, once a week for 13 weeks) with stable medication.	Stable medication alone	UPDRS III, BBS,TUG, TS, OLS, gait (backward FAP, backward stride length, backward velocity, forward FAP, forward stride length, forward velocity), SMW, PPS.

Notes: UPDRS III, Unified Parkinson's Disease Rating Scale Part III; TUG, Timed Up and Go test; PDQ-39/8, Parkinson's Disease Questionnaire-39/8; PDQ-39SI, PDQ-39 Summary Index; BBS, Berg Balance Scale; FRT, Functional reach test; TS, Tandem stance test; OLS, One-leg stance test; FAP, Functional ambulation profile; SMW, Six minute walk; PPS, Post-program survey; DSB-WMS, Digit Span Backward Subtest from Wechsler Memory Scale; LVF, Letter Verbal Fluency; CVF, Category Verbal Fluency; SCWT, Stroop Color Word Test; Trail A–B, Trails A and B; Tinetti's FE, Tinetti's Falls Efficacy Scale; RTLS, reaction time upon light signal; VPS, Vitality Plus Scale; UPDRS-ME, Modified Unified Parkinson's Disease Rating Scale Motor Examination.

or healthcare providers. All trials used independent outcome assessors who were unaware of intervention assignment, except patient-reported outcomes. All trials reported a low drop-out rate and provided a clear description of reasons for drop out, but AE might result in missing data in five trials [35–39]. Important outcome measurement data were not reported in two trials [32,38], but the other trials demonstrated consistency of methods and results. Unreliable randomization was found in one trial [31], control group lacking validation occurred in four trials [33,36–38] and extremely small sample size existed in two trials [30,35]. The summary assessments of risk of bias are presented in Figure 2.

4. Data available for analysis

Of the ten included studies, only nine trials [30–37,39] with 409 participants had data available for meta-analysis because one [38] did not report its single outcome data. Data from two articles [32,34] reporting different outcomes of the same trial were synthesized as one trial in the meta-analysis. The number of patients practicing Tai Chi was divided up and 2 independent comparisons (labeled as comparison 1 and 2) were finally included into the data analysis for the trial with 3 groups [32,34]. Standard mean difference (Std.MD) was presented in the effect of HRQOL and Gait for different scales or units were used. The results of falls, PPS and adverse events were presented with paragraph description rather than statistical synthesis due to the varied measuring methods. Publication bias was not detected because none of the groups included more than 10 studies.

5. Primary outcome

UPDRS III was reported in seven trials [30,33,34,36,37,39] and subgroup analysis was performed. Reduction of total UPDRS III score was greater for Tai Chi plus medication than other exercise plus medication and medication alone (MD: −4.34, 95% CI: −6.67–−2.01). But there was no difference between Tai Chi without medication and no intervention and qigong alone (MD: 2.55, 95% CI: −0.23–5.32) (Figure. 3).

6. Secondary outcomes

6.1. Balance and mobility function. BBS was reported in four trials [35–37,39] and subgroup analysis was performed. Increase in total BBS score was greater for Tai Chi plus medication than other exercise plus medication and with medication alone (MD: 4.25, 95% CI: 2.83–5.66), and the improvement was also greater for Tai Chi without medication

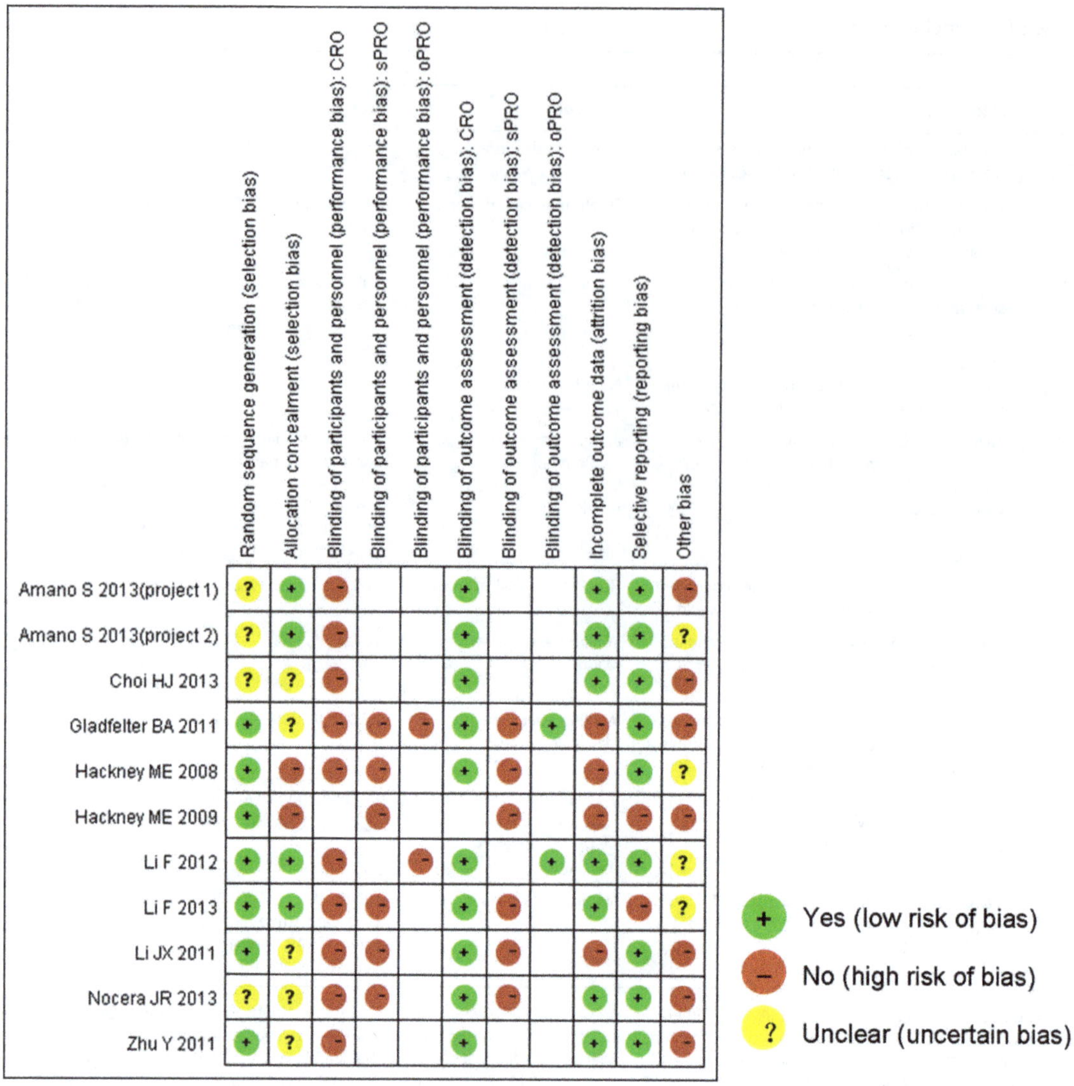

Figure 2. Risk of bias summary. The article [33] reported two independent trials that are labeled as project 1 and 2. Blank entries mean that the outcome was not reported. CRO, clinician-reported outcome; sPRO, subjective patient-reported outcome; oPRO, objective patient-reported outcome.

than other exercise alone (MD: 9.33, 95% CI: 3.06–15.60) (Figure. 4).

FRT was reported in two trials [34,35] and subgroup analysis was performed. Increase in maximal reach distance was greater for Tai Chi plus medication than other exercises plus medication (MD: 3.89, 95% CI: 1.73–6.04), and the improvement was also greater for Tai Chi without medication than with other exercise alone (MD: 3.05, 95% CI: 2.04–4.06) (Figure. 5).

TUG was reported in four trials [30,34,35,39] and subgroup analysis was performed. Reduction in TUG time was greater for Tai Chi plus medication than other exercise plus medication and medication alone (MD: −0.75, 95% CI: −1.30–−0.21), but there was no significant difference between Tai Chi without medication and other exercise alone (MD: −1.54, 95% CI: −8.63–5.55) (Figure. 6).

6.2. HRQOL. HRQOL was reported in four trials [31,32,35,37] and subgroup analysis was performed. Three trials [31,32,35] reported the total score of PDQ-39 (long or short version) and one [37] introduced PDQ-39SI, so SMD was used for data analysis. Improvement of HRQOL was greater for Tai Chi plus medication than other exercise plus medication and medication alone (SMD: −1.10, 95% CI: −1.81–−0.39), but there was no significant difference between Tai Chi without medication and other exercise alone (SMD: −0.09, 95% CI: −0.86–1.04) (Figure. 7).

6.3. Gait. Gait velocity was reported in four trials [33,34,39] and subgroup analysis was performed. Different units were introduced to report gait velocity in the four trials, therefore SMD was used for data analysis. There was no significant difference in the change in gait velocity between Tai Chi plus medication and other exercise plus medication and medication alone (SMD: 0.41, 95% CI: −0.37–1.19) or between Tai Chi without medication and no intervention and other exercise alone (SMD: −0.12, 95% CI: −0.72–0.48) (Figure. 8).

Stride length was reported in four trials [33,34,39] and subgroup analysis was performed. Different units were introduced to report stride length in the four trials, so SMD was used for data analysis. The increase in stride length was greater for Tai Chi plus medication than other exercise plus medication and medication alone (SMD: 0.56, 95% CI: 0.03–1.09), but there was no

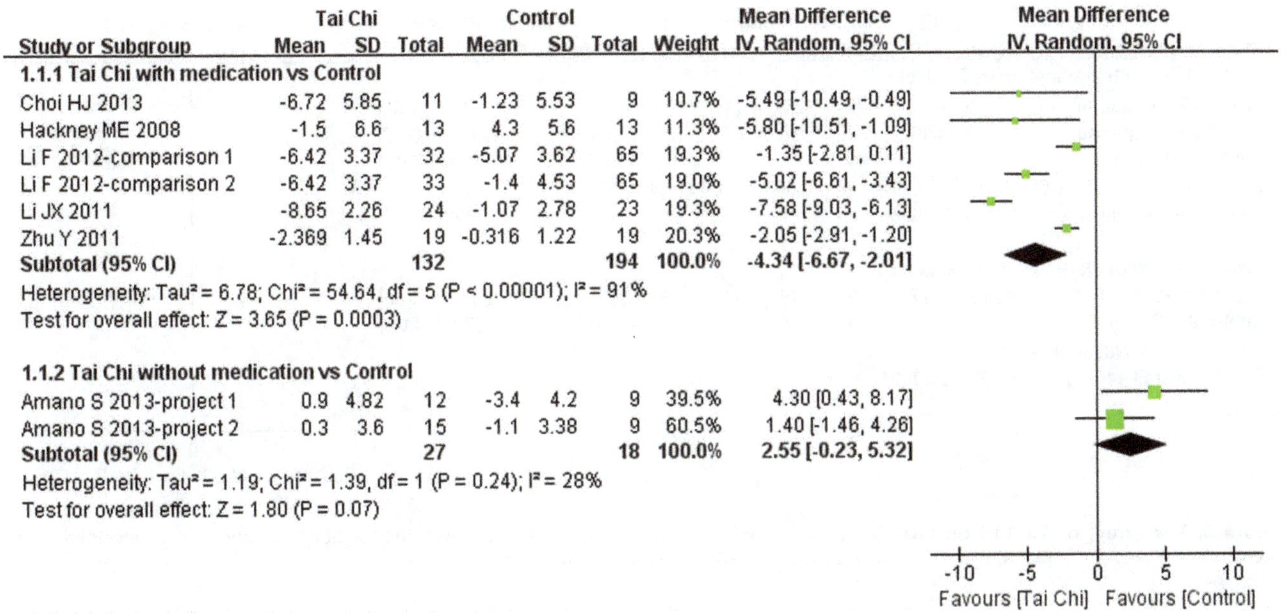

Figure 3. The effect of Tai Chi on UPDRS III score. Subgroup analysis was performed according to whether or not medications were included in the intervention. A random model was used to address the high heterogeneity. UPDRS III, Unified Parkinson's Disease Rating Scale Part III.

difference between Tai Chi without medication and no intervention and other exercise alone (SMD: −0.13, 95% CI: −0.73–0.47) (Figure. 9).

6.4. Falls. Falls data were obtained by patient self-report diaries in two trials [34,35]. Patients were provided with a clear definition of falls before the intervention and required to record any falls they experienced. Patients [34] who received a 6 month Tai Chi intervention with stable medication had 67% fewer falls than patients who received a 6 month stretching intervention with medication (incidence-rate ratio: 0.33, 95% CI: 0.16–0.71), and marginally fewer falls than patients who received a 6 month resistance training intervention with medication (incidence-rate ratio: 0.47, 95% CI: 0.21–1.00). However, patients [35] who received a 12 week Tai Chi intervention without medication reported a similar rate of falls as patients who received no intervention.

6.5. PPS. A PPS was conducted in two trials [35,39] but different questionnaires were used to assess opinions on the experience of Tai Chi and the improvement in physical well-being. Patients [39] who received a 13 week Tai Chi intervention with medication enjoyed the class and somewhat agreed that the intervention improved balance, walking, co-ordination, endurance and mood, but did not agree that the intervention increased strength. Patients [35] who received a 12 week Tai Chi intervention supported and enjoyed the exercises.

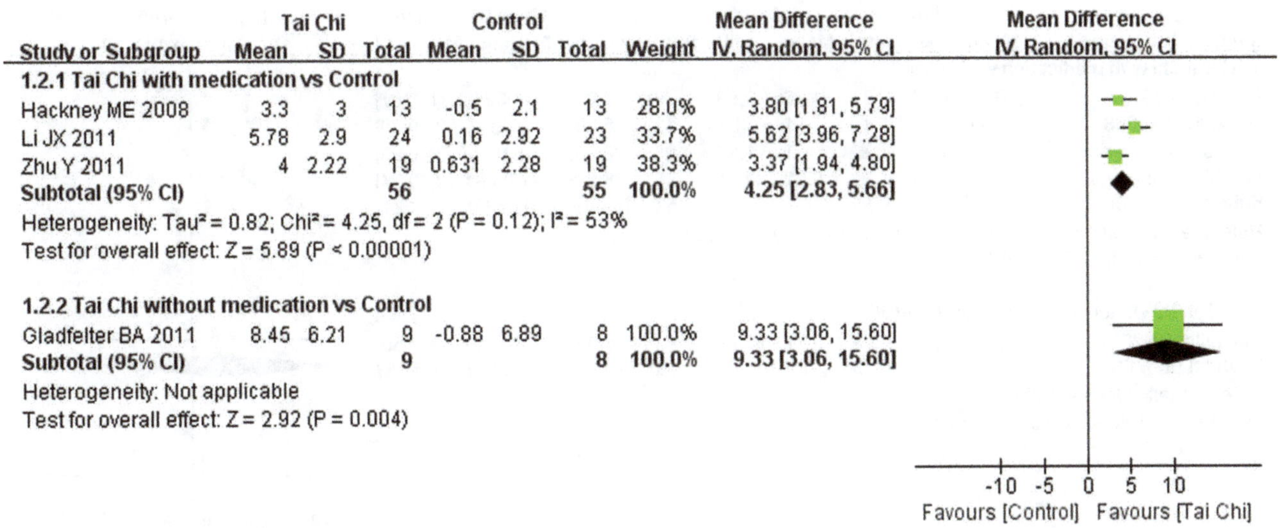

Figure 4. The effect of Tai Chi on BBS score. Subgroup analysis was performed according to whether or not medications were included in the intervention. A random model was used to address the high heterogeneity. BBS, Berg Balance Scale.

Study or Subgroup	Tai Chi Mean	Tai Chi SD	Tai Chi Total	Control Mean	Control SD	Control Total	Weight	Mean Difference IV, Random, 95% CI
1.3.1 Tai Chi with medication vs Control								
Li F 2012-comparison 1	5	4.14	32	2.2	4.11	65	50.5%	2.80 [1.05, 4.55]
Li F 2012-comparison 2	5	4.14	33	0	4.62	65	49.5%	5.00 [3.20, 6.80]
Subtotal (95% CI)			**65**			**130**	**100.0%**	**3.89 [1.73, 6.04]**
Heterogeneity: Tau² = 1.60; Chi² = 2.95, df = 1 (P = 0.09); I² = 66%								
Test for overall effect: Z = 3.53 (P = 0.0004)								
1.3.2 Tai Chi without medication vs Control								
Gladfelter BA 2011	2.67	1.27	9	-0.38	0.84	8	100.0%	3.05 [2.04, 4.06]
Subtotal (95% CI)			**9**			**8**	**100.0%**	**3.05 [2.04, 4.06]**
Heterogeneity: Not applicable								
Test for overall effect: Z = 5.90 (P < 0.00001)								

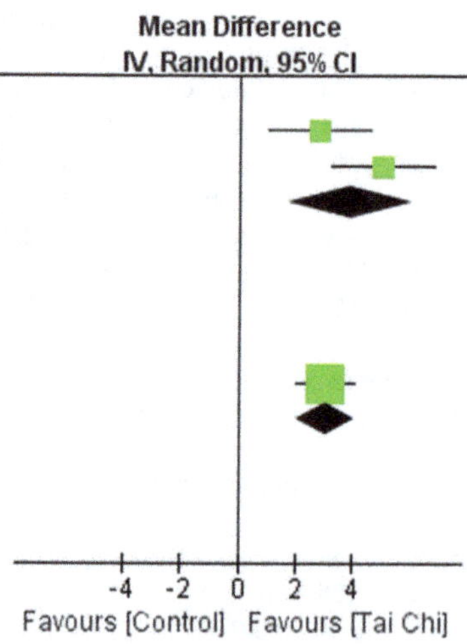

Figure 5. The effect of Tai Chi on FRT. Subgroup analysis was performed according to whether or not medications were included in the intervention. A random model was used to address the high heterogeneity. FRT, functional reach test.

6.6. AE. Only one trial [32,34] reported safety as a planned outcome. Six trials [34–39] reported AEs and four trials [30,31,33] did not report AE. None of the trails further defined the AE as adverse effects of Tai Chi. No serious AEs such as hospitalization, disability or death were noted, but minor AEs including pain, falls, dizziness and other symptoms were reported in the small population.

Discussion

Tai Chi has been recommended as a regimen of life promotion [40] and falls reduction [41] in China and other countries. However, the efficacy of Tai Chi on PD is not well known. This is the first systematic review and meta-analysis to address the effect of Tai Chi in the management of PD and provides a new level of evidence for clinical professionals.

Our primary finding was that Tai Chi plus medication resulted in significantly greater benefit in terms of general motor symptoms, balance, mobility, and stride length, with few AE. Rigidity is one of the main manifestations of PD, leading to impairments in postural stability, balance and gait performance, and these symptoms do not respond well to either first-line or sub-optimal medications [42]. The movements of Tai Chi include weight shift, body rotation, slow strides and single-leg standing in different positions, requiring delicate joint control with muscle co-ordination [40]; therefore Tai Chi possibly trains postural stability and balance. This suggests that the combination of Tai Chi and medications may be optimal for PD patients who are partially insensitive to the pharmacologic treatment alone, especially if they have poor mobility and balance.

UPDRS III is most widely used for both clinical and research purposes to assess the motor function of PD patients [27] and we set it as our primary outcome in this systematic review. It has been previously reported that the minimal clinical relevant difference (MCRD) of UPDRS III is the improvement by 2.3–2.7 points [43] or by 5 points [44]. In our meta-analysis, a significant

Study or Subgroup	Tai Chi Mean	Tai Chi SD	Tai Chi Total	Control Mean	Control SD	Control Total	Weight	Mean Difference IV, Random, 95% CI
1.4.1 Tai Chi with medication vs Control								
Choi HJ 2013	-0.36	0.57	11	1.26	2.53	9	9.0%	-1.62 [-3.31, 0.07]
Hackney ME 2008	-1	0.1	13	-0.1	1.1	13	35.3%	-0.90 [-1.50, -0.30]
Li F 2012-comparison 1	-1.05	1.78	32	-1	1.69	65	28.9%	-0.05 [-0.79, 0.69]
Li F 2012-comparison 2	-1.05	1.78	33	-0.02	2.11	65	26.8%	-1.03 [-1.82, -0.24]
Subtotal (95% CI)			**89**			**152**	**100.0%**	**-0.75 [-1.30, -0.21]**
Heterogeneity: Tau² = 0.13; Chi² = 5.16, df = 3 (P = 0.16); I² = 42%								
Test for overall effect: Z = 2.70 (P = 0.007)								
1.4.2 Tai Chi without medication vs Control								
Gladfelter BA 2011	-1.33	1.15	9	0.21	10.17	8	100.0%	-1.54 [-8.63, 5.55]
Subtotal (95% CI)			**9**			**8**	**100.0%**	**-1.54 [-8.63, 5.55]**
Heterogeneity: Not applicable								
Test for overall effect: Z = 0.43 (P = 0.67)								

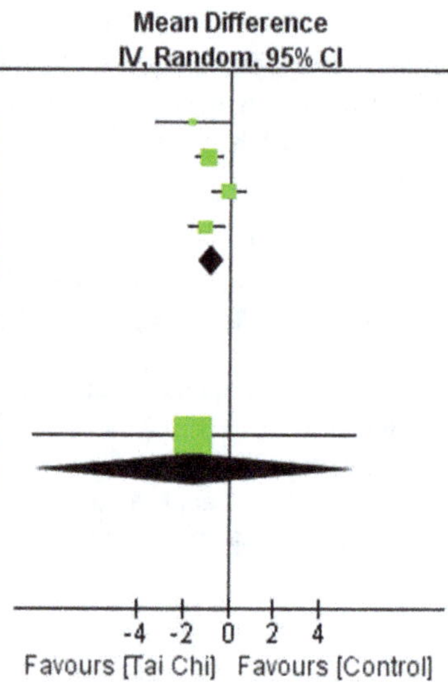

Figure 6. The effect of Tai Chi on TUG. Subgroup analysis was performed according to whether or not medications were included in the intervention. A random model was used to address the high heterogeneity. TUG, Timed Up and Go test.

Study or Subgroup	Tai Chi Mean	Tai Chi SD	Tai Chi Total	Control Mean	Control SD	Control Total	Weight	Std. Mean Difference IV, Random, 95% CI
1.5.1 Tai Chi with medication vs Control								
Li F 2013-comparison 1	-9.66	10.3	32	-3.89	8.86	65	28.4%	-0.61 [-1.04, -0.18]
Li F 2013-comparison 2	-9.66	10.3	33	-0.09	10.09	65	28.3%	-0.93 [-1.37, -0.49]
Li JX 2011	-7.23	2.9	24	-0.14	2.92	23	23.2%	-2.40 [-3.16, -1.63]
Nocera JR 2013	1.1	12.62	15	9	18.77	6	20.0%	-0.52 [-1.49, 0.44]
Subtotal (95% CI)			**104**			**159**	**100.0%**	**-1.10 [-1.81, -0.39]**
Heterogeneity: Tau² = 0.41; Chi² = 16.87, df = 3 (P = 0.0008); I² = 82%								
Test for overall effect: Z = 3.05 (P = 0.002)								
1.5.2 Tai Chi without medication vs Control								
Gladfelter BA 2011	-0.21	7.38	9	-0.88	6.89	8	100.0%	0.09 [-0.86, 1.04]
Subtotal (95% CI)			**9**			**8**	**100.0%**	**0.09 [-0.86, 1.04]**
Heterogeneity: Not applicable								
Test for overall effect: Z = 0.18 (P = 0.85)								

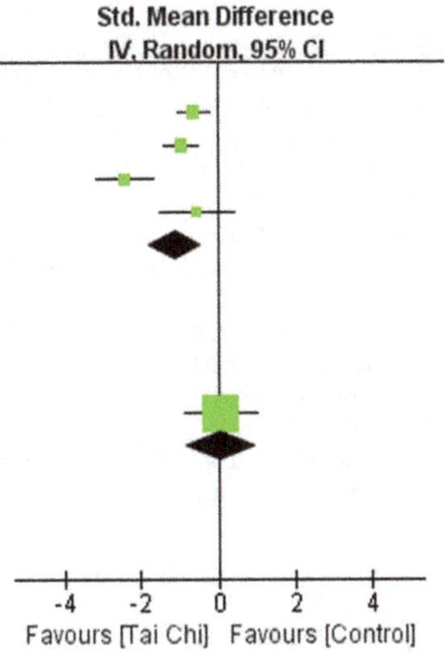

Figure 7. The effect of Tai Chi on HRQOL. Subgroup analysis was performed according to whether or not medications were included in the intervention. Standardized mean difference was calculated for PDQ-39 (short and long versions) and PDQ-39SI scores. HRQOL, health-related quality of life; PDQ-39, Parkinson's Disease Questionairre-39; PDQ-39SI, PDQ-39 Summary Index.

improvement of UPDRS III by 4.34 points in the group of Tai Chi plus medication was observed after pooled analysis, which is approaching the MCRD. This similarity means that the evidence of Tai Chi to improve motor symptoms of PD could be put in a real clinical situation.

The patients included in this review all had PD of mild-to-moderate severity, so the positive effect of Tai Chi cannot be extrapolated outside of this population. Tai Chi is one type of active physical exercise that can be used in place of passive rehabilitation strategies, but patients must have a basic ability to stand and move independently for certain duration. PD patients who are in the latter stages of the disease or in the "off" period of medication may not complete a Tai Chi intervention because of severe rigidity [45]. Therefore, the initiation of a Tai Chi program has to be carefully timed after the assessment of the disease severity and overall patient conditions.

Patient enjoyment and support for a therapy should be considered when deciding on a medical intervention [46]. We found a high satisfaction rate for Tai Chi intervention in the studies included in this review, which suggests that Tai Chi is feasible in clinical settings.

HRQOL reflects the overall influence of a disease on patients' physical mobility, daily activity, social functioning, psychological wellbeing and cognition [47], and is assessed from the point of view of the patient. Our research found that Tai Chi plus medications resulted in a greater improvement in HRQOL than other exercise plus medication and medication alone. This suggests that Tai Chi has an additional beneficial effect or better interaction with medication regarding PD-related health status, which is important for patients. However, knowledge of the assigned intervention may impact on patient-reported outcomes and the estimated effect has been observed to be more biased in trials with more subjective outcomes [48]. Based on the fact that it

Study or Subgroup	Tai Chi Mean	Tai Chi SD	Tai Chi Total	Control Mean	Control SD	Control Total	Weight	Std. Mean Difference IV, Random, 95% CI
1.6.1 Tai Chi with medication vs Control								
Hackney ME 2008	0.105	19.80084	13	0.05	19.31386	13	28.8%	0.00 [-0.77, 0.77]
Li F 2012-comparison 1	10.5	13.45	33	9.9	15.67	65	35.9%	0.04 [-0.38, 0.46]
Li F 2012-comparison 2	10.5	13.45	32	-4.5	13.33	65	35.3%	1.11 [0.66, 1.57]
Subtotal (95% CI)			**78**			**143**	**100.0%**	**0.41 [-0.37, 1.19]**
Heterogeneity: Tau² = 0.39; Chi² = 13.23, df = 2 (P = 0.001); I² = 85%								
Test for overall effect: Z = 1.03 (P = 0.30)								
1.6.2 Tai Chi without medication vs Control								
Amano S 2013-project 1	0.01	0.13	12	0.04	0.19	9	47.7%	-0.18 [-1.05, 0.68]
Amano S 2013-project 2	0.01	0.18	15	0.02	0.1	9	52.3%	-0.06 [-0.89, 0.76]
Subtotal (95% CI)			**27**			**18**	**100.0%**	**-0.12 [-0.72, 0.48]**
Heterogeneity: Tau² = 0.00; Chi² = 0.04, df = 1 (P = 0.84); I² = 0%								
Test for overall effect: Z = 0.39 (P = 0.70)								

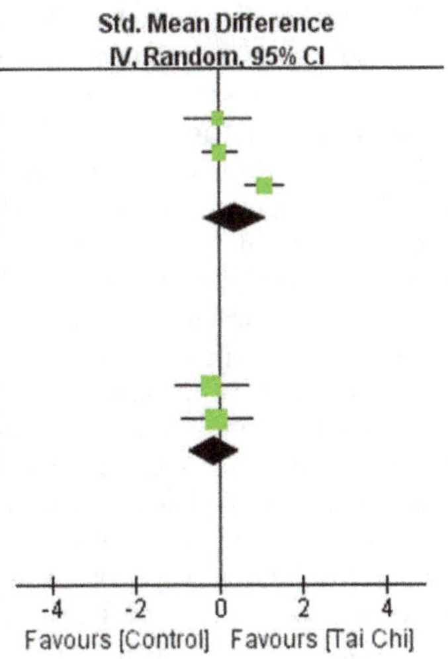

Figure 8. The effect of Tai Chi on gait velocity. Subgroup analysis was performed according to whether or not medications were included in the intervention. Standardized mean difference was used for different units of velocity.

Study or Subgroup	Tai Chi Mean	Tai Chi SD	Tai Chi Total	Control Mean	Control SD	Control Total	Weight	Std. Mean Difference IV, Random, 95% CI
1.7.1 Tai Chi with medication vs Control								
Hackney ME 2008	0.1	20.42974	13	0.015	18.9206	13	24.5%	0.00 [-0.76, 0.77]
Li F 2012-comparison 1	10.3	12.66	33	4.3	13.22	65	38.3%	0.46 [0.03, 0.88]
Li F 2012-comparison 2	10.3	12.66	32	-2.1	11.73	65	37.2%	1.02 [0.57, 1.47]
Subtotal (95% CI)			**78**			**143**	**100.0%**	**0.56 [0.03, 1.09]**
Heterogeneity: Tau² = 0.14; Chi² = 6.12, df = 2 (P = 0.05); I² = 67%								
Test for overall effect: Z = 2.06 (P = 0.04)								
1.7.2 Tai Chi without medication vs Control								
Amano S 2013-project 1	-0.01	0.05	12	0.01	0.09	9	47.5%	-0.28 [-1.14, 0.59]
Amano S 2013-project 2	0.01	0.08	15	0.01	0.04	9	52.5%	0.00 [-0.83, 0.83]
Subtotal (95% CI)			**27**			**18**	**100.0%**	**-0.13 [-0.73, 0.47]**
Heterogeneity: Tau² = 0.00; Chi² = 0.20, df = 1 (P = 0.65); I² = 0%								
Test for overall effect: Z = 0.43 (P = 0.67)								

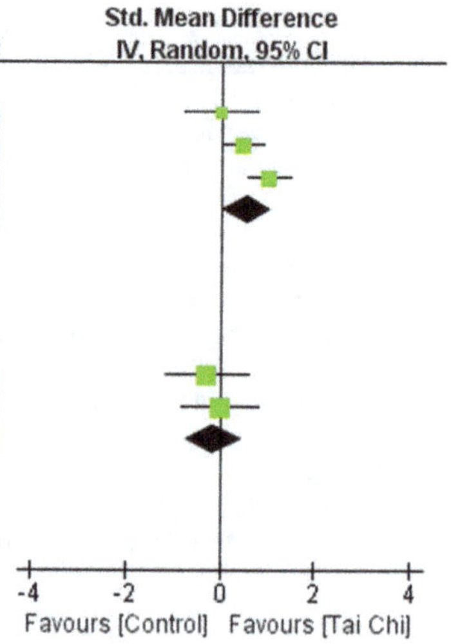

Figure 9. The effect of Tai Chi on stride length. Subgroup analysis was performed according to whether or not medications were included in the intervention. Standardized mean difference was used for different units of stride length.

is not easy to blind participants practicing Tai Chi, it is therefore important to draw a conclusion in real situations considering both HRQOL reported by patients and other types of outcomes (such as objective outcomes and outcomes reported by caregivers or clinicians).

Falls are common and sometimes life threatening for PD patients [49]. A high score in the Freezing of Gait Questionnaire, older age, and the presence of falls in medical history are independent risk factors for falls [50]. We found that the reduction in falls was greater after a long-term (e.g. 6 months) Tai Chi program plus stable medications than other exercise plus medication, but that the reduction in falls after a short Tai Chi program without medication was not different from other exercise alone. However, the inconsistent results of Tai Chi in falls prevention were only obtained from two trials with small sample sizes, distinct designs and lack of comparative information. Therefore, the only conclusion we can draw is that the combination of Tai Chi with medications may be more effective for fall prevention, but further studies are needed on this topic.

However, performance of Tai Chi program without medication only had a beneficial effect on BBS and FRT, indicating that Tai Chi is not strong enough to combat all aspects of PD impairments.

Limitations for the review

There are five main limitations to this review. First, the trials included had a small sample size and were conducted in only a few centers, which may bias the conclusions and further updates are needed to synthesize newly published eligible studies. Second, information recording the dosage and course of medications and evidence on whether Tai Chi reduces complications and side effects of long-term medications were not reported in any study, and these issues raise some uncertainty when recommending Tai Chi for PD patients. Third, long-term outcome of Tai Chi on PD was not investigated based on current evidence and further RCTs focusing on the effect of Tai Chi over a much longer period are needed for PD is a long-term disease [51]. Fourth, the logistics of balancing the benefits of Tai Chi with its economic cost and service availability were not analyzed in any study. Last, little evidence was found in this review as to whether the effects of Tai Chi are specific or non-specific, whether the promising effects are additive or synergistic with medication, and whether the effects can be attributed to a complex system rather than a single exercise [52–53].

Difference from existing studies

Up to now, there are two systematic reviews trying to evaluate the effect of Tai Chi for PD [23, 54]. However, both of them only describe the outcomes rather than performing a meta-analysis to provide a pooled effect, which is not enough for new evidence.

Conclusions

Tai Chi program performed with medication resulted in promising gains in mobility and balance and it was safe and popular among PD patients at an early stage. These results provide new evidence for PD management. More multi-center RCTs with a large sample size that carefully address blinding and prudently select outcomes are needed to confirm these results and to assess the feasibility of Tai Chi intervention for different medical situations. Research on the mechanism by which Tai Chi benefits PD patients is also required.

Author Contributions

Conceived and designed the experiments: XN XG XS. Performed the experiments: XN SL FL XG. Analyzed the data: XN SL FL. Contributed reagents/materials/analysis tools: SL. Wrote the paper: XN. Interpreting the data as a clinical professional: XS. Interpreting the data as a clinical epidemiologist: XG.

References

1. National Collaborating Centre for Chronic Conditions (UK) (2006) Parkinson's disease: National clinical guideline for diagnosis and management in primary and secondary care. NICE Clinical guideline No. 35. Available: http://publications.nice.org.uk/parkinsons-disease-cg35/introduction. Accessed: 1 July 2013.
2. World Health Organization (2006) Neurological Disorders: Public Health Challenges. Geneva: WHO Press. 153p.
3. Zhang ZX, Roman GC, Hong Z, Wu CB, Qu QM, et al. (2005) Parkinson's disease in China: prevalence in Beijing, Xian, and Shanghai. Lancet 365:595–597.
4. Ossig C, Reichmann H (2013) Treatment of Parkinson's disease in the advanced stage. J Neural Transm 120:523–529.
5. Pahwa R, Lyons KE (2009) Levodopa-related wearing-off in Parkinson's disease: identification and management. Curr Med Res Opin 25:841–849.
6. Antonini A, Tolosa E (2009) Apomorphine and levodopa infusion therapies for advanced Parkinson's disease: selection criteria and patient management. Expert Rev Neurother 9:859–867.
7. Okun MS, Foote KD (2010) Parkinson's disease DBS: what, when, who and why? The time has come to tailor DBS targets. Expert Rev Neurother 10:1847–1857.
8. Pedrosa DJ, Timmermann L (2013) Review: management of Parkinson's disease. Neuropsychiatr Dis Treat 9:321–340.
9. Tomlinson CL, Patel S, Meek C, Herd CP, Clarke CE, et al. (2012) Physiotherapy intervention in Parkinson's disease: systematic review and meta-analysis. BMJ 345:e5004.
10. National Center for Complementary and Alternative Medicine (2006) Tai Chi for health purposes (update 2010). Available: http://nccam.nih.gov/health/taichi/introduction.htm. Accessed: 1 July 2013.
11. Li F, Harmer P, Glasgow R, Mack KA, Sleet D, et al. (2008) Translation of an effective tai chi intervention into a community-based falls-prevention program. Am J Public Health 98:1195–8.
12. Wang J, Feng B, Yang X, Liu W, Teng F, et al. (2013) Tai chi for essential hypertension. Evid Based Complement Alternat Med 2013:215254.
13. Yeh GY, Roberts DH, Wayne PM, Davis RB, Quilty MT, et al. (2010) Tai chi exercise for patients with chronic obstructive pulmonary disease: a pilot study. Respir Care 55:1475–1482.
14. Caminiti G, Volterrani M, Marazzi G, Cerrito A, Massaro R, et al. (2011) Tai chi enhances the effects of endurance training in the rehabilitation of elderly patients with chronic heart failure. Rehabil Res Pract 2011:761958.
15. Wayne PM, Kiel DP, Buring JE, Connors EM, Bonato P, et al. (2012) Impact of Tai Chi exercise on multiple fracture-related risk factors in post-menopausal osteopenic women: a pilot pragmatic, randomized trial. BMC Complement Altern Med 12:7.
16. Wang C, Bannuru R, Ramel J, Kupelnick B, Scott T, et al. (2010) Tai Chi on psychological well-being: systematic review and meta-analysis. BMC Complement Altern Med 10:23.
17. Irwin MR, Olmstead R, Motivala SJ (2008) Improving sleep quality in older adults with moderate sleep complaints: A randomized controlled trial of Tai Chi Chih. Sleep 31:1001–1008.
18. Hall AM, Maher CG, Latimer J, Ferreira ML, Lam P (2008) A randomized controlled trial of tai chi for long-term low back pain (TAI CHI): study rationale, design, and methods. BMC Musculoskelet Disord 10:55.
19. Ding M (2012) Tai Chi for stroke rehabilitation: a focused review. Am J Phys Med Rehabil 91:1091–1096.
20. Wang C (2011). Tai chi and rheumatic diseases. Rheum Dis Clin North Am 37:19–32.
21. Wang C, Schmid CH, Rones R, Kalish R, Yinh J, et al. (2010) A randomized trial of tai chi for fibromyalgia. N Engl J Med 363:743–754.
22. Chang JY, Tsai PF, Beck C, Hagen JL, Huff DC, et al. (2011) The effect of tai chi on cognition in elders with cognitive impairment. Medsurg Nurs 20:63–70.
23. Lee MS, Lam P, Ernst E (2008) Effectiveness of tai chi for Parkinson's disease: a critical review. Parkinsonism Relat Disord14:589–594.
24. Antman EM, Lau J, Kupelnick B, Mosteller F, Chalmers TC (1992) A comparison of results of meta-analyses of randomized control trials and recommendations of clinical experts: Treatments for myocardial infarction. JAMA 268: 240–248.
25. Oxman AD, Guyatt GH (1993) The science of reviewing research. Annals of the New York Academy of Sciences 703: 125–133.
26. J. P. T. . Higgins and S. . Green, eds (2011) Cochrane Handbook for Systematic Reviews of Interventions Version 5.1.0, chapter 9, Cochrane Collaboration.
27. Movement Disorder Society Task Force on Rating Scales for Parkinson's Disease (2003) The Unified Parkinson's Disease Rating Scale (UPDRS): status and recommendations. Mov Disord 18:738–750.
28. Moher D, Liberati A, Tetzlaff J, Altman DG, The PRISMA Group (2009) Preferred Reporting Items for Systematic Reviews and Meta-Analyses: The PRISMA Statement. PLoS Med 6: e1000097.
29. Schulz KF, Weeks L, Sterne JA, Cochrane Bias Methods Group, Cochrane Statistical Methods Group (2011) The Cochrane Collaboration's tool for assessing risk of bias in randomised trials. BMJ 343:d5928.
30. Choi HJ, Garber CE, Jun TW, Jin YS, Chung SJ, et al. (2013) Therapeutic effects of tai chi in patients with Parkinson's disease. ISRN Neurol 2013:548240.
31. Nocera JR, Amano S, Vallabhajosula S, Hass CJ (2013). Tai Chi Exercise to Improve Non-Motor Symptoms of Parkinson's Disease. J Yoga Phys Ther. doi: 10.4172/2157-7595.1000137.
32. Li F, Harmer P, Liu Y, Eckstrom E, Fitzgerald K, et al.(2013) A randomized controlled trial of patient-reported outcomes with tai chi exercise in Parkinson's disease. Mov Disord. Epub.doi: 10.1002/mds.25787.
33. Amano S, Nocera JR, Vallabhajosula S, Juncos JL, Gregor RJ, et al. (2013) The effect of Tai Chi exercise on gait initiation and gait performance in persons with Parkinson's disease. Parkinsonism Relat Disord. 19:955–960.
34. Li F, Harmer P, Fitzgerald K, Eckstrom E, Stock R, et al. (2012) Tai chi and postural stability in patients with Parkinson's disease. N Engl J Med 366:511–519.
35. Gladfelter BA (2011) The Effect of Tai Chi Exercise on Balance and Falls in Persons with Parkinson's. Evidence-Based Practice Project Reports. 2p. Available: http://scholar.valpo.edu/ebpr/2. Accessed 1 July 2013.
36. Zhu Y, Li JX, Li N, Jing HZ, Hua L, et al. (2011) Effect of Taijiquan on Motion Control for Parkinson's Disease at Early Stage. Chin J Rehabil Theory Pract 17: 355–358.
37. Li JX (2011) The motion control effect of Parkinson's disease patients treating by Taijiquan with madopar. Nanjing University of Chinese Medicine. http://192.168.0.2:8000/D/Thesis_Y1945441.aspx Accessed 1 July 2013.
38. Hackney ME, Earhart GM (2009) Health-related quality of life and alternative forms of exercise in Parkinson disease. Parkinsonism Relat Disord 15:644–648.
39. Hackney ME, Earhart GM (2008) Tai Chi improves balance and mobility in people with Parkinson disease. Gait Posture 28:456–460.
40. Lan C, Chen SY, Lai JS, and Wong AM (2013) Tai Chi Chuan in Medicine and Health Promotion Evidence-Based Complementary and Alternative Medicine 2013: 502131.
41. Panel on Prevention of Falls in Older Persons, American Geriatrics Society and British Geriatrics Society (2011) Summary of the Updated American Geriatrics Society/British Geriatrics Society clinical practice guideline for prevention of falls in older persons. J Am Geriatr Soc 59:148–157.
42. Ossig C, Reichmann H (2013) Treatment of Parkinson's disease in the advanced stage. J Neural Transm 120:523–529.
43. Shulman LM, Gruber-Baldini AL, Anderson KE, Fishman PS, et al. (2010) Weiner WJ. The clinically important difference on the unified Parkinson's disease rating scale. Arch Neurol 67:64–70.
44. Schrag A, Sampaio C, Counsell N, Poewe W (2006) Minimal clinically important change on the unified Parkinson's disease rating scale. Mov Disord 21:1200–1207.
45. Higginson IJ, Gao W, Saleem TZ, Chaudhuri KR, Burman R, et al. (2010) Symptoms and quality of life in late stage Parkinson syndromes: a longitudinal community study of predictive factors. PLoS One 7:e46327.
46. Tang JL, Glasziou P (2010) Fundamentals of Evidence Based Medicine. Beijing: Perking University Medical Press. 12p.
47. Soh SE, McGinley JL, Watts JJ, Iansek R, Morris ME (2012) Health-related quality of life of australians with Parkinson disease: a comparison with international studies. Physiother Can 64:338–346.
48. Wood L, Egger M, Gluud LL, Schulz KF, Jüni P, et al. (2008) Empirical evidence of bias in treatment effect estimates in controlled trials with different interventions and outcomes: meta-epidemiological study. BMJ 336:601–605.
49. Kerr GK, Worringham CJ, Cole MH, Lacherez PF, Wood JM, et al. (2010) Predictors of future falls in Parkinson disease. Neurology 75:116–124.
50. Rudzińska M, Bukowczan S, Stożek J, Zajdel K, Mirek E, et al. (2013) The incidence and risk factors of falls in Parkinson disease: prospective study. Neurol Neurochir Pol 47:431–437.
51. Tanner CM, Meng CC, Ravina B, Lang A, Kurlan R, et al. (2014) A practical approach to remote longitudinal follow-up of Parkinson's disease: The FOUND study. Mov Disord. Epub. doi: 0.1002/mds.25814.
52. Wayne PM, Kaptchuk TJ (2008) Challenges inherent to t'ai chi research: part I—t'ai chi as a complex multicomponent intervention. J Altern Complement Med 14:95–102.
53. Wayne PM, Kaptchuk TJ (2008) Challenges inherent to t'ai chi research: part II-defining the intervention and optimal study design. J Altern Complement Med 14:191–197.
54. Toh SFM (2013) A Systematic Review on the Effectiveness of Tai Chi Exercise in Individuals with Parkinson's Disease from 2003 to 2013. Hong Kong J Occup Ther 23:69–81.

Physical and Perceptual Cooling with Beverages to Increase Cycle Performance in a Tropical Climate

Florence Riera*, **Than Tran Trong**, **Stéphane Sinnapah**, **Olivier Hue**

Laboratoire ACTES - EA 3596, Université des Antilles et de la Guyane Campus de Fouillole, Point à Pitre, France

Abstract

Purpose: This study compares the effects of neutral temperature, cold and ice-slush beverages, with and without 0.5% menthol on cycling performance, core temperature (T_{co}) and stress responses in a tropical climate (hot and humid conditions).

Methods: Twelve trained male cyclists/triathletes completed six 20-km exercise trials against the clock in 30.7°C±0.8°C and 78%±0.03% relative humidity. Before and after warm-up, and before exercise and every 5 km during exercise, athletes drank 190 mL of either aromatized (i.e., with 0.5 mL of menthol (5 gr/L)) or a non-aromatized beverage (neutral temperature: 23°C±0.1°C, cold: 3°C±0.1°C, or ice-slush: −1°C±0.7°C). During the trials, heart rate (HR) was continuously monitored, whereas core temperature (T_{co}), thermal comfort (TC), thermal sensation (TS) and rate of perceived exertion (RPE) were measured before and after warm-up, every 5 km of exercise, and at the end of exercise and after recovery.

Results: Both the beverage aroma ($P<0.02$) and beverage temperature ($P<0.02$) had significant and positive effects on performance, which was considerably better with ice-slush than with a neutral temperature beverage, whatever the aroma ($P<0.002$), and with menthol *vs* non-menthol ($P<0.02$). The best performances were obtained with ice-slush/menthol and cold/menthol, as opposed to neutral/menthol. No differences were noted in HR and T_{co} between trials.

Conclusion: Cold water or ice-slush with menthol aroma seems to be the most effective beverage for endurance exercise in a tropical climate. Further studies are needed to explore its effects in field competition.

Editor: Naoyuki Hayashi, Tokyo Institute of Technology, Japan

Funding: The authors have no support or funding to report.

Competing Interests: The authors have declared that no competing interests exist.

* Email: florence.riera@gmail.com

Introduction

Cyclic aerobic exercise performance is negatively affected by a hot environment; this has been demonstrated for running [1] and cycling, although it depends somewhat on the race [2]. The negative effects are even more marked in a hot and humid environment (i.e., the so-called tropical climate) because the evaporative processes are limited [3,4]. Although the exact causes are not well known, explanations related to hyperthermia and/or dehydration have been proposed. During exercise, if heat storage cannot be limited (because of the failure of evaporative processes), the core temperature may limit the exercise [5] or the brain may provoke a voluntary cessation of effort – or a reduction of its intensity – to maintain thermal homeostasis [6]. A large volume of sweat loss can also gradually reduce blood and stroke volumes if not replaced, which tends to limit muscle blood flow [7].

Pre-cooling and cooling protocols, such as water immersion and cold air exposure, are among the strategies used to decrease the deleterious effect of the hot environment on aerobic performance. Although they may be successful, they are time-consuming and logistically very difficult to apply in real sports contexts [8,9]. Thus in order to reduce core temperature [10], cold fluid consumption thus may be the most appropriate strategy [8] in a hot environment. In a systematic review, Burdon et al. [11] noted that, although the findings are mixed, cold fluids generally seem to attenuate the core temperature and improve exercise performance in the heat. Recently, studies have demonstrated a more efficient effect of ice slurry (*vs* cold water) on running and cycling performances [8,12] and this may be a practical and effective pre-competition maneuver to improve performance in warm and humid conditions [13].

Menthol is a compound of plant origin (Mentha) that specifically stimulates cold receptors and, when applied to the skin and mucosal surfaces, exerts a cooling sensation similar to the action of spraying cold water on the face [14]. The mucous membranes of the oropharyngeal cavity are especially sensitive to menthol. When administered orally, menthol enhances cold sensations in the mouth and modulates taste-receptor activity [15]. It has been suggested that by stimulating the major palatine nerve, oral administration of menthol might also directly influence the nasal sensation of airflow [16]. Indeed, oral administration of a menthol lozenge caused a subjective sensation of improved airflow without actual changes in airway resistance [14]. Eccles [17] summarized these findings by noting that menthol may influence thirst, the drive to breathe and arousal due to its effects on oral and nasal cold receptors. Menthol might therefore also be used to help exercise performance in a hot climate [18]. It was recently demonstrated that swilling an L(-) menthol solution increased the exercise cycling time, suggesting that a change in oropharyngeal temperature perception during exercise in the heat positively affects endurance capacity [18] and the sense of effort. However, the cumulative effects of cold water/ice-slush and menthol ingestion on performance in the heat have never been studied.

In the present study, we thus tested the hypothesis that an ice-slush/menthol or a cold/menthol beverage would improve performance in the heat more than non-cumulative drinks (cold, ice-slush, neutral or menthol drinks).

Methods

Subjects

Twelve heat-acclimated trained (i.e., living and training in Guadeloupe) male cyclists and triathletes participated in the study (age = 42±13 years; body mass = 74.0±6.1 kg; height = 180.0± 8.3 cm; $\dot{V}O2_{max}$ = 59.9±10.4 mL.min^{-1}.kg^{-1}; peak power output at $\dot{V}O2_{max}$ = 340±42 W). The athletes were training at least 10 hours per week at the time of study. The study was approved by the Ethics Committee of the Centre Médico-Sportif in Guadeloupe (Ministry of Youth and Sports) and the Ethics Committee of the Training and Research in Sport Science Unit in Guadeloupe (Ministry of Higher Education and Research). All athletes completed a medical screening questionnaire and gave written informed consent prior to the study, which was accepted by the University Ethics Committee and was conducted according to the Declaration of Helsinki.

Preliminary measurements

On the athletes' first visit to the laboratory, maximum aerobic capacity ($\dot{V}O2_{max}$) was measured during an incremental exercise test on an electronically braked cycle ergometer (TECHMED, TM 4170, Besancon, France). The initial workload was 30 W and increased by 30 W every minute until volitional fatigue. Gas exchange was measured throughout the entire test (ZAN Ferraris, Cardiorespiratory System, Oberthulba, Germany). The $\dot{V}O2_{max}$ was achieved when two of the following criteria were met: (1) $\dot{V}O2$did not increase with an increase in intensity, (2) a clear plateau in oxygen uptake was seen, (3) HR was within 10 beats.min^{-1} of the age-predicted maximum of 220 - age, and (4) the respiratory exchange ratio (RER) was greater than 1.05. All the triathletes and cyclists were accustomed to this type of test but nevertheless participated in a trial to familiarize themselves with the protocol for the experimental trials, using their own bicycle fixed on a cycle trainer (Tacx Satori T1856, Tacx BV, Wassenaar, the Netherlands). The familiarization trial was performed under neutral environmental conditions (23°C±0.5°C and 59.9±9% relative humidity (RH)).

Experimental design

The experimental trials were separated by 3–7 days and were undertaken in a randomized crossover design. Athletes were also asked to limit their exercise to 60 minutes of light-intensity exercise the day before each trial. At the start of the trial days, the athletes consumed a standard breakfast that included food and 600 mL of beverage. The trials began at the same time of day for each athlete (between 14:00 and 16:30) to control for circadian variations in T_{co} and digestion control. During the trials, the athletes wore cycling shorts, a chest-strapped heart rate monitor, a cycling jersey, socks and shoes.

Experimental procedures

The experimental trials were performed in a laboratory in the tropical conditions of Guadeloupe, French West Indies (mean ± SD temperature in laboratory: 30.7°C±0.8°C and 78% ±0.03% RH). During the sessions, athletes were not subjected to any flow of ambient air. Heart rate (HR) was monitored continuously using a portable telemetry unit (Suunto Memory Belt, Suunto, Vantaa, Finland) recording it every 5 seconds, and the data were analyzed with Suunto software. The core temperature (T_{co}) was assessed via the gastrointestinal temperature using ingestible temperature measurement pills (CorTemp, HQ, Inc., Palmetto, FL, USA). Athletes were instructed to ingest these pills 8 to 10 h before all experimental trials to ensure the pill was out of the stomach, thereby avoiding variability in T_{co} due to pill movement or fluid/ food consumption. The experimental trial included 15 min of warm-up, with cycling at a freely chosen cadence against a resistance related to the mean power output noted at the first ventilatory threshold (i.e., 178 W±45 W), followed by 20 km of exercise at the fastest possible speed against a resistance related to their mean power output noted at the second ventilatory threshold (i.e., 335 W±90 W), and then 15 min of recovery at the warm-up resistance level. Subjects were required to cycle in a cadence-independent mode. During the experimental trial, T_{co} was measured before and after warm-up, every 5 km during the 20-km cycle time trial, at the end of cycling, and after the recovery phase.

During the experimental trials, athletes were asked to drink 190 mL of a randomly assigned beverage as fast as possible before warm-up, at the beginning of the time trial, every 5 km of exercise, at the end of the trial and at the end of the recovery. The six experimental trials were as follows: a neutral or a menthol aroma beverage at one of three temperatures: (1) neutral (23°C±0.1°C), (2) cold (3°C±0.1°C) or ice-slush (−1°C±0.7°C). The menthol beverages used a 0.01% natural menthol aroma (% vol: 86.0% ±1.0%; dosage: 0.50/g/L) (Robertet, Grasse, France).

The ice-slush was produced with an ice-slush machine (Brema, GB 902A, Professional Slush Machine, Ice Makers, Germany). Although ice expands in volume, we carefully ensured that the volume of ice-slush (in mL of water) was precisely the same as the volume of cold water. The temperature of each beverage was measured with a digital thermometer (YSI 409B, Yellow Springs Instruments, OH, USA). A spoon was provided to aid ingestion of the ice-slush.

Measurements

Before and after warm-up and every 5 km of the trial, $T_{co,}$ perceived exertion (RPE), perceived thermal sensation (TS), and perceived thermal comfort (TC) were recorded. Before the athletes drank 190 mL of neutral, cold or ice-slush beverage (with or without menthol), T_{co} was recorded and they were asked to rate their perceived exertion on the 15 grades of the Borg perceived exertion scale [19]. Perceived thermal sensation and perceived thermal comfort were determined on seven-point (a modified 7-point scale ranging from "extremely cold" (1) to "extremely hot" (7)) and four-point (a modified 4-point scale ranging from "comfortable" (1) to "very uncomfortable" (4)) scales adapted from Hodder and Parsons [20]. The RPE, TS and TC were assessed every 5 km and immediately at the end of the trial. Nude body mass was assessed (±0.1 kg) before and after the 20-km sessions (Tanita SC 330P, Tanita, Amsterdam, the Netherlands). An indication of hydration status throughout the experimental

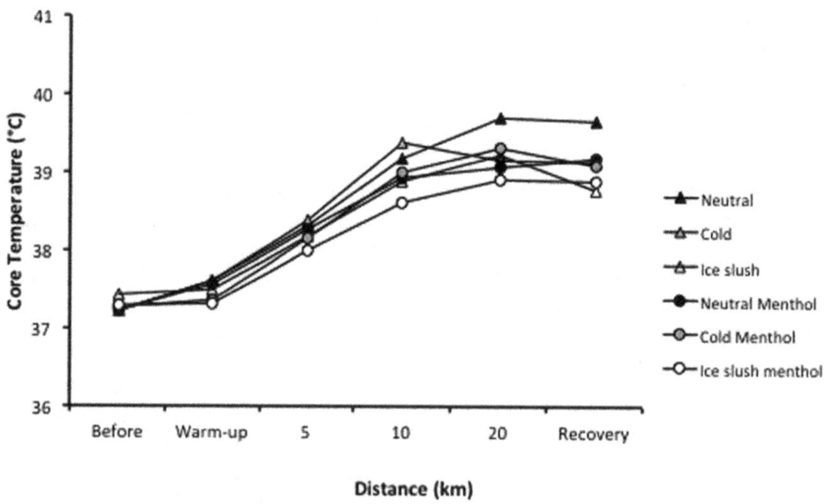

Figure 1. Core temperature (°C) before and after warm-up; at 5-km, 10-km and 20-km of the experimental trials; and during recovery. Mean values are shown.

trials was later determined by changes in nude body mass. During the session, athletes drank 1140 mL of beverage.

Statistical analyses

We tested for normality using Skewness and Kurtois tests, with acceptable Z values not exceeding +1 or −1. Once the assumption of normality was confirmed, parametric tests were performed. The following variables: T_{co}, performance, HR, TC, TS and RPE, were examined along with three-way analyses of variance (ANOVA) with repeated measures (beverage condition x beverage temperature x time). Scheffe's post-hoc tests were used when required. Data analysis was performed using the Statistical Package for Social Sciences (SPSS) (Chicago, IL, USA). Significance was set at the $P<0.05$. All data are presented as mean ± SD.

Results

Core temperature (T_{co})

There was no significant difference in the mean T_{co} noted in the six experimental sessions before exercise (37.3±0.1°C), during warm-up (37.5±0.1°C) or during recovery (39.1±0.3°C) (Figure 1). There was no aroma or temperature effect on T_{co} but a tendency ($P<0.07$) toward a temperature x time effect, with T_{co} increasing less in the ice-slush than the neutral condition (Figure 1).

When the delta T_{co} (i.e., the increase in T_{co} with time) was analyzed, it showed a tendency toward a beverage temperature effect ($P<0.06$) with a significantly lower delta T_{co} in ice-slush *vs* neutral condition ($P<0.05$). Moreover, a significant aroma x temperature x time effect was noted ($P<0.02$) for the delta T_{co} (Figure 2).

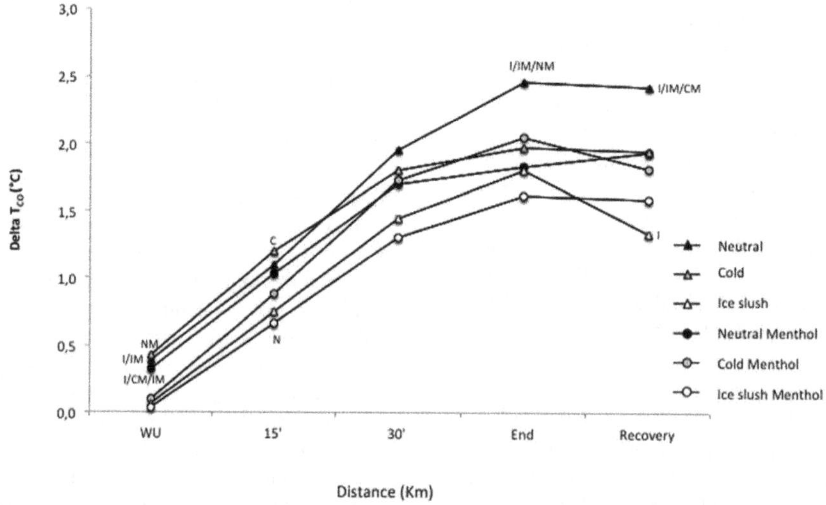

Figure 2. Delta core temperature (°C) after warm up; at 5-km, 10-km and 20-km of the experimental trials; and during recovery. Significant ($P<0.05$) differences are represented by letters (N: different from neutral, C: different from cold, I: different from Ice, NM: different from Neutral-Menthol, IM: different from Ice-Menthol, CM: different from Cold-Menthol, I/IM: different from both Ice and Ice-Menthol, I/NM/IM: different from Ice, Neutral-Menthol and Ice-Menthol, I/CM/IM: different from Ice, Cold-Menthol and Ice-Menthol).

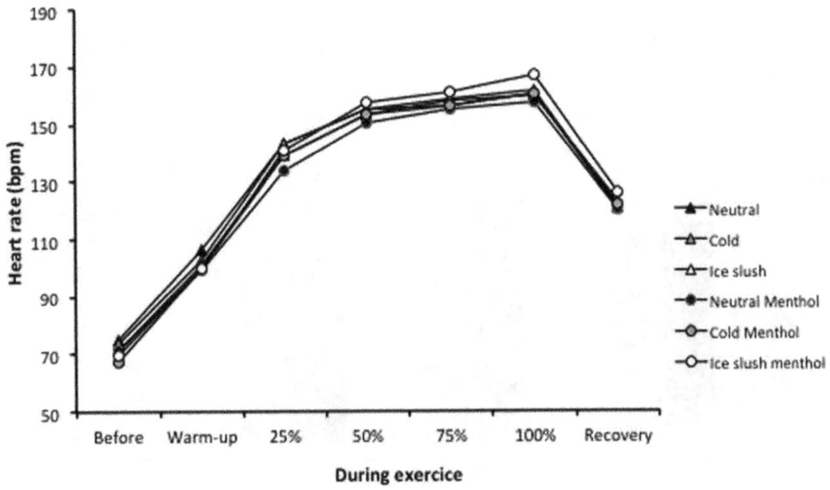

Figure 3. Heart rate (beats·min^{-1}) before and during warm-up; at 25%, 50%, 75% and 100% of the cycling times; and during recovery.

Heart rate

HR increased significantly from warm-up until the end of exercise (20 km) and then decreased similarly in the six conditions (time effect $P<0.001$). HR was significantly affected by aroma x time ($P<0.05$) (Figure 3).

Performance

Mean performance was significantly affected by both the aroma condition (performance (time in seconds): 2130±246 s and 2250±288 s, in menthol and non-menthol, respectively; $P<0.02$) and the temperature condition ($P<0.02$), with a significant difference ($P<0.002$) between neutral (2253±240 s) and ice-slush (2100±280 s) (Figure 4).

The post-hoc analysis demonstrated significantly better performance for both cold/menthol and ice-shush/menthol as opposed to neutral ($P<0.05$ and $P<0.03$, respectively), neutral/menthol ($P<0.05$ and $P<0.007$, respectively) and cold ($P<0.003$ and $P<0.007$, respectively) (Figure 4). When analyzed by 5-km bouts (Figure 4), performance, which was significantly better in the menthol condition ($P<0.04$), was affected by both time ($P<0.02$) and temperature ($P<0.005$) with significantly better results in ice-slush *vs* neutral condition ($P<0.003$). As noted in Figure 2, performance showed a significant aroma x time effect ($P<0.01$), with the time over the 5-km bouts increasing, except in the cold/menthol and ice-slush/menthol conditions.

Environmental conditions, weight and hydration status

The mean ± SD ambient temperature was similar between trials (30.7°C±0.8°C), as was relative humidity (78% ±0.03%). Athletes were instructed to consume 190 mL of beverage before exercise, 760 mL during the 20 km, and 190 mL after the recovery. The athletes' body mass was not different before sessions (mean sessions ± SD: 72.0±3.2 kg) but decreased similarly after sessions (mean sessions ± SD: 70.6±0.3 kg).

Thermal sensation, comfort sensation and RPE

There were no significant differences in TS, CS, or RPE, with all of them increasing with time. TS was significantly affected by aroma x time (means ± SD at the end of exercise; no menthol: 3.5±0.5; menthol: 3.7±0.3; $P<0.02$).

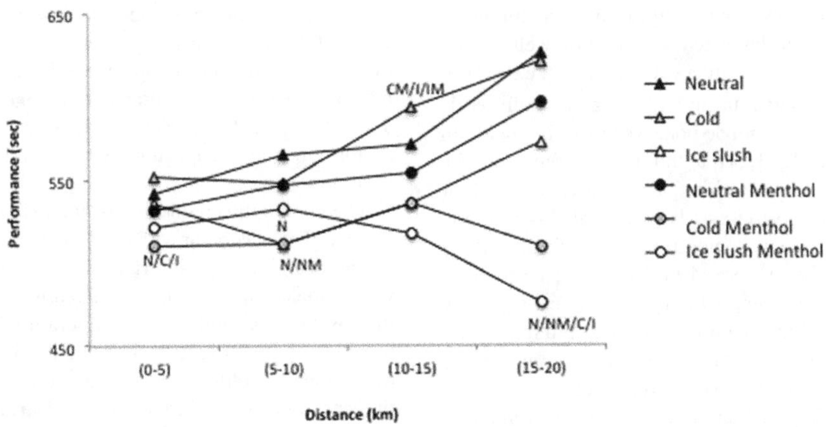

Figure 4. Mean cycling distance (km) by 5-km blocks. Differences are represented by letters (N: different from neutral, C: different from cold, I: different from Ice, NM: different from Neutral-Menthol, IM: different from Ice-Menthol, CM: different from Cold-Menthol, I/IM: different from both Ice and Ice-Menthol, I/NM/IM: different from Ice, Neutral-Menthol and Ice-Menthol, I/CM/IM: different from Ice, Cold-Menthol and Ice-Menthol).

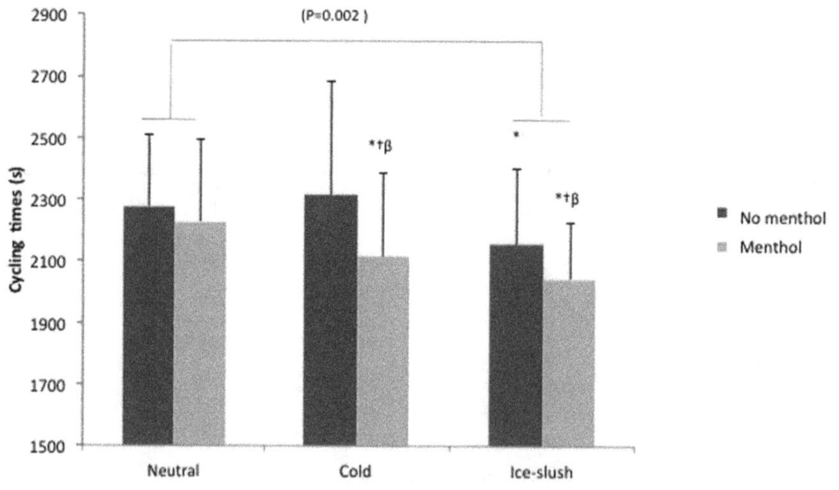

Figure 5. Cycling times (seconds) for the 20-km trial with ingestion of water at neutral, cold and ice-slush temperatures, with or without the water containing 0.05% L(-) menthol. Mean values and SD are shown. * significantly different from Neutral ($P<0.01$), † significantly different from Neutral-Menthol ($P<0.01$), and β significantly different from water Cold-Menthol ($P<0.01$).

Discussion

The most important findings of our study were that (1) performance was better using ice-slush than neutral temperature beverage, whatever the aroma, (2) performance was better with menthol, whatever the beverage temperature, and (3) the best performances were obtained with combinations of either ice-slush with menthol or cold water with menthol.

Water temperature effect

The lack of a significant difference in performance between the effects of cold and neutral water has not been fully elucidated. Indeed, Lee et al. [21] demonstrated longer exercise times and lower rectal temperatures when subjects drank cold water (4°C) as opposed to warm beverages [37°C] during cycling to exhaustion in a hot environment. Burdon et al. [22] noted a positive effect of cold beverages on cycling performance, and in a recent review Burdon et al. [11] concluded that cold beverages attenuate core temperature rise and improve exercise performance in the heat. However, other studies have failed to observe any difference between cold water and ambient water intake [23,24].

The explanations for the lack of significant results are numerous and include the use of unacclimatized and/or not well-trained athletes [25], insufficient exercise intensity stimulus (i.e., <60% $\dot{V}O2_{max}$), insufficient environmental stress [11], and insufficiently cold water [11]. The effect of a single bolus versus serial ingestion seems less clear: Lee et al. [1,21] found no difference in the exercise performance of subjects drinking 400 mL of 10°C or 37°C fluids every 15 min of exercise or 1L in a single bolus at 50–60 min of exercise, but they demonstrated significant effects following the intake of a beverage at 4°C drunk in a large bolus before exercise and 100 mL every 10 min of exercise [24]. Very recently, we demonstrated significant effects on core temperature and HR in swimmers drinking 190 mL of 1.3°C water (i.e., vs 26.5°C) every 15 min of steady-pace exercise. The most likely explanation for our findings is that studies using fixed-intensity exercise have usually noted an increase in performance with cold water [18,24,], whereas studies using self-paced exercise have not [23,24]. Indeed, our athletes were well trained ($\dot{V}O2_{max}$ of 59.9 $ml.min^{-1}.kg^{-1}$), the 20-km exercise was performed at a power output of 335±90 W, and the environmental stress was high.

The performance was increased with ice-slush compared with neutral temperature water. Moreover, the ice-slush tended to increase performance more than the cold beverage. This agrees with the literature: Siegel et al. [26] demonstrated that a pre-cooling beverage of −1°C ice slurry increased submaximal endurance running time in the heat, compared with a pre-cooling beverage of 4°C water. Ihsan et al. [8] noted the same for 40-km cycling time-trial performance and Yeo et al. [13] for 10-km outdoor running. However, whereas these authors [20,36,39] noted lower core temperature before or during the first parts of exercise, we failed to see any significant difference between ice-slush or cold and neutral temperature water ingestion before and during exercise. This confirms the recent findings of Morris et al. [27], who observed no change in rectal or aural canal temperature when subjects were given that subjects either had to drink or were directly given in the stomach water at different temperatures to drink or water delivered directly to the stomach, and confirms the limitations of using thermometry to estimate body heat storage during exercise [28]. We can therefore also hypothesize that because performance was increased with the ingestion of ice-slush, the metabolic rate also increased, with the subjects producing more heat than during slower sessions. The combined effect of increased performance and ice-slush ingestion was a constant T_{co}. This also strongly suggests that ice-slush could increase exercise performance in a tropical climate without any detectable changes in T_{co}.

The cooling mechanism with the help of an icy beverage is the same as that of cooling with a cold beverage: a truly cold (very cold or ice-slush) beverage interferes with the rise in core temperature, which makes it possible to increase exercise intensity without increasing HR and core temperature, as partially noted in previous works [8,13,29]. The smaller increase in core temperature, due to cold/ice-slush ingestion (i.e., *vs* neutral or cold) prevents immediate blood flow redistribution to the skin, thus allowing greater blood flow to the exercising muscles. This effect could be more powerful with an ice-slush ingestion, as noted by Siegel [26], because (1) the larger heat sink created by the ingestion of the ice slurry yields bigger heat-storing capacity than liquid H_2O alone [12] and (2) given that an ice slurry is ingested through the mouth, it has been hypothesized that it might increase brain cooling via direct heat exchange with blood in the carotid arteries [12], thus delaying the critically high brain temperatures that start both the inhibitory signal to motor control centers [30] and the cardiovascular adjustments due to T_{co} increase. However, such a mechanism was recently contested by Morris et al. [27], who suggested that a more likely mechanism would be that the thermoreceptors independently modulating sudomotor output probably reside in the abdominal area (i.e., the stomach). The significant effect of ice-slush would therefore be the following: with a temperature lower than that of cold water, ice-slush creates a larger heat sink and thus better reducing whole-body water loss, as has been suggested [27]. This in turn would positively influence the thermoreceptors in the stomach and limit the blood flow redistribution that accompanies the sudomotor activity, thereby allowing greater blood flow for exercising muscles. However, because we did not measure sweating or skin blood flow, this explanation remains speculative. A potential sensory effect of ice-slush in the mouth or oropharyngeal area may also explain the benefits of ice-slush. Indeed, although Morris et al. [27] demonstrated that local sweat production was activated following fluid delivered directly to the stomach, but not when the beverage was swilled, suggesting that, independently of core and skin temperature, the thermoreceptors modulating the sudomotor output during fluid ingestion probably reside in the abdominal area and not in the mouth, Eccles [31] reported that cold water increased thirst satiety via sensory cold receptors in the oropharynx and Guest *et al.* demonstrated that responsive regions of the humain brain are also activated by intra-oral thermal stimulation [32].

In our study, it might further be hypothesized that the rate of the core temperature increase was a primary signal for pacing the cycling trials, as this rate was lowest in the ice-slush trial (Figure 5). However, the literature has reported similar rates (but better performance) with and without pre-cooling [33].

The present study is the first to demonstrate a significant effect of menthol use (i.e., as drink administration) on sports performance, whatever the beverage temperature. Other researchers have demonstrated the beneficial effects of menthol in subjects swilling an L(-) menthol solution during exercise in the heat [18], while still others have recorded subject reports of feeling cooler [34]. Yet the mechanism of the menthol effect is far from evident. Green [15] postulated that when administered orally, menthol provokes the sensation of cooling by making subsequent stimuli (inspired air, water consumed) feel cool, and oral administration of a menthol lozenge caused a subjective sensation of improved airflow. Eccles [17] also suggested that menthol may mimic the cool stimulus associated with ingestion of cold water. One of the possible mechanisms that would explain the better performance using menthol versus neutral aroma is that menthol provided a cooling sensation that was perceived as refreshing and stimulating [18], thus decreasing the RPE. One might also point out that if menthol indeed enhances sensation airflow [16], it could prevent heat-induced hypocapnia and the reduction in cerebral blood flow [30] usually has a positive effect on central fatigue. Indeed, there is some evidence that heat stress results in hyperventilation, which lowers the carbon dioxide tension and consequently reduces the cerebral blood flow [30], inducing cerebral fatigue. Inhibiting the drive to breathe because of its interaction with airway cold receptors [17], menthol may therefore limit hyperventilation, reducing hypocapnia, and by extension cerebral fatigue. However, it is difficult to explain how athletes were able to obtain better performances with menthol without any change in their HR. Although heat sensations did not prevent them from cycling (i.e., menthol provokes cold sensations), cycling at higher intensity should have induced an increase in HR (i.e., given that the water intake, the environmental conditions and the water losses were the same in all trials). We suggest that thermoreceptors in the hypothalamus do not detect increases in temperature because of these menthol effects and thus no inhibitory signal is sent to the motor control centers [30]. This might also prevent the redistribution of blood from the core to the periphery, with adequate cardiac output being maintained. The result would be better performance than during the non-menthol condition without any change in HR (the cardiac output not being maintained in the non-menthol condition due to hyperthermic afferences). If this hypothesis is correct, we should have noted higher T_{co} in the menthol conditions (the menthol would trick the hypothalamic thermoreceptors, giving the sensation of cold, but not prevent the core temperature from increasing), which was not the case.

Sensations

Psychological effects have a strong influence [35] on performance in a warm environment. Although some studies have demonstrated lower rates of perceived exertion or lower thermal sensations using ice [12,13] or cold water cooling or menthol [18], others have not [29]. In the present study, we observed no significant difference in thermal sensation, thermal comfort or RPE across beverage temperatures, aroma, or beverage temperature x aroma, with these three parameters increasing over time. One explanation is that, despite the lower thermal sensation, thermal comfort and RPE under conditions of menthol and/or ice-slush beverage, with the increases in exercise intensity/performance, these three parameters remained unchanged, as hypothesized by Wegmann [35].

Specifically, the lack of change in RPE despite significantly better performance suggests an effect of both menthol and ice as physiological and/or psychological signals that combine to produce self-paced effort. Indeed, RPE has been demonstrated to be a powerful feed-forward control mechanism [36] that linearly increases with intensity in controlled conditions.

Menthol x temperature beverages

Post-hoc analysis demonstrated significantly better performance in two conditions, ice-slush/menthol and cold/menthol beverages, indicating a strong and significant effect of combined low temperature/menthol on performance in tropical environment. When compared with the neutral condition (i.e., neutral temperature with no menthol), ice-slush/menthol and cold/menthol increased performance times by 10.2% and 7.1%, respectively, which is substantial compared with the effects of other cooling strategies in similar time-trial exercise (i.e., 1.3% for Ross et al. [37] and 6.5% for Ihsan et al. [8] during cycling; 0.5% for Yeo et al. [13] for running). This better time performance was overexpressed in the last part of the exercise (i.e., between the 15th and 20th kilometer, with 24.1% and 18.6% increases for ice-slush/menthol and cold/menthol, respectively, compared with neutral). The use of cold/menthol or ice-slush/menthol beverages during time trials in a tropical climate thus seems a good strategy to enhance performance. However, the debate remains open about the amount of water that should be drunk. As reported by Burdon et al. [11], fluid ingestion protocols vary widely, from regular consumption of a standardized bolus not adjusted for body weight or body surface [22,23] to ad libitum consumption [29] or a large single bolus at one point during exercise [24]. From a physiological point of view, consuming large amounts of cold fluid is believed to create a heat sink, which should theoretically result in the attenuation of the heat accumulated over exercise and reduce the rise in T_{co}. However, athletes do not usually drink large volumes of water in one bolus but instead drink intermittently over the course of the exercise [38]. Moreover, it has been demonstrated that emptying is more rapid with smaller volumes [8], resulting in more rapid rehydration, as in the present study.

Conclusion

The present study demonstrated an increase in performance using menthol or ice-slush beverage, the best performances being obtained with cold/menthol and ice-slush/menthol solutions. The mechanisms involved in these results remain undiscovered because, as noted by Cheung [39], "understanding or defining the signal, or signals, that becomes integrated to produce self-paced effort is a difficult problem to elucidate, as it is most likely an amalgam of physiological and psychological sources and further mediated by individual factors and core temperature itself would appear to be an obvious signal.".

Further studies are needed to elucidate the performance increase induced by menthol.

Acknowledgments

The authors would like to acknowledge and thank the athletes for their generous time commitment and effort throughout the study.

Author Contributions

Conceived and designed the experiments: FR. Performed the experiments: TT. Analyzed the data: OH. Contributed reagents/materials/analysis tools: SS. Contributed to the writing of the manuscript: FR.

References

1. Maughan RJ (2010) Distance running in hot environments: A thermal challenge to the elite runner. Scand J Med Sci Sports 20 Suppl 3: 95–102.
2. Nybo L (2010) Cycling in the heat: Performance perspectives and cerebral challenges. Scand J Med Sci Sports 20 Suppl 3: 71–9.
3. Hue O (2011) The challenge of performing aerobic exercise in tropical environments: Applied knowledge and perspectives. Int J Sports Physiol Perform 6: 443–54.
4. Voltaire B, Galy O, Coste O, Recinais S, Callis A, et al. (2002) Effect of fourteen days of acclimatization on athletic performance in tropical climate. Can J Appl Physiol 27: 551–62.
5. González-Alonso J, Teller C, Andersen SL, Jensen FB, Hyldig T, et al. (1999) Influence of body temperature on the development of fatigue during prolonged exercise in the heat. J Appl Physiol 86: 1032–9.
6. Noakes TD (1998) Maximal oxygen uptake: "Classical" versus "contemporary" viewpoints: A rebuttal. Med Sci Sports Exerc 30: 1381–98.
7. González-Alonso J (2007) Hyperthermia impairs brain, heart and muscle function in exercising humans. Sports Med 37: 371–3.
8. Ihsan M, Landers G, Brearley M, Peeling P (2010) Beneficial effects of ice ingestion as a precooling strategy on 40-km cycling time-trial performance. Int J Sports Physiol Perform 5: 140–51.
9. Marino FE (2002) Methods, advantages, and limitations of body cooling for exercise performance. Br J Sports Med 36(2):89–94.
10. Hue O, Monjo R, Lazzaro M, Baillot M, Hellard P, et al. (2013) The effect of time-of-day on cold water ingestion by high-level swimmers in tropical climate. Int J Sports Physiol Per 8: 442–451.
11. Burdon CA, O'Connor HT, Gifford JA, Shirreffs SM (2010) Influence of beverage temperature on exercise performance in the heat: A systematic review. Int J Sport Nutr Exerc Metab 20: 166–74.
12. Siegel R, Laursen PB (2012) Keeping your cool: possible mechanisms for enhanced exercise performance in the heat with internal cooling methods. Sports Med 42: 89–98.
13. Yeo ZW, Fan PW, Nio AQ, Byrne C, Lee JK (2012) Ice slurry on outdoor running performance in heat. Int J Sports Med 33: 859–66.
14. Eccles R, Jawad MS, Morris S (1990) The effects of oral administration of L(-) menthol on nasal resistance to airflow and nasal sensation of airflow in subjects suffering from nasal congestion associated with the common cold. J Pharm Pharmacol 42: 652–4.
15. Green BG (1985) Menthol modulates oral sensations of warmth and cold. Percept Psychophys 38: 110–4.
16. Naito K, Komori M, Kondo Y, Takeuchi M, Iwata S (1997) The effect of l-menthol stimulation of the major palatine nerve on subjective and objective nasal patency. Auris Nasus Larynx 24:159–62.
17. Eccles R, (2000), Role of cold receptors and menthol in thirst, the drive to breathe and arousal. Appetite 34: 29–35.
18. Mündel T, Jones DA (2010) The effects of swilling an L (-)-menthol solution during exercise in the heat. Eur J Appl Physiol 109: 59–65.
19. Borg G (1970) Perceived exertion as an indicator of somatic stress. Scand J Rehabil Med 2(2): 92–8.
20. Hodder SG, Parsons K (2007) The effects of solar radiation on thermal comfort. Int J Biometeorol 51: 233–50.
21. Lee JK, Shirreffs SM, Maughan RJ (2008) Cold drink ingestion improves exercise endurance capacity in the heat. Med Sci Sports Exerc 40: 1637–44.
22. Burdon CA, O'Connor HT, Gifford JA, Shirreffs SM, Chapman P, et al. (2010) Effect of drink temperature on core temperature and endurance cycling performance in warm, humid conditions. J Sports Sci.
23. Lee JK, Maughan RJ, Shirreffs SM (2008) The influence of serial feeding of drinks at different temperatures on thermoregulatory responses during cycling. J Sports Sci 26:583–90.
24. Lee JK, Shirreffs SM (2007) The influence of drink temperature on thermoregulatory responses during prolonged exercise in a moderate environment. J Sports Sci 25:975–85.
25. Hopkins WG, Hewson DJ (2001) Variability of competitive performance of distance runners. Med Sci Sports Exerc 33: 1588–92.
26. Siegel R, Maté J, Brearley MB, Watson G, Nosaka K, et al. (2010) Ice slurry ingestion increases core temperature capacity and running time in the heat. Med Sci Sports Exer. 42: 717–25.
27. Morris NB, Bain AR, Cramer MN, Jay O (2014) Evidence that transient changes in sudomotor output with cold and warm ingestion are independently modulated by abdominal, nut not oral thermoreptors. J Appl Physiol 116(8): 1088–95.
28. Jay O, Reardon FD, Webb P, Ducharme MB, Ramsay T, et al. (2007) Estimating changes in mean body temperature for humans during exercise using core and skin temperatures is inaccurate even with a correction factor. J Appl Physiol 103: 443–451.
29. Mündel T, King J, Collacott E, Jones DA (2006) Drink temperature influences fluid intake and endurance capacity in men during exercise in a hot, dry environment. Exp Physiol 91: 925–33.
30. Nybo L (2008) Hyperthermia and fatigue. J Appl Physiol 104: 871–8.
31. Eccles R (1994) Menthol and related cooling compounds. J Pharm Pharmacol 46: 618–30.
32. Guest S, Grabenhorst F, Essick G, Chen Y, Young M, et al. (2007) Physiology and behaviour 94: 975–984.
33. Cotter JD, Sleivert GG, Roberts WS, Febbraio MA (2001) Effect of pre-cooling, with and without thigh cooling, on strain and endurance exercise performance in the heat. Comp Biochem Physiol A Mol Integr Physiol 128: 667–77.
34. Gillis DJ, House JR, Tipton MJ (2010) The influence of menthol on thermoregulation and perception during exercise in warm, humid conditions. Eur J Appl Physiol 110: 609–18.
35. Wegmann M, Faude O, Poppendieck W, Hecksteden A, Fröhlich M, et al. (2012) Pre-cooling and sports performance: A meta-analytical review. Sports Med 42: 545–64.
36. Crewe H, Tucker R, Noakes TD (2008) The rate of increase in rating of perceived exertion predicts the duration of exercise to fatigue at a fixed power output in different environmental conditions. Eur J Appl Physiol 103: 569–77.
37. Ross ML, Garvican LA, Jeacocke NA, Laursen PB, Abbiss CR, et al. (2011) Novel precooling strategy enhances time trial cycling in the heat. Med Sci Sports Exerc 43: 123–33.
38. Hunt JN, MacDonald I (1954) The influence of volume on gastric emptying. J Physiol 126: 459–74.
39. Cheung SS (2007) Neuropsychological determinants of exercise tolerance in the heat. Pro Brain Res 162: 43–60.

Prevalence of Anxiety and Depressive Symptoms and Related Risk Factors among Physicians in China

Yanhong Gong[1]◑, Tieguang Han[2]◑, Wei Chen[3], Hassan H. Dib[4], Guoan Yang[2], Runsen Zhuang[2], Yuqi Chen[2], Xinyue Tong[1], Xiaoxv Yin[1]*, Zuxun Lu[1]*

1 Department of Social Medicine and Health Management, School of Public Health, Tongji Medical College, Huazhong University of Science and Technology, Wuhan, Hubei, P. R. China, **2** Shenzhen Health Education and Promotion Center, Shenzhen, Guangdong, P. R. China, **3** Department of Occupational Health, Laiwu Municipal Center for Disease Control and Prevention, Laiwu, Shandong, P. R. China, **4** National Center for AIDS/STD Control and Prevention, Chinese Center for Disease Control and Prevention, Beijing, P. R. China

Abstract

Background: Physicians' poor mental health not only hinders their professional performance and affects the quality of healthcare provided but also adversely affects patients' health outcomes. Few studies in China have evaluated the mental health of physicians. The purposes of this study are to quantify Chinese physicians' anxiety and depressive symptoms as well as evaluate associated risk factors.

Methods: In our study, 2641 physicians working in public hospitals in Shenzhen in southern China were recruited and interviewed by using a structured questionnaire along with validated scales testing anxiety and depressive symptoms. Multivariable logistic regression models were used to identify risk factors for anxiety and depressive symptoms.

Results: An estimated 25.67% of physicians had anxiety symptoms, 28.13% had depressive symptoms, and 19.01% had both anxiety and depressive symptoms. More than 10% of the participants often experienced workplace violence and 63.17% sometimes encountered it. Among our study population, anxiety and depressive symptoms were associated with poor self-reported physical health, frequent workplace violence, lengthy working hours (more than 60 hours a week), frequent night shifts (twice or more per week), and lack of regular physical exercise.

Conclusions: Our study demonstrates that anxiety and depressive symptoms are common among physicians in China, and the doctor-patient relationship issue is particularly stressful. Interventions implemented to minimize workload, improve doctor-patient relationships, and assist physicians in developing healthier lifestyles are essential to combat anxiety and depressive symptoms among physicians, which may improve their professional performance.

Editor: Diane M. Harper, University of Missouri Kansas City School of Medicine, United States of America

Funding: This project was funded by the Shenzhen Health Education and Promotion Center. The funders had no role in study design, data collection and analysis, decision to publish, or preparation of the manuscript.

Competing Interests: The authors have declared that no competing interests exist.

* Email: zuxunlu@yahoo.com (ZL); hnyinxiaoxv@126.com (XY)

◑ These authors contributed equally to this work.

Introduction

Physicians are vulnerable to some mental disorders such as anxiety, depression, and occupational burnout, likely owing to their exposure to high levels of occupational stress [1,2]. Adverse mental health among physicians can hinder their professional performance and affect the quality of healthcare provided [3–5]. These issues will inevitably have negative effects on patients' health and the development of healthcare system based on manpower sources [6,7]. Therefore, interest in the psychological well-being of physicians has increased recently, warranting further research regarding factors that influence the mental health of physicians [8].

Several studies have evaluated the mental health of doctors in developed countries such as the US, Britain, Canada, Norway, Japan, and Dutch. Previous studies indicated that the prevalence of depressive symptoms among physicians ranged from 10% to 15% in the US, Britain, Norway, and Japan [9–14]. A recent Dutch investigation concluded that anxiety and depressive symptoms were prevalent in 24% and 29% of physicians, respectively [15]. Researchers in China did not examine mental health and psychological well-being among physicians until the beginning of the 21st century. In recent years, a few studies in China focused on anxiety or depressive symptoms among physicians with varying results [16–19]. For example, one study showed that the prevalence of depressive symptoms among physicians was 31.7%, while in another study the prevalence of depressive symptoms reached 65.3% [17,19]. Considering that social, cultural, and economic factors have significant effects on mental health [20,21], it is necessary to perform additional studies in different regions of a socially and economically diverse country such as China. Furthermore, anxiety and depression symptoms are the two most common mental disorders and commonly occur together [22]. A study that focuses on these two classes of symptoms simultaneously can provide a comprehensive evaluation of their prevalence and identify common potential risk factors. Consequently, we conducted an investigation to quantify Chinese physicians' anxiety and depressive symptoms as well as evaluate associated risk factors that predispose them to anxiety and depressive symptoms.

Methods

Ethics Statement

The study protocol was approved by the Research Ethics Committee in Tongji Medical College, Huazhong University of Science and Technology, Wuhan, China. All the participants read the purpose statement of the investigation and each provided a written informed consent.

Participants and sampling

This study implemented a cross-sectional survey. Data were collected from June 2009 to October 2009 in the city of Shenzhen-Guangdong Province (Southern China). There were 59 public hospitals in Shenzhen in 2009, and all these hospital enrolled in this study. One quarter of physicians with more than one year of work experience were randomly sampled from the 59 public hospitals. Of 10952 eligible subjects, 2738 physicians were randomly selected, 92 (3.36%) refused to participate, and finally 2646 participants were interviewed through self-administered anonymous questionnaires. Of the 2646 questionnaires distributed, five were discarded because of too many missing data. Finally, 2641 physicians were qualified for this study, with an overall response rate of 96.46%.

Measurement

The questionnaire includes four sections: socio-demographic information, lifestyles, work-related characteristics, and self-reported health status. Socio-demographic information included gender, age, education level, and marital status. Lifestyle items comprised of sleeping time, physical exercise, and smoking status. Work-related characteristics contained hospital grade, job title, work department, working hours per week, night shift rotation period, and the frequency of doctor-patient conflicts and violence (i.e. "Over the past 12 months, how often did you encounter verbal abuse, threats, intimidation or physical violence by patients and their families?"). Self-reported health status covered two parts: self-perceived physical health and mental health. Self-perceived physical health was measured using a single 5-point Likert scale question ranging from "very bad" to "very good" and coded in the form of values from 1 to 5. Mental health condition comprised of intensified anxiety and depressive symptoms that are measured by the Zung Self-Rating Anxiety Scale (SAS) and the Zung Self-Rating depression Scale (SDS), respectively [23,24]. Each scale has 20 items presented in a multiple-choice format, and each item is given a severity score from 1 (where very seldom the anxiety/depression symptoms are present) to 4 (where anxiety/depression symptoms are present most of the time). The total score was computed as an original score, and then multiplied by 1.25 to get the standard score with higher scores representing higher intensity of the relevant symptoms. As for the Chinese norm of SAS, a score of more than 50 is considered anxiety symptom. In regards to the Chinese norm of SDS, depressive symptom is defined as a score of 53 or higher [25,26]. In our research, SAS and SDS have demonstrated high internal consistency; their Cronbach's alpha coefficient was 0.88 and 0.89, respectively. Additionally their Chinese version has been extensively validated [27,28].

To reduce information loss, all missing SAS and SDS values were replaced with the calculated mean of a given subject's complete response to other questions of the respectively scale [29]. For example, if a participant has 2 missing responses in SDS, the values are filled with the calculated average of the remaining completed 18 questions of SDS. However, there were still a few missing items among the categorized variables that were not filled in, such as gender, educational level, and marital status and so on.

Statistical analysis

All statistical procedures were performed using the Statistical Package for Social Sciences Version 12.0 for Windows. Descriptive analysis was carried out for socio-demographics data, lifestyle items, work-related characteristic variables and self-perceived physical health status. Prevalence of anxiety and depressive symptoms were calculated and compared to socio-demographic characteristics, lifestyles, personal physical health, and work-related characteristics. Chi-square tests were conducted to compare the prevalence of anxiety and depressive symptoms between groups. Multivariable logistic regression analysis was used to analyze the risk factors of anxiety and depressive symptoms (demographic variables, lifestyles, work-related characteristic variables, and self-perceived physical health as the independent variables). Adjusted odds ratios (ORs) and 95% confidence intervals (CIs) for each variable were calculated. For all comparisons, differences were tested using two-tailed tests and p-values less than 0.05 were considered statistically significant.

Results

The study's participants had a mean age of 39.76 (SD = 9.13) years. More than half of physicians were males (54.71%) and about 70% of physicians had bachelor or post-graduate degree. Almost one third of physicians (35.75%) reported a good self-perceived physical health status, while 13.56% reported poor physical health. Only 20.53% of physicians regularly performed physical exercise, and 30.42% of male physicians were current smokers. With respect to exposure to violence at work, more than 10% of the participants often experienced workplace violence and 63.17% sometimes encountered it (Table 1).

The mean standard score of SAS and SDS was 43.09 (SD = 11.10) and 46.08 (SD = 12.04). Overall, there was an estimated of 25.67% physicians with anxiety symptoms, 28.13% with depressive symptoms and 19.01% with both anxiety symptoms and depressive symptoms. Associations between sample characteristics and anxiety or depressive symptoms were assessed using Pearson chi-square tests and the results were displayed in Table 1. Almost all work-related characteristic variables and lifestyle items (except smoking) were associated significantly with anxiety and depressive symptoms. In addition, there were associations between age, gender, work department and anxiety/depressive symptoms.

Table 2 demonstrated the adjusted ORs and 95% CIs for anxiety and depressive symptoms. Compared with male physicians, females physicians had higher odds for anxiety (OR = 1.81, 95% CI: 1.37–2.38) and depressive symptoms (OR = 1.57, 95% CI: 1.21–2.03). Risk factors such as worse self-reported physical health, more violence exposure at work, lack of regular physical

Table 1. Descriptive statistics for the characteristics and associations with anxiety and depressive symptoms of the participants.

Variables	Physician		Anxiety symptoms		Depressive symptoms	
	N	%	%	P	%	P
Total	2641	100	25.67	-	28.13	-
Age, mean (SD[a])	39.76 (9.13)		39.26 (8.14)	0.0947[b]	38.67 (8.25)	0.0001[b]
Gender				<0.0001		0.0002
Male	1445	57.94	22.01		25.61	
Female	1049	42.06	30.79		32.51	
Education level				0.0745		0.0514
High school or less	118	4.48	20.34		23.73	
Vocational School	466	17.68	21.46		24.68	
Bachelor degree	1538	58.35	27.37		30.23	
Master degree	389	14.76	25.19		27.25	
Doctor degree	125	4.74	26.40		22.40	
Marital status				0.0998		0.5690
Married/cohabitation	2184	83.01	26.33		27.98	
Single/widow/divorced	447	16.99	22.60		29.31	
Self-perceived Health Status				<0.0001		<0.0001
Very good	135	5.13	7.41		11.85	
Good	806	30.62	8.93		12.90	
Fair	1334	50.68	26.91		29.84	
Bad/very bad	357	13.56	65.55		62.18	
Job title				0.2626		0.0691
Elementary or less	733	28.19	23.60		28.65	
Intermediate	807	31.04	26.15		30.98	
Senior	1060	40.77	26.98		26.13	
Work department				<0.0001		<0.0001
Internal medicine	436	16.51	24.31		27.29	
Surgery	441	16.70	26.98		28.57	
Obstetrics and gynecology	322	12.19	35.71		36.96	
Pediatrics	174	6.59	31.03		35.63	
Intensive care	147	5.57	35.37		37.41	
others	1121	42.45	20.70		23.37	
Hospital grade				0.0035		0.6288
1	280	10.60	21.07		25.71	
2	1490	56.42	24.30		28.52	
3	871	32.98	29.51		28.24	
Frequency of conflicts and violence				<0.0001		<0.0001
None	629	23.98	9.54		13.67	
Sometimes	1657	63.17	25.53		28.18	
Often	337	12.85	56.97		54.60	
Working hours/week				<0.0001		<0.0001
35–44	788	30.16	16.75		19.16	
45–59	993	38.00	22.76		25.88	
60–69	542	20.74	34.87		36.53	
≥70	290	11.10	42.41		44.14	
Shift work/week				<0.0001		<0.0001
0	938	36.17	19.19		20.26	
1	1177	45.39	28.21		32.03	
≥2	478	18.43	32.85		34.73	

Table 1. Cont.

Variables	Physician		Anxiety symptoms		Depressive symptoms	
	N	%	%	*P*	%	*P*
Sleeping times (hours)				<0.0001		<0.0001
≥8	357	13.56	11.20		19.33	
6–8	2126	80.78	26.43		28.08	
<6	149	5.66	49.66		51.01	
Physical exercise				<0.0001		<0.0001
Yes	539	20.53	13.73		16.70	
No	2086	79.47	28.72		31.11	
Smoking				0.0991		0.0017[c]
Male, No	1002	69.58	20.86	c	23.45	
Male, Yes	438	30.42	24.20		30.59	
Female, No	1021	98.74	30.36		32.13	
Female, Yes	13	1.26	46.15		53.85	

Note: *P* values are associated with Chi-square tests.
[a]SD is standard deviation.
[b]*P* value is associated with analysis of variance.
[c]*P* value is associated with Cochran-Mantel-Haenszel statistics.

exercise, more than sixty working hours per week, and twice or more night shifts per week were associated with anxiety or depressive symptoms. In addition, participants having insufficient sleep were more likely to experience anxiety symptoms than their counterparts. The participants with depressive symptoms were more prone to be current smokers (OR = 1.57, 95% CI: 1.18–2.09).

Discussion

Prevalence of anxiety and depressive symptoms among physicians

Our study demonstrated that anxiety and depression symptoms were common among physicians. Our results confirm previous findings regarding Chinese physicians' anxiety or depression symptoms. Regarding anxiety symptoms, the mean standard SAS score among our study participants (43.09) was close to that reported by a previous study that applied SAS to assess anxiety symptoms among physicians (46.8 in male physicians and 46.7 in female physicians) [18]. With respect to depressive symptoms, the prevalence among physicians in our study (28.13%) was similar to that reported in a Shanghai-based study among primary-care physicians (31.7%), which used an identical evaluation method [17]. However, the prevalence of depressive symptoms among hospital physicians in the Liaoning Province study was much higher (65.3%) [19]. Our results may differ owing to the participants' differences in terms of age, gender, and place of residence; additionally this variation might be due to differences in the study design and assessment of anxiety or depressive symptoms. Even though variation existed, in comparison with the Chinese general population, the status of anxiety and depressive symptoms among physicians were significantly higher [30,31].

The mental health of Chinese physicians participating in our study was poorer than that in some other countries. For example, the prevalence of depressive symptoms among physicians in the US, Britain (intensive care unit physicians), Canada, Norway, Japan, and Benin were 11.3%, 12%, 15.5%, 11%, 8.8%, and 14%, respectively [9–14]. The relatively poor mental health status among physicians in China may be attributed to various reasons. The workload of physicians in China continues to increase owing to the aging population, universal health care, and inadequate growth in the number of physicians [32,33]. Additionally, the doctor-patient relationship in China is perceived as unsatisfactory and medical disputes often occur within healthcare facilities [34]. Finally, physicians' income in China is lower than that of physicians in many Western countries, and there exists a mismatch between high workload and relative low reward among physicians in China.

Associated factors of anxiety and depressive symptoms among physicians

The present study indicated that physical health, lifestyles, and work-related conditions are the primary risk factors for anxiety and depressive symptoms among physicians in China. The positive association between physical health and psychological well-being is well documented [35,36]. Moreover, poor self-perceived physical health status has the largest effect on physicians' anxiety and depressive symptoms in our fully adjusted statistical model.

With regards to work-related conditions, workplace violence was a significant predictor of physician's mental health in our fully adjusted model. Physicians who often experienced workplace violence were nearly seven times more likely to be anxious and four times more likely to be depressed compared to those who seldom or never encountered it. Previous studies in Poland and Turkey also demonstrated that workplace violence increases the prevalence of psychological conditions such as anxiety and depression among exposed employees [37,38]. In our study, more than three-quarters of participants sometimes or often encountered workplace violence. Consequently, the doctor-patient relationship should be improved by the implementation of several measures, including introducing and implementing malpractice insurance for physicians and enhancing doctor-patient communication.

Table 2. Logistic regression analysis of anxiety and depressive symptoms with mutually adjusted odds ratios and 95% confidence intervals.

Variables	Anxiety symptoms	Depressive symptoms
Age	1.00 (0.98–1.02)	0.99 (0.98–1.01)
Gender (Ref[a]: Male)		
Female	1.81 (1.37–2.38)***	1.57 (1.21–2.03)***
Education level (Ref: Vocational School or below)		
Bachelor degree	0.92 (0.67–1.27)	1.07 (0.79–1.43)
Post-graduate degree	0.79 (0.52–1.18)	0.84 (0.58–1.23)
Marital status (Ref: Married)		
Single/widow/divorced	0.90 (0.65–1.24)	1.17 (0.88–1.57)
Self-perceived Health Status (Ref: Very good)		
Good	0.90 (0.44–1.86)	1.03 (0.56–1.91)
Fair	2.57 (1.29–5.11)**	2.52 (1.39–4.57)**
Bad/very bad	10.03 (4.87–20.67)***	7.44 (3.95–14.04)***
Job title (Ref: Elementary or less)		
Intermediate	0.85 (0.63–1.16)	1.21 (0.91–1.61)
Senior	0.87 (0.57–1.33)	1.06 (0.71–1.57)
Work department (Ref: Internal medicine)		
Surgery	1.14 (0.77–1.70)	0.98 (0.68–1.42)
Obstetrics and gynecology	1.51 (1.00–2.28)	1.29 (0.88–1.90)
Pediatrics	1.24 (0.77–2.00)	1.26 (0.81–1.97)
Intensive care	1.28 (0.75–2.19)	1.30 (0.79–2.13)
others	1.20 (0.86–1.68)	1.02 (0.75–1.39)
Hospital grade (Ref: 1)		
2	1.04 (0.7–1.53)	0.98 (0.69–1.39)
3	1.2 (0.79–1.82)	0.85 (0.58–1.24)
Frequency of conflicts and violence (Ref: None)		
Sometimes	2.36 (1.67–3.32)***	1.73 (1.29–2.32)***
Often	6.72 (4.38–10.30)***	3.95 (2.69–5.82)***
Working hours/week (Ref: 35–44 hours)		
45–59	1.04 (0.77–1.40)	1.10 (0.83–1.44)
60–69	1.74 (1.24–2.43)**	1.56 (1.14–2.13)**
≥70	1.94 (1.30–2.90)**	1.90 (1.31–2.77)***
Shift work/week (Ref: No)		
1	1.14 (0.85–1.52)	1.27 (0.97–1.66)
≥2	1.52 (1.08–2.14)*	1.40 (1.02–1.93)*
Sleeping (Ref: ≥8 hours)		
6–8	1.76 (1.17–2.66)**	0.99 (0.71–1.37)
<6	2.70 (1.51–4.83)***	1.58 (0.95–2.64)
Physical exercise (Ref: Yes)		
No	1.53 (1.10–2.13)*	1.39 (1.03–1.86)*
Smoking (Ref: No)		
Yes	1.18 (0.86–1.62)	1.57 (1.18–2.09)**

[a]Ref is reference.
*P<0.05;
**P<0.01;
***P<0.0001 (two-tailed test).

Additionally, our results indicated that physicians who work at least 60 hours per week or who work night shifts twice or more per week were at greater risk of experiencing anxiety and depressive symptoms, which confirms the findings of previous studies demonstrating a significant positive association between lengthy working hours or frequent shift work and anxiety or depressive symptoms [39,40]. The documented positive associations between very long working hours (more than 60 hours per week) or too frequent night shifts (twice or more a week) within a short period of time and symptoms of anxiety or depression should be carefully considered by hospital administrators or other parties responsible for scheduling physicians.

Lifestyle parameters, such as physical exercise, smoking, and sleeping, were important risk factors for developing anxiety or depression symptoms [36,41]. Physical exercise serves to restore personal stamina and has been shown to be effective at relieving stress. In addition, there is evidence that regular exercise can improve tolerance towards working shifts, and moderate physical exercise at least three to four hours before sleep is recommended [5,42,43]. Approximately one-fifth of physicians in our study exercised regularly, which is lower than the proportion of the general Chinese population that often performs physical activities (28.2%) [44]. On the basis of our results, we suggest that hospitals provide more support in establishing exercise facilities for healthcare workers and encourage them to get involved in exercise activities.

Our study is consistent with a previous study exploring the associations between smoking and symptoms of anxiety or depression [36]. There is evidence that physicians who are current smokers are more likely to experience fewer anxiety symptoms because nicotine can effectively reduce anxiety episodes [45], but there are no data regarding the association between nicotine and depressive symptoms. Additionally, previous studies have indicated that people with sleeping problems were predisposed to psychological disorders such as depression, anxiety disorder, and suicide attempts [46]. In our study, sleeping time was significantly associated with anxiety symptoms, but physicians with fewer than six hours of sleep per day had a tendency to experience depressive symptoms ($P = 0.08$) [47].

This study has a few limitations that must be acknowledged. First, because this is a cross-sectional study, we cannot establish causality between anxiety or depressive symptoms and their related risk factors. Future longitudinal studies should be conducted to confirm the conclusions from our study. Furthermore, study participants were limited to physicians working in public hospitals in a large city, and the conclusions of this study need to be verified in other areas (e.g., rural areas) and in other types of health facilities (e.g., private clinics) in China. However, our large sample size may increase the validity. Finally, previous studies have shown a moderate correlation between depressive symptoms and occupational burnout [48–50], which renders it difficult to distinguish burnout symptoms from those of depressive symptoms and increases the possibility of overestimation of the prevalence of depressive symptoms among physicians.

Conclusion

We have shown that physicians are at high risk of experiencing anxiety and depressive symptoms. The doctor-patient relationship was a potent source of stress and is strongly associated with physicians' psychological health. Lengthy working hours and frequent night shifts are also risk factors affecting the psychological health of physicians. In addition, the lifestyles of physicians (including physical activity, smoking, and sleep habits) were shown to significantly affect the risk of anxiety and depressive symptoms. Therefore, interventions implemented to minimize workload, improve doctor-patient relationships, and encourage physicians to develop a healthier lifestyle are essential to combat anxiety and depressive symptoms among physicians, which will improve their professional performance and health outcomes.

Acknowledgments

The authors thank the Health, Population and Family Planning Commission of Shenzhen Municipality for supporting. The authors also thank all study participants who have been involved and contributed to the procedure of data collection.

Author Contributions

Conceived and designed the experiments: GAY RSZ YQC ZXL. Analyzed the data: YHG TGH WC XYT XXY. Wrote the paper: YHG TGH HHD.

References

1. Wallace JE (2012) Mental health and stigma in the medical profession. Health (London) 16: 3–18.
2. Arnetz BB (2001) Psychosocial challenges facing physicians of today. Social Science and Medicine 52: 203–213.
3. Tsai YC, Liu CH (2012) Factors and symptoms associated with work stress and health-promoting lifestyles among hospital staff: a pilot study in Taiwan. BMC Health Serv Res 12: 199.
4. Fahrenkopf AM, Sectish TC, Barger LK, Sharek PJ, Lewin D, et al. (2008) Rates of medication errors among depressed and burnt out residents: prospective cohort study. BMJ 336: 488–491.
5. Ahmed-Little Y (2007) Implications of shift work for junior doctors. BMJ 334: 777–778.
6. Landrigan CP, Rothschild JM, Cronin JW, Kaushal R, Burdick E, et al. (2004) Effect of reducing interns' work hours on serious medical errors in intensive care units. New England Journal of Medicine 351: 1838–1848.
7. Lockley SW, Cronin JW, Evans EE, Cade BE, Lee CJ, et al. (2004) Effect of reducing interns' weekly work hours on sleep and attentional failures. New England Journal of Medicine 351: 1829–1837.
8. Devi S (2011) Doctors in distress. Lancet 377: 454–455.
9. Coomber S, Todd C, Park G, Baxter P, Firth-Cozens J, et al. (2002) Stress in UK intensive care unit doctors. British Journal of Anaesthesia 89: 873–881.
10. Lloyd S, Streiner D, Shannon S (1994) Burnout, depression, life and job satisfaction among Canadian emergency physicians. Journal of Emergency Medicine 12: 559–565.
11. Ofili AN, Asuzu MC, Isah EC, Ogbeide O (2004) Job satisfaction and psychological health of doctors at the University of Benin Teaching Hospital. Occup Med (Lond) 54: 400–403.
12. Schwenk TL, Gorenflo DW, Leja LM (2008) A survey on the impact of being depressed on the professional status and mental health care of physicians. Journal of Clinical Psychiatry 69: 617–620.
13. Vaglum P, Falkum E (1999) Self-criticism, dependency and depressive symptoms in a nationwide sample of Norwegian physicians. J Affect Disord 52: 153–159.
14. Wada K, Yoshikawa T, Goto T, Hirai A, Matsushima E, et al. (2011) Association of depression and suicidal ideation with unreasonable patient demands and complaints among Japanese physicians: a national cross-sectional survey. Int J Behav Med 18: 384–390.
15. Ruitenburg MM, Frings-Dresen MH, Sluiter JK (2012) The prevalence of common mental disorders among hospital physicians and their association with self-reported work ability: a cross-sectional study. BMC Health Serv Res 12: 292–298.
16. Li J, Yang W, Cho SI (2006) Gender differences in job strain, effort-reward imbalance, and health functioning among Chinese physicians. Social Science and Medicine 62: 1066–1077.
17. Shen LL, Lao LM, Jiang SF, Yang H, Ren LM, et al. (2012) A survey of anxiety and depression symptoms among primary-care physicians in China. Int J Psychiatry Med 44: 257–270.
18. Sun W, Fu J, Chang Y, Wang L (2012) Epidemiological study on risk factors for anxiety disorder among Chinese doctors. J Occup Health 54: 1–8.
19. Wang, Sun W, Chi TS, Wu H, Wang L (2010) Prevalence and associated factors of depressive symptoms among Chinese doctors: a cross-sectional survey. Int Arch Occup Environ Health 83: 905–911.
20. Donisi V, Tedeschi F, Percudani M, Fiorillo A, Confalonieri L, et al. (2013) Prediction of community mental health service utilization by individual and ecological level socio-economic factors. Psychiatry Research.

21. Amaddeo F, Jones J (2007) What is the impact of socio-economic inequalities on the use of mental health services? Epidemiologia e Psichiatria Sociale 16: 16–19.
22. Russell GF, De Silva P (1983) Observations on the relationship between anxiety and depressive symptoms during the course of depressive illnesses. British Journal of Clinical Pharmacology 15 Suppl 2: 147S–153S.
23. Zung WW (1965) A self-rating depression scale. Arch Gen Psychiatry 12: 63–70.
24. Zung WW (1971) A rating instrument for anxiety disorders. Psychosomatics 12: 371–379.
25. Liu Y, Maier M, Hao Y, Chen Y, Qin Y, et al. (2013) Factors related to quality of life for patients with type 2 diabetes with or without depressive symptoms - results from a community-based study in China. J Clin Nurs 22: 80–88.
26. Kong LP, Cui Y, Qiu YF, Han SP, Yu ZB, et al. (2013) Anxiety and depression in parents of sick neonates: a hospital-based study. J Clin Nurs 22: 1163–1172.
27. Wang Chi (1984) Self-rating depression scale (SDS). Shanghai Archives of Psychiatry (in Chinese): 71–72.
28. Wang Chi (1984) Self-rating anxiety scale (SAS). Shanghai Archives of Psychiatry (in Chinese): 73–74.
29. Shrive FM, Stuart H, Quan H, Ghali WA (2006) Dealing with missing data in a multi-question depression scale: a comparison of imputation methods. BMC Med Res Methodol 6: 57.
30. Wang, Fang P, Fu X, Chen J (2012) Epidemilogy of anxiety disorder among urban residents and their attitudes toward utilization of mental care service in central China. Medicine and Society (in Chinese) 25: 74–76.
31. Zhu DF, Xu SY, Yang Q, Wu QQ, Wang L, et al. (2010) Prevalence of anxiety and depressive symptoms and their influencing factors among urban residents of Zhejiang province. Chin J Public Health (in Chinese) 26: 429–431.
32. Liu Y, Rao K, Wu J, Gakidou E (2008) China's health system performance. Lancet 372: 1914–1923.
33. National Health and Family Planning Commission of the People's Republic of China (2012) Statistics Bulletin of Development of Health Service in China, 2008–2011 (in Chinese). Available from: http://www.moh.gov.cn/zwgkzt/pgb/list.shtml. Accessed 29 April 2012.
34. Zhao M (2011) Evaluation of the third-party mediation mechanism for medical disputes in China. Medicine and Law 30: 401–415.
35. Osborn DP, Fletcher AE, Smeeth L, Stirling S, Bulpitt CJ, et al. (2003) Factors associated with depression in a representative sample of 14 217 people aged 75 and over in the United Kingdom: results from the MRC trial of assessment and management of older people in the community. Int J Geriatr Psychiatry 18: 623–630.
36. Averina M, Nilssen O, Brenn T, Brox J, Arkhipovsky VL, et al. (2005) Social and lifestyle determinants of depression, anxiety, sleeping disorders and self-evaluated quality of life in Russia–a population-based study in Arkhangelsk. Soc Psychiatry Psychiatr Epidemiol 40: 511–518.
37. Aytac S, Dursun S (2012) The effect on employees of violence climate in the workplace. Work 41 Suppl 1: 3026–3031.
38. Merecz D, Drabek M, Moscicka A (2009) Aggression at the workplace–psychological consequences of abusive encounter with coworkers and clients. International Journal of Occupational Medicine and Environme tal Health 22: 243–260.
39. Virtanen M, Kivimaki M (2012) Saved by the bell: does working too much increase the likelihood of depression? Expert Rev Neurother 12: 497–499.
40. Bannai A, Tamakoshi A (2014) The association between long working hours and health: a systematic review of epidemiological evidence. Scandinavian Journal of Work, Environment and Health 40: 5–18.
41. Henwood T, Tuckett A, Turner C (2012) What makes a healthier nurse, workplace or leisure physical activity? Informed by the Australian and New Zealand e-Cohort Study. J Clin Nurs 21: 1746–1754.
42. Costa G (2003) Factors influencing health of workers and tolerance to shift work. Theoretical Issues in Ergonomics Science 4: 263–288.
43. Harma M (1996) Ageing, physical fitness and shiftwork intolerance. Appl Ergon 27: 25–29.
44. General Administration of Sport of China (2008) Bulletin of the status of physical exercise in China in 2007. Available: http://www.sport.gov.cn/n16/n33193/n33208/n33418/n33598/1010427.html. Accessed 29 December 2012.
45. Pomerleau OF, Pomerleau CS (1990) Behavioural studies in humans: anxiety, stress and smoking. Ciba Foundation Symposium 152: 225–235; discussion 235–229.
46. Ribeiro JD, Pease JL, Gutierrez PM, Silva C, Bernert RA, et al. (2012) Sleep problems outperform depression and hopelessness as cross-sectional and longitudinal predictors of suicidal ideation and behavior in young adults in the military. Journal of Affective Disorders 136: 743–750.
47. Takahashi M, Iwasaki K, Sasaki T, Kubo T, Mori I, et al. (2012) Sleep, fatigue, recovery, and depression after change in work time control: a one-year follow-up study. Journal of Occupational and Environmental Medicine 54: 1078–1085.
48. McKnight JD, Glass DC (1995) Perceptions of control, burnout, and depressive symptomatology: a replication and extension. Journal of Consulting and Clinical Psychology 63: 490–494.
49. Iacovides A, Fountoulakis KN, Kaprinis S, Kaprinis G (2003) The relationship between job stress, burnout and clinical depression. Journal of Affective Disorders 75: 209–221.
50. Glass DC, McKnight JD, Valdimarsdottir H (1993) Depression, burnout, and perceptions of control in hospital nurses. Journal of Consulting and Clinical Psychology 61: 147–155.

23

Personnel and Participant Experiences of a Residential Weight-Loss Program

Unni Dahl[1,2], Marit By Rise[2]*, Bård Kulseng[3], Aslak Steinsbekk[2]

1 Central Norway Health Authority, Stjørdal, Norway, **2** Department of Public Health and General Practice, Norwegian University of Science and Technology, Trondheim, Norway, **3** Regional Centre for Obesity Treatment, St. Olav's University Hospital, Trondheim, Norway

Abstract

Background: Residential weight-loss programs aim to help persons with obesity lose weight and maintain a long-term healthy lifestyle. Knowledge is needed on the different actors' perceptions and experiences from such programs. The aim of this study was to describe how personnel argued for and perceived a residential weight-loss program, to investigate how the participants experienced the program, and to contrast these perspectives.

Methods: This qualitative study took place in an 18-week residential weight-loss program. Exercise, diet, and personal development were the main components in the program. Data was collected through participant observation and individual and focus group interviews with participants and personnel.

Results: Program personnel characterized persons with obesity in specific terms, and these formed the basis of the educational aims, teaching principles, and content of the program. According to personnel, persons with obesity typically had problems acknowledging their own resources, lived unstructured lives, had a distorted relationship to food, experienced a range of social problems and featured a lack of personal insight. Program participants reported enthusiasm about their experiences of exercise and appreciated measures of success with the exercise program. They had, however, very different experiences regarding the usefulness and appropriateness of the parts of the program focused on social and personal development. Some felt that weight loss required an engagement with personal development while others viewed it as unnecessary and inappropriate.

Conclusion: The reliance in personnel accounts on particular characteristics of persons with obesity as a rationale for the program might lead to stigmatizing and stereotyping. Program activities focused on social and personal development need to be better understood by participants if they are to be viewed as helpful. To achieve this personnel must carefully consider how these parts of the program are communicated and conducted.

Editor: Christy Elizabeth Newman, The University of New South Wales, Australia

Funding: The authors have no support or funding to report.

Competing Interests: The authors have declared that no competing interests exist.

* E-mail: marit.b.rise@ntnu.no

Introduction

Obesity is a growing problem in the Western world [1], and many diseases and illnesses accompany it [2,3]. Recently surgery has become more common to achieve weight-loss. A new systematic review and meta-analysis on the outcomes and risks of bariatric surgery showed that surgery was more effective than non-surgical interventions regarding weight-loss [4]. Although risks of complications exist, death rates were lower than in previous meta-analyses. Meta-analysis of observational studies also indicates that bariatric surgery might lead to a reduced risk of cardiovascular disease and mortality for persons with obesity [5], but this has yet to be investigated in clinical trials. Martins and colleagues compared bariatric surgery to three conservative treatments - including the weight-loss camp that served as the setting for this qualitative study [6]. They found that although all treatments led to significant weight-loss, patients who had undergone bariatric surgery had lost significantly more weight one year after the interventions.

Although weight-loss surgery is increasingly used, the combination of exercise, diet, and behaviour therapy in comprehensive weight-loss programs seems to be the most commonly available intervention [7,8]. Although many clinical studies of weight-loss programs show that the participants lose weight during and after the intervention [9–13], some authors have stated that non-surgical treatments of obesity are generally ineffective in long-term weight-control [4]. One study investigating the long-term maintenance of weight-loss after an extensive lifestyle intervention - at the weight-loss camp investigated in the qualitative study presented here - showed for example that a 15% weight reduction after the intervention was reduced to 5.3% reduction of the initial body weight 2–4 years afterwards [12]. Thus, one of the main challenges in weight-loss programs is to achieve long-term sustainable changes.

Soderlund and colleagues [8] conducted a systematic review of randomized controlled trials investigating long-term effects of physical exercise with or without behavior-change therapy and/or dieting. The authors conclude that the programs with the best results involve different professional groups, and include a combination of diet, behavioral-modification therapy, and exercise. Other studies have also shown that adding exercise or behavior therapy to diet improved weight-loss and reduced the health risk factors connected to obesity [9,11,14].

Weight-loss programs thus aim to help the participants modify their health behaviors. The main argument for residential programs is to fortify a sustainable long-term lifestyle change. Residential weight-loss programs constitute a rather new approach [7], and research on the effects of such programs on adults is scarce [15]. Weight-loss programs include behaviour therapies that aims to help the participants achieve the necessary skills to reach a more healthy weight [16]. Lifestyle interventions usually include many behavioural techniques such as self-monitoring, modelling, environmental restructuring, and support, both in groups and individually [13]. Other central terms are self-regulation, goal setting, and problem solving [17,18]. This makes it difficult to recognize the particular elements which might be supporting learning and behavioural changes. In addition, most behaviour therapy interventions are poorly defined and described in the literature [8]. Many authors have emphasized that interventions in general often are implemented without a deep understanding of how different initiatives are supposed to lead to change [19]. More detailed knowledge about the content of weight-loss programs is therefore required, as well as a deeper understanding of what really happens in lifestyle interventions for persons with obesity.

A residential program differs from out-patient intervention by length and intensity, and in that the participants are removed from their everyday lives. A residential program also offers more time for communication between participants and personnel [20]. Therefore, residential weight-loss programs are arenas for close interaction between participants and personnel, and with a broad range of opportunities provided for personnel to teach and support participants in their endeavour to change behaviour. Although lifestyle-modification programs often combine exercise, diet and behaviour change activities, a good relationship that allows for open communication is generally recommended [21]. Several have also emphasized the importance of motivation to make lifestyle changes [8,17,18]. Since motivation to alter lifestyle is crucial to achieve long-term changes, support and help from personnel during such programs would be important [8]. Many have argued that personnel skills and attitudes should be characterized by trust, respect and acceptance when caring for persons with chronic diseases [22,23]. Respect has been described as unconditionally recognizing the patient as a valuable person, and as an integral part of health professionals' work [24].

Very little research has explored different actors' perceptions of and experiences from weight-loss programs. It has been emphasized that to achieve good results different stakeholders in an intervention should share an understanding of how change is supposed to be implemented and sustained [25]. Including both personnel and participants in the same study would contribute to the understanding of the stakeholders' rationale for an intervention, as well as their views on potential outcome. Therefore, the aim of this study was to describe how personnel argued for and perceived a residential weight-loss program, to investigate how the participants experienced the program, and to contrast these perspectives.

Methods

Ethics Statement

The Regional Ethics Committee for Research in Medicine in Central Norway approved of the study. All participants received oral and written information about the study and signed a written consent form. None of the authors have any contact with or interest in the Danish weight-loss camp outside this research project.

Design

This was a qualitative study consisting of on-site participant observation, in-depth semi-structured individual interviews, and focus group interviews. A combination of methods was chosen to ensure data triangulation. Observation was chosen to provide data on real life interaction between participants and personnel and to gain insight into the participants' immediate reactions to the program. Focus group interviews were conducted to explore the interaction and discussions between participants regarding their experiences and views of the program. Individual interviews were also employed to explore in more depth the ways in which personnel articulated their arguments for and experiences of providing the program, and to delve deeper into the individual experiences of a selected subset of participants.

The study formed part of a Norwegian clinical investigation on the effectiveness of different interventions (weight-loss program versus surgery) for persons with obesity. The study was registered in Clinicaltrials.gov with registration number NCT00239850. An effect study from this program is published elsewhere [6].

Setting

The study took place at a Danish residential weight-loss centre (Ebeltoft kurcenter), which offers an 18-week on-site program. A total of 80 participants were at the centre at the time of the data collection. This study focused on 30 participants who were referred to this program due to taking part in a Norwegian study on the effect of different weight-loss approaches [6].

Most of the activities at the centre were organized and conducted in groups. The program consisted of group-based intensive exercise, diet (individual calorie intake was based on energy calculations for a normal weight person with a sedentary activity level), and an educational program. Structured group exercise and educational sessions took place from Monday to Friday every week. Exercise was compulsory three times per day. Typical exercise activities were badminton, ball games, aerobics, and swimming. In addition, participants were encouraged to be physically active on their own. Program participants were advised to start on an individually suitable exercise level and to focus on the activities that they liked the most.

Participants lived together in groups in small houses with sleeping and cooking facilities, and they cooked their own dinners with provided groceries. Breakfast, lunch, and in-between meals were served in a buffet. The different types of food were marked with labels of energy content. The diet contained 55–60% carbohydrates, 15% protein, and less than 30% fat. At the beginning of the program, each participant learned to calculate their energy intake by counting calories and weighing the food. If necessary, diet plans were adjusted individually according to weight measurements during the program.

The educational program comprised lessons about nutrition, monitoring of food intake and instruction in behavioral techniques from cognitive therapy. The personal development component included a minimum of two individual conversations with one of the psychotherapists, motivational meetings for all participants, and "family meetings" (for all residents in each house) to discuss and resolve problems regarding the living arrangements. In addition, mandatory group therapy classes in personal development were held one hour per week. Classes in personal development were led by a psychotherapist. The goals of this component of the program were to gain insight into personal problems and to consider how these problems may be associated with the obesity. The overall aim of the personal development component was to help the participants live a mentally healthy life as an important part of the process of lifestyle change.

Participants and Personnel

The participants in this qualitative study also participated in a clinical study investigating the effect of different types of weight-loss interventions, including a stay at the residential weight-loss centre [6]. A total of 30 (21 female and 9 male) Norwegian participants took part and stayed at the centre. These participants were between 22 and 56 years old, their body mass index was between 40 and 63, and the group's mean body weight was 144 kg. All those who were referred to the program from Norway also participated in a Norwegian effect study [6] in addition to this qualitative study. The inclusion criteria for the effect study were ages between 18 and 60 years old and a BMI over 40 kg/m^2 or a BMI over 35 kg/m^2 including comorbidities. There were no additional inclusion criteria for the qualitative study.

The personnel were recruited among the staff at the centre. Since an important aim was to explore the rationale for the choice of program content and structure, key personnel with responsibility for providing the program were recruited to individual interviews.

Data Collection

For the purpose of achieving immersion in the field of inquiry, the first author (UD) took part in the program over the three week period and observed and interviewed personnel and participants. A data collection period was predefined to two periods totaling to three weeks and was conducted during the 1st, 2nd, and 14th weeks of the 18-week program. These weeks were chosen to ensure that the initial expectations and experiences (the first two weeks), as well as the experiences from most of the stay (week 14), were captured. During this period, thematic saturation was reached, and no new experiences, discussions, or perceptions emerged in the last interviews or observation.

Observation. The first author (UD) participated in all activities as an ordinary participant during the three weeks of data collection, that is, she took part in exercise, classes, and social life. The participants were informed before arrival at the weight-loss camp that the researcher would be present during some of the program, and that this was a part of the larger research project. This period of overt participant observation provided an opportunity to observe real life settings and the interaction between personnel and participants. It also provided insights that were used to inform the development of the question guide that was subsequently used in the focus groups and interviews. The observation also involved informal conversations between the researcher and those personnel and participants who did not later participate in interviews. Field notes were written during observation and at the end of every day. Summaries were developed at several points during the three weeks of data collection. Video and audio recording was not used during observation. The field notes were used to record facts about the program and to write reflections during observations and interviews. Field notes were also used as background for focus group interviews and were later compared with the interview transcripts.

Interviews. Those who took part in interviews were asked directly by the first author (UD) and all agreed to participate. A total of 10 Norwegian participants took part in interviews (8 in focus groups and 2 individually). The age and weight range for these 10 persons were the same as for the total sample. Six personnel participated in individual interviews. All interviews were conducted by the first author (UD).

Semi-structured interview guides were employed during focus groups and individual interviews. The guides were used as a memo list to ensure that all the topics were covered in all interviews. The interviewer introduced themes from the interview guide if the participants did not spontaneously talk about them. The participants were also free to talk about issues and topics outside the guide. The main opening question in all interviews was "What are your experiences with taking part in/providing this program?" Additionally, the personnel were asked to describe the content of the program and the rationale for it. Other important topics in interviews with personnel were how personnel attitudes might influence the participants, and how they motivated persons with obesity to change their life-styles.

Each interview lasted from 45 to 90 minutes and was audio taped. All interviews were subsequently transcribed verbatim and de-identified. Redundant words and pauses were removed, and local dialect was changed to written Norwegian.

A strategic sample of eight of the participants, three men and five women, were recruited to focus group interviews. The sampling strategy aimed to achieve some variation in experiences, BMI, age and gender. Focus group participants were interviewed two times, in the 1st and the 14th weeks of the program. The topics discussed in the first interview were immediate perceptions and experiences with the program: overall setting, exercise, living arrangements, and food. The second interviews focused more on the positive and negative experiences that participants reported of the program.

Two female participants were interviewed individually in depth in the first and second weeks of the program. The interviews were conducted to elaborate on specific issues discussed in the focus group interviews. The two participants were selected based on observations of their role in the group of Norwegian participants. During interactions and discussions they had expressed clear views and had provided rich descriptions that offered the potential for meaningful further exploration of key topics in a one-on-one interview. Topics discussed in these interviews included how to make sustainable lifestyle changes, overall approach to weight-loss, and collaboration between the personnel.

Six personnel (2 males and 4 females) took part in individual in-depth interviews. These were considered to be key personnel; the director, the administrative executive, and the leaders of the main areas diet, exercise and personal development. The personnel were selected because they strongly influenced the content and form of the program. Five personnel were interviewed during the first and second weeks. In week 14, three of these were interviewed a second time. In addition, one substitute personnel member was added in week 14 since one of the members had a leave of absence. The second interviews were done to elaborate on the topics discussed in the first interview, and to discuss personnel experiences with the current class of participants.

Data Analysis

Interview transcripts and fields notes were analysed together. The focus of the analysis was to explore the connections between the personnel rationale for the program and the participant experiences of the program. The analysis was inductive and thematically based. The interview transcripts and field notes were read and the main themes generated. The first and fourth author (UD and AS) read all transcripts and made separate analyses. These analyses were subsequently discussed in a group including the third author (BK), and finally with the second author to get a different point of view and to look for alternative interpretations. It was observed that the personnel articulated several recurrent descriptions or characterisations of people with obesity. These perceptions were described by personnel as forming the basis of the rationale for the program, and so perceptions were employed as a coding structure to categorise and interpret the findings. The validity of the results was cross-checked by re-reading the interviews. To illustrate the main themes the most illustrative and comprehensive quotes were chosen. Quotes were translated from Norwegian to English by the first (UD) and second author (MR) and controlled by the fourth author (AS). Quotes from participants used in the result presentation are identified by interview number and gender. Quotes from personnel are not identified to ensure anonymity.

Results and Discussion

A total of 10 participants and six personnel participated in interviews. In addition, observation included 30 participants and approximately 10 personnel.

During the analysis of data from interviews and observations, it became clear that there were important differences between how the personnel and participants experienced and perceived the purpose and activities of the weight-loss program. The personnel were very consistent in their perceptions, while the participant experiences and reactions were more diverse. Personnel described very similar rationales for the aims of the program, and for the content and teaching principles used to achieve these aims. Participants had, on the other hand, experiences that ranged from joy and excitement to feeling the program was a struggle and waste of time.

During the analysis, the personnel rationale for the program was categorised into five recurrent themes in their characterization of people with obesity: lack of acknowledgement of resources, lack of structure, a distorted relationship to food, social problems, and lack of personal insight. The program was seen to be intended to change these five characterisations, and the program content and teaching principles were selected deliberately in order to achieve these changes. However, interviews and observation both revealed that participants viewed the program content very differently to the personnel. All participants were very enthusiastic about the exercise program and complied with the strict structures and routines involved in the exercise and diet program. The participants were, however, divided on the usefulness of the parts of the program concerning social and personal development. Division was particularly strong on the usefulness and necessity of the personal development classes.

In the following section, the five characterisations of participants that personnel believed had to be changed in order for participants to achieve and maintain weight-loss, are discussed in more detail. Quotes that describe participant experiences and reactions to the program content are woven into these sections in order to be contrasted with personnel views. Quotes from personnel and participants are used to illustrate and support the findings.

1. Lack of Acknowledgement of Resources

The first characterisation ascribed to participants by personnel was the perceived lack of acknowledgement of their own resources in being physically active and sticking to a diet. This was said to be due mainly to low self-efficacy beliefs and low self-confidence. Personnel emphasised the importance of strengthening participants' self-confidence by ensuring experiences of success in their efforts to exercise and eat properly during the program. Personnel thus highlighted the importance of compulsory and regular exercise and of setting achievable goals.

> *The participants shall first and foremost get confirmation that they can do a hundred times more than they believe they can.* [...] *It is about transferring the joy of success from one situation to another.* (Personnel).

Participants confirmed this practice by reporting that even small efforts were praised regularly by personnel, and that personnel also frequently encouraged participants individually during group exercise. This was also confirmed during observation. In the interviews, participants confirmed that personnel supported and respected them. This attitude was described as strengthening their motivation, self-confidence, and sense of self-worth.

> *That is how they* [the personnel] *build our self-confidence. We are all of a sudden humans again and not just the chubby clown.* (Female, first focus group interview).

When it came to the exercise part of the program participants confirmed personnel claims that success experiences encouraged participants to keep working towards weight-loss. The positive experience of exercise was highlighted both in the observation and interviews from the beginning, and was in fact the most striking finding of the research. The participants were enthusiastic about learning and managing new activities, or activities that they had not engaged in for years or had never tried before. They were also very enthusiastic about improving their physical condition and achieving new goals.

> *My first victory* [...] *was that I managed to ride a bike for 15 kilometres. I think I walked on air for four days after that experience.* (Female, second focus group interview).

This attitude towards exercise remained stable through the program. In the 14th week of the program, participants unanimously agreed that exercise was fun, increased their energy, and instilled in them a desire to be active in the future.

2. Lack of Structure

The second characterisation that personnel attributed to persons with obesity was that they generally lead unstructured lives. Personnel reported a belief that many things in obese persons' lives were seen to happen by chance, such as when and what to eat, and what activities to engage in.

> *Our experience is that many obese people are incredibly unstructured and live extremely unstructured lives. Such as keeping appointments and being stringent and sharp in the things you do.* (Personnel).

According to the personnel, the program schedule had to be very strict. They described that their strictness was important to provide the participants with a daily structure that they could then seek to maintain at home.

And those who succeed, those we know maintain their weight-loss... they are those who have a structured life afterwards. Those who eat at fixed times and who get out of bed at approximately the same time each day, and those who know what they want with themselves. (Personnel).

This strict structure was evident across all program activities. All participants had to be present at the morning meetings, group exercises, and at six meals every day (at fixed hours). Other activities, like teaching classes and the weekly weighting, were also scheduled. According to the participants, adhering to the structure was an effort they felt they had to do to comply with the program. Although there were several who compared the program to military training and being back at school with very little freedom, both observation and interviews showed that the participants all agreed that a strict schedule was appropriate to initiate lifestyle change.

You are supposed to learn some things while you are here. It is like school... subjects are mandatory. And when you know that you have to be ticked off on a list to be registered [by an employee] *you show up. There's no alternative. And if it hadn't been like that the activity would not have been very great. If you are not there at eight o'clock in the morning they call you and ask: "Where are you?"* (Female, Individual interview).

3. Distorted Relationship to Food

The third characterisation articulated by personnel proposed that people with obesity have a distorted relationship to food.

Those with a really high BMI have a behaviour that fully can be compared with an alcoholic or a drug addict. They have no control over food. They always have their form of drug lying around in small storages on secret places so they always know that they are close to the food and they become insecure if it is not in the house. (Personnel)

According to the personnel, most persons with obesity were addicted to food and would have to live with an eating disorder for the rest of their lives. The program was designed to give the participants the practical experience of eating like a standard weight person and, through that, to change their relationship towards food.

I tell the participants that they all have a normal weight person inside. They shall hold on to this person and from now on leave the decisions to the standard weight person. [...] *This is not a treatment; it is four months of practice in living as a standard weight person.* (Personnel).

In the beginning of the program, it was observed that participants talked a lot about how to manage the new diet chart, frequency of eating and the amount of food, and the result of their latest weighing. Although there was a consensus among participants about the necessity of managing new eating habits, the experience of enthusiasm and success were less apparent in discussions about diet than about the exercise program. The participants expressed the belief that changing eating habits and adhering to the diet regime was laborious. At the end of the program this was, however, a theme the participants talked less about. When asked, the participants said that following a diet plan had become an automatic behaviour.

In the beginning I was strictly adhering to the written diet chart, but now I have noticed that I am composing the diet based on my energy target. (Female, second focus group interview).

4. Social Problems

The fourth characterisation of people with obesity highlighted by personnel was a belief that they often have poor social skills. Personnel expressed that persons with obesity often had felt like an outsider and therefore had adopted unfavourable approaches to handle this. Examples of approaches mentioned by the personnel were taking on the comedian role, social isolation, avoiding conflict, and not recognizing or acknowledging their own needs. The housing structure during the program, in which people share apartments and house work and cooking takes place in groups, was deliberately chosen to give the participants practice in socializing with other people.

Quite a few experience social isolation. So groups are a way to get out of isolation and learn to associate with others. (Personnel).

The main approach to managing conflict between participants was in line with this focus on social training. Personnel facilitated problem-solving techniques by asking participants what they believed they could do themselves. According to the personnel, this was intended to assist participants with focusing their skills and abilities.

If two persons share a flat and have different habits... If one of them stays up at night to watch TV and the other person wants to sleep but can't. Then one is forced to say: "Do you know what, I need to sleep. Could you be so kind as to turn off the TV?" [...] *Then there are two people learning. One is the person who gets the message and the other is the person giving the message. They both learn how it is to enter a conflict.* (Personnel).

The participants had different experiences with the social development component of the program. Some participants described that living closely together was a very positive experience and that they had made friends for life. Others described it as challenging and difficult, and said that they hardly talked with the other participants in their group.

They have strong emphasis on the mental part, and it is very important... and I feel that I have come a long way [...] *and at the same time... I don't want to participate so much because... well, there is a lot of gossip here. And if you open up with sensitive stuff you cannot be sure whether it is on every corner afterwards. So I have... I told them* [the personnel] *that this was my decision, and it was fine. This part of the program should have been different. I don't think all will benefit from it.* (Female, second focus group interview).

5. Lack of Personal Insight

The fifth characterisation described by personnel asserted that persons with obesity lack insight into their personal problems. Personnel expressed the belief that lifestyle change require a development in personal insight, and that participants have to reflect on their own behaviour to achieve this. Therefore, the program included classes in personal development. During these group classes, participants were urged to identify underlying factors that may have influenced their obesity problem, such as family relations, working conditions, or economic contexts. The personnel believed such personal development was crucial to enable participants to implement and maintain lifestyle changes.

> *It is important that they become aware of what in their life makes a difference in being obese or not. They have some enemies out there and some accomplices* [...] *Not only persons... it might also be their work. But to get control over them you first have to be conscious of what they are.* (Personnel).

The participants were clearly divided in their perceptions of the usefulness of the personal development program and views on whether personal development classes should be compulsory. Some strongly disagreed, while others shared personnel views about the importance of personal development. Some participants even asked for more individual sessions with the psychotherapists.

> *I think we get tools to gain self-insight and retrieve things we have forgotten... also things that you might not want to touch.* [...] *And suddenly* [...] *you have changed as a person. And you experience things and perceive things quite differently and you get a different outlook in life.* (Female, second focus group interview).

Other participants saw losing weight, not as a matter of personal development and psychological factors, but rather as a matter of changing bad habits - to eat less and exercise more. These participants were more likely to avoid or refuse to engage in the process of identifying any underlying factors, either by not attending the personal development classes, or by not participating in the discussions during class.

> *It is about the personal* [development] *part... I cannot benefit from it. I will never open up in that room and talk among the others. I will not do that.* (Male, second focus group interview).

According to the personnel, those who withdrew from classes or discussions were the persons most in need of attending. Personnel expressed the belief that they were prepared for the type of conflicts that arose, e.g., participants not showing up to classes due to feeling alienated from the content. Personnel explanations of this type of reaction drew on their understandings of some of the potential mechanisms underlying obesity, such as having an eating disorder or a lack of self-insight.

> *There are some who do not want to attend our classes. There are some who do anything to avoid them. But they are mandatory. And this is because sometimes you have to hear things more than once before it sticks* [...]. *Those who do not bother to attend the lessons are often those who need it the most.* (Personnel).

Personnel perceptions of persons with obesity as persons in need of insight and personal development were noticed by the participants. Some of the participants expressed the view that these generalised characterisations were demeaning, and explained that this could make them feel misunderstood and not treated as individuals.

> *...they talk to us like we are all the same.* [...] *As if we are flawed.* [...] *And as if we all have the same problems."* (Male, second focus group interview).

Discussion of Results

According to the participants, the best part of the program was the strict and intensive exercise regime, which was overwhelmingly embraced. Here, the participants and personnel also interacted without any noteworthy conflicts. The participants were very enthusiastic, and the major reason for this was in accordance with the personnel rationale for the program: the experience of success. Experiencing success to strengthen self-confidence and self-efficacy is a well-known approach [26], and such experiences are also recommended to give persons with obesity faith in their own capacity to make healthier choices [27]. Experiencing self-efficacy regarding exercise has also been shown to increase success when trying to lose weight [28]. Experiences of receiving support from personnel were also highlighted by the participants. This is in line with previous findings in which support and encouragement from personnel have been described by persons with obesity as important facilitators for change [29,30].

The rationale of the program was explained and justified in personnel accounts by articulating a series of claims about the most common characteristics of persons with obesity. The personnel viewed this population as typically resourceful, even if people with obesity didn't always find this easy to acknowledge themselves, and also lacking in structure, social skills, and personal insight. It was a clear finding that the stereotyping helped the personnel build a joint understanding among themselves regarding both the objectives of and activities in the program. Stereotypes also seemed to help the personnel to remain focused and firm during the program. There are some similarities between the personnel views and the negative attitudes and stigmas that persons with obesity are likely to experience both in society and among health care professionals [31,32]. Some of the more typical obesity-related stigmas are laziness, non-compliance, and being more overindulgent and less successful than persons without obesity [31,32]. Persons with obesity have reported experiences of stigmatization on a regular basis, and even more so for those most obese [33]. Inappropriate comments from doctors are in fact among the most common stigmatizing experiences for persons with obesity [34]. Health personnel also attribute obesity to negative characteristics, such as a lack of willpower, sloppiness and laziness [35], lack of discipline, lack of motivation, denial of eating wrongly, and psychological problems [36].

Personnel attitudes observed in the present study might be in conflict with the ideal of building a relationship of trust and acceptance [22]. It would be problematic if the very common negative attitudes towards persons with obesity [33,34,37,38] also exist among the professionals who are supposed to help and support. It is also reasonable to believe that if the personnel perceptions border on stigmatizing, the result for participants will be poor. Obesity stigma has, for instance, been found to negatively influence the motivation to exercise [37] and to increase consumption of calories [34,39]. Therefore, stigma will most likely not be a facilitator for weight-loss. Personnel in this study are thus likely to walk on a very fine line in perpetuating these ideas for the purpose of supporting participants. One the one hand, it was found that their rationale for the program resembles the same topics as is noticed in the literature on stigma. On the other hand, it was found both in the observation and interviews that the participants for the most part felt that personnel respected them. Therefore, a very clear awareness among personnel also, or especially, at residential weight-loss centres is needed.

According to the personnel in this study, characteristics of persons with obesity were also described as the reasons for being obese, and changing these characteristics was described as a potential way towards a healthier lifestyle. Some studies have shown that persons with obesity agree that determination, commitment, and discipline are necessary to change diet and exercise [29]. To maintain weight-loss, attitudes have been described as important [40], for instance, taking responsibility for one's life, caring about appearance, self-confidence, and believing that success is possible. Maintaining weight-loss has also been linked to determination, commitment, and patience [41]. Persons with obesity have also confirmed that eating habits can be linked to sadness, lack of motivation, lack of control [29], and negative emotions [42], and obesity has been connected to depression and mood disorders [40]. The mandatory social training in the housing arrangement and the personal development classes in the program were meant to help strengthen participants' social skills and increase their personal insight. The results showed, however, that some of the participants strongly disagreed with personnel on the usefulness and appropriateness of this approach, especially the personal development classes. Personnel did not see the resistance and objections from some of the participants as an indication that they should rethink and revise the program. Neither did they see the reactions as relating to their own attitudes, but rather as a confirmation that personal development was needed.

Most agree that making changes in exercise and diet is essential to losing weight. The idea that personal development is important to achieve and maintain weight-loss is less well recognised or understood. Claiming that a person with obesity has to change internal factors such as self-knowledge and self-acceptance is also a more sensitive topic than claiming that more exercise and healthy food is necessary to lose weight. Yet personnel argued consistently that personal development was especially important to maintaining lifestyle changes long-term. Studies have also confirmed that knowledge about how to eat healthy is not always sufficient to be able to change eating behaviours long-term [42]. A possible explanation for the participant responses to the different parts of the program could be the length of time between taking part in an activity to experiencing results [43]. While the exercise gave almost immediate results and experiences of success, the area of personal development, with its focus on increasing self-insight to prepare for a lasting lifestyle change, can be seen as more abstract and remote. A focus on the positive outcomes from lifestyle changes are important [44], and the reward for strengthening social skills and gaining personal insight can appear too distant and indistinct.

It could also be important to discuss the criteria of success in weight-loss programs. While successful obesity treatment can be related to absolute weight-loss, another main focus could be to reduce the risk of cardiovascular and metabolic diseases [7]. Although successful long-term weight-loss has been defined as losing 10% of initial weight and maintaining this for one year or more [45], studies have shown that even modest weight-loss can improve psychosocial problems [40]. In addition, moderate changes and the experience of success can motivate persons with obesity to maintain lifestyle changes [46]. This was confirmed by the participants in the present study. Research has, however, also shown that persons with obesity tend to choose immediate rewards over long term benefits [47], and they tend to overestimate the reward from the immediate fulfilment of a need [48]. To wait for long-term reward can be extra challenging, and the connection between the input (personal development classes) and output (weight-loss) would be more challenging, yet imperative, to communicate.

Strengths and Limitations

The strength of this study is that it is the first to explore and contrast personnel and participant perspectives in a residential weight-loss program that has been reported to be successful [12]. The program has been developed and modified over time according to experiences made in a real-world setting [16]. There are, however, some limitations. The observation took place in 3 out of 18 weeks. A somewhat different picture might have emerged if the whole length of the program had been observed.

The interviews partially revealed situations that were not observed, and in our judgement, we achieved a good overview of the main picture through quite extensive observation and long interviews. However, this study only collected data from a limited group of participants in this program. Although the personnel confirmed that the participants taking part in this study did not differ substantially from other groups, the results could have been different if a different group was studied.

Conclusion

Personnel characterisation of persons with obesity as a rationale for the design and delivery of a weight-loss program could lead to stigmatizing and discrimination, and thereby less adherence to the program. Participants embraced and adapted to the exercise part of the program. However, the personnel claim that social training and personal development is necessary to lose weight and to maintain weight was not supported by all participants. The social and personal development part of the program is therefore likely to be the most challenging and controversial part of residential weight-loss programs.

Acknowledgments

We thank the personnel and participants at Ebeltoft Kurcenter for participating in the study.

Author Contributions

Analyzed the data: UD MBR BK AS. Wrote the paper: UD MBR BK AS.

References

1. Jeffery RW, Harnack LJ (2007) Evidence implicating eating as a primary driver for the obesity epidemic. Diabetes 56: 2673–2676. db07-1029 [pii];10.2337/db07-1029 [doi].
2. Must A, Spadano J, Coakley EH, Field AE, Colditz G et al. (1999) The disease burden associated with overweight and obesity. JAMA 282: 1523–1529. joc81719 [pii].
3. Calle EE, Thun MJ, Petrelli JM, Rodriguez C, Heath CW Jr (1999) Body-mass index and mortality in a prospective cohort of U.S. adults. N Engl J Med 341: 1097–1105. MJBA-411501 [pii];10.1056/NEJM199910073411501 [doi].
4. Chang SH, Stoll CR, Song J, Varela JE, Eagon CJ et al. (2014) The Effectiveness and Risks of Bariatric Surgery: An Updated Systematic Review and Meta-analysis, 2003–2012. JAMA Surg 149: 275–287. 1790378 [pii];10.1001/jamasurg.2013.3654 [doi].
5. Kwok CS, Pradhan A, Khan MA, Anderson SG, Keavney BD et al. (2014) Bariatric surgery and its impact on cardiovascular disease and mortality: A systematic review and meta-analysis. Int J Cardiol. S0167-5273(14)00379-9 [pii];10.1016/j.ijcard.2014.02.026 [doi].
6. Martins C, Strommen M, Stavne OA, Nossum R, Marvik R et al. (2011) Bariatric surgery versus lifestyle interventions for morbid obesity–changes in body weight, risk factors and comorbidities at 1 year. Obes Surg 21: 841–849. 10.1007/s11695-010-0131-1 [doi].
7. Rossner S, Hammarstrand M, Hemmingsson E, Neovius M, Johansson K (2008) Long-term weight loss and weight-loss maintenance strategies. Obes Rev 9: 624–630. OBR516 [pii];10.1111/j.1467-789X.2008.00516.x [doi].
8. Sodlerlund A, Fischer A, Johansson T (2009) Physical activity, diet and behaviour modification in the treatment of overweight and obese adults: a systematic review. Perspect Public Health 129: 132–142.
9. Nicholson F, Rolland C, Broom J, Love J (2010) Effectiveness of long-term (twelve months) nonsurgical weight loss interventions for obese women with

polycystic ovary syndrome: a systematic review. Int J Womens Health 2: 393–399. 10.2147/IJWH.S13456 [doi].
10. Romanova M, Liang LJ, Deng ML, Li Z, Heber D (2013) Effectiveness of the MOVE! Multidisciplinary weight loss program for veterans in Los Angeles. Prev Chronic Dis 10: E112. 10.5888/pcd10.120325 [doi];E112 [pii].
11. Foster-Schubert KE, Alfano CM, Duggan CR, Xiao L, Campbell KL et al. (2012) Effect of diet and exercise, alone or combined, on weight and body composition in overweight-to-obese postmenopausal women. Obesity (Silver Spring) 20: 1628–1638. oby201176 [pii];10.1038/oby.2011.76 [doi].
12. Christiansen T, Bruun JM, Madsen EL, Richelsen B (2007) Weight loss maintenance in severely obese adults after an intensive lifestyle intervention: 2- to 4-year follow-up. Obesity (Silver Spring) 15: 413–420.
13. Powell LH, Calvin JE, III, Calvin JE, Jr. (2007) Effective obesity treatments. Am Psychol 62: 234–246. 2007-04834-009 [pii];10.1037/0003-066X.62.3.234 [doi].
14. Avenell A, Broom J, Brown TJ, Poobalan A, Aucott L et al. (2004) Systematic review of the long-term effects and economic consequences of treatments for obesity and implications for health improvement. Health Technol Assess 8: iii-182. 99-02-02 [pii].
15. Douketis JD, Macie C, Thabane L, Williamson DF (2005) Systematic review of long-term weight loss studies in obese adults: clinical significance and applicability to clinical practice. Int J Obes (Lond) 29: 1153–1167.
16. Foster GD, Makris AP, Bailer BA (2005) Behavioral treatment of obesity. Am J Clin Nutr 82: 230S–235S.
17. Middleton KM, Patidar SM, Perri MG (2012) The impact of extended care on the long-term maintenance of weight loss: a systematic review and meta-analysis. Obes Rev 13: 509–517. 10.1111/j.1467-789X.2011.00972.x [doi].
18. Foster GD, Makris AP, Bailer BA (2005) Behavioral treatment of obesity. Am J Clin Nutr 82: 230S–235S. 82/1/230S [pii].
19. Grol R, Wensing M (2004) What drives change? Barriers to and incentives for achieving evidence-based practice. Med J Aust 180: S57–S60. gro10753_fm [pii].
20. Bleich SN, Huizinga MM, Beach MC, Cooper LA (2010) Patient use of weight-management activities: A comparison of patient and physician assessments. Patient Education and Counseling 79: 344–350.
21. Shay LE (2008) A concept analysis: adherence and weight loss. Nurs Forum 43: 42–52.
22. Anderson RM, Funnell MM (2008) The art and science of diabetes education: a culture out of balance. Diabetes Educ 34: 109–117.
23. Maldonato A, Piana N, Bloise D, Baldelli A (2010) Optimizing patient education for people with obesity: possible use of the autobiographical approach. Patient Educ Couns 79: 287–290.
24. Beach MC, Duggan PS, Cassel CK, Geller G (2007) What does 'respect' mean? Exploring the moral obligation of health professionals to respect patients. J Gen Intern Med 22: 692–695. 10.1007/s11606-006-0054-7 [doi].
25. May CR, Mair F, Finch T, MacFarlane A, Dowrick C et al. (2009) Development of a theory of implementation and integration: Normalization Process Theory. Implement Sci 4: 29. 1748-5908-4-29 [pii];10.1186/1748-5908-4-29 [doi].
26. Bandura A (2004) Health promotion by social cognitive means. Health Educ Behav 31: 143–164.
27. Cochrane G (2008) Role for a sense of self-worth in weight-loss treatments: helping patients develop self-efficacy. Can Fam Physician 54: 543–547.
28. Byrne S, Barry D, Petry NM (2012) Predictors of weight loss success. Exercise vs. dietary self-efficacy and treatment attendance. Appetite 58: 695–698. S0195-6663(12)00006-2 [pii];10.1016/j.appet.2012.01.005 [doi].
29. Jones N, Furlanetto DL, Jackson JA, Kinn S (2007) An investigation of obese adults' views of the outcomes of dietary treatment. J Hum Nutr Diet 20: 486–494. JHN810 [pii];10.1111/j.1365-277X.2007.00810.x [doi].
30. Chan RS, Lok KY, Sea MM, Woo J (2009) Clients' experiences of a community based lifestyle modification program: a qualitative study. Int J Environ Res Public Health 6: 2608–2622. 10.3390/ijerph6102608 [doi].
31. Fabricatore AN, Wadden TA (2003) Psychological functioning of obese individuals. Diabetes spectrum 16: 245–252.
32. Puhl RM, Heuer CA (2009) The Stigma of Obesity: A Review and Update. Obesity 17: 941–964.
33. Myers A, Rosen JC (1999) Obesity stigmatization and coping: relation to mental health symptoms, body image, and self-esteem. Int J Obes Relat Metab Disord 23: 221–230.
34. Puhl RM, Brownell KD (2006) Confronting and coping with weight stigma: an investigation of overweight and obese adults. Obesity (Silver Spring) 14: 1802–1815. 14/10/1802 [pii];10.1038/oby.2006.208 [doi].
35. Foster GD, Wadden TA, Makris AP, Davidson D, Sanderson RS et al. (2003) Primary care physicians' attitudes about obesity and its treatment. Obes Res 11: 1168–1177. 10.1038/oby.2003.161 [doi].
36. Ferrante JM, Fyffe DC, Vega ML, Piasecki AK, Ohman-Strickland PA et al. (2010) Family physicians' barriers to cancer screening in extremely obese patients. Obesity (Silver Spring) 18: 1153–1159. oby2009481 [pii];10.1038/oby.2009.481 [doi].
37. Vartanian LR, Novak SA (2011) Internalized societal attitudes moderate the impact of weight stigma on avoidance of exercise. Obesity (Silver Spring) 19: 757–762. oby2010234 [pii];10.1038/oby.2010.234 [doi].
38. Sikorski C, Luppa M, Kaiser M, Glaesmer H, Schomerus G et al. (2011) The stigma of obesity in the general public and its implications for public health - a systematic review. BMC Public Health 11: 661. 1471-2458-11-661 [pii];10.1186/1471-2458-11-661 [doi].
39. Schvey NA, Puhl RM, Brownell KD (2011) The impact of weight stigma on caloric consumption. Obesity (Silver Spring) 19: 1957–1962. oby2011204 [pii];10.1038/oby.2011.204 [doi].
40. Elfhag K, Rossner S (2005) Who succeeds in maintaining weight loss? A conceptual review of factors associated with weight loss maintenance and weight regain. Obes Rev 6: 67–85. OBR170 [pii];10.1111/j.1467-789X.2005.00170.x [doi].
41. Byrne SM (2002) Psychological aspects of weight maintenance and relapse in obesity. J Psychosom Res 53: 1029–1036. S0022399902004877 [pii].
42. Christiansen B, Borge L, Fagermoen MS (2012) Understanding everyday life of morbidly obese adults-habits and body image. Int J Qual Stud Health Well - being 7: 17255. 10.3402/qhw.v7i0.17255 [doi];QHW-7-17255 [pii].
43. Reach G (2009) Obstacles to patient education in chronic diseases: a trans-theoretical analysis. Patient Educ Couns 77: 192–196.
44. Bandura A (2004) Health promotion by social cognitive means. Health Educ Behav 31: 143–164. 10.1177/1090198104263660 [doi].
45. Wing RR, Hill JO (2001) Successful weight loss maintenance. Annu Rev Nutr 21: 323–341. 10.1146/annurev.nutr.21.1.323 [doi];21/1/323 [pii].
46. Penn L, Moffatt SM, White M (2008) Participants' perspective on maintaining behaviour change: a qualitative study within the European Diabetes Prevention Study. BMC Public Health 8: 235. 1471-2458-8-235 [pii];10.1186/1471-2458-8-235 [doi].
47. Mobbs O, Crepin C, Thiery C, Golay A, Van der Linden M (2010) Obesity and the four facets of impulsivity. Patient Education and Counseling 79: 372–377.
48. Mobbs O, Crepin C, Thiery C, Golay A, Van der Linden M (2010) Obesity and the four facets of impulsivity. Patient Educ Couns 79: 372–377. S0738-3991(10)00119-9 [pii];10.1016/j.pec.2010.03.003 [doi].

24

Irisin Levels Are Lower in Young Amenorrheic Athletes Compared with Eumenorrheic Athletes and Non-Athletes and Are Associated with Bone Density and Strength Estimates

Vibha Singhal[1,2¶], Elizabeth A. Lawson[1¶], Kathryn E. Ackerman[1,3], Pouneh K. Fazeli[1], Hannah Clarke[1], Hang Lee[4], Kamryn Eddy[1,5], Dean A. Marengi[1], Nicholas P. Derrico[6], Mary L. Bouxsein[6,7], Madhusmita Misra[1,2]*

1 Neuroendocrine Unit, Massachusetts General Hospital and Harvard Medical School, Boston, Massachusetts, United States of America, **2** Pediatric Endocrine Unit, Massachusetts General Hospital for Children and Harvard Medical School, Boston, Massachusetts, United States of America, **3** Division of Sports Medicine, Boston Children's Hospital, Boston, Massachusetts, United States of America, **4** Department of Biostatistics, Massachusetts General Hospital and Harvard Medical School, Boston, Massachusetts, United States of America, **5** Harris Center, Massachusetts General Hospital, Boston, Massachusetts, United States of America, **6** Endocrine Division, Massachusetts General Hospital and Harvard Medical School, Boston, Massachusetts, United States of America, **7** Department of Orthopedic Surgery, Beth Israel Deaconess Medical Center and Harvard Medical School, Boston, Massachusetts, United States of America

Abstract

Irisin and FGF21 are novel hormones implicated in the "browning" of white fat, thermogenesis, and energy homeostasis. However, there are no data regarding these hormones in amenorrheic athletes (AA) (a chronic energy deficit state) compared with eumenorrheic athletes (EA) and non-athletes. We hypothesized that irisin and FGF21 would be low in AA, an adaptive response to low energy stores. Furthermore, because (i) brown fat has positive effects on bone, and (ii) irisin and FGF21 may directly impact bone, we hypothesized that bone density, structure and strength would be positively associated with these hormones in athletes and non-athletes. To test our hypotheses, we studied 85 females, 14–21 years [38 AA, 24 EA and 23 non-athletes (NA)]. Fasting serum irisin and FGF21 were measured. Body composition and bone density were assessed using dual energy X-ray absorptiometry, bone microarchitecture using high resolution peripheral quantitative CT, strength estimates using finite element analysis, resting energy expenditure (REE) using indirect calorimetry and time spent exercising/week by history. Subjects did not differ for pubertal stage. Fat mass was lowest in AA. AA had lower irisin and FGF21 than EA and NA, even after controlling for fat and lean mass. Across subjects, irisin was positively associated with REE and bone density Z-scores, volumetric bone mineral density (total and trabecular), stiffness and failure load. FGF21 was negatively associated with hours/week of exercise and cortical porosity, and positively with fat mass and cortical volumetric bone density. Associations of irisin (but not FGF21) with bone parameters persisted after controlling for potential confounders. In conclusion, irisin and FGF21 are low in AA, and irisin (but not FGF21) is independently associated with bone density and strength in athletes.

Editor: Yi-Hsiang Hsu, Harvard Medical School, United States of America

Funding: This study was funded by NIH Grants UL1 RR025758, R01 HD060827, K23 MH092560; K24HD071843; and Massachusetts General Hospital Claflin Distinguished Scholar Award. The funders had no role in study design, data collection and analysis, decision to publish, or preparation of the manuscript.

Competing Interests: The authors have declared that no competing interests exist.

* E-mail: mmisra@partners.org

¶ E-mail: These authors are joint first authors on this work.

Introduction

Irisin and FGF21 are novel hormones implicated in the modulation of energy homeostasis [1], and more recently with bone metabolism. A recently discovered myokine and adipokine, irisin has been proposed to be an important mediator of the beneficial metabolic effects of exercise [2]. It is released systemically from skeletal muscle and induces the "browning" of subcutaneous white adipocytes, uncoupling protein 1 (UCP1)-mediated thermogenesis, and increased energy expenditure [2]. Irisin secretion also increases in men who exercise [2,3]. However, the impact of *chronic* exercise on irisin in over-exercising females has not been examined, and the impact of associated hypothalamic amenorrhea is unknown.

FGF21 is secreted into the circulation from the adipocytes and liver, and is expressed in fat, skeletal muscle and the pancreas. FGF21 regulates carbohydrate and lipid metabolism, resulting in improved glucose homeostasis and lipid parameters, and reduces body weight in animal models. Like irisin, FGF21 promotes conversion of white to beige adipose tissue, activation of UCP1-

driven thermogenesis and energy expenditure, although this may represent an autocrine/paracrine rather than endocrine effect [4,5]. A positive relationship between FGF21 and physical activity has been described [6], and initiation of an exercise regimen in sedentary young women leads to increased FGF21 [7].

In addition, both irisin and FGF21 have been implicated in bone metabolism. Brown adipose tissue is an independent predictor of bone density in women [8], and the volume and activity of brown adipose tissue is positively associated with total and cortical bone cross-sectional area in young children and adolescents [9]. In rodent models, irisin increases trabecular and cortical thickness as well as trabecular density through increased osteoblast activation and inhibition of RANKL mediated osteoclastogensis [10]. Effects of FGF21 on bone are still being defined, with one study demonstrating deleterious effects on bone through inhibition of osteoblastogenesis in favor of adipogenesis [11] whereas a study in adult females reported a positive association between FGF21 and bone density [12] supported by *in vitro* data [13]. Thus irisin and FGF21 may impact bone both through induction of brown adipogenesis, as well as through direct effects. Data are lacking regarding associations of irisin and FGF21 with bone parameters in athletes and non-athletes, and the impact of a hypogonadal state (in athletes with functional hypothalamic amenorrhea) on these associations.

Although exercise may increase irisin and FGF21 levels in healthy individuals, we hypothesized that levels of irisin and FGF21 would be low in amenorrheic athletes, signaling an adaptive response to an overall state of energy deficit. In addition, we hypothesized that irisin and FGF21 levels would be positively associated with measures of bone density, structure and strength in athletes and non-athletes.

Subjects and Methods

Subjects

We studied 85 adolescent women [38 amenorrheic athletes (AA), 24 eumenorrheic athletes (EA) and 23 non-athletes] between 14–21 years of age enrolled in an ongoing study, all of whom were >85% ideal body weight based on the 50th percentile for BMI for age. Clinical characteristics of a subgroup of these women have been previously reported [14,15,16,17]. However, levels of irisin and FGF21, and the relationship between irisin and FGF21 levels and measures of bone metabolism have not been previously described. All study participants were recruited from the community through advertisements and referrals from healthcare providers. We defined 'amenorrhea' as absence of menses for 3 months in a 6-month period of oligo-amenorrhea (cycle length greater than 6 weeks) or absence of menses at ≥15 years (upper limit of normal for menarche), after other causes of amenorrhea were ruled out. Duration since last menses in AA (median and interquartile range) was 165 (24–360) days. We defined eumenorrheic athletes as those who had had ≥9 menses in the previous year. Three athletes (all less than 17 years old) had not attained menarche, and other causes of menarchal delay (other than excessive exercise) were ruled out in these athletes.

Inclusion criteria for athletes included ≥4 hours of aerobic weight-bearing activity or ≥20 miles of running weekly for the preceding 6 months. Inclusion criteria for non-athletes included < 2 hours per week of weight-bearing activities. Per study design, no subject met criteria for anorexia nervosa at study enrollment, although 34% of AA and 4% of EA had a past or current history of some form of disordered eating behavior. The racial distribution included 81.0% White or Asian, 13.1% Mixed and 6.0% Black, while the ethnic distribution included 95.2% non-Hispanic and 4.8% Hispanic. Race and ethnic distribution did not differ significantly across groups.

Subjects were recruited from local area high schools and colleges and referrals from pediatricians, adolescent medicine physicians, endocrinologists, nutritionists and sports medicine physicians. All subjects who met inclusion criteria were included in the study in a consecutive fashion.

Ethics Statement

The study was approved by the Institutional Review Board (IRB) of the Partners HealthCare system (Protocol 2009-P-000353). Per IRB guidelines and using IRB approved consent and assent forms, (i) informed written consent was obtained from subjects ≥18 years old and parents of subjects <18 years, and (ii) informed written assent was obtained from subjects <18 years.

Study Design

Subjects were seen in the Clinical Research Center of Massachusetts General Hospital. The screening visit included a history and physical examination, and laboratory evaluations to rule out conditions other than excessive exercise accompanied by inadequate caloric intake that may cause hypothalamic amenorrhea. We thus ruled out hyperprolactinemia, primary ovarian failure, polycystic ovarian syndrome (PCOS) and thyroid dysfunction.

Qualifying subjects underwent a history and physical examination, assessment of hours per week of physical activity (averaged over a year) and measurement of fasting resting energy expenditure using the VMAX Encore 29 metabolic cart (Viasys Healthcare, Carefusion; San Diego, CA) [18,19]. Subjects did not alter their usual food intake in the days preceding the study visit. Similarly, exercise activity on the days preceding the study visit was not curtailed to allow for usual levels of physical activity. However, fasting morning blood for irisin and FGF-21 levels was drawn before any exercise activity. EA and non-athletes were assessed in the early to mid follicular phase of their cycles (based on menstrual history). All subjects had assessment of (i) body composition and areal bone density (spine, hip and whole body) using dual energy x-ray absorptiometry (DXA), and a subset were assessed for (ii) bone microarchitecture and estimates of strength at the distal radius (site of non-weight bearing bone) using high resolution peripheral quantitative computed tomography (HRpQCT) and finite element analysis (FEA) using published methods [14,15,16]. FEA-derived estimates of failure load using these methods are strongly correlated ($r^2 = 0.75$) with experimentally measured failure loads that produce Colles' fractures in human cadaveric radii. HR-pQCT data were acquired on a single instrument by one operator, who performed standard evaluations (periosteal contouring). All finite element analyses (endosteal contouring) were also performed by one blinded investigator [15].

Biochemical Analysis

We used an ELISA to measure irisin (Adipogen; Liestal, Switzerland; intra-assay coefficient of variation (CV) 6.9%, inter-assay CV 9.07%, detection limit 0.001 mcg/mL) and FGF21 (R&D Systems; Minneapolis, MN; intra-assay CV 3.4%, inter-assay CV 7.5%, detection limit 4.67 pg/mL). For the irisin assay, the laboratory evaluated thee different assay kits on the number of standards (assay range), sample type (serum or plasma), sample volume, sample dilution, assay range, sensitivity, assay time and cost. The Adipogen assay was chosen because it had the greatest detection range (0.001–5 ug/mL), required the least volume of sample, and was the most sensitive (0.001 mcg/mL). This was important given the limited studies of irisin in the pediatric age group, and some uncertainty regarding expected values in a pediatric population. Of note, this assay reports irisin levels that are an order of magnitude higher than the Phoenix Pharmaceuticals assay [20]. All samples were processed immediately and stored at −80 degrees Celsius until they were analyzed to minimize peptide degradation, and contrary to one study that demonstrated inverse associations of irisin levels with duration of sample storage [21], we found no such inverse association of irisin or FGF-21 levels with duration of storage. In fact, another study found no impact of repeated freeze thaw cycles on irisin levels [22], suggesting relative stability of this peptide hormone.

A chemiluminescent immunoassay was used to measure 25-hydroxyvitamin D (DiaSorin, Stillwater, MN; intraassay CV 2.9–5.5%, interassay CV 8%; sensitivity 4 ng/ml). A subset of at least 55 subjects were assessed for P1NP, CTX, testosterone, SHBG and estradiol levels. We used an RIA to measure P1NP (Orion Diagnostics, Espoo, Finland; intra-assay CV 3.5–5.3%, inter-assay CV 3.6–5.4%), lower limit of detection 0.7 ng/ml), and an IRMA to measure CTX (Immunodiagnostics Systems, Fountain Hills, AZ; intra-assay CV 5.2–6.8%, inter-assay CV 5.6–7.4%, lower limit of detection 0.02 ng/ml). Testosterone was measured by RIA (Diagnostic Products Corp, Los Angeles, CA; intra-assay CV 5·1–9·8%, inter-assay CV 8.2%, limit of detection 12 ng/dl), SHBG by IRMA (Diagnostic Products Corp, intra-assay CV 2·8–5·3%, inter-assay CV 8.2%, limit of detection 3 nmol/l), and estradiol by ultrasensitive ELISA (ALPCO Diagnostics, Salem, NH; intra-assay CV of 6.36% and inter-assay CV of 7.6%, minimum level of detection 1.4 pg/mL). Free androgen index (FAI) was calculated using the following formula: [total testosterone (nmol/l) × 100]/SHBG (nmol/l) [23]. All blood samples were spun immediately after collection, and the serum separated and stored in −80 degree Celsius freezers until analysis in duplicate.

Statistical Analysis

JMP Statistical Discoveries (version 10.0; SAS Institute, Inc., Cary, NC) was used for statistical analyses. Our sample size had > 80% power for detecting a significant difference between AA and control groups for irisin and FGF21 respectively at an alpha level of 0.05 based on published data [24,25]. Clinical characteristics, hormone levels and bone parameters were compared across the three groups (AA, EA and non-athletes) using analysis of variance (ANOVA). Irisin and FGF21 levels were logarithmically transformed prior to analyses to approximate a normal distribution. When the overall ANOVA had a significant p-value, the Tukey Kramer test was used to compare differences between groups while controlling for multiple comparisons. For non-parametric comparisons of three groups, we used the Kruskal-Wallis test followed by the Steel-Dwass method for between group comparisons.

We used Pearson or Spearman correlations (depending on data distribution) to determine associations of hormones with bone measures, body composition and REE. Because irisin is a myokine, associations of irisin with these measures may differ in chronically exercising athletes compared with non-athletes. In addition, amenorrhea may modify associations of irisin with various parameters within athletes. For these reasons, we performed exploratory analyses of associations of irisin and FGF21 not only for the group as a whole, but also within AA, EA, all athletes (AA+EA), and non-athletes. Multivariate least-square analyses were constructed to control for confounders and to test interactions between subject group and hormone levels. Significance was defined as a two-tailed p-value <0.05. Data are reported as mean ± SD.

Results

Subject Characteristics

Subject characteristics are presented in Table 1. AA were slightly older than the other groups, although bone age and Tanner stage did not differ among groups. Mean duration since the last menstrual cycle in AA was 9.7±2.4 months, and menarchal age was older in AA than in EA and non-athletes. BMI was lower in AA than EA. Total fat mass was lower in AA than EA and non-athletes, and lean mass was higher in EA than in non-athletes. Percent body fat was lower in both groups of athletes versus non-athletes and in AA compared to EA. By design, hours of weekly exercise were higher in AA and EA than non-athletes (with no difference between AA and EA). Resting energy expenditure (REE) was higher in EA than AA and non-athletes. After controlling for lean mass, resting energy expenditure remained higher in EA than AA. REE/lean mass was lowest in AA.

Bone parameters are shown in Table 2 and have been previously reported for a subset of 50 subjects [14,15,16]. Spine BMD Z-scores were lower in AA than EA, whereas hip and whole body BMD Z-scores were highest in EA. Trabecular and cortical volumetric BMD (vBMD), cortical thickness, stiffness and failure load were lower and cortical porosity higher in AA than in non-athletes, and percent cortical area was lower in both groups of athletes compared with non-athletes. Differences among groups remained significant for most parameters after controlling for age, and for age and race (Table 2). Levels of P1NP (a bone formation marker) and CTX (a bone resorption marker) were available for a subset of 55 subjects. P1NP levels did not differ across groups (88.1±37.9, 98.4±55.2 and 83.8±38.3 ng/ml in AA, EA and non-athletes respectively, $p = 0.60$). CTX levels trended higher in the athletes (1.06±0.33, 1.16±0.39 and 0.91±0.30 ng/ml in AA, EA and non-athletes respectively, $p = 0.09$). Estradiol levels and the free androgen index (while lowest in AA) did not differ significantly across groups.

Hormone Levels

Table 1 and Figure 1 demonstrate levels of irisin and FGF21 across the groups. Irisin and FGF21 levels were significantly lower in AA than EA and non-athletes, and these differences persisted after controlling for age ($p = 0.0001$ for both for the overall ANOVA), or for body fat and lean mass ($p < 0.05$), while there were no differences in hormone levels between EA and non-athletes. Log irisin and log FGF21 correlated positively with each other within athletes ($r = 0.26$, $p = 0.04$), but the association was inverse in non-athletes ($r = -0.50$, 0.01). Within individual athlete groups, associations were weaker, and mostly driven by AAs (AA: Spearman Rho = 0.28, $p = 0.09$; EA: Spearman Rho = 0.13, $p = 0.54$). Our results remained similar when we excluded the three athletes who had not attained menarche from the analysis.

Relationship between Hormone Levels, Measures of Energy Expenditure and Measures of Body Composition

Associations of irisin with measures of energy expenditure and body composition are shown in Table 3. Irisin was positively associated with resting energy expenditure in the group as a whole, within athletes and also non-athletes. However, associations were not significant for AA and EA analyzed separately. We found no associations of irisin with hours/week of exercise or fat mass in any of the groups. Log irisin was positively associated with lean mass in all athletes and within AA, but not in EA, non-athletes or the group as a whole.

Table 1. Clinical characteristics of amenorrheic athletes (AA), eumenorrheic athletes (EA) and non-athletes (NA).

	AA N = 38	EA N = 24	NA N = 23	ANOVA P-value	AA vs. EA P-value	AA vs. NA P-value	EA vs. NA P-value
Age (years)	19.3±2.0	18.0±2.0	19.1±1.7	**0.04**	**0.03**	0.86	0.16
Bone age (years)	17.4±1.0	17.2±1.2	17.5±1.1	0.49	0.60	0.91	0.50
Tanner stage distribution (T2, 3, 4, 5)	2.6%, 10.5%, 15.8%, 71.1%	0%, 4.2%, 20.8%, 75.0%	0%, 8.7%, 0%, 91.3%	0.31	0.66	0.17	0.06
Age at menarche (y)	14.0±1.8	12.8±1.4	12.2±1.5	**0.0004**	**0.02**	**0.0004**	0.45
Days since last menses	165 (24–360)	-	-	-			
BMI (kg/m^2)	20.3±2.2	22.4±2.3	21.5±2.5	**0.005**	**0.004**	0.15	0.43
Height (cm)	165.7±6.7	165.7±8.2	162.6±7.2	0.23	0.98	0.37	0.35
Fat mass (kg)	11.7±3.7	15.1±4.4	16.0±4.9	**0.0004**	**0.009**	**0.001**	0.79
Lean mass (kg)	43.5±5.7	46.3±7.7	40.5±4.4	**0.006**	0.18	0.15	**0.004**
Percent body fat	20.3±5.1	23.5±3.8	27.0±5.2	**<0.0001**	**0.03**	**<0.0001**	**0.04**
Hours/week of exercise	10.4±5.6	11.0±4.9	0.8±0.7	**<0.0001**	0.87	**<0.0001**	**<0.0001**
Resting energy expenditure (calories)	1247±183	1444±218	1255±193	**0.0005**	**0.0007**	0.99	**0.004**
REE/lean mass (cal/kg)	28.9±3.8	31.6±5.3	31.2±4.9	**0.04**	**0.06**	0.13	0.95
History of fractures	50%	16.7%	8.7%	**0.0007**	**0.01**	**0.0009**	0.67
25(OH) vit D (ng/ml)	38.3±12.5	30.5±13.8	21.1±7.8	**<0.0001**	**0.04**	**<0.0001**	**0.03**
Irisin (mcg/ml)§	3.20 (2.58–3.53)	3.85 (3.50–4.80)	3.60 (3.30–4.20)	**0.0004**	**0.001**	**0.009**	0.83
FGF21 (pg/ml)§	54.5 (32.3–102.3)	94.5 (60.3–189.8)	132.0 (109.0–230.0)	**0.0001**	**0.02**	**<0.0001**	0.26

Mean ± SD or Median (Interquartile Range); FGF21: fibroblast growth factor 21; AA: amenorrheic athletes; EA: eumenorrheic athletes; NA: non-athletes.
§P values reported for log converted data.

Table 2. Areal (DXA) and volumetric (HRpQCT) bone density measures, cortical microarchitectural parameters, and strength estimates (FEA) in amenorrheic athletes (AA), eumenorrheic athletes (EA) and non-athletes (NA).

	AA N=38	EA N=24	NA N=23	ANOVA P-value	AA vs. EA P-value	AA vs. NA P-value	EA vs. NA P-value
Spine aBMD (g/cm^2)[†]	0.91 (0.83–1.02)	0.99 (0.87–1.08)	0.96 (0.84–1.08)	**0.04[a]**	0.07[b]	0.12	1.00
Spine aBMD Z-scores	−0.75±1.25	0.03±0.98	−0.25±0.97	**0.02[a]**	**0.02[a]**	0.21	0.66
Total hip aBMD (g/cm^2)	0.96±0.13	1.04±0.12	0.95±0.09	**0.01[a,c]**	**0.03[a,c]**	0.89	**0.02[a,c]**
Total hip aBMD Z-scores	0.05±1.10	0.81±0.90	−0.28±0.70	**0.0009[a,c]**	**0.01[a,c]**	0.40	**0.0009[a,c]**
Femoral neck aBMD (g/cm^2)[†]	0.83 (0.76–0.93)	0.88 (0.82–0.98)	0.81 (0.74–0.89)	0.09[b]	0.16	0.91	0.12[b,d]
Femoral neck aBMD Z-scores	−0.19±1.22	0.34±1.03	−0.59±0.80	**0.02[a,c]**	0.16	0.35	**0.01[a,c]**
Whole body aBMD (g/cm^2)[†]	1.05 (0.99–1.12)	1.11 (1.04–1.18)	1.07 (0.99–1.13)	0.09[a,c]	0.09[a,d]	0.78	0.36[d]
Whole body aBMD Z-scores	−0.48±1.12	0.38±1.12	−0.39±0.99	**0.01[a,c]**	**0.01[a,c]**	0.95	**0.049[a,c]**
Total vBMD ($mgHA/cm^3$)	294.0±62.2	305.8±51.4	332.3±72.9	0.08[b]	0.76	0.07[b]	0.33
Trabecular vBMD ($mgHA/cm^3$)[†]	161.2 (134.5–177.5)	189.6 (155.3–203.4)	176.7 (149.2–203.4)	**0.048[b]**	0.095	0.12	0.93
Cortical vBMD ($mgHA/cm^3$)[†]	923.7 (876.2–947.5)	934.1 (876.9–947.9)	950.8 (911.7–987.6)	**0.04[a,c]**	0.99	**0.046[a,c]**	0.13
Total cross-sectional area (mm^2)	272.4±49.9	284.7±45.7	257.3±43.5	0.21	0.65	0.49	0.19
% Cortical area	19.6±5.0	18.8±3.8	22.9±4.5	**0.02[a,c]**	0.85	**0.04[a,d]**	**0.03[a,d]**
Cortical thickness (mm)	0.82±0.20	0.82±0.14	0.94±0.16	**0.04[b]**	0.99	**0.049[b,d]**	0.10
Cortical porosity (%)	1.10±0.78	0.70±0.44	0.66±0.40	**0.02[a,c]**	0.09[a,c]	**0.04[a,c]**	0.98
Stiffness (kN/m)[§]	69.4 (57.2–88.2)	80.8 (73.5–86.5)	78.1 (68.4–92.3)	**0.03[a,d]**	0.11[b,d]	**0.049[b]**	0.98
Failure load (kN)[§]	3.56 (2.97–4.52)	4.09 (3.73–4.40)	3.97 (3.53–4.61)	**0.03[a,d]**	0.10[b,d]	**0.05[b]**	0.99

Mean ± SD or Median (Interquartile Range);
[†]Kruskal Wallis test;
[§]p value reported for log converted data;
[a]$p<0.05$ after controlling for age,
[b]$p<0.10$ after controlling for age,
[c]$p<0.05$ after controlling for age and race (Black vs. non-Black),
[d]$p<0.10$ after controlling for age and race.
AA: amenorrheic athletes; EA: eumenorrheic athletes; NA: non-athletes; aBMD: area bone mineral density; vBMD: volumetric bone mineral density.

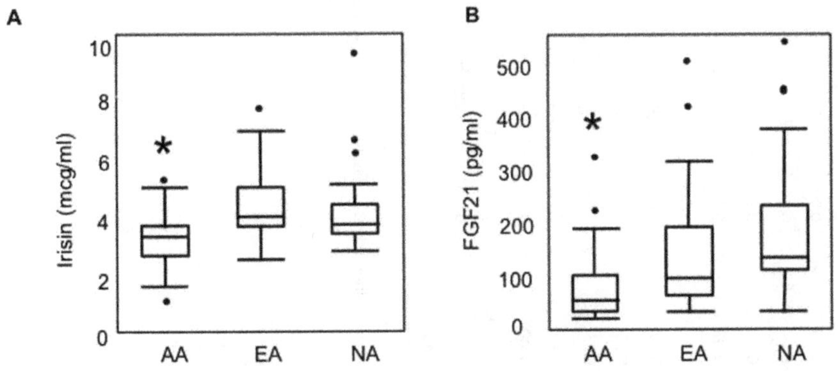

Figure 1. Irisin and FGF21 levels in athletes and non-athletes. (A) Irisin and (B) FGF21 levels were lower in amenorrheic athletes (AA) compared to eumenorrheic athletes (EA) and non-athletes (NA) (ANOVA for three-group comparison for log converted values, followed by the Tukey Kramer test to compare any two groups). *, $p<0.05$ vs. EA and NA.

Associations of FGF21 with measures of energy expenditure, body composition are shown in Table 4. Log FGF21 was associated inversely with resting energy expenditure in EA and non-athletes, but not in the other groups. Across all groups, there were negative associations between log FGF21 and with hours/week of exercise, and positive associations with body fat content. Within individual groups, we found no associations of log FGF21 with hours/week of exercise, or percent body fat mass. There were no associations of log FGF21 with lean mass. Irisin and FGF21 levels were overall not associated with age ($p=0.52$ and 0.85 respectively), or bone age ($p=0.89$ and 0.61).

Relationship between Hormone Levels and Sex Steroids

Log irisin levels were associated positively with the free androgen index in AA ($r=0.63$, $p=0.002$), and with estradiol in non-athletes (rho = 0.46, $p=0.05$). Log FGF21 was associated positively with the free androgen index in AA ($r=0.55$, $p=0.009$) and inversely with estradiol levels in non-athletes ($r=-0.63$, $p=0.005$). Associations of irisin and FGF21 with the free androgen index (but not estradiol) remained significant after controlling for fat mass or lean mass.

Relationship between Hormone Levels and Bone Parameters

Across all groups, irisin levels were positively associated with spine, femoral neck and whole body BMD Z scores (Table 3). Irisin levels were also associated with total and trabecular vBMD, and with bone strength estimates, including stiffness and failure load. All associations appeared to be driven mostly by the athletes taken together (AA and EA). Associations within AA and EA groups were weaker. Table 3 also shows associations that remained significant after controlling for (i) lean mass, (ii) lean mass and activity levels, and (iii) lean mass, fat mass and activity levels. In contrast, the only associations observed between FGF21 and bone parameters were a positive association with cortical volumetric BMD, and an inverse association with cortical porosity for all groups taken together, and inverse associations with total and trabecular vBMD in non-athletes.

We tested for interactions between subject groups and irisin and FGF21 in determining associations of irisin with bone parameters across groups, and our analysis did not show strong evidence that the patterns of irisin effects on bone outcomes were different across subgroups.

Across all groups, the association of irisin with whole body BMD Z-scores, total and trabecular vBMD, percent cortical area, cortical thickness, stiffness and failure load were significant after controlling for FGF21 and lean mass ($p=0.01$, 0.04, 0.02, 0.05, 0.04, 0.02, 0.02 and 0.04 respectively). In addition, spine and whole body BMD Z-scores, stiffness and failure load remained significantly associated with irisin after controlling for FGF21, lean mass and hours/week of exercise ($p=0.03$, 0.01, 0.05 and 0.04 respectively), and for FGF21, lean and fat mass and hours/week of exercise ($p=0.04$, 0.01, 0.06 and 0.04 respectively). Within athletes, the association between irisin and spine and whole body BMD Z-scores remained significant after controlling for FGF21, lean and fat mass, and hours/week of exercise. A trend persisted for the negative association between FGF21 and cortical porosity after controlling for irisin and lean mass ($p=0.08$), but not after controlling for hours/week of activity and/or fat mass. Our results were similar when we excluded the three premenarchal athletes from our analysis.

Discussion

This is the first study to demonstrate low levels of irisin and FGF-21 in adolescent amenorrheic athletes, which we speculate represents an adaptive response to conserve energy in these young women. Irisin levels were associated with resting energy expenditure and FGF-21 with body fat content. Importantly, irisin levels were associated with measures of areal and volumetric bone density and strength estimates in athletes, and associations with bone density and strength measures persisted after controlling for potential confounders. In contrast, FGF21 levels were associated with only a few bone parameters.

Irisin and FGF-21 promote the "browning" of white adipose tissue, resulting in "beige fat", a metabolically favorable fat capable of burning energy through thermogenesis. This specialized tissue has features of brown fat, including multilocular fat cells, an abundance of mitochondria, and UCP-1, an enzyme that uncouples oxidative phosphorylation from ATP production, leading to energy release as heat [2,4].

Irisin levels have not been previously reported in adolescent female athletes. One study suggested that in moderately trained young healthy male athletes, plasma irisin levels are increased 30 minutes after sprinting, but this effect is not seen after eight weeks of training [3]. In another study, initiation of an endurance exercise routine in sedentary men led to a two-fold rise in plasma irisin levels at ten weeks [2], while a third study in adults reported

Table 3. Associations of irisin (log converted values) with areal (DXA) and volumetric (HRpQCT) bone density measures, cortical microarchitectural parameters, and strength estimates (FEA) in all subjects (All), amenorrheic athletes (AA), eumenorrheic athletes (EA), all athletes (ATH) and all non-athletes (NA).

	All		AA		EA		ATH		NA	
	r	p	r	p	r	p	r	p	r	p
Energy Status and Body Composition										
Resting energy expenditure (calories)	**0.39**	**<0.0001**	0.24	0.15	0.25	0.25	**0.46**	**0.0002**	**0.49***	**0.02**
Hours/week of exercise activity	−0.10	0.34	0.20	0.23	0.27	0.22	0.18	0.16	0.07	0.74
Lean mass (kg)	−0.01	0.94	**0.34**	**0.04**	−0.09	0.67	**0.26***	**0.04**	−0.07	0.76
Fat mass (kg)	0.03	0.76	0.11	0.51	−0.11	0.62	0.21	0.11	−0.37	0.08
Bone Parameters										
Spine BMD Z-scores	**0.21**	**0.03**[a,b,c]	0.03	0.84	0.28	0.19	**0.33**	**0.008**[b,c]	−0.20	0.35
Total hip BMD Z-scores	0.05	0.63	0.05	0.77	0.19	0.39	**0.31**	**0.02**	−0.11	0.6
FN BMD Z-scores	0.12	0.22	0.05	0.78	0.25	0.24	**0.30**	**0.02**	0.09	0.7
Whole body BMD Z-scores	**0.21**	**0.04**[a,b,c]	0.18	0.30	0.11	0.63	**0.36**	**0.005**[a,b,c]	0.24	0.27
Total vBMD (mgHA/cm^3)	**0.30**	**0.007**[a]	0.25	0.15	**0.43***	**0.04**[a,b]	**0.28**	**0.03**	0.14	0.53
Trabecular vBMD (mgHA/cm^3)	**0.31**	**0.005**[a]	0.10	0.54	0.38	0.08	**0.30**	**0.02**	0.23	0.30
Cortical vBMD (mgHA/cm^3)	0.16	0.19	0.24	0.18	0.04	0.87	0.18	0.2	−0.18	0.44
Total cross-sectional area (mm^2)	0.07	0.58	0.07	0.69	0.17	0.51	0.15	0.29	0.03	0.90
Cortical area/total area	0.15	0.21	0.08	0.66	0.27	0.30	0.06	0.55	0.02	0.90
Cortical thickness (mm)	0.18	0.13	0.09	0.60	**0.51***	**0.04**[a]	0.14	0.33	0.08	0.70
Cortical porosity (%)	−0.16	0.18	−0.23	0.18	−0.04	0.87	−0.23	0.10	0.18	0.44
Stiffness (kN/m)	**0.34**	**0.004**[a,b]	0.25	0.15	0.32	0.22	**0.37**	**0.007**	0.12	0.63
Failure load (kN)	**0.34**	**0.003**[a,b,c]	0.23	0.18	0.26	0.32	**0.38**	**0.006**	0.13	0.59
P1NP (ng/ml)	0.05	0.71	−0.16	0.53	0.02	0.95	−0.12	0.47	**0.60***	**0.008**[a,b,c]
CTX (ng/ml)	−0.03	0.84	0.06	0.82	−0.31	0.20	−0.13	0.46	0.16*	0.52

Spearman correlations; *Pearson correlations;
For bone parameters: [a]$p<0.05$ after controlling for lean mass; [b]$p<0.05$ after controlling for lean mass and activity; [c]$p<0.05$ after controlling for lean mass, activity and fat mass; BMD: bone mineral density; FN: femoral neck; vBMD: volumetric bone mineral density.
All: all subjects; AA: amenorrheic athletes; EA: eumenorrheic athletes; ATH: all athletes; NA: non-athletes.
P values ≤ 0.05 are bolded.

Table 4. Associations of FGF-21 (log converted values) with areal (DXA) and volumetric (HRpQCT) bone density measures, cortical microarchitectural parameters, and strength estimates (FEA) in all subjects (All), amenorrheic athletes (AA), eumenorrheic athletes (EA), all athletes (ATH) and all non-athletes (NA).

	All		AA		EA		ATH		NA	
	r	p	r	p	r	p	r	p	r	p
Energy Status and Body Composition										
Resting energy expenditure (calories)	−0.04	0.72	0.16	0.35	**−0.40**	**0.05**	0.19	0.14	**−0.47**	**0.02**
Hours/week of exercise activity	0.04	0.70	−0.09	0.58	−0.02	0.94	−0.05	0.71	−0.05	0.83
Lean mass (kg)	0.02	0.86	−0.01	0.96	−0.34	0.10	−0.05	0.72	−0.20	0.36
Fat mass (kg)	**0.34**	**0.0004**	0.16	0.34	0.01	0.95	0.22	0.09	0.32	0.14
Bone Parameters										
Spine BMD Z-scores	0.07	0.48	−0.01	0.94	0.02	0.94	0.15	0.25	−0.06	0.80
Total hip BMD Z-scores	0.03	0.76	−0.04	0.80	0.04	0.85	0.14	0.28	0.04	0.85
FN BMD Z-scores	0.04	0.72	0.03	0.87	0.003	0.99	0.15	0.23	−0.12	0.58
Total vBMD (mgHA/cm^3)	0.04	0.73	−0.01	0.94	0.14	0.51	0.09	0.52	**−0.45**	**0.03**[a,b,c]
Trabecular vBMD (mgHA/cm^3)	0.006	0.96	−0.05	0.77	0.09	0.69	0.11	0.40	**−0.52**	**0.01**[a,b,c]
Cortical vBMD (mgHA/cm^3)	**0.25**	**0.04**	0.20	0.26	0.12	0.64	0.17	0.23	0.04	0.87
Total cross-sectional area (mm^2)	−0.06	0.64	−0.03	0.86	−0.07	0.79	0.03	0.86	0.08	0.73
Cortical area/total area	0.04	0.71	−0.11	0.54	0.20	0.43	−0.03	0.84	−0.24	0.31
Cortical thickness (mm)	0.08	0.49	−0.11	0.53	0.27	0.29	0.01	0.94	−0.27	0.25
Cortical porosity (%)	**−0.24***	**0.04**[a]	−0.03	0.84	−0.36	0.16	−0.16	0.25	−0.11	0.63
Stiffness (kN/m)	0.099	0.41	0.005	0.98	0.03	0.90	0.15	0.28	−0.30	0.19
Failure load (kN)	0.09	0.43	−0.01	0.95	0.06	0.82	0.15	0.29	−0.27	0.26
P1NP (ng/ml)	−0.07	0.62	0.11	0.67	−0.21	0.39	−0.05	0.77	−0.06	0.80
CTX (ng/ml)	0.05	0.71	−0.04	0.86	0.14	0.58	0.11	0.51	0.08	0.75

Spearman correlations;
[a]$p<0.05$ after controlling for lean mass;
[b]$p<0.05$ after controlling for lean mass and activity;
[c]$p<0.05$ after controlling for lean mass, activity and fat mass; BMD: bone mineral density; FN: femoral neck; vBMD: volumetric bone mineral density.
All: all subjects; AA: amenorrheic athletes; EA: eumenorrheic athletes; ATH: all athletes; NA: non-athletes.
P values ≤0.05 are bolded.

an increase in irisin following acute exercise, but a decrease in irisin after a 12-week period of endurance and strength training [26]. We found that irisin levels were lower in AA compared to EA and non- athletes, and these differences persisted after controlling for fat and lean mass. Our data likely reflect the effects of chronic exercise on irisin levels, in contrast to some previous studies that examined effects of short-durations of exercise on irisin secretion. Our data are consistent with a study of adult men that reported inverse associations of irisin with regular exercise related physical activities [27]. Furthermore, irisin levels were positively associated with resting energy expenditure. Irisin levels did not differ between EA and non-athletes in our study, suggesting that chronic exercise does not affect irisin levels in the setting of eumenorrhea and preserved energy stores. Decreased irisin levels in AA likely represent an adaptive response in chronic exercisers to reduce REE and conserve energy by reducing brown adipogenesis. This is corroborated by reports of lower irisin levels [25] and lower occurrence of brown fat in conditions of extreme malnutrition, such as anorexia nervosa [28], reductions in circulating irisin following marked weight loss in patients after bariatric surgery [22], and increased levels in obesity [25].

We did not assess brown fat in our subjects, and this is an area of future study. Of note, although our AA subjects had lower BMI than EA, their BMI was not as low as in girls with anorexia nervosa. Thus, these AA subjects are in a state of subtle energy deficit as indicated by their reduced fat mass and lower resting energy expenditure after correcting for lean mass, but not in the state of extreme energy deficit observed in anorexia nervosa. Another small study in patients with anorexia nervosa assessed irisin levels in those reporting moderate vs. high levels of physical activity, and found no differences in BMI, REE or irisin levels across groups, although the higher activity group had higher total energy expenditure [29]. These data suggest that irisin drives changes in REE (or vice versa), but not in total energy expenditure, consistent with irisin being an inducer of brown adipogenesis (and driver of REE), and the positive associations of irisin with REE in our subjects.

In addition, consistent with irisin being a myokine and with other studies that have reported positive associations of irisin with muscle mass [22,25,30], we observed positive associations of irisin with lean mass in athletes. Other studies have reported positive associations of irisin with nutritional markers such as BMI, fat mass, IGF-1 and insulin, and with markers of the metabolic syndrome such as higher blood pressure, insulin resistance and lipid levels, [22,25,27]. Higher irisin levels in obesity, and in patients with the metabolic syndrome may represent a physiological response to improve glucose tolerance and lipid parameters in these individuals [25,26,27]. One study reported lower irisin levels in patients with type 2 diabetes than controls of similar BMI, which may represent a failure of this physiological response leading to diabetes [31]. However, a study in obese children reported an increase (rather than a decrease in irisin levels after a year of exercise and lifestyle intervention [32]. These seemingly conflicting data speak to the complexity of irisin interactions with metabolic endpoints, and the need for further studies to clarify the role of irisin as a regulator of metabolism. We found no associations of irisin with fat mass in our study, maybe because we assessed only lean individuals in our cohort.

Of interest, irisin levels were higher in our study than reported in many previous studies, likely consequent to differences in the specific assay used for analysis [20] and the younger age of our subjects. Some studies have reported inverse associations of irisin with age [22,33], and several fold higher irisin levels in young adult men compared with middle aged women [22].

Moreover, irisin has a potential role in modulating bone metabolism through direct [10,34] and indirect (brown fat mediated) effects. A recent study demonstrates that irisin may affect osteoblastogenesis via the Wnt/beta-catenin pathway downstream of the BMP receptor signal, and also inhibits osteoclast differentiation [10]. Furthermore, *in vivo* studies indicate that irisin increases bone trabecular volume and cortical thickness in mice [10]. Our data are consistent in that irisin levels predicted trabecular volumetric BMD measures in addition to other measures of bone density and strength estimates in athletes. Effects of irisin on bone may also be mediated via induction of brown adipogenesis given reports of associations of brown fat with bone strength estimates in women [8], and with cortical thickness in children and adolescents [9]. In adult women, lower irisin levels have been associated with a higher risk of osteoporotic fractures [33].

Similar to irisin, FGF21 levels increase with acute or short durations of exercise [35,36], decrease with regular exercise and caloric restriction in animals and humans [37,38], decrease in extreme states of malnutrition (as in anorexia nervosa) related to BMI [24], and increase in obesity and the metabolic syndrome related to fat mass [39,40,41]. Given known effects of FGF21 in inducing brown adipogenesis [4,5] and increasing REE, these changes likely represent an adaptive response to decrease brown adipogenesis and conserve energy in anorexia nervosa, and to increase brown adipogenesis and expend energy in obesity. Conversely, these changes may also signal an FGF21 resistant state. Consistent with the study in women with anorexia nervosa [24], we found that FGF21 levels were low in AA compared to EA and non athletes and inversely associated with hours per week of exercise, likely again an adaptive response to conserve energy. In contrast, a study of sedentary healthy young women reported an increase in FGF-21 levels after two-weeks of exercise [24], suggesting that short-term energy expenditure in sedentary women may result in increases in FGF-21 whereas longer-term chronic energy expenditure leads to decreased FGF-21 to preserve energy. FGF21 also impacts bone metabolism, although available reports are contradictory with some studies indicating beneficial [12,13], and others indicating deleterious [11] effects of FGF21 on bone. In our study, FGF21 was associated positively with cortical volumetric BMD and inversely with cortical porosity for the group taken together, consistent with a beneficial effect of FGF21 on bone. However, associations were lost after controlling for irisin, body composition and exercise activity. Further studies are needed to clarify effects of FGF-21 on bone.

Few studies have examined associations of irisin and FGF21 with the sex steroids. We observed positive associations of both hormones with the free androgen index in AA. However, associations of these hormones with estradiol were conflicting, with positive associations noted with irisin and inverse associations with FGF21 in non-athletes. Of interest, positive associations of FGF21 with testosterone levels have been reported in women with polycystic ovarian syndrome (PCOS) [42], and positive associations of irisin and FGF21 with testosterone levels may reflect associations of these hormones with components of the metabolic syndrome. Although one study reported higher FGF21 levels in women with PCOS than in those without this condition, another study found no differences in FGF21 across groups [43].

Conclusions

We report low levels of irisin and FGF-21 in young amenorrheic athletes compared with eumenorrheic athletes and non-athletes, even after taking into account fat and lean mass. In addition, we demonstrate that irisin levels are a determinant of measures of areal and volumetric bone mineral density and bone strength estimates in athletes, but not non-athletes. While this is the first study to report levels of irisin and FGF21 in adolescent female athletes and non-athletes, it is a cross-sectional study and therefore causality cannot be inferred from our data. Further research regarding the role of these hormones in regulating bone metabolism will be important.

Author Contributions

Conceived and designed the experiments: MM. Performed the experiments: VS KEA HC KE DAM NPD MLB MM. Analyzed the data: VS EAL HL MM. Wrote the paper: VS EAL PKF MM.

References

1. Lee P, Linderman JD, Smith S, Brychta RJ, Wang J, et al. (2014) Irisin and FGF21 are cold-induced endocrine activators of brown fat function in humans. Cell Metab 19: 302–309.
2. Bostrom P, Wu J, Jedrychowski MP, Korde A, Ye L, et al. A PGC1-alpha-dependent myokine that drives brown-fat-like development of white fat and thermogenesis. Nature 481: 463–468.
3. Huh JY, Panagiotou G, Mougios V, Brinkoetter M, Vamvini MT, et al. FNDC5 and irisin in humans: I. Predictors of circulating concentrations in serum and plasma and II. mRNA expression and circulating concentrations in response to weight loss and exercise. Metabolism 61: 1725–1738.
4. Fisher FM, Kleiner S, Douris N, Fox EC, Mepani RJ, et al. FGF21 regulates PGC-1alpha and browning of white adipose tissues in adaptive thermogenesis. Genes Dev 26: 271–281.
5. Lee P, Brychta RJ, Linderman J, Smith S, Chen KY, et al. Mild cold exposure modulates fibroblast growth factor 21 (FGF21) diurnal rhythm in humans: relationship between FGF21 levels, lipolysis, and cold-induced thermogenesis. J Clin Endocrinol Metab 98: E98–102.
6. Cuevas-Ramos D, Almeda-Valdes P, Gomez-Perez FJ, Meza-Arana CE, Cruz-Bautista I, et al. Daily physical activity, fasting glucose, uric acid, and body mass index are independent factors associated with serum fibroblast growth factor 21 levels. Eur J Endocrinol 163: 469–477.
7. Cuevas-Ramos D, Almeda-Valdes P, Meza-Arana CE, Brito-Cordova G, Gomez-Perez FJ, et al. Exercise increases serum fibroblast growth factor 21 (FGF21) levels. PLoS One 7: e38022.
8. Lee P, Brychta RJ, Collins MT, Linderman J, Smith S, et al. (2012) Cold-activated brown adipose tissue is an independent predictor of higher bone mineral density in women. Osteoporos Int 24: 1513–1518.
9. Ponrartana S, Aggabao PC, Hu HH, Aldrovandi GM, Wren TA, et al. (2012) Brown adipose tissue and its relationship to bone structure in pediatric patients. J Clin Endocrinol Metab 97: 2693–2698.
10. Zhang J, Cheng J, Tu Q, Chen J (2013) Effects of Irisin on Bone Metabolism and its Signal Transduction ASBMR 2013 Book of Abstracts.
11. Wei W, Dutchak PA, Wang X, Ding X, Bookout AL, et al. (2012) Fibroblast growth factor 21 promotes bone loss by potentiating the effects of peroxisome proliferator-activated receptor gamma. Proc Natl Acad Sci U S A 109: 3143–3148.
12. Lee P, Linderman J, Smith S, Brychta RJ, Perron R, et al. (2013) Fibroblast growth factor 21 (FGF21) and bone: is there a relationship in humans? Osteoporos Int.
13. Ishida K, Haudenschild DR (2013) Interactions between FGF21 and BMP-2 in osteogenesis. Biochem Biophys Res Commun 432: 677–682.
14. Ackerman KE, Nazem T, Chapko D, Russell M, Mendes N, et al. (2011) Bone microarchitecture is impaired in adolescent amenorrheic athletes compared with eumenorrheic athletes and nonathletic controls. J Clin Endocrinol Metab 96: 3123–3133.
15. Ackerman K, Putman M, Guereca G, Taylor A, Pierce L, et al. (2012) Cortical Microstructure and Estimated Bone Strength in Young Amenorrheic Athletes, Eumenorrheic Athletes and Non-Athletes. Bone In Press.
16. Lawson EA, Ackerman KE, Estella NM, Guereca G, Pierce L, et al. (2013) Nocturnal oxytocin secretion is lower in amenorrheic athletes than nonathletes and associated with bone microarchitecture and finite element analysis parameters. Eur J Endocrinol 168: 457–464.
17. Fazeli PK, Ackerman KE, Pierce L, Guereca G, Bouxsein M, et al. (2013) Sclerostin and Pref-1 have differential effects on bone mineral density and strength parameters in adolescent athletes compared with non-athletes. Osteoporos Int 24: 2433–2440.
18. Harris JA, Benedict FG (1918) A Biometric Study of Human Basal Metabolism. Proc Natl Acad Sci U S A 4: 370–373.
19. Weir JB (1949) New methods for calculating metabolic rate with special reference to protein metabolism. J Physiol 109: 1–9.
20. Peter PR, Park KH, Huh JY, Wedick NM, Mantzoros CS (2014) Circulating irisin levels are not affected by coffee intake: a randomized controlled trial. PLoS One 9: e94463.
21. Hecksteden A, Wegmann M, Steffen A, Kraushaar J, Morsch A, et al. (2013) Irisin and exercise training in humans - results from a randomized controlled training trial. BMC Med 11: 235.
22. Huh JY, Panagiotou G, Mougios V, Brinkoetter M, Vamvini MT, et al. (2012) FNDC5 and irisin in humans: I. Predictors of circulating concentrations in serum and plasma and II. mRNA expression and circulating concentrations in response to weight loss and exercise. Metabolism 61: 1725–1738.
23. Miller KK, Rosner W, Lee H, Hier J, Sesmilo G, et al. (2004) Measurement of free testosterone in normal women and women with androgen deficiency: comparison of methods. J Clin Endocrinol Metab 89: 525–533.
24. Dostalova I, Kavalkova P, Haluzikova D, Lacinova Z, Mraz M, et al. (2008) Plasma concentrations of fibroblast growth factors 19 and 21 in patients with anorexia nervosa. J Clin Endocrinol Metab 93: 3627–3632.
25. Stengel A, Hofmann T, Goebel-Stengel M, Elbelt U, Kobelt P, et al. (2013) Circulating levels of irisin in patients with anorexia nervosa and different stages of obesity–correlation with body mass index. Peptides 39: 125–130.
26. Norheim F, Langleite TM, Hjorth M, Holen T, Kielland A, et al. (2014) The effects of acute and chronic exercise on PGC-1alpha, irisin and browning of subcutaneous adipose tissue in humans. FEBS J 281: 739–749.
27. Park KH, Zaichenko L, Brinkoetter M, Thakkar B, Sahin-Efe A, et al. (2013) Circulating irisin in relation to insulin resistance and the metabolic syndrome. J Clin Endocrinol Metab 98: 4899–4907.
28. Bredella MA, Fazeli PK, Freedman LM, Calder G, Lee H, et al. (2012) Young women with cold-activated brown adipose tissue have higher bone mineral density and lower Pref-1 than women without brown adipose tissue: a study in women with anorexia nervosa, women recovered from anorexia nervosa, and normal-weight women. J Clin Endocrinol Metab 97: E584–590.
29. Hofmann T, Elbelt U, Ahnis A, Kobelt P, Rose M, et al. (2014) Irisin Levels are Not Affected by Physical Activity in Patients with Anorexia Nervosa. Front Endocrinol (Lausanne) 4: 202.
30. Kurdiova T, Balaz M, Vician M, Maderova D, Vlcek M, et al. (2014) Effects of obesity, diabetes and exercise on Fndc5 gene expression and irisin release in human skeletal muscle and adipose tissue: in vivo and in vitro studies. J Physiol 592: 1091–1107.
31. Moreno-Navarrete JM, Ortega F, Serrano M, Guerra E, Pardo G, et al. (2013) Irisin is expressed and produced by human muscle and adipose tissue in association with obesity and insulin resistance. J Clin Endocrinol Metab 98: E769–778.
32. Bluher S, Panagiotou G, Petroff D, Markert J, Wagner A, et al. (2014) Effects of a 1-year exercise and lifestyle intervention on irisin, adipokines, and inflammatory markers in obese children. Obesity (Silver Spring).
33. Anastasilakis AD, Polyzos SA, Makras P, Gkiomisi A, Bisbinas I, et al. (2014) Circulating irisin is associated with osteoporotic fractures in postmenopausal women with low bone mass but is not affected by either teriparatide or denosumab treatment for 3 months. Osteoporos Int 25: 1633–1642.
34. Colaianni G, Cuscito C, Mongelli T, Oranger A, Mori G, et al. (2014) Irisin enhances osteoblast differentiation in vitro. Int J Endocrinol 2014: 902186.
35. Kim KH, Kim SH, Min YK, Yang HM, Lee JB, et al. (2013) Acute exercise induces FGF21 expression in mice and in healthy humans. PLoS One 8: e63517.
36. Cuevas-Ramos D, Almeda-Valdes P, Meza-Arana CE, Brito-Cordova G, Gomez-Perez FJ, et al. (2012) Exercise increases serum fibroblast growth factor 21 (FGF21) levels. PLoS One 7: e38022.
37. Fletcher JA, Meers GM, Laughlin MH, Ibdah JA, Thyfault JP, et al. (2012) Modulating fibroblast growth factor 21 in hyperphagic OLETF rats with daily exercise and caloric restriction. Appl Physiol Nutr Metab 37: 1054–1062.
38. Yang SJ, Hong HC, Choi HY, Yoo HJ, Cho GJ, et al. (2011) Effects of a three-month combined exercise programme on fibroblast growth factor 21 and fetuin-A levels and arterial stiffness in obese women. Clin Endocrinol (Oxf) 75: 464–469.
39. Reinehr T, Woelfle J, Wunsch R, Roth CL Fibroblast growth factor 21 (FGF-21) and its relation to obesity, metabolic syndrome, and nonalcoholic fatty liver in children: a longitudinal analysis. J Clin Endocrinol Metab 97: 2143–2150.
40. Zhang X, Yeung DC, Karpisek M, Stejskal D, Zhou ZG, et al. (2008) Serum FGF21 levels are increased in obesity and are independently associated with the metabolic syndrome in humans. Diabetes 57: 1246–1253.
41. Shen Y, Ma X, Zhou J, Pan X, Hao Y, et al. (2013) Additive relationship between serum fibroblast growth factor 21 level and coronary artery disease. Cardiovasc Diabetol 12: 124.
42. Gorar S, Culha C, Uc ZA, Dellal FD, Serter R, et al. (2010) Serum fibroblast growth factor 21 levels in polycystic ovary syndrome. Gynecol Endocrinol 26: 819–826.
43. Sahin SB, Ayaz T, Cure MC, Sezgin H, Ural UM, et al. (2014) Fibroblast growth factor 21 and its relation to metabolic parameters in women with polycystic ovary syndrome. Scand J Clin Lab Invest.

Awareness, Treatment, Control of Diabetes Mellitus and the Risk Factors: Survey Results from Northeast China

Chang Wang[1], Yaqin Yu[1], Xiangyang Zhang[2], Yong Li[1], Changgui Kou[1], Bo Li[1], Yuchun Tao[1], Qing Zhen[1], Huan He[1], Joseph Sam Kanu[1], Xufeng Huang[3], Mei Han[3], Yawen Liu[1]*

1 Department of Epidemiology and Biostatistics, School of Public Health, Jilin University, Changchun City, Jilin Province, P.R. China, **2** Beijing Hui-Long-Guan hospital, Peking University, Beijing, P.R. China, **3** Illawarra Health and Medical Research Institute, University of Wollongong, Wollongong, Australia

Abstract

Background: The awareness, treatment and control of diabetes mellitus (DM) can effectively reflect on the social status of diabetes conditions. Although several researchers have investigated the awareness, treatment and control rates of diabetes mellitus in China, little is known about their association with risk factors. This study aims to examine the relationship between risk factors and awareness, treatment and control of diabetes mellitus in northeast China.

Methods: A cross-sectional survey was conducted in 2012. Multistage stratified random cluster sampling design was used to select participants aged 18 to 79 years old. The analysis was based on a representative sample of 1,854 adult subjects. Multivariable logistic regression analysis was used to examine socio-demographic factors associated with the levels of awareness, treatment and control of diabetes mellitus.

Results: The awareness, treatment, and control rates of diabetes mellitus were 64.1%, 52.9% and 44.2%, respectively. In the multivariable logistic regression analysis, family history of diabetes was significantly positively associated with awareness (OR, 2.145; 95% CI, 1.600–2.875) and treatment (OR, 2.021; 95% CI, 1.559–2.619) of diabetes mellitus, while negatively associated with control (OR, 0.671; 95% CI, 0.529–0.951). Cigarette smokers and alcohol drinkers were less likely than non-smokers and non-drinkers to be aware of their blood glucose levels (OR, 0.895, 0.614; 95% CI, 0.659–1.216, 0.446–0.844, respectively). Participants who frequently exercise were more likely to be aware of their diabetic conditions than people who never or rarely exercise (OR, 2.003; 95% CI, 1.513–2.651).

Conclusions: We found that the awareness and treatment of diabetes mellitus were positively associated with age and were high in participants with a family history of diabetes and those who exercise frequently, but low for cigarette smokers and alcohol drinkers. Participants with a family history of diabetes had their diabetic condition poorly controlled.

Editor: Stephen L. Atkin, Weill Cornell Medical College Qatar, Qatar

Funding: This work was supported by the Scientific Research Foundation of the Health Bureau of Jilin Province, China (Grant Number: 2011Z116). The funders had no role in study design, data collection and analysis, decision to publish, or preparation of the manuscript.

* Email: ywliu@jlu.edu.cn

Introduction

With rapid economic development, population ageing and urbanization, DM has become an important medical problem in nearly all countries [1,2,3]. It is estimated that the number of people with DM is expected to rise to 552 million by 2030, with a 69% increase from 2010 to 2030 for developing countries, compared to 20% for developed countries [4,5]. DM has become a heavy economic burden for every country.

China's prevalence of DM has been ranked second in the world, and has the largest absolute disease burden that is due to increasing prevalence and low awareness, treatment and control of DM [1,6]. It is estimated that the age-standardized prevalence of total DM in China is 9.7% (10.6% among men and 8.8% among women) [7]. Early detection of high blood glucose levels and a comprehensive care of diabetes are effective for improving clinical outcomes and quality of life for DM. Therefore, China critically needs government-initiated primary prevention measures for DM, which focuses on the risk factors of the awareness, treatment and control.

The awareness, treatment and control of DM can effectively reflect on the social status of diabetes conditions. Although several researchers have investigated the awareness, treatment and control rates of DM in China [8,9], little is known about their association with risk factors.

Jilin province is located in northeast China and has a population of about 27 million people. Jilin Department of Health and Jilin University jointly investigated the prevalence of DM and risk factors for awareness, treatment and control of DM in Jilin province in 2012. We used data from this investigation to examine the distribution of awareness, treatment, and control of DM among adult residents in northeast China, as well as how risk factors relate to the awareness, treatment and control of DM.

Materials and Methods

Study population

We carried out a large-scale community-based cross-sectional health interview and examination survey on permanent residents aged 18 to 79 years old who had lived in Jilin province for more than six months. The survey respondents were asked to answer each question face-to-face with investigators who had been uniformly trained.

Sampling method

Five-stage stratified random cluster sampling was used to select the study sample. In the first stage, 32 districts/counties were identified in proportion to population, geographic location and ethnicity, form 9 cities (Changchun, Jilin, Siping, Liaoyuan, Tonghua, Baishan, Songyuan, Baicheng and Yanbian). At the second stage, three or four towns (depending on the size of the district) were selected by stratified random sampling to guarantee the representativeness of each sample. In the third stage, three neighborhood committees were chosen by stratified random sampling from each of the towns previously selected. In the fourth stage, one village from each chosen neighborhood committee was selected by simple random sampling. In the final stage, cluster random sampling was used to identify individuals aged 18 to 79 years old from each of the villages selected for the study.

Data collection and measurement

A strict quality control system was implemented at each stage of the data collection to ensure uniformity and accuracy of the data. Before the formal investigation, a pre-investigation was conducted to explore the design of the questionnaire. In addition, systematic training for all investigators was organized to teach them on how to administer the screening questionnaire, and how to take anthropometric measurements. Before the interview, the identity of each participant was confirmed by the investigator. The validity of each answered questionnaire was examined by the interviewer after the participant had completed the questionnaire in order to ascertain whether the responses were consistent with the real situation. After the fieldwork, all data were processed by parallel double entry. Three verifications were carried out to check for incomplete or inconsistent responses, and then deleted the missing data that cannot be repaired.

The data collection included an intensive investigation and household survey. The purpose of the investigation was explained to the participants before the interview, and then given the option to sign an informed consent form, and only those who consented to participate in the study proceeded to answering the questions and doing the further investigations. The study was approved by the Institutional Review Board of the School of Public Health, Jilin University, Jilin, China. The demographic information collected included gender, age, family income, level of education, occupation, smoking, drinking, exercise, diagnosis and treatment of diabetes, and self-reported family history of diabetes. In addition, anthropometric measurements including height, weight, and fasting blood sugar were taken.

During the interview, weight and height were determined though standardized protocol and measured in light indoor clothing without shoes. Body mass index (BMI) was calculated as weight in kilograms divided by height in meters squared (kg/m^2). Fasting plasma glucose (FPG) levels were measured using the Bayer Bai Ankang fingertip blood glucose monitor machine by taking a small drop of blood from a finger onto a strip of paper in the morning after participants fasted for 10 or more hours overnight.

Definitions

DM was defined as a FPG ≥7.0 mmol/L or self-reported use of anti-diabetic medications during the 2 weeks prior to the examination. Diagnosed diabetes was defined as those meeting the standards for DM [10] or participants reported he/she had previous diagnosis of diabetes by a medical doctor in a hospital above the county level. Individuals with diabetes were considered to be aware of diabetes if they reported having a previous diagnosis of diabetes by medical doctors. Individuals with diabetes were classified as being taking treatment for diabetes if they reported using anti-diabetic medications during the 2 weeks prior to the examination. Among treated diabetes, diabetes was considered to be controlled if FPG≤ 7.0 mmol/L.

Education was divided into three (3) levels: junior school (including those who never attended school, those who attained elementary schooling only, and those who attained junior school); high school (including those who attained high school and a 3-year secondary vocational schooling); and tertiary level of education (including undergraduate and graduate levels of education). Manual labor occupation included production workers, farmers and service workers. Mental labor included office and other technical staffs. Other occupations included students, unemployed and retirees. Body Mass Index (BMI) was classified as: underweight, BMI<18.5 kg/m^2; normal weight, 18.5≤BMI< 24 kg/m^2; overweight, 24≤BMI<28 kg/m^2; and obese, BMI≥ 28 kg/m^2 [11]. Smoker was defined as a person who smoked more than one cigarette per day in the past 30 days. Drinker was defined as a person who consumed an average of more than one alcoholic drink per week, whether spirits, beer, wine or other forms of alcohol. Participants who were classified as "sometimes exercise" were defined as persons who exercised one or two times a week; those who exercised more than three times a week were defined as "exercise frequently" ; while those don't or seldom exercise were defined as "never exercise" or "rarely exercise".

Statistical analysis

All statistical analyses were weighted to represent the total adult population of Jilin province. The sampling weights were obtained from the 2010 China population census data, and were calculated based on four factors: regional, urban/rural, gender, and age in Jilin province. Frequency distributions were used to describe the awareness, treatment, and control with the categories of participants' characteristics. The Rao-Scott Chi-square tests corrected for complex sampling design were used to compare the awareness, treatment and control of diabetes in the different groups. Multivariable logistic regressions were used to examine the socio-demographic factors associated with the levels of diabetes awareness, treatment and control, and the odds-ratio (OR) and 95% confidence intervals (CI) were calculated. Sampling errors were estimated by using the primary sampling units and strata provided in the data set. The standard errors of these estimates were corrected for the clustering used in the five-stage stratified random clustering sampling procedure. Data were analyzed using the complex samples function of SPSS version 21.0 and $P \leq 0.05$ was considered to be statistically significant.

Results

Of the 18260 participants, a total of 1854 (8.2% after weighted) were diagnosed with DM. The analyzed sample included 1,854 participants, which consisted of 941 women and 913 men. As shown in Table 1, participants aged 55–64 years were the largest age group (29.9%), 63.6% only attained junior school education, 26.1% had a high school education, and 34.0% had a family monthly income of 1000–2000 Yuan. Table 1 also shows that manual labor had a higher percentage than mental labor (46.1% vs. 16.3%); 29.0% had a family history of diabetes; and 30.7% were cigarette smokers at the time of the study; 31.6% were alcohol drinkers.

Table 2 shows the awareness, treatment and control (among treated) rates of DM in relation to the various socio-demographic factors. The awareness, treatment and control percentages of DM were 64.1%, 52.9% and 44.2% respectively. Women had a greater awareness (74.2% vs. 56.4%) and treatment (62.2% vs. 45.7%) of DM than men. The awareness, treatment and control rates increased with advancing age ($P<0.05$). Levels of educations were not significantly associated with control of DM ($P>0.05$). Manual laborers had greater awareness (58.9% vs. 54.8%) and treatment (47.6% vs. 41.2%) of DM compared to mental workers. People with a family history of diabetes (73.0% vs. 60.5%, $P<0.001$) were more likely to be aware of their diabetic conditions and to be treated with anti-diabetic medications than those without the family history (61.4% vs. 49.4%, $P<0.001$), but the percentage of control was significantly higher in those having no family history of diabetes compared to those having family history (47.6% vs. 37.5%, $P=0.005$). There were no statistically significant associations between BMI and awareness, treatment or control of DM.

Table 1. Demographic characteristics between different socio-demographic factors.

Category	Subcategory	Frequency (n = 1854)	Percentage (%)	Estimated population
Gender	Female	941	43.4	653
	Male	913	56.6	850
Age (years)	18~34	50	7.5	113
	35~44	200	15.0	226
	45~54	565	28.7	430
	55~64	681	29.9	448
	65~79	358	18.9	284
Education	<Junior school	1221	62.6	940
	High school	452	26.1	392
	Undergraduate	181	11.3	170
Income (Chinese Yuan)	<500	463	21.3	321
	500~	378	19.5	292
	1000~	610	34.0	511
	2000~	260	16.1	242
	3000~	143	9.1	137
Occupation	Manual labor	883	46.1	693
	Mental labor	260	16.3	244
	Other	711	37.6	565
Family history	No	1330	71.0	1066
	Yes	524	29.0	436
Region	Rural	923	44.4	667
	Urban	931	55.6	835
BMI*	Normal	546	29.1	432
	Underweight	28	1.4	21
	Overweight	816	44.8	665
	Obesity	446	24.8	368
Smoker	Never	1082	55.9	840
	Now	533	30.7	461
	Once	239	13.4	202
Drinker	No	1326	68.4	1028
	Yes	528	31.6	475
Exercise	Never or rare	635	34.3	515
	Sometimes	332	19.3	290
	Frequently	887	46.4	697

*BMI, Body mass index. Percentage did not add up to 100% due to missing data.

Table 2. Comparison of awareness, treatment and control of diabetes between various factors [n (%)].

Category	Subcategory	Awareness		Treatment		Control among treated	
		%(n)	Estimated population	%(n)	Estimated population	%(n)	Estimated population
Total		64.1(1245)	963	52.9(1056)	794	44.2(466)	351
Gender	Female	74.2(696)	484	62.2(596)	406	45.8(277)	186
	Male	56.4(549)	479	45.7(460)	388	42.5(189)	165
	P value	<0.001		<0.001		0.338	
Age (years)	18~34	27.4(13)	31	4.7(3)	5	10.4(1)	1
	35~44	48.8(100)	110	39.4(81)	89	35.8(30)	32
	45~54	62.7(359)	270	53.5(305)	230	41.2(120)	95
	55~65	73.5(500)	330	63.2(432)	283	43.1(190)	122
	65~79	78.3(273)	222	65.6(235)	186	54.6(125)	102
	P value	<0.001		<0.001		0.006	
Education	<Junior school	67.5(841)	634	55.7(714)	524	43.9(312)	230
	High school	59.4(293)	233	48.4(250)	190	44.8(113)	85
	Undergraduate	56.6(111)	96	47.1(92)	80	44.4(41)	36
	P value	0.011		0.035		0.975	
Income (Chinese Yuan)	<500	70.2(341)	225	59.7(290)	191	39.4(112)	75
	500~	64.7(242)	189	50.0(197)	146	43.1(86)	63
	1000~	62.3(398)	319	51.8(341)	265	47.1(163)	125
	2000~	66.4(183)	161	54.7(156)	132	43.3(70)	57
	3000~	51.3(81)	70	43.5(72)	59	51.3(35)	31
	P value	0.017		0.042		0.374	
Occupation	Manual labor	58.9(552)	408	47.6(461)	330	38.1(180)	126
	Mental labor	54.8(155)	134	41.2(121)	101	42.9(51)	43
	Other	74.6(538)	422	64.3(474)	363	50.1(235)	182
	P value	<0.001		<0.001		0.005	
Family history	No	60.5(836)	645	49.4(704)	526	47.6(331)	251
	Yes	73.0(409)	318	61.4(352)	268	37.5(135)	100
	P value	<0.001		<0.001		0.005	
Region	Rural	65.8(636)	439	52.7(533)	352	41.1(221)	145
	Urban	62.8(609)	524	53.0(523)	442	46.6(245)	206
	P value	0.300		0.929		0.105	
BMI	Normal	62.8(364)	271	50.4(305)	218	44.8(136)	98
	Underweight	53.6(17)	11	41.8(14)	9	23.5(3)	2
	Overweight	64.1(543)	427	54.0(468)	359	43.7(203)	157
	Obesity	66.5(309)	245	55.2(260)	203	45.3(121)	92

Table 2. Cont.

Category	Subcategory	Awareness		Treatment		Control among treated	
		%(n)	Estimated population	%(n)	Estimated population	%(n)	Estimated population
	P value	0.621		0.420		0.570	
Smoker	Never	68.2(769)	573	56.0(652)	470	46.0(304)	216
	Now	52.8(300)	243	44.6(262)	205	39.1(101)	80
	Once	73.1(176)	147	58.7(142)	118	46.0(61)	54
	P value	<0.001		<0.001		0.228	
Drinker	No	70.9(968)	728	59.3(833)	610	45.5(380)	277
	Yes	49.5(277)	235	38.9(223)	185	40.0(86)	74
	P value	<0.001		<0.001		0.186	
Exercise	Never or rare	53.4(368)	275	43.9(310)	226	42.2(131)	95
	Sometimes	58.2(207)	169	46.8(176)	136	43.1(77)	59
	Frequently	74.6(670)	520	62.0(570)	432	45.6(258)	197
	P value	<0.001		<0.001		0.660	

Data are presented as % (n).

Table 3 shows the results of multivariate logistic regressions for the awareness, treatment and control rates of DM. These were performed to determine whether the statistically significant factors found in the univariate analysis were associated with awareness, treatment and control.

After controlling for potential confounding factors of socio-demographic variables, the analyses showed that older individuals have greater probability of being aware of their diabetic conditions and seek medical treatment than younger individuals, and this is presented in Table 3. A family history of diabetes was significantly associated with awareness (OR, 2.145; 95% CI, 1.600–2.875) and treatment (OR, 2.021; 95% CI, 1.559–2.620) of DM, and participants with a family history of diabetes were less likely than those without to have their diabetes controlled (OR, 0.671; 95% CI, 0.529–0.951). Cigarette smokers and alcohol drinkers were less likely than non-smokers and non-drinkers to be aware of their blood glucose levels (OR, 0.895, 0.614; 95% CI, 0.659–1.216, 0.446–0.844, respectively). Participants who exercise frequently were more likely than those who never or rarely exercise to be aware of their diabetes (OR, 2.003; 95% CI, 1.513–2.651) and take anti-diabetic medication (OR, 1.560; 95% CI, 1.209–2.014).

Discussion

In recent years, there have been efforts to perform epidemiological studies on diabetes, but little data covers the awareness, treatment, and control of DM in China. Knowing the factors associated with awareness, treatment and control of DM can be very useful in reducing the prevalence of this disease in China. To our knowledge, this is the first large representative population-based survey to provide insightful data on awareness, treatment, and control of DM and associated factors in Jilin province in northeast China.

In our study, we found that the awareness and treatment of DM in Jilin province is higher than that reported in a prior study in China [6], but much lower than other countries [12,13]. Our univariate analyses showed the relationships of eleven potential confounding factors (gender, age, education, income level, occupation, family history of diabetes, region, BMI, cigarette smoking, alcohol drinking and exercise) with awareness, treatment and control of DM (Table 2). Multivariate logistic regression analyses showed the relationships between gender, age, education, income level, occupation, family history of diabetes, cigarette smoking, alcohol drinking and exercise with awareness, treatment and control of DM, as well as the relationships between age, income level, occupation, family history of diabetes, alcohol drinking and exercise with treatment of DM (Table 3). Prior work [13,14] found that women were more likely than men to be aware of their risks of diabetes, and take their anti-diabetic medications, and those differences were also significant in this study. We also observed that the awareness and treatment of DM increased concomitantly with age, which is consistent with previous studies [15,16]. This may be partly due to the relatively long course of diabetes, as it gives older people more time to accumulate diabetes knowledge. Moreover, life is relatively more stable for older people after retirement, giving them more energy and time to focus on the disease awareness, prevention and control. Previous studies had shown that high family monthly income may be associated with high awareness and treatment rates of DM [17,18], but our study did not find these associations. The reason for this discrepancy needs further investigation. In addition, we found that participants with family history of diabetes were more likely than other members of the diabetes group to be aware of their blood glucose levels and take their anti-diabetic medications. However, cigarette

Table 3. Multivariate logistic regression for awareness, treatment and control of diabetes mellitus.

Category	Subcategory	Awareness		Treatment		Control among treated	
		OR(95.0% CI)	*P*	OR(95.0% CI)	*P*	OR(95.0% CI)	*P*
Gender	Male v. female	0.640(0.464–0.884)	0.007	0.764(0.572–1.020)	0.068	–	–
Age	35~44 v. 18~34	2.611(1.116–6.108)	<0.001	15.789(2.956–84.347)	<0.001	3.949(0.319–48.895)	0.172
	45~54 v. 18~34	4.328(1.901–9.854)		27.302(5.269–141.477)		4.799(0.401–57.375)	–
	55~64 v. 18~34	5.966(2.597–13.703)		33.474(6.396–175.198)		4.726(0.395–56.494)	–
	65~79 v. 18~34	6.951(2.902–16.653)		33.108(6.279–174.583)		6.766(0.558–82.023)	–
Education	High school v. <Junior school	0.948(0.684–1.313)	0.889	1.014(0.755–1.362)	0.778	–	–
	Undergraduate v. <Junior school	0.884(0.521–1.500)		1.196(0.715–2.003)		–	–
Income	500~ v. <500	0.876(0.604–1.272)	0.049	0.731(0.530–1.007)	0.091	–	–
	1000~ v. <500	0.737(0.530–1.026)		0.793(0.584–1.079)		–	–
	2000~ v. <500	1.278(0.819–1.994)		1.178(0.780–1.780)		–	–
	3000~ v. <500	0.740(0.436–1.255)		0.864(0.509–1.469)		–	–
Occupation	Mental labor v. manual labor	0.989 (0.630–1.550)	0.747	0.789 (0.517–1.181)	0.043	1.228 (0.783–1.927)	0.096
	other v. manual labor	1.212 (0.824–1.526)		1.283 (0.986–1.670)		1.403 (1.030–1.910)	
Family history	Yes v. no	2.145(1.600–2.875)	<0.001	2.021(1.559–2.619)	<0.001	0.710 (0.529–0.951)	0.022
Smoker	Now v. never	0.895(0.659–1.216)	0.007	1.088(0.817–1.450)	0.217	–	–
	Once v. never	1.699(1.147–2.517)		1.373(0.962–1.985)		–	–
Drinker	Yes v. no	0.614(0.446–0.844)	0.003	0.551(0.409–0.742)	<0.001	–	–
Exercise	Sometimes v. never or rare	1.377(0.952–1.991)	<0.001	1.259(0.905–1.752)	0.003	–	–
	Frequently v. never or rare	2.003(1.513–2.651)		1.560(1.209–2.014)		–	–

Results are expressed as Odd Ratio and (95% confidence interval).
–, not retained in the model.

smokers and alcohol drinkers were more likely to be unaware of their risks of diabetes, and this is consistent with prior studies [14,19]. Our results suggest that cigarette smokers and alcohol drinkers should pay more attention to their blood glucose levels. The results of study also showed a pronounced relationship between frequent exercise and awareness and treatment of DM. Because we used a cross-sectional design in this our study, our ability to draw causal inference is limited. Therefore, we were unable to explain whether people who exercise more frequently will be more concerned about their blood glucose level or those who are aware of the diabetes condition will take anti-diabetic medications and exercise more frequently. However, it is certain that exercise is a behavioral intervention that DM patients usually undertake to control their high blood glucose levels [20,21].

Although the univariate analyses of diabetes control showed that control among treated diabetes was associated with age, occupation and family history of diabetes, the multivariate analyses model only observed the relationship between mental labor, family history and diabetes control. Our study did not show statistically significant gender differences related to controlling glycemia. This finding agrees with other studies [22,23,24]. Importantly, we found that a family history of diabetes was associated with poor glycemic control and high diabetes treatment, and this is consistent with a prior study [25]; therefore, there is a need for increased public concern and regular surveillance for those who have a family history of diabetes.

In our study, the large sample size and precise physical measurements improved the validity of our results. Furthermore, the study contributed to meaningful insights concerning the current situation and associated risk factors of awareness, treatment and control of DM in northeast China. However, there are some limitations of this present study that should be mentioned. First, the awareness of diabetes was based on self-reported diagnosed DM. Second, the cross-sectional design might limit the ability to draw causal inference between the risk factors and DM. Third, the results in our study were from Jilin province, which may limit our ability to generalize the results to the whole of northeast China.

In summary, we observed that awareness and treatment rates of DM increased with age and higher in participants with a family history of diabetes and those who exercises frequently. The low control rate of diabetes among treated individuals was related to family history of the disease, which contributes to a high incidence of diabetes. Our results suggest that attempts to prevent diabetes should focus on the factors that lead to neglect of heath status; and effective preventive strategies should concentrate on young people and those who have a family history of diabetes, and include decreasing or cessation of alcohol consumption, smoking cessation or doing more exercise.

Acknowledgments

The authors would like to thank Yanhua Wu, Yuan Tang, Zhihui Yan, Le Lv, Huihui Zhang and Fanyu Liu for their participations in this study.

Author Contributions

Conceived and designed the experiments: CW YY Y. Li CK BL YT QZ Y. Liu. Performed the experiments: CW YY Y. Li CK BL YT QZ Y. Liu. Analyzed the data: CW. Contributed reagents/materials/analysis tools: YY Y. Li CK BL YT QZ Y. Liu. Contributed to the writing of the manuscript: CW HH JSK XH MH.

References

1. Chen R, Song Y, Hu Z, Brunner EJ (2012) Predictors of diabetes in older people in urban China. Plos One 7: 1–11.
2. Nyenwe EA, Odia OJ, Ihekwaba AE,Ojule A, Babatunde S (2003) Type 2 diabetes in adult Nigerians: a study of its prevalence and risk factors in Port Harcourt, Nigeria. Diabetes Res Clin Pract 62: 177–185.
3. Engelgau MM, Geiss LS, Saaddine JB, Boyle JP, Benjamin SM, et al. (2004) The evolving diabetes burden in the United States. Ann Intern Med 140: 945–950.
4. Shaw JE, Sicree RA, Zimmet PZ (2010) Global estimates of the prevalence of diabetes for 2010 and 2030. Diabetes Res Clin Pract 87: 4–14.
5. Whiting DR, Guariguata L, Weil C, Shaw J (2011) IDF diabetes atlas: global estimates of the prevalence of diabetes for 2011 and 2030. Diabetes Res Clin Pract 94: 311–321.
6. Hu D, Fu P, Xie J, Chen CS, Yu D, et al. (2008) Increasing prevalence and low awareness, treatment and control of diabetes mellitus among Chinese adults: the InterASIA study. Diabetes Res Clin Pract 81: 250–257.
7. Yang W, Lu J, Weng J, Jia W, Ji L, et al. (2010) Prevalence of diabetes among men and women in China. N Engl J Med 362: 1090–1101.
8. Wu YF, Xie GQ, Li Y, Zhao LC, Zhou BF (2005) The current status on the prevalence, awareness, treatment and control of diabetes mellitus in several Chinese subpopulations. Chinese Journal of Epidemiology 26: 564–568.
9. Yifeng L, Aiguo Y, Ying G, Junwei L, Weidong Z, et al. (2008) Prevalence, awareness and treatment of type 2 diabetes mellitus in rural residents of Henan. Journal of Medical Forum 29: 23–25+27.
10. American Diabetes Association (2008) Diagnosis and classification of diabetes mellitus. Diabetes care 31: S55–S60.
11. Zhou BF (2002) Predictive values of body mass index and waist circumference for risk factors of certain related diseases in Chinese adults-study on optimal cut-off points of body mass index and waist circumference in Chinese adults. Biomed Environ Sci 15: 83–96.
12. Sims M, Diez Roux AV, Boykin S, Sarpong D, Gebreab SY, et al. (2011) The socioeconomic gradient of diabetes prevalence, awareness, treatment, and control among African Americans in the Jackson Heart Study. Ann Epidemiol 21: 892–898.
13. Kaiser A, Vollenweider P, Waeber G, Marques-Vidal P (2012) Prevalence, awareness and treatment of type 2 diabetes mellitus in Switzerland: the CoLaus study 29: 190–197.
14. McDonald M, Hertz RP, Unger AN, Lustik MB (2009) Prevalence, awareness, and management of hypertension, dyslipidemia, and diabetes among United States adults aged 65 and older. J Gerontol A Biol Sci Med Sci 64: 256–263.
15. Alkerwi A, Pagny S, Lair ML, Delagardelle C, Beissel J (2013) Level of unawareness and management of diabetes, hypertension, and dyslipidemia among adults in Luxembourg: findings from ORISCAV-LUX study. PLoS One 8: 1–7.
16. Pei-an L, Peipei C, Jiaxi Y, Lei Z, Ning Z, et al. (2010) A survey on the prevalence rate, awareness rate, treatment rate and control rate of diabetes mellitus in Xuzhou. Chin J Mod Nurs 16: 2371–2374.
17. Le C, Jun D, Zhankun S, Yichun L, Jie T (2011) Socioeconomic differences in diabetes prevalence, awareness, and treatment in rural southwest China. Trop Med Int Health 16: 1070–1076.
18. Brown AF, Ettner SL, Piette J, Weinberger M, Gregg E, et al. (2004) Socioeconomic position and health among persons with diabetes mellitus: a conceptual framework and review of the literature. Epidemical Rev 26: 63–77.
19. Toljamo M, Hentinen M (2001) Adherence to self-care and glycaemic control among people with insulin-dependent diabetes mellitus. Journal of Advanced Nursing 34: 780–786.
20. Zhou Y, Liao L, Sun M, He G (2013) Self-care practices of Chinese individuals with diabetes. Experimental and therapeutic medicine 5: 1137–1142.
21. Wong CK, Lo YY, Wong WH, Fung CS (2013) The associations of body mass index with physical and mental aspects of health-related quality of life in Chinese patients with type 2 diabetes mellitus: results from a cross-sectional survey. Health and quality of life outcomes 11: 1–9.
22. Mendes AB, Fittipaldi JA, Neves RC,Chacra AR, Moreira ED Jr. (2010) Prevalence and correlates of inadequate glycaemic control: results from a nationwide survey in 6,671 adults with diabetes in Brazil. Acta Diabetol 47: 137–145.
23. Fox KM, Gerber Pharmd RA, Bolinder B, Chen J, Kumar S (2006) Prevalence of inadequate glycemic control among patients with type 2 diabetes in the United Kingdom general practice research database: a series of retrospective analyses of data from 1998 through 2002. Clin Ther 28: 388–395.
24. Shah BR, Hux JE, Laupacis A, Mdcm BZ, Austin PC, et al. (2005) Diabetic patients with prior specialist care have better glycaemic control than those with prior primary care. J Eval Clin Pract 11: 568–575.
25. Ong KL, Cheung BM, Wong LY, Wat NM, Tan KC, et al. (2008) Prevalence, treatment, and control of diagnosed diabetes in the U.S. National Health and Nutrition Examination Survey 1999–2004. Ann Epidemiol 18: 222–229.

PERMISSIONS

All chapters in this book were first published in PLOS ONE, by The Public Library of Science; hereby published with permission under the Creative Commons Attribution License or equivalent. Every chapter published in this book has been scrutinized by our experts. Their significance has been extensively debated. The topics covered herein carry significant findings which will fuel the growth of the discipline. They may even be implemented as practical applications or may be referred to as a beginning point for another development.

The contributors of this book come from diverse backgrounds, making this book a truly international effort. This book will bring forth new frontiers with its revolutionizing research information and detailed analysis of the nascent developments around the world.

We would like to thank all the contributing authors for lending their expertise to make the book truly unique. They have played a crucial role in the development of this book. Without their invaluable contributions this book wouldn't have been possible. They have made vital efforts to compile up to date information on the varied aspects of this subject to make this book a valuable addition to the collection of many professionals and students.

This book was conceptualized with the vision of imparting up-to-date information and advanced data in this field. To ensure the same, a matchless editorial board was set up. Every individual on the board went through rigorous rounds of assessment to prove their worth. After which they invested a large part of their time researching and compiling the most relevant data for our readers.

The editorial board has been involved in producing this book since its inception. They have spent rigorous hours researching and exploring the diverse topics which have resulted in the successful publishing of this book. They have passed on their knowledge of decades through this book. To expedite this challenging task, the publisher supported the team at every step. A small team of assistant editors was also appointed to further simplify the editing procedure and attain best results for the readers.

Apart from the editorial board, the designing team has also invested a significant amount of their time in understanding the subject and creating the most relevant covers. They scrutinized every image to scout for the most suitable representation of the subject and create an appropriate cover for the book.

The publishing team has been an ardent support to the editorial, designing and production team. Their endless efforts to recruit the best for this project, has resulted in the accomplishment of this book. They are a veteran in the field of academics and their pool of knowledge is as vast as their experience in printing. Their expertise and guidance has proved useful at every step. Their uncompromising quality standards have made this book an exceptional effort. Their encouragement from time to time has been an inspiration for everyone.

The publisher and the editorial board hope that this book will prove to be a valuable piece of knowledge for researchers, students, practitioners and scholars across the globe.

LIST OF CONTRIBUTORS

Eduardo Gómez-Gómez, Martín Efrén Ríos-Martínez, Elena Margarita Castro-Rodríguez, Jesús Muñiz-Murguía and Mario Ramírez-Flores
Centro Universitario de Investigaciones Biomédicas, Universidad de Colima, Colima, Colima, México

Mario Del-Toro-Equíhua, Luz Margarita Baltazar-Rodríguez, Gilberto Velasco-Pineda and Ivan Delgado-Enciso
Facultad de Medicina, Universidad de Colima, Colima, Colima, México

Ana Lilia Pérez-Huitimea
Educación Física y Deporte. Facultad de Ciencias de la Educación, Universidad de Colima, Colima, Colima, México

Todd A. Astorino
Department of Kinesiology, California State University San Marcos, San Marcos, California, United States of America

Matthew M. Schubert
School of Allied Health Sciences, Griffith University, Gold Coast, Queensland, Australia

Igor Lucas Gomes-Santos, Julio César Ayres Ferreira-Filho and Vera Maria Cury Salemi
Heart Institute (InCor-HCFMUSP), University of São Paulo Medical School, São Paulo, Brazil

Tiago Fernandes, Patricia Chakur Brum and Edilamar Menezes de Oliveira
School of Physical Education and Sport, University of São Paulo, São Paulo, Brazil

Gisele Kruger Couto and Luciana Venturini Rossoni
Department of Physiology and Biophysics, Institute of Biomedical Science, University of São Paulo, São Paulo, Brazil

Fernanda Barrinha Fernandes and Dulce Elena Casarini
Division of Nephrology, Kidney and Hypertension Hospital, Federal University of São Paulo, São Paulo, Brazil

Carlos Eduardo Negrao
Heart Institute (InCor-HCFMUSP), University of São Paulo Medical School, São Paulo, Brazil
School of Physical Education and Sport, University of São Paulo, São Paulo, Brazil

Willem J. R. Bossers, Tibor Hortobágyi and J. G. van Heuvelen
University of Groningen, University Medical Center Groningen, Center for Human Movement Sciences, Groningen, The Netherlands

Erik J. A. Scherder
University of Groningen, University Medical Center Groningen, Center for Human Movement Sciences, Groningen, The Netherlands
VU University, Department of Clinical Neuropsychology, Amsterdam, The Netherlands

Froukje Boersma
University of Groningen, University Medical Center Groningen, Department of General Practice, Elderly Care Medicine, Groningen, The Netherlands

Lucas H. V. van der Woude and Marieke
University of Groningen, University Medical Center Groningen, Center for Human Movement Sciences, Groningen, The Netherlands
University of Groningen, University Medical Center Groningen, Center for Rehabilitation, Groningen, The Netherlands

Caiyue Liu
Department of Plastic and Reconstructive Surgery, Changzheng Hospital, Second Military Medical University, Shanghai, China

Patricia J. Ward and Arthur W. English
Department of Cell Biology, Emory University School of Medicine, Atlanta, Georgia, United States of America

Gregory E. P. Pearcey and Kevin E. Power
School of Human Kinetics and Recreation, Memorial University of Newfoundland, St. John's, NL, Canada

Duane C. Button
School of Human Kinetics and Recreation, Memorial University of Newfoundland, St. John's, NL, Canada
Faculty of Medicine, Memorial University of Newfoundland, St. John's, NL, Canada

Trisha D. Scribbans, Brittany A. Edgett, Brendon J. Gurd and Jennifer B. L. Matusiak
School of Kinesiology and Health Studies, Queen's University, Kingston, Ontario, Canada

Kira Vorobej, Andrew S. Mitchell and Joe Quadrilatero
Department of Kinesiology, University of Waterloo, Waterloo, Ontario, Canada

Sophie D. Joanisse and Gianni Parise
Department of Kinesiology, McMaster University, Hamilton, Ontario, Canada

Marie-Kathrin Breyer
Department of Respiratory Medicine, Maastricht University Medical Center + (MUMC+), Maastricht, the Netherlands
Program Development Center (CIRO), Center of expertise for chronic organ failure, Horn, the Netherlands
Department of Respiratory and Critical Care Medicine and Ludwig Boltzmann Institute for COPD and Pulmonary Epidemiology, Otto Wagner Hospital, Vienna, Austria

Martijn A. Spruit, Frits M. E. Franssen, Lowie E. G. W. Vanfleteren, Miriam T. J. Groenen and Erica P. A. Rutten
Program Development Center (CIRO), Center of expertise for chronic organ failure, Horn, the Netherlands

Corrine K. Hanson
Division of Medical Nutrition Education, School of Allied Health Professions, University of Nebraska Medical Center, Ohmaha, Nebraska, United States of America

Piet L. B. Bruijnzeel
Inflammation Neuroscience and Respiratory, AstraZeneca, Molndal, Sweden

Emiel F. M. Wouters
Department of Respiratory Medicine, Maastricht University Medical Center + (MUMC+), Maastricht, the Netherlands
Program Development Center (CIRO), Center of expertise for chronic organ failure, Horn, the Netherlands

Tadej Debevec and Igor B. Mekjavic
Department of Automation, Biocybernetics and Robotics, Jozef Stefan Institute, Ljubljana, Slovenia

Elizabeth J. Simpson and Ian A. Macdonald
MRC/Arthritis Research UK Centre for Musculoskeletal Ageing Research, University of Nottingham Medical School, School of Life Sciences, Queen's Medical Centre, Nottingham, United Kingdom

Ola Eiken
Department of Environmental Physiology, Swedish Aerospace Physiology Centre, Royal Institute of Technology, Stockholm, Sweden

Francesca Lanfranconi, Luca Pollastri, Alessandra Ferri and Giuseppe Miserocchi
Department of Health Sciences, Laboratory of Clinical Physiology and Sport Medicine, University of Milano-Bicocca, Monza, Italy

Donatella Fraschini and Giuseppe Masera
Department of Pediatrics, University of Milano-Bicocca, San Gerardo Hospital, Monza, Italy

Ilaria Croci
The University of Queensland Diamantina Institute, The University of Queensland, Translational Research Institute, Brisbane, Australia
School of Human Movement Studies, University of Queensland, Brisbane, Australia

Fabio Borrani and Davide Malatesta
Institute of Sport Sciences University of Lausanne, University of Lausanne, Lausanne, Switzerland
Department of Physiology, University of Lausanne, Lausanne, Switzerland

Nuala Byrne
Institute of Health and Biomedical Innovation, Queensland University of Technology, Brisbane, Australia
Bond Institute ofHealth and Sport, Bond University, Robina, Australia

Rachel Wood
Institute of Health and Biomedical Innovation, Queensland University of Technology, Brisbane, Australia

Ingrid Hickman
The University of Queensland Diamantina Institute, The University of Queensland, Translational Research Institute, Brisbane, Australia
Department of Nutrition and Dietetics, Princess Alexandra Hospital, Brisbane, Australia
Mater Medical Research Institute, Mater Mother's Hospital, Brisbane, Australia

Xavier Chenevière
Institute of Sport Sciences University of Lausanne, University of Lausanne, Lausanne, Switzerland
Department of Medicine, University of Fribourg, Fribourg, Switzerland

Yu-Shan Yue and Yi Zhu
Second School of Clinical Medical, Nanjing University of Chinese Medicine, Nanjing, Jiangsu, China

Xu-Dong Wang
Institute of Literature in Chinese Medicine, Nanjing University of Chinese Medicine, Nanjing, Jiangsu, China

Bin Xie
First School of Clinical Medical, Nanjing University of Chinese Medicine, Nanjing, Jiangsu, China

Zhong-Han Li
Applied Health Science Department, University of Waterloo, Waterloo, Ontario, Canada

Bing-Lin Chen and Xue-Qiang Wang
Department of Sport Rehabilitation, Shanghai University of Sport, Shanghai, China

Kathryn R. Martin
Epidemiology Group, School of Medicine and Dentistry, University of Aberdeen, Aberdeen, United Kingdom
Medical Research Council Unit for Lifelong Health and Ageing at University College London, London, United Kingdom
Laboratory of Epidemiology and Population Sciences, National Institute of Aging, National Institutes of Health, Bethesda, Maryland United States of America

Rachel Cooper, Rebecca Hardy and Diana Kuh
Medical Research Council Unit for Lifelong Health and Ageing at University College London, London, United Kingdom

Tamara B. Harris
Laboratory of Epidemiology and Population Sciences, National Institute of Aging, National Institutes of Health, Bethesda, Maryland United States of America

Soren Brage
Medical Research Council Epidemiology Unit, School of Clinical Medicine, Institute of Metabolic Science, University of Cambridge, Cambridge, United Kingdom

Xiaoyue Tan
Department of Pulmonary Function Test, Shanghai Pulmonary Hospital Affiliated to Tongji University, Shanghai, China
State Key Laboratory of Cardiovascular Disease, Heart-Lung Function Testing Center, Fuwai Hospital, National Center for Cardiovascular Diseases, Chinese Academy of Medical Sciences and Peking Union Medical College, Beijing, China

Wenlan Yang, Jian Guo and Changwei Wu
Department of Pulmonary Function Test, Shanghai Pulmonary Hospital Affiliated to Tongji University, Shanghai, China

Yan Zhang
Department of Pulmonary Function Test, Shanghai Pulmonary Hospital Affiliated to Tongji University, Shanghai, China
Respiratory Division, Hangzhou, Zhejiang Provincial Hospital of traditional Chinese Medicine, The First Affiliated Hospital of Zhejiang Chinese Medicine University, Hangzhou, China

Rikesh Sapkota, Shailendra Prasad Kushwaha and Sugang Gong
Department of Pulmonary Circulation, Shanghai Pulmonary Hospital Affiliated to Tongji University, Shanghai, China

Xingguo Sun
State Key Laboratory of Cardiovascular Disease, Heart-Lung Function Testing Center, Fuwai Hospital, National Center for Cardiovascular Diseases, Chinese Academy of Medical Sciences and Peking Union Medical College, Beijing, China

Jinming Liu
Department of Pulmonary Function Test, Shanghai Pulmonary Hospital Affiliated to Tongji University, Shanghai, China
Department of Pulmonary Circulation, Shanghai Pulmonary Hospital Affiliated to Tongji University, Shanghai, China

Lin Li and Liu Ji
Key Laboratory of Adolescent Health Assessment and Exercise Intervention, Ministry of Education, Shanghai, China
Physical Education and Health School, East China Normal University, Shanghai, China

Wei-Wei Men and Ming-Xia Fan
Shanghai Key Laboratory of Magnetic Resonance, East China Normal University, Shanghai, China

Yu-Kai Chang
Graduate Institute of Athletics and Coaching Science, National Taiwan Sport University, Taiwan

Gao-Xia Wei
Key Laboratory of Mental Health, Institute of Psychology, Chinese Academy of Sciences, Beijing, China
Key Laboratory of Behavioral Science, Institute of Psychology, Chinese Academy of Sciences, Beijing, China

Matthew D. Campbell, Mark Russell, Emma J. Stevenson and Daniel J. West
Department of Sport, Exercise and Rehabilitation, Faculty of Health and Life Sciences, Northumbria University, Newcastle-upon-Tyne, United Kingdom

Mark Walker
Institute of Cellular Medicine, Newcastle University, Newcastle-upon-Tyne, United Kingdom

Michael I. Trenell
Institute for Ageing and Health, Faculty of Medicine, Newcastle University, Newcastleupon-Tyne, United Kingdom

Steven Luzio, Gareth Dunseath and Stephen C. Bain
Diabetes Research Group, College of Medicine, Swansea University Swansea, United Kingdom

Daniel Tuner and Richard M. Bracken
Applied Sports, Technology, Exercise and Medicine Research Centre, College of Engineering, Swansea University, Swansea, United Kingdom

Mette Toftager, Lars B. Christiansen and Jens Troelsen
Institute of Sports Science and Clinical Biomechanics, University of Southern Denmark, Odense, Denmark
Centre for Intervention Research in Health Promotion and Disease Prevention, National Institute of Public Health, University of Southern Denmark, Copenhagen, Denmark

Annette K. Ersbøll and Pernille Due
Centre for Intervention Research in Health Promotion and Disease Prevention, National Institute of Public Health, University of Southern Denmark, Copenhagen, Denmark

Peter L. Kristensen
Institute of Sports Science and Clinical Biomechanics, University of Southern Denmark, Odense, Denmark

Sanna Neselius and Helena Brisby
Department of Orthopaedics, Sahlgrenska University Hospital, Gothenburg, Sweden
Institute for Clinical Sciences, the Sahlgrenska Academy at the University of Gothenburg, Gothenburg, Sweden

Jan Marcusson
Geriatric Section, University Hospital in Linköping, Linköping, Sweden
Institution of Clinical and Experimental Medicine, Linköping University, Linköping, Sweden

Henrik Zetterberg
Clinical Neurochemistry Laboratory, Sahlgrenska University Hospital, Mölndal, Sweden
Institute of Neuroscience and Physiology, Department of Psychiatry and Neurochemistry, the Sahlgrenska Academy at the University of Gothenburg, Gothenburg, Sweden
UCL Institute of Neurology, Queen Square, London, United Kingdom

Kaj Blennow
Clinical Neurochemistry Laboratory, Sahlgrenska University Hospital, Mölndal, Sweden
Institute of Neuroscience and Physiology, Department of Psychiatry and Neurochemistry, the Sahlgrenska Academy at the University of Gothenburg, Gothenburg, Sweden

Thomas Karlsson
Disability Research, Department of Behavioral Sciences and Learning, Linköping University, Linköping, Sweden
Linnaeus Centre HEAD, Linköping University, Linköping, Sweden

Heidi Hintsala
Center for Environmental and Respiratory Health Research, University of Oulu, Oulu, Finland
Medical Research Center Oulu, Oulu University Hospital and University of Oulu, Oulu, Finland

Tuomas V. Kenttä and Heikki V. Huikuri
Medical Research Center Oulu, Oulu University Hospital and University of Oulu, Oulu, Finland
Institute of Clinical Medicine, Department of Internal Medicine, University of Oulu, Oulu, Finland

Mikko Tulppo
Department of Exercise and Medical Physiology, Verve Research, Oulu, Finland
Department of Applied Science, London South Bank University, London, England

Antti Kiviniemi
Department of Exercise and Medical Physiology, Verve Research, Oulu, Finland

Matti Mäntysaari
Institute of Health Sciences, University of Oulu, Oulu, Finland

Sirkka Keinänen-Kiukaannemi
Institute of Health Sciences, University of Oulu, Oulu, Finland
Unit of General Practice, Oulu University Hospital, Oulu, Finland

Risto Bloigu
Medical Informatics and Statistics Research Group, University of Oulu, Oulu, Finland

Karl-Heinz Herzig
Institute of Biomedicine, Department of Physiology and Biocenter of Oulu, University of Oulu, Oulu, Finland
Department of Psychiatry, Kuopio University Hospital, Kuopio, Finland

Riitta Antikainen
Medical Research Center Oulu, Oulu University Hospital and University of Oulu, Oulu, Finland
Institute of Health Sciences, University of Oulu, Oulu, Finland Oulu City Hospital, Oulu, Finland

Hannu Rintamä ki
Institute of Biomedicine, Department of Physiology and Biocenter of Oulu, University of Oulu, Oulu, Finland
Finnish Institute of Occupational Health, Oulu, Finland

Jouni J. K. Jaakkola
Center for Environmental and Respiratory Health Research, University of Oulu, Oulu, Finland
Medical Research Center Oulu, Oulu University Hospital and University of Oulu, Oulu, Finland
Institute of Health Sciences, University of Oulu, Oulu, Finland
Department of Medicine, Oulu University Hospital, Oulu, Finland

Tiina M. Ikäheimo
Center for Environmental and Respiratory Health Research, University of Oulu, Oulu, Finland
Medical Research Center Oulu, Oulu University Hospital and University of Oulu, Oulu, Finland
Institute of Health Sciences, University of Oulu, Oulu, Finland

Xiaojia Ni
Research and Development Department of New Drugs, Guangdong Provincial Hospital of Chinese Medicine, Guangzhou, Guangdong Province, China
The Second College of Clinical Medicine, Guangzhou University of Chinese Medicine, Guangzhou, Guangdong Province, China

Shaonan Liu and Xinfeng Guo
Key Unit of Methodology in Clinical Research, Guangdong Provincial Hospital of Chinese Medicine, Guangzhou, Guangdong Province, China

Fuchang Lu
The Second College of Clinical Medicine, Guangzhou University of Chinese Medicine, Guangzhou, Guangdong Province, China

Xiaogeng Shi
Department of Neurology, Guangdong Provincial Hospital of Chinese Medicine, Guangzhou, Guangdong Province, China

Florence Riera, Than Tran Trong, Stéphane Sinnapah, Olivier Hue
Laboratoire ACTES - EA 3596, Université des Antilles et de la Guyane Campus de Fouillole, Point á Pitre, France

Yanhong Gong, Xinyue Tong, Xiaoxv Yin and Zuxun Lu
Department of Social Medicine and Health Management, School of Public Health, Tongji Medical College, Huazhong University of Science and Technology, Wuhan, Hubei, P. R. China

Tieguang Han, Guoan Yang, Runsen Zhuang and Yuqi Chen
Shenzhen Health Education and Promotion Center, Shenzhen, Guangdong, P. R. China

Wei Chen
Department of Occupational Health, Laiwu Municipal Center for Disease Control and Prevention, Laiwu, Shandong, P. R. China

Hassan H. Dib
National Center for AIDS/STD Control and Prevention, Chinese Center for Disease Control and Prevention, Beijing, P. R. China

Unni Dahl
Central Norway Health Authority, Stjørdal, Norway
Department of Public Health and General Practice, Norwegian University of Science and Technology, Trondheim, Norway

Marit By Rise and Aslak Steinsbekk
Department of Public Health and General Practice, Norwegian University of Science and Technology, Trondheim, Norway

Bård Kulseng
Regional Centre for Obesity Treatment, St. Olav's University Hospital, Trondheim, Norway

Vibha Singhal and Madhusmita Misra
Neuroendocrine Unit, Massachusetts General Hospital and Harvard Medical School, Boston, Massachusetts, United States of America

Pediatric Endocrine Unit, Massachusetts General Hospital for Children and Harvard Medical School, Boston, Massachusetts, United States of America

Elizabeth A. Lawson, Pouneh K. Fazeli, Hannah Clarke and Dean A. Marengi
Neuroendocrine Unit, Massachusetts General Hospital and Harvard Medical School, Boston, Massachusetts, United States of America

Kathryn E. Ackerman
Neuroendocrine Unit, Massachusetts General Hospital and Harvard Medical School, Boston, Massachusetts, United States of America
Division of Sports Medicine, Boston Children's Hospital, Boston, Massachusetts, United States of America

Hang Lee
Department of Biostatistics, Massachusetts General Hospital and Harvard Medical School, Boston, Massachusetts, United States of America

Kamryn Eddy
Neuroendocrine Unit, Massachusetts General Hospital and Harvard Medical School, Boston, Massachusetts, United States of America
Harris Center, Massachusetts General Hospital, Boston, Massachusetts, United States of America

Nicholas P. Derrico
Endocrine Division, Massachusetts General Hospital and Harvard Medical School, Boston, Massachusetts, United States of America

Mary L. Bouxsein
Department of Orthopedic Surgery, Beth Israel Deaconess Medical Center and Harvard Medical School, Boston, Massachusetts, United States of America

Chang Wang, Yaqin Yu, Yong Li, Changgui Kou, Bo Li, Yuchun Tao, Qing Zhen, Huan He, Joseph Sam Kanu and Yawen Liu
Department of Epidemiology and Biostatistics, School of Public Health, Jilin University, Changchun City, Jilin Province, P.R. China

Xiangyang Zhang
Beijing Hui-Long-Guan hospital, Peking University, Beijing, P.R. China

Xufeng Huang and Mei Han
Illawarra Health and Medical Research Institute, University of Wollongong, Wollongong, Australia

Index

N

O

P

R

S

T

W

www.ingramcontent.com/pod-product-compliance
Lightning Source LLC
LaVergne TN
LVHW082126200926
848484LV00008B/2009